D0140618

THE
POLITICS
OF
HEALING

Histories of Alternative Medicine
in Twentieth-Century North America

Robert D. Johnston

Editor

Routledge
New York & London

Published in 2004 by
Routledge
29 West 35th Street
New York, NY 10001
www.routledge-ny.com

Published in Great Britain by
Routledge
11 New Fetter Lane
London EC4P 4EE
www.routledge.co.uk

Copyright © 2004 by Routledge
Routledge is an imprint of the Taylor & Francis Group.

Printed in the United States of America on acid-free paper.

10 9 8 7 6 5 4 3 2 1

Library of Congress Cataloging-in-Publication Data

The politics of healing : histories of alternative medicine in
twentieth-century North America / [edited by] Robert D. Johnston.
     p. cm.
    ISBN 0-415-93338-2 (hardcover : alk. paper) — ISBN 0-415-93339-0
(pbk. : alk. paper)
   1. Alternative medicine—North America—History—20th century. 2.
Alternative medicine—North America—Political aspects—20th century.
I. Johnston, Robert D.
  R733.P65 2003
  615.5'097'0904—dc21

                                 2003011930

FOR ISAAC

who, with his infectious laughter,
has always provided the most wonderful healing

CONTENTS

ACKNOWLEDGMENTS

I WOULD LIKE TO THANK, above all, my family for being willing to take a trip of personal as well as intellectual adventure through some of the worlds of alternative medicine. Thank you, Isaac, Sandy, and my dearest Anne!

Karen Wolny and Brendan O'Malley were critical to shepherding this project at Routledge, while Jaclyn Bergeron has made sure that the book stayed on track even when it seemed that it might derail. Matt Guglielmi, Bethany Moreton, Jay Nelson, and Amy Nickel provided terrific research and logistical support for the volume.

My former colleagues in the History of Medicine section at the Yale Medical School provided me with considerable courage and intellectual inspiration to continue with this project, and I want to thank, in particular, Sue Lederer, Naomi Rogers, and John Warner. Also, Nadav Davidovitch has been my mentor in many of these matters, whether in a seminar room in New Haven or on a motorbike in the streets of Tel Aviv.

The authors deserve great credit, not just for their excellent contributions to the volume but for their good cheer amid many uncertainties. And for helping find the authors, I very much appreciate the efforts especially of Norman Gevitz and Charles Rosenberg.

Finally, my foremost thanks go to Greg Field. We conceived of this book together, and he deserves credit for many of the ideas here. In the end, the pull of family, as well as the politics of healing, drew him away from this project. But his thoughtfulness and intelligence are reflected throughout.

INTRODUCTION
The Politics of Healing

Robert D. Johnston

OVER THE PAST DECADE, alternative medical therapies have played an increasingly prominent role in American health care. In the nation's grocery stores, homeopathic treatments and over-the-counter herbal remedies crowd aisles that were once largely devoted to analgesics, sore throat lozenges, and fruit-flavored, animal-shaped children's vitamins. Eager to fill their beds and their coffers, hospitals advertise—even celebrate—the inclusion of nontraditional medical practices. Medical schools, too, embrace this development with curricular reforms aimed at teaching prospective physicians about alternative forms of healing. With attention turning toward a range of mind-body and holistic treatments, health care in the United States seems more full of variety than has been the case since the establishment of modern medical authority in the early 1900s. Indeed, the emergence in the medical lexicon of a well-recognized acronym, CAM (for "complementary and alternative medicine"), is suggestive of how these alternatives are becoming a visible, and increasingly significant, current within the medical mainstream.

At first glance, it would appear that the burgeoning interest in alternative healing has appeared almost phoenix-like, at the tail end of a century that started with the near-extinction of such alternatives. Decades had passed, it seemed, since the mainstream medical practitioners drove out the "irregulars," tarnishing the alternatives as—at best—based on unsound science and—at worst—fraudulent quackery. The standard narrative of the rise of allopathic medical care in the United States suggests that the Progressive era was the crucial period, during which physicians successfully established their institutional and therapeutic authority. For example, in his epic and influential award-winning account, *The Social Transformation of American Medicine* (1982), Paul Starr described the period from the 1890s to the 1920s as a time when M.D.'s were able to sway most Americans to their cause, thereby gaining the hegemonic control necessary for the establishment of a state-sponsored monopoly of health care in the United States. Lacking both institutional power and scientific legitimacy, nonorthodox therapies retreated to the margins. Few people sought out alternatives because people came to rely on the medical model, trusting their physicians' claims to a regime of expert knowledge, and becoming skeptical—if not outright disdainful—of different voices. In this grand narrative, the central issues confronting American medicine by the late twentieth century were administrative in scope: in particular, whether doctors would be able to maintain their professional autonomy against incursions by corporate cost accountants. The therapeutic authority of the mainstream apparently remained unchallenged, indeed monolithic. As Starr himself puts it, by the end of the 1920s "[p]hysicians finally had medical practice pretty much to themselves."[1]

Yet the apparent renaissance of alternative therapies in recent years should instead lead us to consider that the central assumptions of this narrative are inadequate. No longer can we simply assume a decades-long belief in the epistemological legitimacy of the medical model, to the exclusion of therapeutic alternatives. Nor can we take for granted the marginality of non-orthodox treatments as if their continued existence was for so many years merely a story of vestigial curiosities, oddities to be pulled off the shelf and gawked at much like an exhibit from an early natural history museum. These tenets now fail us, and our task no longer is to account for the recent explosions of interest in CAM, but rather to explain unexpected continuities. Instead, only a more complex rendering of American medical history in the twentieth century can shake off the ahistorical surprise that accompanies so many accounts of alternative medicine's "comeback."[2]

The Politics of Healing has two main goals. First, this collection seeks to document a number of the ways that practitioners and laypeople conceptualized and practiced alternative medicine throughout the twentieth century, including during the midcentury so-called golden age of regular medicine. Examination of a range of therapies and medical ideologies—from homeopathy through irregular treatments for polio to anti-vaccinationism—can demonstrate how alternative healing remained vital over the decades of supposed disestablishment. This range suggests as well how older treatments changed and new systems developed, challenging the notion that the entire regime of alternatives was frozen in social and intellectual disrepute.

The second primary purpose of the volume is to emphasize that the survival of alternative medicine was not merely a matter of individual choice or professional competition, but at its heart was also a matter of *politics*. These essays therefore represent a purposeful step beyond the traditional boundaries within the historical profession that have separated the study of medicine and the study of the political realm. To be sure, part of this story is a simple matter of interest-group rivalry, with mainstream medicine using the powers of state licensure to legitimate its practice and criminalize irregulars. We need, though, to greatly expand our conception of the political in medical matters. As many of the articles in *The Politics of Healing* show, alternative therapeutic regimes often forged integral connections to oppositional political cultures. The history of homeopathy, for example, is inextricably linked to the fate of feminism. Anti-fluoridationism has intimate ties to anti-communism, but also to the movement for consumer rights. The ferment of black nationalism nurtured Afrocentric healing methods. And we cannot separate those who have opposed orthodox medicine over the past two decades either from radical social movements spawned by the New Left or from conservative movements inspired by the growth of evangelical Christianity. When ordinary people take to the streets or to the halls of Congress, they take their bodies—and complex accompanying reflections on healing—with them.[3]

Some rough and basic numbers that place the last decade in historical context should be enough to establish the chronological fluidity of twentieth-century alternative medicine. The work of Harvard Medical School researcher David Eisenberg and his associates has become commonplace both in the popular media and in the scholarly literature. An initial study in the *New England Journal of Medicine* jolted the medical profession to attention by reporting that a full one-third of adult Americans used at least one alternative therapy in 1990. Eisenberg and his colleagues found that "the estimated number of visits made in 1990 to providers of unconventional therapy was greater than the number of total visits to primary care medical doctors nationwide, and the amount spent out of pocket on unconventional therapy was comparable to the amount spent out of pocket by Americans for all hospitalizations." A follow-up study was even more dramatic, providing evidence of a substantial increase in the number of Americans using alternative healing methods and visiting non-allopathic practitioners between 1990 and 1997. By the latter date, an estimated *half* of all those age thirty-five to forty-nine used at least one of a host of methods ranging from acupuncture to therapeutic touch to biofeedback.[4]

Yet the absence of historical analysis in these studies—partly the result of a lack of data, but even more the consequence of a simple inattention to the past—produced a much greater sense of novelty than warranted. Take a look at roughly analogous studies from the age when orthodox medicine had supposedly carried all before it. The most authoritative survey comes from 1932, when social scientist Louis Reed conducted a study of "sectarian" medical practices for the Establishment-oriented Committee on the Costs of Medical Care. Reed's *The Healing Cults* reported findings of broadly similar import to those of Eisenberg. Reed warned of the 36,000 nonmedical healers amid 142,000 "trained and licensed physicians." These irregulars received $125 million annually for their services.[5]

To be sure, the first three decades of the century had witnessed a radical decline in the number of homeopaths and "eclectic" healers. Still, according to Reed, the remarkable rise of osteopaths, chiropractors, naturopaths, and Christian Scientists—not to mention astral healers and practitioners of quartz therapy and Jewish Science—more than made up for the disappearance of older forms of alternative healing. In many western states, nonorthodox healers rivaled the number of regular physicians. Yet alternative medicine was by no means a product of the isolated frontier. Reed also duly noted an Illinois Medical Society–sponsored investigation of six thousand Chicagoans. A full 87 percent of respondents had at some point in their lives "dabbled in [a] cult," with wealthier residents more likely to use "doubtful healing practices" than less prosperous immigrants. Windy City citizens resented physicians' perceived "graft," lack of responsiveness to questions, "set[ting] themselves up as wiser and less fallible than other people," and ignorance of and intolerance toward alternative healing methods. No wonder that different establishment medical figures during the 1920s commented that—in the words of the president of the American Public Health Association—"there has never been a time when the people had less confidence" in doctors, worried about the public's "wholesale desertion of the medical profession," and despaired because "it is generally conceded that the medical profession is losing its grip upon the people." George Vincent, the president of the Rockefeller Foundation, even warned that without proper vigilance, "the medical profession in this country will be swamped by the cults and societies ranged against it."[6]

Perhaps we will discover, as we continue much-needed investigations on a much-neglected topic, that the more things changed in the twentieth century, the more they stayed substantially the same.

Arguably the most powerful symbol of the recent coming of age of alternative medicine in the United States was the establishment of the Office of Alternative Medicine (OAM) within the National Institutes of Health. The two legislators with the greatest responsibility for the growth of this office, and for the overall nurturing of alternative medicine within the vast medical-governmental complex, have been Senators Tom Harkin and Orrin Hatch. Such a seemingly strange pairing—an extremely liberal agricultural rebel from Iowa and an extremely conservative Mormon free-enterpriser from Utah—should, in turn, help provide us with crucial insight into the complex politics of healing in America.[7]

This leftist and rightist team remains unapologetic in its advocacy of unconventional medicine. Because of the relief that it has provided for his allergies, Harkin is a fervent promoter of bee pollen, and he credits acupuncture with making his terminally ill brother more comfortable. Hatch is a strong supporter of chiropractors, and even more of the dietary supplement industry. In 1994 the two senators pushed through Congress the Dietary Supplement and Health Education Act, which helped keep the regulatory hands of the Food and Drug Administration off supplement makers. Harkin and Hatch then successfully sought the upgrade of the OAM into a wealthier and more powerful "center"; in 1998 it became the National Center for Complementary and Alternative Medicine. The dynamic duo combined again in 2000 to lobby for the creation of a White House Commission on Complementary and Alternative Medicine. Once again, their efforts were crowned with victory.[8]

Why are such ideological non-bedfellows working so closely, and so well, together? Sociologist Michael Goldstein provides an elegant answer that clarifies the distinctive politics of alternative healing in America. As he argues, a

> potentially pivotal characteristic of alternative medicine is that it draws on ideologies associated with both the political "right" and "left," thereby transcending common political categories. Many of its basic criticisms of mainstream medicine emerge from a left perspective that opposes the dominance of professionals as well as excess profit-making in medicine. Alternative medicine also encompasses a strong countercultural component whose roots are on the left. Yet, the strong focus on enhanced individual responsibility for health, along with an emphasis on nongovernmental solutions to health problems, often gives alternative medicine a distinctly rightward cast.

In other words, Harkin and Hatch are by no means loners or eccentrics who literally got a bee in their bonnet and decided to run with their own crankish agenda. Rather, they are expressing a basic pattern in modern American civic life, one that moves "beyond left and right" and expresses a powerful politics of the body that we need to grapple with and not simply dismiss.[9]

Another pair of curious companions further reveals the promise of moving beyond left and right as we seek to understand the complex political roots of alternative medicine: Phyllis Schlafly and Michael Lerner. Schlafly has been one of the most powerful women in postwar American politics. Most of her efforts have been directed not within the realm of the politics of healing, but rather at forging a modern and militant conservatism. One of the most important of Barry Goldwater's publicists, breaking onto the national scene with the 1964 publication of *A Choice Not an Echo*, this Catholic housewife and activist became even more famous when she—more than any other single individual—helped to defeat the Equal Rights Amendment. Schlafly then went on to found the Eagle Forum, a right-wing grassroots women's organization that fights against cultural and political liberalism and for American military strength.[10]

Yet Schlafly has in recent years also come into her own as a crusader against the medical establishment. For example, Schlafly rails against Ritalin, seeing this medicine not as a benign aid helping children with attention deficit disorder to live more normal lives. Rather, Ritalin is, to Schlafly, a government-mandated drug that is overprescribed and that is leading many children toward drug addiction. Schlafly is even more opposed to compulsory vaccination. She views mandated immunizations as the hand of a Big Brother government, reaching into the lives of citizens who should be able to decide for themselves how to treat themselves and their families. Schlafly indicts what she sees as the poor science behind vaccination testing, and she accuses government regulators of conflicts of interest because of their relationship with vaccine manufacturers. Both Schlafly's Web page and that of her son Roger contain many links to organizations resisting compulsory vaccination, and hers also includes a section titled "How to Legally Avoid School Immunizations."[11]

In terms of mixing oppositional politics and nonconventional medical perspectives, Phyllis Schlafly has an avid counterpart on the left side of the political spectrum. Again, Michael Lerner's politics primarily revolve around nonmedical issues. Lerner is arguably the most prominent left-wing Jewish intellectual in the United States. Or, rather, he is the most identifiably Jewish of left-wing intellectuals, seeking to integrate a renewed brand of Jewish spirituality with progressive politics. Since 1986 editor of *Tikkun* magazine, Lerner has been at the center of debates about how to honor Palestinian rights while working for a secure Israel, and also (through a highly publicized partnership with Cornel West) how to help reconcile African Americans and Jews. Lerner's primary season in the sun, though, came when First Lady Hillary Rodham Clinton adopted his phrase "the politics of meaning" to suggest the need to bring a greater concern for ethical issues into the public realm. Conservative commentators such as Rush Limbaugh attacked Lerner as Hillary's dangerous left-wing guru, and the Clintons soon distanced themselves from the radical rabbi.[12]

In invoking a "politics of meaning," Lerner actually went far beyond Clinton. Lerner sought something that might, on the surface, please Schlafly and Hatch: a "politics in the image of God" that would recognize "our connection to a higher ethical and spiritual purpose that gives meaning to our lives." Lerner decried fundamental leftist materialist assumptions that focused only on bringing more prosperity to more people. Instead, using feminism as a model for bringing together the public and private dimensions of politics, Lerner emphasized the need to make all areas of life meaningful, in order to satisfy the "hunger to serve the common good" that he found among "middle Americans." Lerner sought above all to make everyday work more purposeful by challenging the economic and political power of corporations, by providing employees with a much greater voice in the workplace, and by reducing the workweek to thirty hours—all thereby allowing ordinary citizens to escape "a world governed by a money-oriented ethos" and presenting the possibility of a renewed "alliance between middle-income people and the poor."[13]

Yet Lerner also made a new orientation toward medicine an integral part of his larger political message. At a time when a great variety of schemes for socializing the *cost* of medicine were in the air, Lerner insisted that the *kind* of care available was just as important as its availability. Proclaiming that "[t]hroughout history, much human sickness has been produced by the disruption of the spiritual and ethical ecology of the universe," Lerner railed against the "mechanistic and materialistic principles" of modern medicine. Seeking to reunite mind and body in the service of healing people—not just fighting particular diseases—Lerner called for a dramatic overhaul of medical education. "Practicums for medical professionals," he announced, "should focus as much on how to develop one's own inner spirituality and healing capacities as on how to master various medical techniques." Lerner proposed that hospitals hold "a daily gathering of the healers to take some time for meditation, and for ritual recommitment to the patients' health and to the nobility of the healing enterprise."[14]

There surely are countless different paths into the politics of alternative medicine other than through the specific ideas of Tom Harkin or Orrin Hatch, Phyllis Schlafly or Michael Lerner. Continued exploration of the strong feminist strains within the historical tradition of North American alternative medicine would, for example, certainly prove valuable. So would a focus on populism as a mode of political thinking and action that challenges elites of all kinds. Yet the examples of Harkin, Hatch, Schlafly, and Lerner—all powerful political figures even though they inhabit the margins of the political mainstream—should begin to suggest the critical significance of the politics of healing to the general politics of democracy.[15]

The Politics of Healing contains five parts. The first, "Precursors: The Years in the Wilderness," explores, for the most part, the decades before World War II. These were the years when established medicine was supposedly taking all before it, the years when the tremendous ferment of the nineteenth-century alternative medicine world sickened and died. Yet as Nadav Davidovitch, Anne Kirschmann, Barbara Clow, and Michael Ackerman compellingly demonstrate, alternative medicine survived this mean era, laying an impressive foundation for those who would take up its legacy later in the century. But alternatives did not just survive; they often thrived. Davidovitch and Kirschmann, for example, explore the ways that homeopathy—supposedly the classic case of the co-optation of nineteenth-century heterodox medicine—continued to provide many occasions for dissent across the twentieth century. Ackerman, in turn, reveals how our current celebration of whole foods has roots more than a half century deep. And Clow shows that those who opposed established medicine had deep popular support and significant political power. These essays, in particular, will dramatically reshape the chronology of North American alternative medicine.

In the second section, "Intersections: Allopathic Medicine Meets Alternative Medicine," Otniel Dror and Wade Davies make it clear that we can draw no effective intellectual, cultural, or political dividing lines between orthodox and heterodox medicine. Whether on the Navajo reservation or in the august halls of Harvard University, both laypeople and intellectuals wrestled with the relationship between the visible and the invisible, the "Western" and the "non-Western." In the process, they created legacies that speak forcefully to the ways we might think about race and power, as well as the ways we might think about the relationship between the body and the mind.

"Contesting the Cold War Medical Monopoly" is the book's third section. Here politics, in the more standard sense of politicians fighting it out in the halls of Congress or citizens fighting it out in their local communities, becomes most evident. During the supposed postwar nadir of alternative medicine, according to Naomi Rogers, Michelle Nickerson, and Gretchen Reilly, a wide variety of activists struggled against the medical establishment over issues such as mental health, polio, and fluoridation. Sister Elizabeth Kenny forged a remarkable popularity, as well as significant political support, with her populist crusades against the polio establishment. Right-wing California housewives deluged Congress with mail expressing their fears that liberal psychiatrists and government officials would set up an American Siberia to silence political opposition. Anti-fluoridationists won referendum after referendum in communities concerned about a supposed poison in their water supply, but even more about a loss of their political liberties. Scholars have written these battles off as the product of extremist cranks. But these Cold War anti-establishment activists were much more powerful, and in fact considerably more rational, than we have been led to believe.

The largest section of the volume, "Contemporary Practices/Contemporary Legacies," places the renaissance of alternative healing practices over the last three decades in full historical and political perspective. The unity in the essays of Amy Sue Bix, Georgina Feldberg, Velana Huntington, Sita Reddy, David Hess, Matthew Schneirov, and Jonathan Geczik comes from their authors' thorough embedding of alternative medical practices and ideologies within vigorous—and generally oppositional—political and cultural movements. Feminism has effectively institutionalized many alternative medical practices, as Bix shows for the national level and Feldberg for the local. In turn, changing political cultures of race have, according to Huntington and Reddy, been crucial to the development of Orisha and Ayurveda healing practices. Finally, Hess, Schneirov, and Geczik emphasize the ways that a democratic public culture influences alternative healing practices, often in ways that break down traditional political divides.

Two concluding essays take us back through the twentieth century and up to the very present. Populist crusades against compulsory mass vaccination have changed in fundamental ways, Robert Johnston shows, even as they have retained many similarities to movements a century ago. So-called anti-vaccinationists have, for instance, become much more favorably disposed toward science, even to some extent accommodating themselves to vaccinations themselves. In the process, those we can now call "vaccine safety advocates" have found a new, quite remarkable legitimacy in the eyes of the media and political establishment. Whorton, in turn, supplies an elegant synthesis of the coming of age of alternative medicine. Whorton, the most influential historian of alternative medicine, shows that therapies such as osteopathy, chiropractic, and naturopathy have become so successful that they have veered toward becoming mainstream themselves. Indeed, one might conclude that in the coming decades it will become increasingly difficult to distinguish any genuine alternatives within medicine, as the buzzword of the day becomes "integrative."

All of the authors in this volume are respectful toward their subjects; most are overtly sympathetic to medical pluralism. Yet this does not mean that the scholars' attitudes are by any means predictable. For example, Michael Ackerman is skeptical of his food reformers, while Anne Kirschmann clearly cheers for her homeopathy advocates. Sita Reddy finds substantial fault with the tendency within the New Age Ayurveda community to use long-established Orientalist ideas of an exotic and mystical "East" to further goals that are as much insular as communitarian, while Robert Johnston celebrates anti-vaccinationists as populist democratic reformers. Amy Bix even combines these viewpoints within the same essay. On one hand, Bix celebrates the many crucial victories won by feminists opposed to orthodox medicine. Yet she also warns that an uncritical embrace of alternative medicine could ultimately victimize as much as empower women.

In the end, regardless of their own perspectives, all the authors who have contributed to this volume believe that the historical study of alternative medicine is crucial to understanding the development not just of medicine but of democracy in our current age. They thus seek to provide a contribution to public culture, as well as to scholarship. Therefore *The Politics of Healing*, while designed primarily for a scholarly audience, should also be of considerable interest to healing professionals and ordinary citizens alike. Each essay is accessible to both general and academic audiences. For all, then, who are concerned with the development of the multiple choices historically available to North Americans as they have tried to live the healthiest lives possible, these pioneering essays could even help empower us—citizens and scholars alike—as we ourselves engage in today's politics of healing.

PRECURSORS: THE YEARS IN THE WILDERNESS

NEGOTIATING DISSENT

Homeopathy and Anti-Vaccinationism at the Turn of the Twentieth Century

Nadav Davidovitch

I

The hegemonic status of vaccinations in the world of medicine today is an impressive feat. Vaccinations occupy a place of honor parallel to achievements such as antibiotics as well as improvements in sanitation and water quality, considered as a leading cause of the drop in death rates from contagious diseases and the rise in longevity that has been registered in the course of the twentieth century.[1] Yet while vaccinations are considered a paradigm of success, at the same time they have encountered fierce criticism and unparalleled opposition throughout the history of medicine. In many places opposition to vaccination has reached the scope of civil insurrection, with closure of schools and places of employment. Massive political mobilization against these medical interventions has also been common.[2] To this day, especially with the recent reintroduction of immunization against smallpox, vaccination continues to be an issue steeped in controversy.[3]

The history of opposition to vaccination is protracted and can be traced back to Edward Jenner's publication in 1798 on the possibility of immunization against smallpox. Jenner's suggestions raised immediate and strong controversy both in the medical community and among the public at large.[4] Still, one cannot regard opposition to vaccination as a uniform phenomenon. Vaccinations themselves have undergone many changes, both in manufacturing techniques and in the social and legal context of their administration. The character of opposition has varied over the years and from country to country. Yet despite this, those opposed to vaccination have generally been portrayed in monolithic terms as irrational groups, tied primarily to the radical fringes of alternative medicine. Such a tendency is in fashion not only in current medical publications, but also in writings within the realm of the history of medicine.[5] Yet as of late there has finally been recognition of the great intellectual and civic potential embodied in historical research on opposition to vaccinations, as well as in the ability of this issue to serve as a vehicle for gaining a better understanding of the politics of the body and of the relations among health, culture, and society.[6]

This article focuses on the discourse of vaccinations at the turn of the twentieth century, a period when public health officials deepened their influence in the medical world and in daily life. My discussion does not focus on the "regular" perspective of conventional medicine; rather, it seeks to examine the attitude toward vaccination of one of the medical establishment's chief alternatives, homeopathy. Homeopaths, who constituted an important and powerful force in the medical world of the nineteenth-century United States, had to grapple—as did conventional doctors—with significant changes in matters of health and society in their attempts to establish their professional status and define their professional identity. Homeopaths vigorously discussed the place of vaccination in their practices, along with the more general question of the proper social role of public health.

Too often, though, scholars have treated homeopaths in monolithic terms, assuming a clear and intimate connection between unconventional medicine and opposition to vaccination.[7] A closer look, however, demonstrates that there was no uniform homeopathic "voice" in the question of vaccinations, just as there was not a clear uniform voice in conventional medicine. The closing years of the nineteenth century and early years of the twentieth century were a period in which the worlds of medicine and public health as we know them today were still in their formative stages. In this era's medical world, the laboratory and its products did indeed gain considerable stature. As scholars have shown, however, this was a complex process, and we still know far too little about the contests that were at the very center of the process by which regular medicine gained its dominance in twentieth-century America. By putting our focus on homeopaths, we can begin to see modern medicine as having a plurality of perspectives and being a place where the boundary between alternative and orthodox becomes much more difficult to establish.[8]

The debates among homeopaths over vaccination were important not only in the realm of medicine and its history. They speak to questions of democracy that we continue to grapple with. How, for example, should the state intervene in the lives of its citizens? How can it inculcate practices that it deems to be for the greater public good? Indeed, how can a government claim custodianship over the bodies of its citizens in the first place? Homeopaths during the early twentieth century provided responses to these difficult issues that went far beyond the standard caricature of them as irrational and deluded. Analyzing their reaction to the rising power of vaccination and public health can inform our understanding of the proper role of a democratic citizenry in the formulation of public health policy.

II

What is vaccination? It is the introduction of the crude morbific products of disease into the tissue of the healthy organism.[9]

This all absorbing topic of vaccine, toxin, and serum therapy to my mind is a version of Hahnemann's "psora" and "vital force" theories. It is all summed up in one word: "immunity."[10]

These comments on vaccination, read by homeopaths during discussion of vaccination in homeopathic societies, exemplify the wide spectrum of opinions expressed by homeopathic practitioners. Most historical analyses of the resistance to vaccination tend to characterize alternative healers indiscriminately as anti-vaccinationists.[11] Indeed, a significant number of members in anti-vaccination movements *were* alternative practitioners—including homeopaths. However, a deeper look at homeopathic discussions on the issue of vaccinations reveals a more complex picture—both in terms of differences of opinion regarding the nature of the practice, and in terms of different ways of positioning vaccination in the wider context of the rise of the laboratory.

As Eberhard Wolff has demonstrated, homeopathic treatment of the vaccination issue has always varied. Attitudes among homeopaths toward vaccination ranged from enthusiastic embrace to total rejection. Some homeopaths viewed vaccination as proof of the homeopathic law of similars. Others accepted vaccination as an effective treatment irrespective of homeopathic principles. Only a minority of homeopathic physicians totally rejected the principle of vaccination, not only because they viewed vaccination as a medical procedure opposed to homeopathic principles, but also because it was considered a dangerous practice involving serious side effects.[12]

Samuel Hahnemann, the founder of homeopathy, in fact regarded vaccination in a positive light. In the first four editions of the *Organon*, the homeopathic bible, he viewed the procedure as, in essence, a homeopathic treatment since it is based on the principle of administering a remedy similar to the disease, which can then intervene in physical processes. In a letter to Dr. Schreeter of Lemberg on December 19, 1831, Hahnemann wrote: "In order to provide the dear little Patty with the protective cow pox, the safest plan would certainly be to obtain the lymph direct from the cow; but if this cannot be done . . . I would advice you to inoculate another child with the protective pox, and as soon as slight redness of the punctures shows it has taken, I would immediately for two successive days give *Sulphur* l-30, and inoculate your child from the pock that it produced."[13] Dr. Schreeter, in a note to this letter, commented that he found this advice "to be true and acted upon it in vaccination with good results."[14] Yet not all homeopaths agreed. Even while Hahnemann was still alive, several of his followers in Europe came out against the use of vaccinations.

During the first decades of homeopathy in the United States, there was almost no public mention of vaccination among homeopaths. In 1880, only after several British anti-vaccinationists directly questioned Constantine Hering, one of the most outstanding homeopaths in the United States, did Hering published a letter on the issue of vaccination. Hering did not believe in vaccination and considered it detrimental mainly because of its debilitating influence on otherwise healthy children. Yet he did not work publicly to oppose the procedure, and in a later edition of his widely published self-help book *Homeopathic Domestic Physician* he regarded it as the "lesser of two evils."[15] Some homeopaths did not want to raise an unneeded controversy with the "regular" profession. As D. H. Beckwith commented:

> I am sorry that any paper should have been read or any idea should have been introduced into this institute unfavorable to vaccination. It will bring odium on the homeopathic profession at large. All kinds of things will get into the newspapers. It will be bruited abroad that the members of the American Institute of Homeopathy are opposed to vaccination.[16]

Indeed, since vaccination was founded on using cowpox to prevent a similar disease—smallpox—many homeopaths praised vaccinations, regarding them as confirmation of the homeopathic maxim *Simila similibus curentur* ("Let like be cured by like"). Several texts written by homeopaths on the history of vaccination compared the affliction and isolation suffered by Edward Jenner with the affliction visited upon Samuel Hahnemann, the father of homeopathy.[17] Many underscored that it surely was no coincidence that the date given to the "birth of vaccinations"—1796—was the same year of the publication of the *Organon*. There were even some homeopaths who went so far as to turn Pasteur into a homeopath after his discovery of the vaccinations against anthrax and rabies: "In truth, if Pasteur is a physician, he should be elected to membership of the American Institute of Homeopathy for the patient but brilliant, unconscious confirmation of the truth which Hahnemann promulgated."[18] After Koch published his discovery of the use of tuberculin to treat tuberculosis, he too entered the homeopathic shrine. Not only was tuberculin made in keeping with the homeopathic principle of attenuation of the disease matter, Koch also proved his virtue "by courageously proving the poison on himself," as had Hahnemann, who was purported to have initially tested his homeopathic treatments on himself.[19]

A recurrent question in homeopathic discussion of vaccination was whether vaccination is a homeopathic practice. In contrast to homeopathic remedies, vaccines contained material that did not fulfill the basic principles of homeopathic thinking. They had not undergone "dilution" and, especially, had not undergone the process of "proving" (being given to healthy people in order to test what symptoms it produced). As a result, many homeopaths viewed vaccination as isopathic, not homeopathic—meaning that it was an effective treatment, using disease matter to cure, but not based on homeopathic principles. As a consequence, homeopaths developed what they called "homeopathic vaccinations"—extracting a substance from a diseased tissue, preparing the remedy by dilution and potentiating the material according to homeopathic methods, and then administering it via the mouth. The attractiveness of this last practice was that homeopathic principles were applied, and the procedure did not lead to blood poisoning—a major concern among anti-vaccinationists. Some homeopaths were in fact so convinced of the success of their own oral vaccinations that they issued certificated verifying vaccination, should they be required for a child's entry to school.[20]

In contrast to orthodox medical writing, even pro-vaccination homeopaths were well aware of the side effects of vaccination. A perusal of homeopathic domestic health manuals shows that the side effects of the smallpox vaccination were known and were generally allocated a chapter entitled "Vaccinosis." One homeopathic author, favorable to vaccination, wrote, "Vaccination . . . has been sufficiently tested . . . to demonstrate, beyond all reasonable question, its efficacy in altogether modifying the course and severity of smallpox in those who contract that disease, and in acting as a distinct preventive against it." Yet he admitted, "Vaccination unquestionably, in some constitutions, has the effect of rousing dormant dyscrasia; and, as a result, we have skin disease, and sometimes, but very rarely, some scrofulous affection, the fault being not in vaccination, which, after all, has only anticipated what the course of years would unfailingly have developed."[21]

Others, while still recommending the practice of vaccination, tried to keep their objectivity. The widely circulated book *Vaccinosis and Its Cure by Thuja, with Remarks on Homœoprophylaxis,* by J. Compton Burnett, starts with the following clarification: "Fear not, critical reader, this is not an anti-vaccination treatise, for the writer is himself in the habit of vaccinating his patients."[22] Indeed, Thuja Occidentalis, a homeopathic remedy, is still recommended today to counteract the side effects of vaccinations.[23] James Tyler Kent, the preeminent American homeopath and a known anti-vaccinationist, considered Thuja as a "strong medicine when you have a trace of animal poisoning in the history, as snake bite, small-pox and vaccination."[24]

Further evidence of openness in regard to the issue of vaccinations was the fact that at the turn of the twentieth century, homeopaths often organized vigorous discussions on the subject of vaccinations. Some of these forums were open well beyond the homeopathic

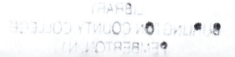

community, so that all sides of the debate could present their positions. In just one example, the Homeopathic Medical County of Philadelphia organized a symposium on smallpox. In this forum a homeopath, a regular physician—a medical inspector from the board of health—and a bacteriologist opposed to vaccination, all were invited to speak.[25] This example of respectful engagement was quite rare in American medical discourse, where orthodoxy tried to erect clear boundaries between scientific medicine and heresy. Homeopaths, however, could take advantage of their unique intermediary position in the American medical scene at the time, especially in the big cities of the East Coast such as New York, Boston, and Philadelphia. We should not overestimate the extent of these interactions; after all, on both sides, many disapproved of the possibility of an open dialogue between the old enemies. Yet an interaction did exist, giving a voice to several factions within homeopathy in the broader American medical discourse through the vaccination debate.[26]

But in my estimation, we must not examine the attitudes of homeopaths to vaccination as simply an internal professional dispute. In order to better understand the reaction to vaccinations at the beginning of the twentieth century, one must first understand the changes—both in terms of medical praxis and discourse—that vaccinations had undergone over the previous century. Until the last third of the 1800s, the smallpox vaccine was the only vaccine in existence.[27] Controversy accompanied the introduction of smallpox vaccinations in various countries. Not all physicians or laypeople approved of the idea of infecting a healthy person with purulent material from a cow. The theoretical foundations behind vaccination were not yet clear, and it would be decades before the germ theory would substantiate the "biological foundations" of vaccination in general.[28] The techniques for manufacturing vaccinations against smallpox did, however, undergo a number of changes during the nineteenth century. Up until then, vaccines were usually "produced" from the arm of an immunized person. Poor levels of sterilization only contributed to side effects, which included tetanus, syphilis, and scrofula.[29] Also, the procedure of vaccination itself was considered as an operation, with various instruments, from scalpels to needles, causing substantial scarification.

With the advent of the germ theory in the 1870s and 1880s, vaccination against smallpox ceased to be the sole subject of immunization, and the context of the debate subsequently changed. The scope of vaccinations enlarged not only to encompass a growing list of bacteria, but also to cover a larger territory of action. Vaccines entered the clinical and preventive medicine realm and also became a hot topic of discussion among public health officers, politicians, and legislators. During this period, in the framework of the bacteriological revolution, researchers such as Pasteur and Koch developed several new vaccines. However, these were not "random" vaccines discovered empirically; they were laboratory-created vaccines based on the germ theory. Vaccines therefore became one of the most significant links between the laboratory and medical practice, part of the paradigm that perceived the world of the laboratory, animal research, and the treatment clinic as a continuum.[30] Vaccines did not, however, remain solely within the inner domain of the medical world. Together with the germ theory, they gradually entered the public sphere. Moreover, they were integrated into popular culture through far-reaching practical implications for everyday life.

One of the new vaccines that dramatically captured public attention was the rabies vaccine. In 1886, for instance, American newspapers reported on several children who had been bitten by rabid dogs and were then sent to France in order to receive the brand-new "miracle cure" against rabies from Pasteur. As historian Bert Hansen has noted, the impact of the extensive publicity the event received went beyond the humanitarian angle, for the newspapers "were also elaborating a story of medical discovery as something useful and exciting to ordinary people. In the process, they were cultivating a sensation about medicine's being newly powerful, about scientific knowledge that makes a difference in a public arena beyond the walls of the medical school and the laboratory."[31] Even John Sutherland, dean of the homeopathic Boston University School of Medicine, wrote on the subject of vaccination in 1901: "Such has been the influence of newspapers and literary-magazine articles on the mind of the laity, that now in the majority of cases a physician is looked upon as culpable by the friends and relatives of the patient if he fails to use 'anti-toxin' as soon as the diagnosis of 'diphtheria' is made."[32]

But during the latter half of the nineteenth century, particularly when attempts were made to make vaccination compulsory and as specific vaccines multiplied, opposition to vaccination gained momentum.[33] A number of anti-vaccination associations mobilized, primarily to fight against the increasingly compulsory nature of vaccination. In 1855, Massachusetts became the first state to enact a law obliging vaccination for every child entering public school. Parents who failed to comply risked a fine or even imprisonment. Other states quickly followed suit. This encroachment of the state into the private domain inspired substantial opposition, as many citizens considered vaccination a harmful intrusion into the body. Opponents described vaccinations as "blood poisoning" and "morbific materials from animal sources."[34] Frequently, the anti-vaccinationists compared vaccinations to bloodletting. Just as bloodletting had earlier served as a potent symbol of the brutal qualities of allopathic medicine, so vaccination now became a barbaric and anachronistic manifestation of the "insanity" of established medicine.[35] The lancet—the very symbol of the bloodletting doctor—became also the symbol of the vaccinating doctor, only this time the physician was penetrating the body of healthy individuals, under the power of the law.

III

As the nineteenth century came to an end, the vaccination issue became more and more controversial within homeopathic circles. A group of homeopaths, mainly university-based, tried to combine the ethos of the laboratory and homeopathic practice. They perceived vaccinations and serum treatments as a golden opportunity to integrate homeopathy, as a respectable scientific discipline, into the world of medicine. A group of homeopathic practitioners, mainly from the Boston University School of Medicine, enthusiastically embraced the research paradigm of the "allopathic" physician and bacteriologist Sir A. E. Wright. Wright, a well-known and respected figure in the world of research and immunology at the beginning of the twentieth century, promoted the theory of the opsonic index. According to Wright, the body secretes material in coping with contagious diseases, and this reaction is measurable. Wright labeled the secretions "opsonin," and the quantitative index of opsonin was termed the "opsonic index." The higher the opsonic index, the better the body's immune system is responding to the illness and the better the patient's chances of recovery.[36]

Several homeopaths eagerly adopted the opsonin theory. Homeopathic researchers such as W. H. Watters of Boston and Eldridge C. Price of Baltimore claimed that use of vaccines prepared from secretions of a patient, and subsequently diluted, would raise the opsonic index of the patient and thus the chances of recovery.[37] This method of preparation was presented as more homeopathic than, and thus far superior to, the use of ready-made and less-diluted vaccine. Examining the writings of these homeopaths, one can discern a clear desire to mobilize vaccination as a platform to enhance the homeopathic image and even transform homeopathy into a leading force in scientific medical research.[38] At the annual meeting of the American Institute of Homeopathy in 1909, Dr. Frank L. Newton of Boston went so far as to introduce a resolution stating that "to the homoeopathic school precedent belongs the credit for introducing the serums, toxins and vaccines in the treatment of disease."[39] This he claimed to be warranted by the fact that "the homoeopathic school was the first to do systematic work in the proving of drugs, that the treatment of opsonins is based on the infinitesimal dosage, which is presented in the principles of the similia."[40] W. H. Watters, another Boston homeopath, went even further. In an essay discussing "what is homœopathy?"—a burning question among homeopaths in the early twentieth century—Watters made a clear relation between homeopathic practice, scientific homeopathic research, vaccination, and immunology:

> The question may now be asked . . . what is your idea of homœopathy? It will be answered as follows: Homœopathy is the term given to a distinct method of using medicinal agents, a method that is based upon sound theories, and one that is yearly becoming more demonstrable by exact science. It is perfectly consistent with known facts, and is probably merely a way of expressing the means employed in reaching the goal of all medicine, the production of immunity.[41]

According to this view, the writings of Samuel Hanhemann on the issue of vital force and its importance in healing processes could be translated scientifically into the languages of immunology and antitoxins.[42] This homeopathic approach did not remain solely in the theoretical realm. In the first decades of the twentieth century, homeopaths in institutions such as the Massachusetts Homeopathic Hospital—a facility tied to the medical school of Boston University—were using vaccines and serums as an integral part of their homeopathic treatment. They believed that vaccination could not only prevent disease, but treat it as well. Reports indicated success primarily in the use of immunization in the treatment of typhoid patients (Figure 1).[43] The growing involvement of Boston University Homeopathic Medical School in vaccine research led to the updating of its curriculum, probably conceived as a way to attract potential students: "In view of the rapidly increasing use of bacterial products in the treatment of many diseases, particularly those of an infectious nature, it seems wise to incorporate into the curriculum a course of instruction in the preparation of vaccines . . . antitoxins, to bacteriolysis and to haemolysis, including the Wasserman reaction and complement fixation test."[44]

These homeopaths still viewed themselves as operating within the homeopathic profession, and it remained important to them to conduct their dialogue in accordance with homeopathic principles: "to find the homeopathic indications for the various serums and toxins in the individual case."[45] And above all, the medical care given to their patients, other than serum and vaccines, consisted of homeopathic remedies. These principles, according to this view, kept the agenda as homeopathic in character. Another "proof" of their homeopathic loyalty was their criticism of high dosages of vaccine and drug companies that combined vaccines, reminiscent of the basic homeopathic criticism Hahnemann had voiced: that medications needed to be highly diluted and materials should not be mixed.

Case 1. Richard D., age 7. Physician reports "a moderately severe case of typhoid fever apparently much benefited by a single inoculation of

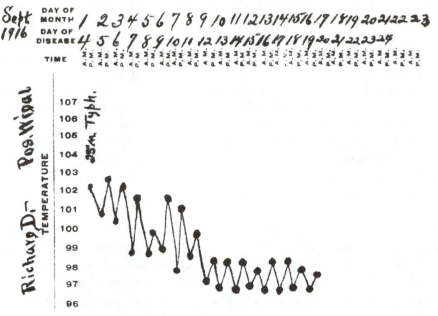

vaccin. Hardest struggle to control the boy's appetite. Felt free from malaise and was crying for something to eat 48 hours following inoculation."

FIGURE 1. From *The New England Medical Gazette,* 1917.

But beyond treatment with "homeopathic" vaccines, homeopaths were also attracted to vaccines by the opportunity they presented to steer their field into the research path of laboratory-based scientific medicine. For these homeopaths the immunological and bacteriological paradigm provided fertile grounds for homeopathic research. This group of mainly university-based homeopaths frequently emphasized its desire to be distinguished from currents within homeopathy and other "irregular" medical practices that they perceived as too extreme, unscientific, and prone to employing overly vociferous rhetoric in their criticism of "organized" medicine. They even believed that collaboration with various parties opposed to "regular" medicine could harm homeopaths.[46] In a typical expression in the *New England Medical Gazette,* a homeopathic journal representing mainly the Boston University Homeopathic Medical School, the editor in 1917 referred to an anti-vaccinationist article published in the *Homœopathic Recorder:*

An interesting, though painful example of the anti-scientific attitude so frequently encountered in some homœopathic periodicals, especially, we regret to say, in the Recorder . . . After delivering himself of this bit of Galenic dogmatism, the author bursts into diatribe against all such "foul mixtures" as sera and vaccins [*sic*] as the causes of innumerable ills (cancer and trachoma *inter alia*) and the cure of none. When our writers can produce case-reports worthy of respect instead of indulging in recriminations and ex cathedra statements, we may reasonably look for a modicum of respect from our allœopathic brethren, but not one moment before.[47]

As can be seen, these homeopaths wanted to remain very cautious, preserving the fine balance between them and conventional doctors. They wanted to operate within the realm of homeopathy, yet be ready to explore new scientific theories and incorporate them into homeopathy. Several homeopaths were even part of campaigns to promote vaccination.[48]

In turn, other "sectarians" strongly condemned the homeopathic interest in vaccination as illegitimately "courting the favor" of conventional doctors. The idea of homeopathic vaccinations, or the trials to integrate serum and vaccine treatments into homeopathic practice, did not impress them: "The homeopathic school has rather straddled the question and wavers between internal vaccination and the real thing—the latter so not to offend their bigger brethren of the drug faith."[49]

Naturally, this approach carried its own price, as the tensions within the homeopathic community escalated as a result of the conflict over vaccination. The price was also social: the voice of homeopathy as an alternative approach, partner to social reforms in matters such as women's status, abolitionism, and freedom of expression, characteristic of the "homeopathic voice" in the mid-nineteenth century, became progressively weaker.[50] The involvement of homeopathy in boards of health or in health legislation, together with conventional physicians, took away much of the radicalism and "alternative" fervor of homeopathy's earlier days. As Naomi Rogers argued, by the end of the nineteenth century "public debates by homeopaths about links between medical and political liberty largely disappeared as neither medical conservatives nor liberals found them a potent symbol in professional debates."[51] The integration of scientific ideology into homeopathic practice, by the promoters of the "new homeopathy," meant that homeopathy should be progressive not so much in the social realm but in its belief in the progress of science.

IV

Indeed, during this period homeopathy produced many vigorous voices that viewed the homeopathic embrace of vaccines as dangerous, leading to the assimilation and destruction of the homeopathic profession. Despite the fact that a significant number of homeopaths supported vaccinations, either enthusiastically or with only slight reservations, a number of homeopaths remained prominent in anti-vaccination associations. Their opposition to vaccinations flowed from sources similar to those that caused the resistance of other anti-vaccinationists: vaccinations did not protect; they caused various diseases, from syphilis to cancer; and they poisoned the blood of the people with animal pollutants. They also argued that vaccinations had not undergone basic homeopathic processes such as "dilution" and "dinamization." Anti-vaccination homeopaths were especially concerned about the administration of vaccinations by injection into the body. In their view, homeopathic vaccination—using diluted disease matter given by mouth—was the only worthwhile vaccination that complied with genuine homeopathic principles. As Stuart Close wrote concerning one of the homeopathic vaccinations:

> In a case requiring the administration of Psorinum . . . shall we use the original crude pus from the sore of a diseased negro, introducing it directly into the circulation, or shall we use a high potency . . . What havoc should we produce if we used Psorinum, Medorrhinum, Syphilinum . . . or any other poisonous drug in the same manner as Vaccininum is used! What wrecked lives; what suffering and death; what outraged feelings; what suits for malpractice.[52]

Beside the clear-cut racism evoked in this piece, not uncommon in both regular and homeopathic American medical circles at the turn of the twentieth century, Close called for a return to original homeopathic principles, such as high potencies and oral treatment. Close represents a different, more militant posture as to how homeopaths should respond to the vaccination issue.

Close was not alone. In 1901, the *Homeopathic Recorder* published an interesting series of letters from homeopaths on the vaccination question. The letters, written by fifteen homeopaths, were sent following the request of William Jefferson Guernsey, a known homeopath from Philadelphia, who wrote a "personal letter to a number of physicians who were known to be good prescribers . . . who had not expressed themselves on the subject."[53] In its introduction Guernsey expressed his disappointment that although the practice of vaccination has become a debatable question, "many physicians have adopted the convenient theory that the easiest way to get rid of temptation is to yield . . . it is assuredly pleasanter and more profitable to do what the numerous political Health Boards require, and to pocket the fee therefore, than to refuse the pecuniary benefit and acquire the reputation of being a 'crank' in the bargain."[54]

Guernsey admitted that while being a recent graduate from medical school, during a smallpox epidemic and owing to lack of patients "he vaccinated of course. Every physician did." His experience with homeopathic vaccination and his growing awareness both of smallpox vaccine side effects and of its compulsion by the state, made him finally "regret to the many vaccinated patients . . . of those who would doubtless have remained well if the enthusiastic young vaccinator had let them alone." When the Philadelphia School Board stopped accepting homeopathic vaccination as an alternative, Guernsey felt the need to ask for the opinion of his homeopathic colleagues. The answers were "so interesting and instructive that it seems like neglecting a duty to hide them from those who might be brought to a study of the question." The letters, written by homeopathic figures such as W. P. Wesselhoeft, Boston; Erastus Case, Hartford, Connecticut; James T. Kent, Chicago; E. B. Nash, Cortland, New York; Edward Rushmore, Plainfield, New Jersey; and G. W. Winterburn, New York City, revealed an interesting spectrum of anti-vaccinationist homeopaths. Although all of them encouraged the use of "internal" homeopathic vaccination, their reaction to "conventional" vaccination ranged from balanced deliberation and even agreement to vaccinate when patients insisted to fierce rhetoric against the "horrible superstition, based upon ignorance and commercialism."[55]

This grand debate was conducted both outside and inside the homeopathic community. Controversy over vaccination was part of a much broader debate over democratic principles, particularly over how citizens and practitioners should relate to the medical establishment in matters of public health. Those homeopaths who opposed vaccination were a minority within their own profession. To understand their stance, we must take into account the context in which the debate took place: the tension that existed at the end of the nineteenth and the beginning of the twentieth centuries between the freedom of the individual and the limits of the power of the state. Various political groups linked their antagonism to vaccination to a more general opposition to the state's intrusion into the private lives of its citizens, only part of which was opposition to intrusion into the body by means of vaccination or other medical procedures. The resistance to vaccinations therefore became part of a wider struggle relating to questions of the extent of state intervention into issues that until then were considered to belong to the private domain, such as family life, education, and religion.

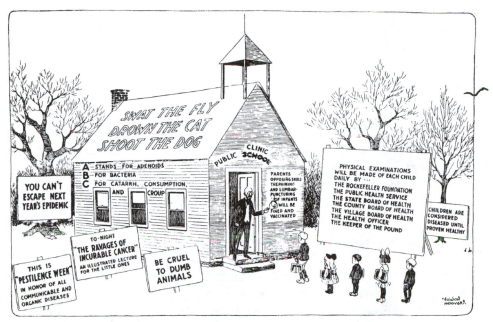

The Little Red, Serumized, Materia-Medicated, Politically-Exploited School-House!

FIGURE 2. From *Life Magazine,* 1904.

As reflected in a 1904 vintage cartoon in *Life* magazine (Figure 2), portraying a line of children entering a public school that becomes a public clinic, anti-vaccinationists fostered a growing sense of uneasiness that public health officials were turning the public schools into experimental medical clinics. In the cartoon, signs planted around the school pointed to a host of issues that concerned those opposed to vaccination and "organized" medicine at the turn of the twentieth century: superfluous operations, pointless experiments on animals, ongoing and accelerated invasion of the private domain by the state, and the tie between big money and research institutions—as exemplified in this case by the Rockefeller Foundation. Such medical intervention into the bodies and souls of children led to the medicalization of the schoolhouse—an institution that critics believed was at the heart of a grassroots democracy and should remain free of interference from the medical establishment. Conventional medicine had come to be viewed as a powerful and dangerous monopoly that sought to dominate and control the health domain, and critics believed that this sphere should remain in the hands of the democratic public.

Life magazine was not the only publication to endorse issues of anti-vaccination, anti-vivisection, and a general resistance to the process of medicalization.[56] At the turn of the twentieth century many articles concerned with the question of vaccinations and what was labeled the "serum craze" were found in various radical journals alongside articles discussing issues from animal experimentation to the growing monopoly of the American Medical Association.[57] Journals such as *Medical Talk for the Home, Homeopathic Envoy, Medical Liberty News, Journal of Zoöphily,* and *The Arena* contained articles fiercely criticizing the medical monopoly of "regular" medicine.[58] Frequent citations from these journals in comparable journals indicate that there was some level of collaboration among editors—a key element in the development of a network of criticism directed at organized medicine in which the vaccination issue assumed a sizable part.

From a reading of these materials one can observe recurring motifs calling for "medical freedom" and linking such liberty to the freedom demanded in matters of religion, politics, and health.[59] Their emphasis was on health issues, stressing the need for people to become wise enough in medical matters to make their own personal decisions and not be forced to conform to the dictates of establishment officials. Lora Little, one of the well-known combatants against vaccinations, defined this task as "the development of health culture."[60] This literature often contained severe social criticism that regarded the germ theory as an unworthy sidetrack, diverting discussion from social inequities such as poverty, inequality, and ignorance. Magic solutions in the form of vaccinations, these critics claimed, were harmful, primarily serving the physicians' interests. As in this fictitious doctor's diary published in *Life*, the usual depiction of physicians was of a greedy creature, caring only for his profits:

> Tuesday: This smallpox scare has helped me out greatly. I vaccinated fourteen swell children yesterday at three dollars each. This is pretty good. Besides, they are all likely to have complications . . . Wednesday: Two cases of diphtheria yesterday. Filled 'em up with serum. Wonder if that serum is any good? Sometime I think it is and sometimes I think it isn't. . . . Saturday: I have just been going over my accounts. Never did such a business before. Why, if this keeps up I shall in future be able to decline all baby cases and devote myself entirely to unnecessary operations.[61]

Another indication of this attitude are the words of the editor of *Medical Talk for the Home*, a journal that came out against what it saw as the tyranny of the medical establishment and supported presentation of information on health issues to the wider public so that everyone could make a personal decision about these issues: "The hunt for microbes is a mania, a terrible mania diverting the doctor's attention from everything else. He has even forgotten to be clean, forgotten to be human, forgotten to be reasonable."[62] The League for Medical Freedom, a short-lived organization established in 1910 to counteract the establishment of a National Health Bureau and other compulsory public health legislation, brought to the fore social and class argumentation:

> The history of civilization is largely the history of struggle of the people against classes seeking mastership, power and wealth at the expenses of the masses. . . . At the present time we are confronted by a powerful, well-organized and aggressive class, seeking from the National government departmental or bureaucratic power for a school of medicine that for half a century has striven with increasing zeal and determination to secure special legislation that would give to the privileged ones such monopoly in the treatment of the sick.[63]

The League, which included several homeopaths among its officers and members, wanted to protect the "sacred . . . right of the individual to choose the physician of his choice for his bodily ills. . . . Political freedom, religious freedom, medical freedom—this sacred trinity must be preserved unless privilege-seeking classes are to be permitted to strike down the sacred rights of man."[64] In an editorial dealing directly with the vaccination question, Flower presented his views on compulsory health legislation:

> While the National League for Medical Freedom does not as a League oppose vaccination or serum therapy, or seek to prevent any persons who wish to have their blood polluted by the

deadly poisons from assuming these risks, it does strenuously oppose compelling those who have no faith in the latest fad of the regular medical profession to have their lives of their children placed in jeopardy through compulsory legislation. . . . The battle of the people against wholesale poisoning of their blood by serums to-day is merely a repetition of the battle against compulsory inoculation of small-pox in the eighteenth century; and the intolerant attitude of the so-called regular doctors and their insistent demand for legal compulsion is the reappearance in the twentieth century of exactly the same spirit that dominated the so-called scientific doctors of the eighteenth century.[65]

Criticism of vaccinations during this period must be viewed as part of a broader social criticism of the "unholy alliance" between law enforcement personnel and physicians in the enforcement of vaccination that was "trespassing" on the vaccinated person's body through the sanction of a legal decree while social reforms that would reduce poverty and improve sanitation were neglected in favor of a "magic bullet" solution. As B. O. Flower commented, giving "organized medicine" the main responsibility in the sanitary field could lead to the wrong solutions: "While in favor of sanitation and cleanliness in the highest degree, we oppose the attempted use of these general principles as a cloak for compulsory medical treatment. We believe that the most eminent sanitary engineers, and not political doctors, should be placed in charge of the sanitary service."[66]

These opposition networks operated not only in regard to vaccinations, but also in other areas of health legislation. The call for medical freedom invoked by those groups coincided with their plea for freedom in religious and political matters, in a period of growing involvement of various state institutions in citizens' life. Citing the *New York Herald* on May 25, 1910, for example, B. O. Flower presented what he saw as the dangerous implications of a growing monopoly of the state in health and other matters:

> Standard Oil is a pulling infant in the way of a trust compared with the gigantic "combine" for which these doctors are working. It would create a monopoly more odious than was ever before conceived, one which would touch and control the life of the people at a thousand points of contact. . . . It would control hygiene, sanitation, food, education, immigration, public and private relief, labor conditions and a dozen other things, besides "research laboratories and equipment." In other words, the American people through their government would be engaged in experimentation upon the living animals—vivisection. Nothing so needless, nothing so audacious in the way of a trust was ever before conceived, much less proposed to be incorporated into the government.[67]

Apart from the political question of who should dictate public health policy, vaccinations carried with them more mundane bodily consequences. Recent scholars have shown how the debates over vaccination were a crucial part of a more general contentious discourse over body politics.[68] In essence, the vaccination—imprinted mainly on the bodies of children at the command of the state—constitutes an excellent case study for the understanding of the politicization of the body. These contests over citizens' bodies helped to shape a classed identity. Vulnerable bodies, such as those of immigrants and the working class, became an object of surveillance and monitoring by the state.

We should remember that the vaccination "operation" did indeed include the penetration of the body and the introduction of a disease agent. For many years prior to the introduction of glycerinated lymph, which made use of vaccine material that was relatively safer compared to vaccine produced from animals, transfer of the vaccine was carried out "arm to arm." Vaccine was produced from the arm of a child who had been not immunized earlier, and the material was then transferred to other children. Thus public health officials used children as a sort of walking laboratory for manufacturing vaccine. We should also remember that at the outset of the twentieth century there was no laboratory capable of establishing whether a child was immunized against smallpox. The procedure was accompanied by pain and, at times, other side effects due to contamination of the wound site. Such complications, and especially the scarification process, were an important component in the rhetoric of vaccination opponents. For example, J. M. Peebles, one of the foremost American anti-vaccinationists, complained: "Every child successfully vaccinated will carry on its body the scar—the brute-caused scar, the grievous sore, the scar of the 'beast' till death."[69] The scar was considered ugly, particularly for girls. For cosmetic reason, in many cases less exposed places such as the thigh or the knee served as vaccination sites for girls, instead of the arm for boys.

But the scar had a practical component, too. During this period, when it was not clear how the vaccination worked and whether a person was vaccinated or not, the only way of knowing was examination of the vaccination site. Indeed, for smallpox vaccination, this is a method used to this day. The only "test" was to examine the scar left on the subject's body, which served as mute proof that the vaccine had taken. The scar appeared several days after the procedure. If there was no sign that the vaccination had taken, the patient had to be revaccinated. Under epidemic conditions, the scar served as a visual form of certification of who was immunized and who was not. There were a number of states in the United States where entrance into public school was contingent on proof of immunization, with those lacking certification barred from school. The medical inspector would examine each child to see if he or she carried the characteristic mark or could produce a certificate from a doctor testifying that the child had been vaccinated or stating the reason the child had not been vaccinated.

One of the ways to get around being vaccinated, however, was to "forge" a scar. Indeed, the network of vaccination opponents did not just engage in theoretical discussions, but also provided instructions how one could escape what opponents perceived as a dangerous procedure:

> Get a little strong nitric acid. It can be got at the drug store. Get the arm ready and have a piece of soft blotting paper handy. Take a match or tooth-pick, dip it into the acid . . . Carefully transfer the drop to the spot on the arm where you wish the sore to appear. . . . After a week or so the spot . . . will begin to turn dark, and in a week or so more it will likely slough out a little piece, leaving a granulated sore underneath. This sore will gradually heal by producing a scar so nearly resembling vaccination that the average physician cannot tell the difference. . . . If a doctor wants to know whether the child has been vaccinated or not, simply show him the scar, and if he is satisfied with the scar well and good. . . . My own children have been treated in this way, and have been examined a great many times in school for vaccination, and the scars have always been regarded as genuine vaccination scars.[70]

The advice appeared in the periodical *Medical Talk for the Home*, edited by C. S. Carr— a known opponent of vaccination who also conducted a struggle against what Carr viewed as the growing monopoly of organized medicine. Carr considered his advice on this and related subjects to be part of a larger "genuine democratization" of health literature. All people, he believed, should have autonomy over their own bodies and the right to choose whether to be vaccinated. Strategies that barred children from public school were a form of intervention by the medical establishment into a private matter. Carr therefore held that citizens had the right to forge a scar that would "satisfy" the authorities. As another anti-vaccinationist wrote: "Every man's house is his castle, and upon the constitutional grounds of personal liberty, no vaccination doctor, lancet in one hand and calf-pox poison in the other, has a legal or moral right to enter the sacred precincts of a healthy home and scar a child's body for life."

The medical establishment responded swiftly and furiously to such evasion. A month after Carr's recommendation, *American Medicine* published a vitriolic editorial entitled "False Vaccination Scars: A Vile Crime Encouraged." The editor even recommended barring opponents of vaccination from hospital facilities, charging:

> The taxpayers have a right to demand it, and the profession through its influence could undoubtedly secure the enactment and execution of the necessary laws. One caution is necessary; the antivaccinationists must not be allowed to defeat the preventive measure by nitric acid sores or other scars made to deceive. If there is no way of detecting the fraud some methods of lessening it should be devised. Should not test questions, and even affidavits, be demanded by the examiners?[71]

The sharp response in *American Medicine* reflects the loathing some of the medical profession harbored toward opponents of vaccination, as well as their feelings that the only way to overcome opposition was, again, through the law.

Clearly, the network of opposition that operated through various print media spread a truly radical and powerful discourse, one that championed free choice in all health matters. Also, names of doctors who were willing to sign vaccination certificates spread by word of mouth as another way of avoiding the legal obligation to undergo immunization. A not insignificant number of homeopaths were also part of this network. As Erastus E. Case, a homeopathic physician from Hartford, Connecticut, admitted, "When compelled to vaccinate by demands of Boards of Health I administer one of the potencies of *Variolin* or *Vaccinin* . . . and scratch the same into the arm, certifying to the fact of vaccination. I do not urge any to be vaccinated, even in this manner; they come to me if conditions necessitate."[72]

The cooperation between homeopathy and other "faddist" organizations such as the League for Medical Freedom infuriated less radical homeopaths. In a typical letter Dr. DeWitt G. Wilcox of Boston wrote to the editor of the *Homœopathic Recorder*: "If we of the homœopathic school are so afraid that the dominant school will legislate us out of existence that we must call to our aid the medical quacks, the Christian Scientists, the poison food squad, and all the other medical sore-heads, then I must say that it is better that we die a respectable death and have a decent burial. For my part I would rather be licked fighting honorably with honest comrades than win by the aid of the Hessians."[73]

V

In 1927 the United States Supreme Court ruled in favor of sterilization of Carrie Buck, a twenty-one-year-old woman institutionalized in a mental health facility as feeble-minded—a psychiatric diagnosis that was common in the medical world at the turn of the twentieth century. The court described Carrie Buck as "the daughter of a feeble-minded mother and the mother of an illegitimate feeble-minded child" and noted "that she may be sterilized without detriment to her general health, and her welfare and that of society will be promoted by her sterilization." In presenting the rationale behind the court's decision to permit forcibly sterilizing the woman against her will, Justice Oliver Wendell Homes wrote: "It is better for all the world, if instead of waiting to execute degenerate offspring for crime, or to let them starve for their imbecility, society can prevent those who are manifestly unfit from continuing their kind. . . . Three generations of imbeciles are enough."[74]

The decision in the *Buck v. Bell* case is usually cited in regard to the history of eugenics,[75] but the decision contains another argument raised by Justice Holmes that is less frequently quoted: "The principle that sustains compulsory vaccination is broad enough to cover cutting the Fallopian tubes."[76] According to Holmes, the same principle that justifies compulsory vaccination—that is, precedence of the public welfare over the rights of the individual in the prevention of infectious diseases—holds in regard to involuntary sterilization as well. While I have no intention to suggest that sterilization and vaccination are acts of equal weight, quoting Justice Holmes' argument—written at the outset of the twentieth century—serves to take vaccination and "defamiliarize" it from its present hegemonic context. Historically there were times when the logic behind vaccination was on the same footing as coercive sterilization, a prerogative that is unquestionably and totally unacceptable today and that reminds us of darker times and deeds that took place not so long after the *Buck v. Bell* decision of 1927.

Vaccination has a unique position in the development of modern medicine and public health policy. At the turn of the century, vaccinations became a crucial part of the emerging public health paradigm. The establishment of a variety of public health practices and legislation, many of which, such as disease notification and infection control, continue to influence us today, had a strong foundation in vaccination ideology—especially its compulsory aspect. The analysis of the vaccination debate from the homeopathic angle can help us to erase simplistic dichotomies, such as between scientific and unscientific medicine or between rational and irrational medical practitioners. Homeopathic criticism of "regular" medicine also included the relationship of orthodoxy to public health authority, and here vaccination played an important part. While the majority of the homeopathic profession was drifting away from homeopathy's original radicalism and embracing the hegemonic scientific language of orthodoxy, many other alternative medicine practitioners—including several factions within homeopathy—tried to present an alternative vision of health and disease.

But the establishment of an alternative "health culture" cannot be disconnected from its political meanings and contexts. Radical criticism of regular medicine and public health measures at the turn of the twentieth century was quite often embedded in a network of dissent against the hegemonic Establishment, whether in politics or medicine. Calls for medical freedom and the right for individual choice in health matters were part of a broader battle for preserving the private sphere out of reach of the state. This network of dissent was composed of various factions, from anti-vivisectionists to anti-vaccinationists, from Christian Scientists to chiropractors. While anti-vaccinationists have been depicted as a monolithic group of unorthodox medical practitioners under the influence of "irrational and unscientific arguments," they were, in fact, composed of both regular and irregular practitioners, as well as laypeople who resisted "progressive" medical ideas imposed by the state. These associations questioned both the efficacy and safety of vaccination, and they attacked coercion as anti-democratic and un-American.

Many homeopathic physicians considered this kind of public condemnation of vaccination as unwise, potentially damaging the professional image of homeopathy. Yet for others, relinquishing the radical qualities of "pure" homeopathy signaled what they feared would be a dangerous process of assimilation and dissolution. For them opposition to vaccination—as with opposition to bloodletting in the past—became the new symbol of struggle against allopathy and the expanding influence of "organized" medicine. Yet the dilemma over definition of the identity of homeopathy was not limited only to professional identity. The vaccination question was broader, including fundamental questions of body politics, since obligatory vaccination undercut the autonomy held by individuals over their bodies to define their own health needs and challenged the traditional relationship between the individual, public health institutions, and the state. The relationship between the period's emerging medical institutions, such as hospitals, medical schools, public health, laboratories, and pharmaceutical firms, were viewed by many citizens as the construction of a dangerous cartel, out to take over their lives.

As part and parcel of the accelerated medicalization of life in general, this monopoly has had far-reaching significance on individuals' daily practices in modern America. Homeopaths on both sides were aware of these trends and struggled to define their position in relation to them. Many of the homeopaths in the United States at the advent of the twentieth century welcomed public health institutions, laboratories, and legislation that established public health as a social institution promoting the public good. Several outstanding homeopathic figures, such as Royal Copeland, the New York health commissioner (1918–1923) and later a U.S. senator, even became part of the public medical Establishment, applying the broad political connections that homeopaths possessed in American politics.[77] On the other hand, homeopaths were also associated with various political groups that expressed sharp criticism against the growing introduction of orthodox medicine and practices into the health domain. The controversy over vaccinations—beyond being a medical question about whether immunization was in keeping with homeopathic principles—was a bitter controversy over the limitations of the state and personal liberty. At the turn of the century, vaccinations became a crucial part of the emerging public health paradigm. The establishment of a variety of public health practices and legislation, many of which, such as disease notification and infection control, continue to influence us today, had a strong foundation in vaccination ideology—especially its compulsory aspect. Criticism of "regular" medicine also included the relationship of orthodoxy to public health authority, and here vaccination played an important part.

Indeed, this debate continues to this day. Despite the great differences both in contemporary vaccines and in the social and cultural context in which medicine operates today, opposition to vaccination is part of a long-standing tradition. Attempts to reduce opposition to an "irrational phenomenon" limited to fringe groups in the unconventional medical community is both shallow and problematic. Opposition to vaccination has many sources, including the desire for self-empowerment as people seek to regain responsibility through custodianship over their bodies. On the other hand, now as then, not all members of the unconventional medical community oppose vaccination. In contrast with the standard narrative of the history of vaccinations that presents this side of the debate as dangerous and irrational, a deeper look reveals its source in divergent groups that sought to establish a dialogue among themselves, parallel to their negotiations with orthodox medicine. A historical examination of the debate surrounding vaccination as a medical procedure carried out on the public in the name of the state and public health agents opens a window through which one can observe processes where medicine, health, and politics intersect. With the recent resurgence of smallpox vaccination programs and the fierce dispute they have created, this historical lesson can help us to listen much more carefully to the parties involved, recognizing their inner rationality as well as their complexity.[78]

MAKING FRIENDS FOR "PURE" HOMEOPATHY

Hahnemannians and the Twentieth-Century Preservation and Transformation of Homeopathy

Anne Taylor Kirschmann

HOMEOPATHS COMMONLY REFER TO the period between 1930 and 1970 in the United States as the "dark ages." Although homeopathy enjoyed considerable popularity in the nineteenth century and was still favored by many patients at the turn of the twentieth, the rapid decline in the numbers of homeopathic medical schools, hospitals, and professional organizations during the first decades of the century did not augur well for its future. Based on the authority of modern biological science, American medicine writ large had resulted in a general consensus in the early decades of the century, affecting the structures of medical education, research, institutions, and labor.[1] Yet homeopathy did not simply disappear. American medicine is also defined by the behavior of individuals—to patronize a particular doctor or healer, to take one drug rather than another, or to refuse drugs altogether. At the personal level, American medicine has been far more eclectic than the hegemony of mainstream medicine suggests.[2]

To understand how and why homeopathy persisted during this period, setting the stage for a revival during the last third of the century, this essay will address several questions: In what ways did homeopathy survive, and in what forms? What was homeopathy's appeal to twentieth-century patients and physicians? And perhaps more importantly, why should answers to these questions be of interest to anyone other than historians of medicine? Taking this last question first, we see that during various periods in its history, homeopathy has played a prominent role in what historian Charles E. Rosenberg calls "Worldview Holism," whereby the body serves as a "tool for thinking about society generally and its state of health or illness."[3] For example, although homeopathy's overriding purpose in the nineteenth century was to radically reform medicine, its popularity was enhanced by its links to various liberal reform movements, including women's rights and anti-racism. Similarly, people's advocacy of homeopathy in the twentieth century was not simply a therapeutic choice but reflected a crisis in values—perceptions that the institutions of modern life were increasingly dominated by technology, bureaucracy, narrowly focused experts, and commercialism.[4] To twentieth-century critics, American medicine epitomized the worst aspects of modern life. To second-wave feminists, it exemplified the public and private subordination and domination of women in society. Thus, homeopathy was both a therapeutic alternative and a form of cultural criticism—an actor in a "morality play directed at modern society and its costs."[5]

Although few in number, homeopaths throughout the twentieth century have been persistent critics of the corporatization of medicine. As such, they were part of a broader twentieth-century insurgency against corporate capitalism. Insisting upon the individual's right and responsibility to make decisions regarding one's own health, homeopaths remonstrated against an erosion of individualism by an increasingly powerful "organized medicine," unduly influenced by the pharmaceutical industry and backed by the state. But to understand the full meaning of homeopaths' insistence upon individualism in the body politic, we must begin with their views about the body itself.

According to homeopathy's founder, Samuel Hahnemann, disease resulted from a disturbed "spirit-like" vital force—an immaterial "being" animating the material organism, manifesting in sensations and functions or "morbid symptoms." Homeopathic physicians prescribed minute doses of particular drugs based on a patient's totality of "symptoms," changes in the health of the body and mind observed by the physician and felt by patients themselves.[6] Patients' emotions and thoughts—like their physical sensations—were part of the anatomy of illness. In "taking the case" physicians paid attention to patients' words, body language, and emotional cues, leading to the selection of the correct remedy. The homeopathic materia medica comprised drugs whose "symptoms" had been determined by testing or "proving" small doses of individual drugs on healthy persons. Based on Hahnemann's Law of Similars (*Similia similibus curantur*), the physician's task was to choose a single drug whose "symptom characteristics" most closely matched a patient's disease symptoms—one "homeopathic" to them. Hahnemann theorized that a similar, artificial disease produced by an infinitesimal dose of the drug substituted itself for the "natural" (original) disease, causing it to disappear. Due to the minuteness of the homeopathic drug, the artificial disease would soon be extinguished by the vital force, "striving to return to the normal state."[7] The homeopathic system of medicine incorporated gentle, pleasant-tasting remedies and a teleological understanding of disease causation and cure. It presumed an interconnected relationship between the mind and body, influencing health and disease, and it incorporated a doctor-patient relationship characterized by shared responsibility—of patients to correctly describe symptoms and of doctors to carefully observe patients and listen to their words.

While some nineteenth-century homeopaths conformed strictly to Hahnemann's teachings, most employed a combination of homeopathic and regular therapeutics. Over time, homeopathy lost its distinctiveness as a separate school of medicine. By the early decades of the twentieth century, the large majority had refashioned homeopathy as a therapeutic field within general medicine, rejecting many of Hahnemann's teachings as outdated.[8] However, a small minority of traditionalists (called Hahnemannians) were determined to maintain homeopathic distinctiveness according to three cardinal principles: prescription of the medicine according to the doctrine of similars, the minimum dose, and the single remedy.[9] In 1921, with homeopathic institutions in decline, Hahnemannians Julia Minerva Green and Julia M. Loos spearheaded efforts to found a joint physician-lay organization to prevent the disappearance of "pure" homeopathy. Incorporated in 1924 as the American Foundation for Homeopathy (AFH), its goals included the establishment of a major research center and hospital, a postgraduate school in homeopathy for physicians, and a national network of lay leagues where patients would study homeopathic principles and philosophy, creating demand for "real" homeopathic physicians. During a period of time when American physicians gradually distanced themselves from patients, the organization united physicians and patients in "making friends [for] pure" homeopathy.[10]

In contrast to the marginalization of women within mainstream medical organizations, women were exceptionally active in organizations to preserve homeopathy. In its heyday, homeopathy had a reputation for being more progressive than regular medicine on the question of women in the profession—a reputation that was enhanced by prominent women's rights activists such as Elizabeth Cady Stanton and Susan B. Anthony, who chose homeopathic physicians and supported women's homeopathic education.[11] Similar to their nineteenth-century roles as founders of medical colleges, teachers, and leaders of homeopathic professional organizations, women were the principal founders of the AFH. They were elected to the board of trustees, taught in the foundation's postgraduate school, and were instrumental in organizing lay leagues.

As founder, first chairperson, and a trustee of the AFH for forty years, Julia Green was one of the organization's guiding lights. A graduate of Wellesley College (1893) and Boston University School of Medicine (1898), Green developed a thriving homeopathic medical practice in Washington, D.C., early in the century. Similar to many professional women of her generation, she was a "social feminist." Believing marriage was incompatible with the demands of a professional career, Green dedicated herself not only to her medical career, but to the advancement of women in society through active participation in the suffrage movement as well as numerous women's professional and civic organizations.[12] A member of the Women's Joint Congressional Committee, founded in 1920 as a lobbyist for social welfare legislation, Green served on the sub-legislative committee on birth control in 1937, corresponding regularly with noted birth control activist and social reformer Mary Ware Dennett. A personal friend of Green's and a longtime advocate of homeopathy, Dennett was employed by the AFH from 1925 to 1927 as Special Lay Representative.

For early-twentieth-century Hahnemannians such as Green and Dennett, the triumph of orthodox medicine was not a scientific victory but a political one. Dennett believed people's freedom to choose health practitioners, like their freedom to make personal decisions regarding sexuality and reproduction, was threatened by the increasing bureaucracy of modern society, and especially by the political power of organized medicine, which she termed a "growing medical monopoly." Dennett resented the "tyranny of experts" who undermined the reasoned opinions and common sense of individuals holding different views. For Green and Dennett, homeopathy was "part of the plan of the universe, of what it means to help work out natural laws and not hinder them."[13] But they also defined homeopathy in the language of Progressivism, calling it a means of "race betterment"—a way to solve the problem of physical and mental illness in individuals, who would then transmit their superior health to future generations. By their lights, homeopathy was a tool of positive eugenics, ideally suited to preventive medicine and public health programs. Hahnemannians throughout the first half of the twentieth century believed their profession was a victim of "deep economic forces affecting all parts of the body politic, tending toward centralization."[14] Claiming that scientific discoveries merely reinforced the power of unseen, nonmaterial life forces, they viewed the rising power and mutual interests of the American Medical Association and the pharmaceutical industry as evidence that pecuniary profit rather than pure science determined medical orthodoxy.

Given the cultural and political dominance of mainstream medicine, AFH trustees believed that patients provided the best hope for keeping homeopathy alive. AFH goals, including the establishment of lay leagues, were based on the premise that patients educated in homeopathic theory and therapeutic principles would create demand for Hahnemannian physicians. Although only twelve lay leagues were organized prior to the 1960s and the numbers of homeopathic advocates remained small up to that time, AFH publications, educational programs, and leagues were a primary link between nineteenth-century traditional homeopathy and what today is called "classical" homeopathy. As a new generation of young people "discovered" homeopathy in the late 1960s and early 1970s, the AFH and affiliated organizations were primary sources of information, education, and support, contributing to the revitalization of homeopathy during the last third of the century.

In sustaining and promoting a different understanding of disease etiology and therapeutics, leagues encouraged the close association of patients and physicians, uniting advocates in a wide-ranging national and even international homeopathic community.[15] Reflecting the diversity and complexity of American society, leagues add to the evidence of a nation divided into discrete segments rather than defined by consolidation and common values.[16] Leagues and the homeopathic community in general constituted a separate society, one in which members could discuss their ideas about medicine, health, and the failures of American democracy without being called crackpots. League members usually met monthly to listen to lectures by homeopathic physicians and participate in discussions on the philosophy and principles of homeopathic medicine. League members actively recruited new doctors, offering them financial aid to attend the AFH postgraduate school and help in establishing medical practices in locations lacking homeopathic doctors. When a physician or medical student expressed interest in homeopathy, organizations in various areas worked together to bring him or her into the homeopathic fold. In addition to helping the newcomer "establish himself in the City or its Suburbs," members promised "a group who will greet you with open arms."[17] As many physicians learned, however, publicly identifying oneself as a homeopath often hindered professional opportunities.

Maisimund Panos, for example, became a physician after the 1947 death of her husband, John Panos.[18] Although both her husband and father had been homeopathic physicians, Panos considered her own knowledge of homeopathy "very basic." Frustrated by her inability to help former patients of her husband's who continued to call her for advice on remedies, she decided to embark upon her own medical career. After receiving her medical degree at Ohio State University and completing an informal preceptorship under a homeopathic physician, Panos took her internship at St. Petersburg City Hospital in Florida. She returned to St. Petersburg after a residency in Ohio with the intention of establishing a medical practice in the city. But according to Panos, the hospital's chief of staff was "chagrined" to learn of her interest in homeopathy, warning her that although he "couldn't keep her out," she should prepare to be ostracized should she continue with it. In 1959 Panos joined the Washington, D.C., practice of Julia M. Green at the invitation of both Green and the local lay league.

Like Panos, Connecticut homeopath Anthony Shupis also transcended the bounds of orthodoxy. In 1948 Shupis lost his privileges at Charlotte Hungerford Hospital in Torrington, Connecticut. Shupis' identity as a homeopath was common knowledge in the area, causing some of his physician friends to advise him to "tone down on the Homeopathy for my own good."[19] But Shupis' public advocacy of homeopathy was only part of the problem. He also violated unspoken rules of professional conduct, criticizing cases of "unwarranted" surgery and expressing anti-immunization views in news columns and letters to editors of papers throughout Connecticut. Shupis believed his expulsion from the staff of the local hospital was the result of his outspoken criticism of local health authorities and medical practices—criticism that was linked to his identity as an "unorthodox" practitioner.[20] The experiences of physicians such as Panos and Shupis became part of the narrative history of homeopathy—examples of the entrenched power of organized medicine to suppress and discredit anyone holding alternative views on health and medicine. Yet by the 1970s, homeopathy's identity as a "persecuted other" was a decided advantage, increasing its appeal to a countercultural and anti-establishment youth movement that viewed American medicine as the embodiment of the worst of mainstream American values.[21]

As Shupis battled with the local medical community, his arguments echoed themes prominent in homeopathic lay and professional publications. From 1920 to 1960, Hahnemannian publications criticized the rising commercialism in medicine influenced by the growing power of pharmaceutical companies. Shupis argued that his ouster was part of a deliberate effort by "the vested drug and surgical interests that control medicine, politics, and medical education in the United States" to silence voices of opposition.[22] Hahnemannians generally agreed that drug companies had "influenced, persuaded, preyed upon, [and] even coerced" physicians, medical organizations, boards of health, and the public into believing the companies were interested in the "welfare of humanity and the protection of the public," whereas their primary interests were "solely for the cold coin of the realm."[23] The pecuniary enrichment of vested interests played a large role in Hahnemannian opposition to serums, antitoxins, and toxoids used to immunize children against tetanus, diphtheria, infantile paralysis (polio), and other communicable diseases.

As Nadav Davidovitch's essay in this volume shows, homeopaths historically were divided on the issue of vaccination, and few homeopaths who had assimilated into mainstream medicine in the twentieth century protested immunization policies. Most twentieth-century Hahnemannians, however, opposed state-mandated vaccination, employing medical as well as political arguments against it.[24] Assisting parents who resisted policies requiring the vaccination of their children, Hahnemannians argued that compulsory vaccination was not only a violation of individual rights, but a prime example of commercialism in medicine, with pharmaceutical companies and doctors the primary beneficiaries of vaccine therapy.[25] More importantly, they argued, vaccinations caused injury to children. Similar to nineteenth-century anti-vaccinationists, twentieth-century Hahnemannians believed that antitoxins and toxoids were dangerous, suppressed an individual's "natural immunity," and were a "mad attempt" by modern medical research to "standardize man."[26] In the 1950s, when public controversy arose over the questions of safety and efficacy of the Salk vaccine as a preventative for polio, articles in homeopathic publications highlighted the cases of 204 children who had developed polio after receiving the vaccine.[27] Homeopaths insisted upon the uniqueness of individuals in the diagnosis and treatment of disease at a time of increasing regimentation of individuals within medical research and health care institutions. Not only did the latter reflect growing conformity and bureaucracy of modern life in general, said homeopaths, but "[t]he profit motive [of immunization] supersedes all other considerations even of personal liberty and the most fundamental of human rights."[28] According to one critic, the inoculation of thousands of people means a new mink coat, for more than one doctor's wife, daughter or girl friend, and new and bigger profits for the very ethical manufacturers of biological products. Were it not for the commercial angle, the profit motive, there would be no such thing as a small-pox scare or mass inoculations for this or any other disease. . . . Remember once and for all that compulsion is incompatible with freedom.[29]

Today, criticism of doctors is often overshadowed by complaints against health insurance providers such as HMOs. However, in other ways, homeopaths' objections sound remarkably current. *The Layman Speaks*, the principal organ of the AFH, cited articles from the United Press, Associated Press, and *Washington Post* criticizing "ineffective drugs," "false and misleading" advertising by drug companies, and iatrogenic disease caused by physicians' improper use of drugs, as well as detrimental side effects of new "wonder drugs" such as penicillin and the sulfonamides.[30] Homeopathic publications featured articles warning of the dangers of biomedical technology such as the X-rays used in treating particular cancers, criticizing the fragmentation of medical care spurred by specialization. They reported on the corrupting influence of commercial interests on doctors, including cases of physicians suspected of overcharging the government for treating veterans and those accused of receiving financial rebates from laboratories, medical supply firms, and druggists.[31] The message was clear. Individuals must be vigilant and educate themselves on matters of health, recognizing that government health agencies, physicians, scientific experts, and others charged with the public's welfare could not be trusted.

No issue better illustrates the magnitude of this belief during the 1950s and '60s than that of fluoridation. The AFH archival file on fluoridation bulges with newsletters, petitions, and testimonials from individuals and organizations opposing the fluoridation of public water supplies, including the National Committee Against Fluoridation, Natural Health Guardian, Massachusetts Citizens Rights Association, and Citizens Medical Reference Bureau, among others.[32] Calling it "mass medication . . . sanctioned by Government," articles in the *The Layman Speaks* and other homeopathic publications argued that fluoridation was a violation of individual constitutional rights, highlighting the opposition and reporting on activities of homeopaths in various locations.[33] In Chicago, Hahnemannian homeopath Arthur H. Grimmer and members of the Chicago Homeopathic Lay League held several meetings to develop strategies opposing the city's plan to fluoridate Chicago's drinking water.[34] In Needham, Massachusetts, Hahnemannian homeopaths and patients led efforts to outlaw fluoridation throughout the Commonwealth. Prior to a referendum on the issue in the town of Needham, homeopathic activists mailed approximately four thousand leaflets to householders, helping to defeat fluoridation in the town by a vote of 3,056 to 1,818.[35]

The foundation staff answered letters requesting information and/or offering advice on ways to effectively thwart what one correspondent called " the most disastrous medically political crime of all time."[36] In reply, AFH publicity director Arthur Green outlined the articles formulated by the Needham Citizens' Rights Association, an organization he helped establish in 1952 when compulsory fluoridation of that town's water supply was first proposed. He called them "our three simple freedoms": "The right of the citizen to a water supply free from any chemical or drug not required for purification; the right of the citizen to freedom of choice in matters concerning his own health, provided this choice does not infringe the rights of others; [and] the right of the professional person—particularly the physician and the Dentist—to investigate freely and speak freely without fear of censor-ship or retribution."[37] According to Green, the issue was not whether fluoride was good or bad; rather, it was a question of freedom of choice in matters pertaining to one's own health. The individual—not doctors, scientists, or public health organizations—experi-enced the consequences (good or bad) of ingesting particular drugs and chemicals. Thus the freedom to choose what entered one's body was not simply a civil right but an ethical issue. As he argued, "it is morally right that the individual choose freely, and morally wrong to strip him of freedom."[38] Green's third point—allowing medically educated professionals to practice freely—reflects the long-standing complaint among homeopaths that "their" professional experts had at best been ignored and at worst faced complete loss of status and professional privilege. This last scenario fueled homeopaths' opposition to anything smacking of "socialized medicine."

Beginning in the 1930s the American Institute of Homeopathy, along with the American Medical Association, opposed government efforts to "socialize medicine," defined as any government-sponsored health insurance programs.[39] By the early 1940s, Hahnemannians joined the chorus of voices opposing revitalized proposals for comprehensive national health insurance, such as the Wagner-Murray-Dingell bill of 1943, which would have made insurance universal, comprehensive, and administered as part of Social Security. During World War II, homeopaths as well as mainstream physicians employed fascism as a symbol in their battle against universal health care, equating the potential results of the Wagner Bill to the "regimentation under the lash of Nazi Germany."[40] The war provided both the lan-guage and the context for homeopaths protesting medical "tyranny" within the United States. "If the enthusiastic advocates of the 'four freedoms' have their way, we may all be en-joying the dubious benefits of socialized medicine and compulsory health insurance by the time the war is over. . . . Compulsion is incompatible with freedom and it is to be hoped that there is enough hard-headed Americanism in the medical profession to resist the inroads of socialized medicine to the utmost."[41]

In 1948 Oscar Ewing, administrator of the Federal Security Agency under Harry Truman, again advanced the subject of national health insurance, stimulating yet another round of debates. And in the changed context of Cold War politics, physicians linked national health care proposals to the creeping and sinister "communist menace" in America.[42] In addition to their symbolic usefulness, totalitarian tropes employed by a medical profession opposed to government-sponsored national health insurance reveal the extent of physicians' fears. They believed (not unreasonably) that agents of the government would use their power to hire and fire doctors, establish rates of pay, prescribe qualifications for specialists, and de-termine what hospitals or clinics should serve particular groups of patients—prerogatives they deemed solely within the purview of physicians. These threats to physician autonomy were even more salient to homeopaths, who believed their profession was already victim-ized by the calculating and politically powerful orthodox profession.[43] Worried that the government—in collaboration with the AMA—would establish therapeutic guidelines and a system of remuneration based on physicians' adherence to "acceptable" medical practices, Hahnemannians viewed government-run health insurance as the possible death knell for homeopathy.[44] Homeopaths urged their colleagues to "practice homoeopathy come what may. Let them call it bootleg medicine, outlaw medicine, black magic, anything they please. All we ask is a square deal, not another raw deal."[45]

In addition to "government intrusion" into private affairs such as state-mandated vaccination and fluoridation of public water supplies, a growing number of people were concerned about harmful medical procedures; food adulterated with artificial flavors, colorings, and preservatives; drug side effects; and the regimentation of individuals within medical research and health care institutions. Letters to the AFH reveal a lack of trust in a society where the usual safeguards or guides, such as government agencies and the courts, could not be relied upon to protect them. Mrs. A. L. Maynard "stayed away" from doctors unless she and her family "had to have one." She used "natural" vitamins to maintain health, turning to the AFH for information on how to locate a homeopathic physician.[46] Dora M. Wilson, who chaired her district Mental Health Club of the National Federation of Women's Clubs, wrote to the foundation for information about homeopathy, stating, "We feel the AMA are monopolistic, dictatorial, and endeavoring to eventually rob us of our liberties as to whom we may wish to help us solve our health problems."[47] Skeptical of the advice proffered by health experts, others solicited "second opinions" from the AFH. Pierre Bouillette of New York City wrote: "[P]eople are warned over the radio, in the newspapers, in offices, etc. about an incoming wave of Asiatic flue [sic] and advised to receive preventive shots. What does Homeopathy recommend? Where can one find the names and addresses of homeopathic physicians in New York City and Northern New Jersey?"[48]

Bouillette's last question touched upon perhaps the greatest threat to homeopathy at this point in time. The AFH postgraduate school had graduated fewer than one hundred physicians from 1924 to 1970, several from foreign countries. With few young doctors replacing those who had retired, homeopathy's own state of health was decidedly precarious. Due to an aging population of patients as well as doctors, long-established leagues in Chicago, Philadelphia, and Boston began to flounder.[49] For example, in 1963, Clara Strodel of the once-large Chicago Lay League reported to the AFH that the new people attending their meetings were elderly patients "expecting us to pull a homoeopath out of a hat because their doctors died or moved away."[50] Even the long-established Washington, D.C., league considered fifteen people at their monthly meeting a good turnout.[51]

Within the next decade, however, homeopathy experienced a dramatic shift in fortunes. One can even mark the precise year and month the turnaround occurred. In February 1969 an article titled "Homoeopathy—A Neglected Medical Art" appeared in *Prevention* magazine. A publication of the Rodale Press, *Prevention* was the bible of self-help health advocates, presenting articles on the role of "natural" foods and vitamins in maintaining health as well as alternative therapeutics in treating disease. But although *Prevention* provided national exposure and linked homeopathy with the rapidly expanding holistic health movement, it was individuals who secured the connections. Many older members of homeopathic lay leagues were members of "health federations" and "natural food" associations. They organized and attended meetings and conventions where topics ran the gamut from the use of laetrile in treating cancer to the superior benefits of raw food.[52] In the 1970s, as lay leagues cast about for new members, they turned to these health organizations, whose own rapid growth was spurred by the interests of a new generation. Members of the Homeopathic Lay League of the Northeast distributed homeopathic literature at various national and regional health food conventions, arranged for homeopathic speakers to appear on their agendas, and placed ads in the growing numbers of health food stores. By 1975 the organization had approximately seven hundred paid members. Other leagues reported equally dramatic success in attracting new members. According to Helen

Pohlmeyer of the New York Homeopathic League, after running monthly ads in the *Village Voice* during the 1970s the organization had so many "young people coming to our meetings that we are hard put to accommodate them in our meeting facilities."[53]

Topics of presentations at league meetings and articles appearing in the homeopathic lay press began to reflect the interests of a new generation of homeopathic advocates. They focused on homeopathy's role in preventive medicine, its "natural" approach to healing, and its relationship to herbs, vitamins, and other methods of healing such as applied kinesiology and acupuncture, both of which posited a role for unseen energy in healing. As the environmental movement gained strength, homeopathic newsletters and publications linked homeopathy with other groups concerned about the potential health hazards associated with hormones and "wonder drugs" in cattle feed, the fluoridation of public water supplies, and the "constant poisoning from supposedly beneficial sprays, fertilizers, preservatives, and purifiers."[54] Although the particular health threats were new, the libertarian and anti-materialist language of an earlier generation of homeopathic advocates resonated with countercultural youth. In her 1960 address as president of the American Institute of Homeopathy, longtime physician Elizabeth Wright decried the "mass medication" of society. She emphasized the constitutional rights of "[w]e, the people, as patients" to "protest exploitation for financial reasons of our individual health." While extolling the benefits of technical progress, efficiency, and legislative efforts to raise standards, Wright argued that they blinded people to the "encroachment of selfish forces," meaning "big business." Calling homeopathy an "enlightened minority," Wright invoked the values of human freedom, the protection of the individual, and the rights of minorities as the "precious heritage" of democracy in its "original Jeffersonian form."[55] With the growth of the civil rights and feminist movements during this period, language defending individual and minority rights acquired new meaning. For a new generation convinced of the moral bankruptcy of established institutions and authority, homeopathy's identity as persecuted minority—outsider to mainstream medicine—greatly enhanced its appeal.

The embrace of homeopathy by the counterculture of the sixties and seventies reflected a desire to revitalize, purify, and unify the individual body as well as the body politic. Heightened awareness of the social and environmental costs of economic and industrial progress, the unpopular war in Vietnam, and racism exposed during the struggle for civil rights led many to conclude that America had lost its moral compass.[56] Many of those drawn to investigate homeopathy were self-described "hippies." In general, they were middle-class whites, opposed to the escalating U.S. involvement in the war in Vietnam, and alienated by an establishment that had given rise to values based on consumerism, patriarchy, runaway technology, and a conformist and market-oriented corporate mentality.[57] They explored various alternative sources of knowledge and ways of organizing work and family life that reflected non-market-oriented values of love, caring, cooperation, service to others, egalitarianism, and self-reliance. Within the next two decades, these newcomers swelled the homeopathic ranks.

For Joe Lillard, homeopathy represented personal freedom, self-reliance, empowerment, and a less expensive alternative to mainstream medicine.[58] After several years as an employee of the federal government, Lillard sought independence, solitude, and the freedom associated with going "back to the land." In 1974, Lillard and some friends jointly purchased a farm outside the Washington, D.C. area. With his friends responsible for the monthly mortgage payments and other expenses, Lillard worked full time maintaining the farm, receiving $40 per month from his co-owners to cover his basic needs. Lillard first learned about homeopathy in 1978 when he suffered a severe cut on his leg from a chain saw, and a local woman who was a homeopathic lay practitioner offered him a remedy to aid in healing the wound. Pleased with the results, Lillard had similar success alleviating his back pain with a homeopathic remedy. For Lillard, homeopathy was a nontechnological and inexpensive alternative to mainstream medicine, in tune with his new self-reliant, low-maintenance approach to life. According to Lillard, learning how to prescribe homeopathically for himself and his farm animals was a form of "empowerment." In the summer of 1979 he attended a course of instruction for lay practitioners offered by the National Center for Homeopathy (NCH), founded in 1974 by the AFH to carry out its educational programs. Lillard and others who attended the school that summer later formed a homeopathic study group in Washington, D.C., and they remain friends to this day.

Beginning in the 1970s, homeopathy was also rejuvenated by a new generation of homeopathic physicians and other health care professionals. All were searching for something beyond what their mainstream medical training and practice offered. They were not necessarily antagonistic toward mainstream medicine; rather, they were discouraged by its methods and disappointed by its limitations. Idealistic, anti-technological, anti-hierarchical, and anti-authoritarian, these professionals were ill fitted for the culture of organized medicine. They were uninspired and even horrified by its practice. Individually they questioned what it meant to be a healer, eventually adopting homeopathy as a philosophical and therapeutic alternative to mainstream medical practice. For many, a large part of homeopathy's appeal was its older model of the doctor-patient relationship, in which physicians spent time listening to patients, and where knowledge of patients' emotional and social lives often influenced therapeutic decisions.[59] But another, more prosaic reason explains why disenchanted medical professionals found their way to homeopathy. It was there to be found. Homeopathy had a body of literature, a few pharmaceutical companies producing homeopathic remedies, a small but dedicated corps of practitioners, and—owing to efforts of the AFH—a means of educating newcomers. Unlike today's plethora of alternative therapies and schools of alternative healing, in the early 1970s homeopathy had the field largely to itself.

Richard Moskowitz graduated from Harvard University in 1959, earning his medical degree from New York University School of Medicine in 1963. Early in his career, Moskowitz was drawn to a personalized and informal way of practicing medicine based on consensus rather than authority. While still in medical school, he developed serious misgivings about practicing medicine the way he had been trained. He shrank from a "culture of entitlement that gives physicians and medical students carte blanche to do as we see fit," compelling patients to "obey and even thank us for it." In his view, such a culture actually propagated disease, "both indirectly by spreading fear and doubt, and directly through overuse of diagnostic and treatment procedures with obvious power to harm."[60] After his internship, Moskowitz took a position as house physician at a small hospital. At that time, the war in Vietnam provided the context for his growing awareness of how concepts of illness and healing were "framed and distorted" by the metaphors and imagery of warfare. With various weapons in their arsenals, physicians attacked disease with antibiotics and other "magic bullets." They employed X rays and chemotherapy to bombard invading cells and bacteria. When an American general rationalized destroying a Vietnamese village in order to save it, Moskowitz recognized the metaphor as having been "lifted almost verbatim from the cancer specialist." He was struck by the knowledge that "what had once seemed like mere figures of speech" in the everyday lives of physicians actually revealed "a systematic philosophy of militarism for its own sake. . . . Trained as a soldier in the endless war against disease, and armed with the latest weapons to shoot down any abnormality that showed itself, I was ready to desert my post and fight no more."[61]

Moskowitz's application for admitting privileges to a local hospital—barely approved by voting physicians—was subsequently overruled by the hospital's board of trustees. In his view, "my antiwar views and unorthodox style of practice had alienated many of the physicians in town." By the end of the decade, Moskowitz was practicing what he called "minimalist medicine," guiding people through the medical system and trying to "protect them from being hurt too badly.[62] He visited patients in their homes, examined them as "non-invasively as possible," and after making a diagnosis allowed a patient's individuality and experience to guide his recommendation. Moskowitz's route to homeopathy was via the "gentle, family-centered atmosphere" of the home birth, whose model of the doctor-patient relationship conformed to his own ideas on the important role of patients in their own healing. Rejecting the authoritarian style that characterized mainstream medicine, Moskowitz said he learned to "sit down, be quiet, and pay attention" during his assistance at over six hundred home births between 1970 and 1982.[63] Seeking subtler and less harmful ways of influencing health than Western medicine allowed, Moskowitz became interested in Oriental medicine and eventually "stumbled" upon homeopathy in 1974, taking a two-week course offered at the NCH. Although he considered the course a barely adequate introduction to homeopathy, the principles of homeopathic practice reinforced what he was already doing, "making a diagnosis but allowing the individuality of the patient to point the way to treatment."[64] Central to his story is the influence of women both on his individual practice and on medicine in general during this period in time. The home birth movement was popularized by women who resented the rigidity of hospital regulations governing labor and delivery as well as the often sexist and paternalistic behavior of male physicians toward women patients.

As Amy Bix's essay in this volume demonstrates, predominately white, middle-class women developed a new style of politics to redress the imbalance of power in both their professional and personal lives. Many rejected the values of the male medical establishment, considering it a unique vehicle of female oppression and domination. As one strand of the feminist revolution of the 1960s, the women's health movement encompassed several goals, including the demystification of medical knowledge and demedicalization of natural life events such as childbirth and menopause. Feminists demanded safer and more effective methods of birth control and sought to remove the control exercised by doctors over reproductive technology. They challenged the superiority of doctors' so-called objective clinical knowledge over subjective knowledge based on women's own experiences of their bodies. Denouncing the authoritarian and elitist values of mainstream medicine, feminists organized self-help groups in which women shared knowledge and validated each other's experiences.[65] The corresponding increase in homeopathic self-study groups comprising mostly women during the 1970s and 1980s was in large part fueled by the politics of feminism.[66]

During her 1980 internship at St. Clare's Hospital in Schenectady, New York, Lisa Harvey acquired a reputation for spending time with people, listening to them—and running behind schedule.[67] Harvey was interested in a type of patient care that paid attention to the nutritional, emotional, psychological, and social needs influencing patients' health. Becoming frustrated with the antibiotics that were "thrown" at people, Harvey said she questioned herself every day about whether she was adhering to the physicians' primary dictum to "first do no harm." In 1982, Harvey moved to Berkeley, California, epicenter of the radical student movement, joining the staff of the Berkeley Women's Health Collective. There she was able to "listen to women's concerns and pay attention to their words." The collective was nonhierarchical, feminist, and cooperative, with all personnel receiving the same pay—approximately $8 per hour. Like Moskowitz, Harvey saw herself not as an "expert" or "boss" but as a teacher and guide to patients. Harvey first heard about homeopathy from several patients who were members of a homeopathic study group in Oakland. At that time, Harvey had become interested in "energetic medicine," which she defined as "a therapy that supports the body's own healing energy through nonmaterial means . . . [working] . . . on an energetic rather than a physical level." Homeopathy's metaphysical principles interested her, and she joined the Oakland study group. Although one member was a nurse and another a nurse practitioner, most were not health professionals. Together they studied cases and developed ideas about appropriate homeopathic remedies. Other homeopathic medical practices also drew inspiration from such feminist values, emphasizing the collaborative nature and lack of hierarchy found in most study groups.

Lia Bello began her career early in the 1970s as a nurse at the Greater Southeast Community Hospital in Washington, D.C. Bello believed she could make a difference in healing by paying attention to patients' words and their emotional needs.[68] However, Bello found little time to listen to and talk with patients amidst her many hospital duties. Idealistic and eager to collaborate with physicians on patient care, she grew frustrated at doctors' lack of interest in what nurses had to say or in the notes they carefully recorded on patients' charts. A self-described "hippie" and feminist, Bello first heard the word *homeopathy* from a clerk in a local health food store. Intrigued, Bello paid a visit to the nearby office of the National Center for Homeopathy. After a program of self-study and attending a course in homeopathy for medical professionals at the NCH, Bello became an apprentice to Washington, D.C., homeopathic physician David Wember. She later joined Wember's practice along with well-known lay prescriber Catherine Coulter, who had studied homeopathy in France. With an emphasis on the patient's emotional state and temperament in prescribing homeopathic remedies, their homeopathic practice corresponded to Bello's own ideas on the role of emotions in healing. Increasingly conscious of herself as a "spiritual being" during this period in her life, Bello found in homeopathy a metaphysical understanding of illness and health. And as part of a team where doctor, nurse, and lay prescriber contributed equally to discussions of patients' cases, homeopathic practice provided the egalitarianism and collaboration for which she had been searching.

During the 1970s and '80s, AFH/NCH-affiliated lay leagues emphasizing patient education in homeopathic principles and philosophy gradually disappeared. In their place arose independent homeopathic study groups focused on self-treatment, whose participants considered themselves practitioners rather than patients. For independent seekers such as Joe Lillard, joining a study group constituted a political act of disengagement from an established medical economy. For professionals such as Moskowitz, Harvey, Bello, and others, homeopathy satisfied a desire for a method of healing that encompassed spiritual and feminist values. With its long history of women's leadership, homeopathy appeared especially progressive compared to the male-dominated medical mainstream. Despite women's prominence in the AFH/NCH, however, the old guard within homeopathy's ranks, includ-

ing women, did not consider themselves feminists. While Julia Green was part of a generation of women physicians who felt more connected to the female community at large,
Maisimund Panos and women professionals of her generation came of age in a cultural climate that downplayed female relationships and rejected public feminism. They had made
it in a man's world, believing individual perseverance and ability were the keys to accom-
plishing one's goals.

When Lia Bello first appeared in the NCH offices in 1974, her general appearance as well
as her feminist ideology set her apart from the center's staff. With her long straight hair, low-
heeled Earth shoes, "natural" cotton clothing, and youth, Bello was in stark contrast to the
"straightness" of the NCH staff. Some of the men were "big guys with cigars," and a few of
the women had "bleached blond hair." According to Bello, their conservatism was oddly appealing, lending homeopathy a kind of established legitimacy.[69] Yet, mirroring the cultural
clashes taking place in society at large, the two generations soon found themselves at odds
over the direction of homeopathy and the goals of the National Center. Indeed, among
homeopaths today, the growing divide between the two groups during the period between
1978 and 1981 continues to be known as the "Great Unpleasantness."

According to Moskowitz, who was director of publications for the NCH in the early
1980s, the 1974 division of the AFH into two separate organizations—one to raise funds
(AFH) and one to carry out homeopathic programs (NCH)—had been "disastrous for
both organizations."[70] The National Center was dependent upon AFH approval and funding of its programs, some of which were turned down by the AFH trustees, who criticized
the center for its "failure to use funds for maximum effectiveness and economy."[71] Although the details are complex, the differences, at bottom, appear both generational and
ideological.[72] Many in the old guard had become used to homeopathy's "outsider" status—
even at times reveling in it. They nevertheless yearned for respectability in the form of
homeopathy's recognition as a legitimate part of American medicine. They discouraged
lay practice, insisting upon the primacy of physicians' authority, and only reluctantly embraced homeopathy's changing identity as part of the holistic health movement. According
to newcomers, they were "defensive," "conservative," and lacked enthusiasm for recruiting
more physicians to the homeopathic ranks. They were satisfied with the status quo in
the center's educational programs, whereas new members wanted to incorporate "exciting" new homeopathic teachers such as George Vithoulkas of Greece.[73] According to
Moscowitz, leaders in the NCH wanted to end their financial dependence on the foundation and, "above all, to get homoeopathy back into the mainstream of the burgeoning
holistic health movement."[74] By all accounts, they succeeded. By the end of the century
homeopathy was transformed into one of the most popular alternatives to mainstream
medicine in the United States.[75]

As cultural critics such as Christopher Lasch, Jackson Lears, and others have shown,
yearnings for the "authentic, the natural, and the real" pervade twentieth-century American
culture. Responding to the fragmentation, sterility, and secularization of modern life and
its "complacent creed of progress," these yearnings have assumed various forms.[76] The
anti-modernism of twentieth-century homeopathy is one expression of such yearnings
within American medicine. Clearly, its proponents and practitioners considered homeopathy useful in preventing illness and managing disease. Homeopathic advocacy, however, was also a tool for conceptualizing and criticizing not only mainstream medicine but
the technological, bureaucratic, and dehumanizing elements within society as a whole.

As a tradition with a moral and spiritual core, upholding decidedly anti-modern values, homeopathy's survival and revival in the twentieth century add to evidence refuting the homogenizing power of America's integrated economy and liberal, secular mass culture.[77] Twentieth-century homeopaths consistently expressed a nineteenth-century-style populist resentment of corporate and state power.[78] They defended their rights as individuals to access a system of healing that was ridiculed by organized medicine—an institution backed by the tremendous authority of modern science and linked closely to government organizations. Homeopaths were, therefore, a small group of insurgents whose "democratic dissidence" was part of an earlier tradition of liberalism that began to lose much of its meaning in the nineteenth century as American society became increasingly interdependent, urban, and industrialized.[79]

Homeopaths' insistence upon individual rights, then, was at cross purposes with both Progressivism and New Deal liberalism, both of which shifted authority from the individual and family to the group and state, subjugating private interest for the good of society. In the context of the first two-thirds of the century, homeopathic advocacy in many ways thus deserves the label "conservative," going against the grain of modern corporate political ideologies. However, when the New Deal political coalition was shattered by the radical populism of the 1960s and 1970s, homeopathy shed its conservative identity. As liberalism was transformed from an ideology legitimated by democratic majoritarianism into one focused on the rights of minorities, homeopathy became part of a "new liberal" order. A young generation resurrected homeopathy's feminist and populist roots, reclaiming and exalting its reformist and anti-orthodox legacy.[80]

Although homeopathy was a relatively minor vehicle for cultural criticism throughout much of the twentieth century, its dissents foreshadowed a growing uncertainty, beginning in the 1970s, of the value and effectiveness of medical care among neoconservatives and liberals alike. Homeopathy's burgeoning popularity, as well as the rapid growth of various medical alternatives during the last third of the century, reflects both a new therapeutic skepticism and a loss of confidence in the institutions of postmodern life more generally. For most of the twentieth century, Hahnemannians likened themselves to Cassandra—issuing warnings no one heeded. At century's end, we should acknowledge their persistent, even providential, role in questioning the meanings and measuring the costs of American progress.

REVISITING THE "GOLDEN AGE" OF REGULAR MEDICINE

The Politics of Alternative Cancer Care in Canada, 1900–1950

Barbara Clow

TYRELL DUECK HAD JUST TURNED thirteen in October 1998 when he slipped in the shower, hurting his right knee.[1] His parents thought the persistent pain was probably the result of a growth spurt or an old soccer injury, but when the knee refused to heal, they consulted their family physician. The doctor, suspecting that Tyrell had cancer, immediately referred him to the Cancer Centre at the Royal University Hospital in Saskatoon, Saskatchewan. In late November, pediatric oncologist Christopher Mpofu delivered the diagnosis: osteogenic sarcoma. Because this type of cancer spreads rapidly and relentlessly, Mpofu recommended an equally aggressive course of treatment: chemotherapy to shrink the tumor, followed by surgery, probably a midthigh amputation. Mpofu believed that swift and decisive intervention would give Tyrell a 65 percent chance of survival, but without treatment, the teenager would die within a year.

Tyrell Dueck's situation, though appalling, was hardly unique. Many others, including Canada's famed Terry Fox, had received the same devastating diagnosis and been given similar odds for beating the disease.[2] Yet Tyrell's story and his suffering made headlines as a result of the treatment choices of his parents and the reactions of the hospital staff, the child welfare authorities, and the courts in Saskatchewan. When Tyrell's parents, Tim and Yvonne Dueck, learned that chemotherapy and amputation were all that conventional medicine could offer their son, they decided to investigate alternatives, including vitamin and dietary therapies available at a clinic in Tijuana, Mexico. As devout, fundamentalist Christians, the Duecks also prayed with other members of their congregation for divine intervention and healing. "The staff worked hard," one journalist commented, "but couldn't convince them that conventional treatment was Tyrell's best chance."[3] In response, the hospital reported the situation to the Department of Social Services on the grounds that Tyrell's life was being placed in jeopardy by his parents. Government officials agreed and petitioned the courts to intervene. On December 11, 1998, a court order granted the Minister of Social Services guardianship over Tyrell Dueck with respect to his medical care. Although Tyrell continued to live at home, his parents were required to bring him to the hospital for chemotherapy notwithstanding their own beliefs and the wishes of the patient. Two full rounds of chemotherapy shrank the tumor, but doctors remained convinced that only amputation held out any real hope of saving the teenager from certain death.

At the end of the following February, Tyrell himself informed Mpofu that he would not undergo further chemotherapy, nor would he submit to amputation of his right leg. Once again, hospital staff and the child welfare authorities appealed to the courts. In an emergency weekend hearing, the presiding judge, Justice Allison Rothery, ordered psychological evaluation to ascertain whether Tyrell was competent to make choices about his health and care. Two psychologists filed different assessments, but Rothery sided with the expert who believed that Tyrell was unduly influenced by an authoritarian father who was not giving him accurate information upon which to make a decision. She consequently ordered the teenager back to the hospital and forbade his parents to accompany him. "This way," she explained, "Dr. Mpofu can bring Tyrell to understand the need for the medical treatment prescribed, and the medical team will be able to provide the psychological preparation and support for . . . treatment that they deem appropriate."[4]

The Duecks' decisions and Rothery's ruling unleashed a storm of controversy as ethicists, activists, laywers, and the public debated the merits of the case. Some were outraged at state interference with parental rights and private choices about health care; others were appalled that the Duecks would refuse treatment that might save their son's life. University of Saskatchewan law professor Ron Fritz also pointed out the practical implications of trying to impose treatment on a thirteen-year-old boy. "What are they going to do?" he asked. "Force him down in order to deliver an anaesthetic and amputate his leg?"[5] Ultimately, Canadians were spared the need to resolve these issues. In March 1999, tests showed that Tyrell's cancer had spread to his lungs, and as a result, doctors estimated that his chances of survival had plummeted to just 10 percent. Hospital and government officials abandoned legal action, and the Duecks were finally free to take their son to the American Biologics Clinic in Tijuana for alternative treatments. Their hopes flared briefly when tests conducted in Mexico indicated that the cancer had not spread, a conclusion allegedly supported by Scripps Hospital in San Diego. Nonetheless, four months later, Tyrell Dueck died.

Media coverage of Tyrell's confrontation with cancer, with health care providers, and with the state provides an illuminating introduction to the political history of alternative medicine in Canada. The Duecks' experiences embodied the most traditional definition of "political"—the willingness and ability of government to intrude into the private lives of citizens and to elicit compliance. Although the family rejected conventional medical therapies, the provincial government and courts required them to accept chemotherapy and, at least in theory, amputation. The Duecks' story also exemplifies the exercise of other types of power by actors other than the state. Government intervention in Tyrell's case, for instance, came at the behest of medical and psychological experts. Although doctors themselves did not have the power to force treatment on Tyrell, their claims to exclusive or superior knowledge of health and healing convinced others to take coercive action. To borrow Paul Starr's terms, the "social authority" of the courts and the government was backed by the "cultural authority" of modern medicine.[6] Indeed, the "cultural authority" of conventional medicine was readily apparent in many of the news features on Tyrell Dueck as well as in the comments of legal and health experts. For example, court-appointed psychologist Josephine Nanson described the "cultural clash" of the "medical community, which is grounded in evidence, versus a family who just doesn't think that way."[7] The media and health professionals also regularly played up the "'right-wing, fundamentalist, faith-healing' Christian world view" of the Duecks despite the fact that the family consistently denied religious convictions were at the heart of their decision to eschew conventional therapy.[8] Here, then, was a predictable, even stereotypical cast of villains and heroes in the history of alternative medicine. As one *Maclean's* reporter concluded, Tyrell's diagnosis "set in train a jarring collision between medical science and Tyrell's Christian fundamentalist parents."[9]

At the same time, the experiences of the Dueck family revealed the power of laypeople. Although Tim and Yvonne were forced to comply with court directives regarding Tyrell's care, they resisted official interference by every means at their disposal, including court appeals. Their cause also evoked considerable popular and political sympathy. According to one reporter, the Duecks "received upwards of 200 calls a day from supportive legislators and parents," many of whom were concerned about the motives of doctors and government officials and about the threat to personal freedom and the sanctity of the family posed by court rulings.[10] Moreover, when provincial authorities and hospital staff suspended legal action after Tyrell's cancer had spread, at least one journalist suggested that public opinion had been instrumental in forcing the hand of the state. An unnamed "government source" allegedly claimed that provincial leaders were anxious to "'unload this whole Tyrell Dueck mess as soon as possible,' partly because the time is ripe for an election call."[11] Tyrell's personal and private battle with disease was thus transformed into a complex political contest as well as a media spectacle.

For many scholars interested in alternative medicine, the Dueck case is explicable as a post–World War II phenomenon. Laypeople, allegedly disenchanted with conventional medicine and empowered by the political activism of the 1960s, have turned increasingly to purveyors of alternative therapies in the last three decades.[12] Press coverage of Tyrell's choices and those of his family in the 1990s seem to support this interpretation. "Perhaps," observed one commentator, "the Duecks' decision and the wider growth of interest in alternative therapies generally reflect not a disbelief in the efficacy of conventional medicine, but a widespread concern that too often human needs are subjected to medical imperatives rather than medical practice serving human needs."[13] Underlying this explanation for the popularity of alternative medicine is the assumption that prior to the Second World War, doctors ruled the health care roost—with the sanction of the state and the public, and with few challenges from unconventional healers. Indeed, historian John Burnham has described the first half of the twentieth century as the "golden age" of conventional medicine.[14]

Although it seems clear that organized, philosophically distinctive alternatives to regular medicine were neither common nor especially robust before World War II, we must not assume that a therapeutic or ideological consensus prevailed in the health care arena. Many medical sects struggled simply to survive after the turn of the century, yet a diverse array of patent medicines and proprietary treatments multiplied and flourished across North America. For many sufferers and their families, as for the Duecks decades later, these therapies and the practitioners who dispensed them constituted a legitimate, viable alternative to conventional care.

More important for a discussion of the politics of healing, the Duecks' struggle for control over Tyrell's care bears some striking affinities with earlier contests over alternative medicine in general, and alternative cancer care in particular. During the 1930s in Ontario, when dozens of unconventional cancer treatments flooded the marketplace, sufferers, the healthy public, regular and alternative practitioners, and provincial legislators found themselves at loggerheads over many of the same principles that defined the Dueck controversy: the limits of personal autonomy, the nature of state and medical authority, and the definition of therapeutic legitimacy. At the same time, the outcome of these battles over alternative cancer care challenges enduring assumptions about the rise and fall of medical monopoly in the twentieth century. While the Duecks tried to resist the power of the government and the medical profession, eventually they were forced to accede to conventional medical prescriptions sanctioned by the state and the courts. By comparison, cancer sufferers in 1930s Ontario often succeeded in limiting governmental, judicial, and professional interference with their health care choices and with the work of alternative practitioners. In other words, lay beliefs and behaviors proved more potent during the "golden age" of conventional medicine than they are today, when public and political confidence in the medical profession have allegedly reached their nadir.[15]

I have divided this article into two main sections. In the first part, I examine the relationships that evolved between the state, the public, and the medical profession in Ontario from the late nineteenth century to the early decades of the twentieth century. This background is crucial for understanding the controversy over alternative cancer care that rocked the province in the 1930s. In the second section, I focus on the life and work of one unconventional cancer practitioner, Rene Caisse, and the attitudes and experiences of her supporters.[16] Caisse, a nurse practicing in a small town north of Toronto, was one of the most popular alternative healers in Ontario during the 1930s, and her herbal treatment for cancer, Essiac, remains one of the most popular—and controversial—alternative therapies for cancer in North America today.[17] Her fight for recognition, especially her dealings with the government, provides a powerful lens through which to view lay attitudes and their impact on the politics of healing during the 1930s. Caisse and her supporters not only disagreed with the medical profession about how best to evaluate Essiac and other alternative treatments for cancer, but also they denounced and defied every attempt to restrict her practice. She never won official acceptance, but popular support for her therapy enabled her to treat thousands of cancer sufferers with impunity, in open defiance of the medical community, the government, and the law.

THE POLITICS OF HEALING IN ONTARIO: SUFFERERS, HEALERS, AND LEGISLATORS

Early in the nineteenth century, doctors practicing in Ontario enjoyed no special privileges in the medical marketplace. Like their counterparts in the United States, "regular" or allopathic practitioners competed with a multiplicity of "irregular" healers, including herbalists, Thomsonians, homeopaths, midwives, and others. Sometimes doctors won the respect and allegiance of patients; sometimes they lost business to their rivals. By the end of the century, however, the regular profession had successfully allied itself with the state, thereby acquiring an unprecedented degree of influence. In 1882, for example, when the provincial authorities founded the first board of health in Ontario, they relied on doctors to formulate and implement policy. Ontario premier Oliver Mowat told the first secretary of the board, Dr. Peter Bryce, "We have passed this health legislation but have little knowledge of just what there is to do, or of its extent . . . its success will depend upon your energies."[18] In the following decades, a variety of public health initiatives, from vaccination programs to the regulation of water supplies, grew directly from professional recommendations to the government.[19] At the same time, regular practitioners dominated all levels of the provincial health administration, from the offices of district health officers and local coroners through to the chair of the board of health. By the 1930s, the convention of appointing a doctor to the position of minister of health had also become deeply entrenched.[20]

Although the Ontario government relied heavily on professional expertise in this period, legislators steadfastly refused to grant doctors a monopoly over the practice of medicine. In the 1860s, for example, regular practitioners vigorously lobbied the provincial government to restrict the activities of medical sects, such as hydropathy, homeopathy, and eclecticism. Rather than banning these irregular practitioners, however, the state sanctioned their activities by making them equal members with doctors in a new regulatory agency, the College of Physicians and Surgeons of Ontario.[21] Principled objections to the notion of monopoly undoubtedly prompted the government's decision, but political sensitivity to public opinion also shaped this policy. As historians R. J. Gidney and W. P. J. Millar have pointed out, "The public interest required that practitioners show proof of medical training and certification by their peers. But there was no compelling justification for conferring exclusive legitimacy on this or that therapeutic doctrine advanced by this or that respectable, trained medical man. . . . In the third quarter of the nineteenth century, what was reputable was still a matter for the laity to decide."[22] Even after the turn of the twentieth century, as the alliance between the state and the medical profession grew stronger, the government remained reluctant to curtail the activities of unconventional healers.[23] In 1921, for instance, Ontario premier E. C. Drury "made it clear that he would not agree to any amendment [to the Medical Act] that would completely prohibit irregulars from practice. He felt that in time of sickness and distress a person was entitled to treatment from those in whom he had placed his confidence."[24] Drury's anti-monopoly sympathies were hardly surprising given the populist roots of his political ideals and the base of his political support in a farm-labor coalition.[25] But political resistance to the aspirations of the medical profession transcended party lines in this period. When Howard Ferguson, head of the business-dominated Conservative Party, succeeded Drury as premier, he adopted a similar stance on medical monopoly. In 1925, Ferguson's administration passed the Drugless Practitioners Act, protecting the rights of osteopaths and chiropractors to practice medicine, as well as the rights and choices of sufferers.[26]

In the early decades of the new century, as the tide of infectious diseases began to recede, a new specter appeared on the horizon: cancer. By 1920, the mortality rates for cancer and tuberculosis were almost identical, and within a decade, tuberculosis and other contagious ailments had been displaced by cardiovascular diseases and cancer as the leading causes of death in Ontario.[27] Noted Canadian scientist Madge Thurlow Macklin concluded that because people "are not dying of infectious disease as they would have done formerly. . . . they have to die of something else."[28] As the Ontario government began to respond to the growing threat posed by neoplastic diseases, provincial cancer care policies embodied the same historic trends that had typified the state's relationship with the public and the medical profession.

On one hand, government officials welcomed advice from the medical community. In 1931, for example, Premier George Henry responded to suggestions from the Ontario Medical Association (OMA) that the government establish a commission to survey the incidence of cancer in the province and report on the value of radiation for the treatment of cancer.[29] The same year, Minister of Health John Robb announced that the time had come to "curb this menace" of cancer in the province, and he concluded that "whatever the solution may be, its success depends upon the education of the public and the cooperation of the medical profession."[30] In 1932, Robb set up formal mechanisms for professional consultation to implement recommendations coming out of the cancer commission, including a special committee of medical experts to "act in an advisory capacity to the Government."[31] The cancer control programs devised for Ontario also bore the stamp of professional opinions and expectations. Although the commissioners had recommended a highly centralized system of cancer institutes, the medical community favored a decentralized approach that would allow surgeons and physicians to continuing treating patients after a diagnosis of cancer. The result of professional influence, as Charles Hayter has concluded, "was a curious hybrid between centralized cancer clinics and community private practice."[32]

On the other hand, political sensitivity to public opinion again worked to moderate governmental deference to medical opinion. For example, legislators steadfastly resisted professional demands for greater control of alternative cancer care. In 1933, when the OMA asked the provincial authorities to undertake an investigation of "non-medically operated" clinics purporting to treat cancer, Minister of Health John Robb dismissed the request, explaining that "the investigation of such institutions only adds to their publicity and would be of very doubtful value."[33] James Faulkner, Robb's successor as minister of health, likewise understood the political implications of popular support for alternative medicine.[34] Consequently, when an unconventional healer applied for a hospital license in 1935, the Department of Health merely denied the request, making no attempt to curtail the practitioner's activities. Moreover, two years later, Faulkner informed Premier Mitchell Hepburn that unconventional cancer therapies "should be thoroughly investigated by competent medical authority so that when this Government makes a pronouncement on the treatment of cancer, we will have such a pronouncement sustained by competent medical authority rather than attacked and made the subject of public controversy."[35] Faulkner was overly sanguine about the influence of medical opinion on the laity; patients and supporters of alternative cancer practitioners did not share the regular profession's contempt for unconventional therapies. Nonetheless, Faulkner had clearly appreciated that public opinion could become a thorn in the government's side when it came to developing policies and programs for the management of cancer. Hepburn too understood the need to appease the electorate. In the fall of 1937, he broke with tradition, naming a lawyer rather than a doctor to head the Department of Health. The medical community, stunned by Hepburn's choice, objected strenuously, but at least a portion of the public found the change encouraging. As one newspaper reported, "the appointment of Harold Kirby, a non-medical man, to the position of Minister of Health, should alter conditions and help ascertain the facts" concerning treatments for cancer.[36]

Ontario's political culture was thus characterized by what we might describe as "constrained collaboration"—at least with respect to the regulation of medical practice and many public health policies. For decades, provincial leaders sought to steer a safe course between their desire for medical expertise in matters of health and healing and their need for public support at the polls and for the implementation of policies and programs. But as is often the case with political compromise, the government's stance did not wholly satisfy either the medical community or the public. Simmering frustrations reached a boil in the middle of the 1930s as the rate of cancer deaths and the number of unconventional practitioners continued to rise. The government's precarious balancing act between patients and practitioners came crashing down as both sides pressed for definitive answers about medical authority and the legitimacy of alternative cancer care. Among all the players in this controversy, Rene Caisse most often occupied center stage.

THE POLITICS OF ALTERNATIVE CANCER CARE: THE CASE OF RENE CAISSE

Born in 1888 in Bracebridge, Ontario, a small town north of Toronto, Rene Caisse trained as a nurse in hospitals in Connecticut and Ontario. She became interested in the treatment of cancer in the 1920s, after encountering a patient who had apparently recovered from breast cancer using only an herbal infusion.[37] Caisse acquired the recipe, tested and refined it, and became convinced that the medicine could provide genuine relief and improvement—sometimes even a cure—for the suffering caused by cancer. She named the herbal treatment "Essiac," her own name spelled backward. As word of this new therapy spread among cancer patients and their families, Caisse found herself inundated with pleas for treatment. Sufferers began lining up outside her apartment in Toronto until the other tenants complained. Eventually, Caisse took up more commodious lodgings in her hometown as her following swelled into the thousands. Both patients and "healthy" supporters extolled the virtues of Essiac.

News of Caisse's work also reached the medical authorities, but unlike patients and supporters, they took a dim view of her therapy. Caisse's views on disease and on the therapeutic action of Essiac were no doubt partly responsible for professional scorn and hostility. As a result of her research and clinical experience, she concluded that the therapy attacked cancer in two ways: one herb targeted the malignant cells, while the other three purged the body of toxins that contributed to the growth of cancer. These explanations resembled humoral theories of disease and treatment, which had long since fallen out of favor with regular practitioners.[38] Biographer Gary Glum maintains that territoriality and jealousy underpinned medical reactions.[39] Whatever the reason, Caisse was apparently harassed by federal and provincial authorities as well as by the medical profession on several occasions in the 1920s and 1930s.[40] In 1926, for example, the federal Department of Health and Pensions sent two officials to investigate Caisse's therapy, and they were authorized to arrest her if she was found to be practicing medicine without a license.[41] Moreover, as her remedy become even more popular during the early 1930s, the medical community stepped up its efforts to curb her activities. The medical authorities had no formal jurisdiction over the nurse, but they pressured private practitioners to impede her work with cancer patients. In the summer of 1937, Caisse informed Premier Hepburn that if the medical profession continued to interfere with her work, she would no longer be able to support his party. "The Liberal Candidate will never be elected in this riding," she warned.[42] Not for the first or last time, Caisse had correctly gauged the mood of her supporters. One patient concluded, "I have not seen the public so much worked up over anything . . . as they are over the report that . . . Miss Caisse will be practically driven out of her native land after all she has accomplished."[43] As the confrontation between the public and the profession became more heated, the government found itself drawn inexorably into the debate over alternative cancer care.

Running true to form, the Ontario government refused to commit itself either to the professional or the popular perspective. Instead Premier Hepburn formed a commission to deal with the controversy aroused by alternative cancer care. In the spring of 1938, the legislature passed the Cancer Remedy Act, establishing the Commission for the Investigation of Cancer Remedies to evaluate unconventional therapies for cancer.[44] The medical community greeted the proposed investigation with considerable enthusiasm, believing that the commission would not only evaluate but also regulate or even eliminate unconventional treatments for cancer.[45] As Robert Noble, registrar of the College of Physicians and Surgeons of Ontario, wrote in 1938, "If ever the saying that 'in unity there is strength' were true, it has been clearly demonstrated in our recent victories over secret cancer remedies, which, in future, will be *controlled* by a Government measure known as 'The Cancer Remedy Act.' "[46] Certainly the powers granted to the commission seemed to justify professional optimism. The commissioners could demand samples, detailed descriptions, and even the formulas of therapies under review. Moreover, failure to comply with the directives of the commission involved stiff sanctions: initial infractions carried fines of up to $500 or thirty days in jail, and repeat offenders faced penalties of up to $2,500 or six months in jail. At the same time, the selection of commissioners encouraged doctors to expect that the methods and standards of "scientific medicine" would prevail in the investigation. With the exception of the chair, Ontario Supreme Court Justice John G. Gillanders, and one other lay member, Ernest A. Collins, a journalist from Copper Cliff, Ontario, doctors and scientists dominated the commission: Robert C. Wallace, principal of Queen's University in Kingston and a distinguished geologist; William Deadman, an influential pathologist from Hamilton; George S. Young, a professor of medicine at the University of Toronto; and two surgeons, Thomas Callahan of Toronto and R. Eugene Valin of Ottawa.[47] For the medical community, the cancer commission seemed to hold out the promise of eradicating unconventional treatments for cancer and the practitioners who preyed upon a desperate or gullible public.

But as in the past, public opinion succeeded in convincing Ontario's political leaders to alter the mandate of the commission and the terms of the investigation. As the medical profession anticipated, the government had originally planned to endow the cancer commission with regulatory as well as investigative powers. But by the time the Cancer Remedy Act made its way to the legislature, it no longer included provisions for controlling unconventional cancer care; the commissioners could still demand information, but they could not proscribe the work of alternative healers.[48] Premier Hepburn's compromise over unconventional cancer care in the 1930s thus bore a striking resemblance to Howard Ferguson's position on drugless practitioners more than a decade earlier. As one official observed, "There is no provision in this Act for requiring the claimant to desist from the use of the material if the report is unfavourable. . . . the patient afflicted with cancer may still receive the treatment he desires."[49]

Popular enthusiasm for Caisse's work exacted further concessions from the government in the weeks and months following the passage of the Cancer Remedy Act. At the end of May 1938, Caisse sent a form letter sent to every patient, explaining that she could not and would not tolerate official interference with her work. "In order not to become subject to this law," she wrote, "I have been obliged to close my clinic, because the bill authorized them to take my discovery from me. The only way I will open my clinic again will be at the request of the Premier."[50] Caisse's announcement incited an immediate reaction from her followers: irate patients swamped government offices with letters of protest; newspapers, especially those in the Bracebridge area, also pressed for action.[51] Whether these supporters feared for their own health or simply objected to encroachments on personal auton-omy, they clearly believed that Caisse should be allowed to continue her work unfettered by either the medical profession or the cancer commission.[52]

Minister of Health Harold Kirby was startled by the public's interpretation of the Cancer Remedy Act as well as by anger over the closure of Caisse's clinic. In dozens of letters and several interviews with the press, he tried to deflect popular criticism by pointing out that Caisse, rather than the government, had made the decision to close her clinic.[53] "If Miss Caisse was half as humane as she claims to be," he told reporters, "her clinic would be open today."[54] Mitchell Hepburn chimed in with his own accusations. "I fail to understand," he wrote to Caisse, "why you are so reluctant to submit your remedy. . . . Surely from a human-itarian point of view one would naturally expect you would give every co-operation to the Government whose only effort is to render some assistance to the people suffering from the dreaded disease of cancer."[55] Unfortunately, this strategy backfired because Caisse's patients and supporters continued to cast the government in the role of villain. "Patients believe that the fault is in the Cancer Act," concluded one man. "If they thought Miss Caisse was being unreasonable they would surely make representation to her."[56]

Kirby continued to criticize Caisse throughout the summer, but he eventually surren-dered to public pressure and amended, albeit informally, the mandate of the commission. At the end of June, he told reporters, "I would frown on any commission walking in and demanding the formula until they have investigated the so-called cures." Nothing in the Cancer Remedy Act required the commissioners to evaluate the clinical results of treat-ment before learning the composition of a therapy. By imposing further conditions on the investigation, Kirby hoped to counter public perceptions of the law as "arbitrary and un-fair."[57] Public outcry had taught him the importance of lay opinion. As one journalist con-cluded, "It [is] unlikely that any commission investigating Cancer treatments will think it wise to provoke a province-wide wave of indignation by demanding Miss Caisse's secret formula."[58]

Despite Kirby's concessions, differences of opinion between the commissioners and Caisse and her followers plagued the investigation. In the fall of 1938, Caisse's lawyer as-serted that she was more than willing to cooperate with the investigation provided the commissioners considered the results of her therapy before she handed over her formula. "I do not say that you have to acknowledge it as a cure," she said, "but that it has benefitted . . . patients." Justice John Gillanders, chair of the commission, pointed out that he and his colleagues could hardly evaluate her work under these conditions. "It would be impracti-cal," he wrote, "to make any investigation without first knowing what substance or method of treatment was being dealt with." But Caisse found it difficult to understand the position of Gillanders and the other commissioners. "It would seem to me," she protested, "that you are taking the attitude of men standing on the shore of a lake who see a man drowning. They see another man throw him a rope and haul him in to safety. They see him safe and well, but they say to the man who saved him, 'We saw it but we will not acknowledge that you saved him unless you can show us what the rope was made of.'"[59] Moreover, many of Caisse's supporters shared her belief that the effects of treatment should take precedence over every other consideration. One reporter summed up lay opinion about Essiac: "The general feeling is that the sole test of her treatment should be 'Does it cure?' and that if it cures it should be nobody's business 'how' or 'why' it cures. . . . When people take a train all they want is to get to their destination and they don't care whether the locomotive runs by steam, electricity or diesel power."[60]

These encounters between Caisse and the commission exposed a conceptual gap that separated many laypeople and alternative healers from the medical community and the government. Patients, healthy supporters, and unconventional practitioners tended to accept the centrality of experience in the evaluation of treatments for cancer; for them, cessation of symptoms provided ample and compelling evidence of health and healing. As one of Caisse's patients asked, "Now in the name of humanity what more proof do the Medical Association and the Government want than a patient fully cured? There are hundreds more who can give you the same proof. Why will you not give this woman what she requires to continue her good work?"[61] But the commissioners—and by implication the politicians who appointed them—did not share this view; at every turn, they privileged medical findings and professional opinions over personal testimony. As Gillanders explained, the value of a particular remedy as well as the state of a patient's health were "questions to be considered in the light of much more evidence than the patient's own belief."[62]

Despite these profoundly different perspectives on alternative cancer care and the commission's insistence that a proper investigation of Caisse's work was not possible without full disclosure of her therapy, the government nonetheless bowed to public opinion. In February 1939, commissioners Robert Wallace and Thomas Callahan were dispatched to Caisse's clinic in Bracebridge as a first step in the evaluation of her work. They spent two days examining patients, observing treatments, and interviewing staff. Given the divergent views held by Caisse and the commissioners, the outcome of the investigation was virtually a foregone conclusion. Dozens of glowing reports from sufferers and supporters did not convince Wallace and Callahan that Essiac was a promising treatment for cancer. They concluded that many of her patients did not have cancer at all and so could not have been cured of the disease, while those who did suffer with cancer had benefited from conventional treatments, such as surgery and radiation therapy, before arriving at the clinic. "We were unable," they reported, "to ascertain any positive evidence in connection with any single case that the Caisse treatments had actually cured cancer. We cannot help feeling that over-confidence in the Caisse treatment before it is a proven cure will only lead to neglect of those cases which might be benefitted by recognized procedures."[63] Caisse and her supporters were stunned and angered by this conclusion, and they continued to pressure the cancer commission and the provincial government to reopen the investigation of Essiac. The commissioners periodically reviewed Caisse's work over the next few years, but they always reached the same conclusions about their methods of evaluation and about her therapy.[64] In their opinion, Essiac was neither a beneficial treatment nor a cure for cancer.

In 1941, after more than a decade of trying to win acceptance and recognition, Caisse closed her clinic doors for the last time. Her retreat would seem to suggest the triumph of the alliance between the government and the medical profession: the tenets of "scientific medicine" had apparently prevailed in the investigation, routing a practitioner who could or would not conform to those standards. Yet for many years—before, during, and after the investigation—lay support for Caisse's work had stayed the hand of the state. Although she had boldly disobeyed the directives of the commission, thereby contravening the provisions of the Cancer Remedy Act, the government never seriously challenged her work with cancer sufferers. She was never fined or jailed for her failure to cooperate with the commission or, indeed, for practising medicine without a license. Moreover, Caisse continued to treat small numbers of cancer sufferers in the decades after World War II until the revival of interest in alternative medicine during the 1960s and 1970s gave her work a new lease on life. Today, twenty-five years after Caisse's death, her therapy continues to generate enthusiasm, apprehension, and controversy.[65]

THE GOLDEN AGE OF MEDICINE: GOING, GOING, GONE

In many ways, popular and professional reactions to Caisse's work in the 1930s resemble lay and medical attitudes revealed by the controversy over Tyrell Dueck's treatment in the 1990s. In both cases, the medical community criticized alternative cancer care. Many doctors felt that cancer sufferers were being fleeced by unscrupulous mountebanks who would rob them of their lives as well as their money. In both cases, laypeople held different opinions about unconventional cancer care. Some sufferers and their families displayed an unshakable faith in alternative medicine, while others were at least willing to entertain the possibility that cancer patients might benefit from both conventional and alternative treatments. More important for this discussion, the public in both eras seemed equally determined to protect patients' rights to choose their treatments and care providers. As one man concluded in 1992, "The medical profession should stop playing God and allow us cancer patients to use the treatment of our choice."[66]

While the public espoused patients' rights in both periods, its ability to influence the medical profession, the courts, and the state, diminished rather than increased over time. During the 1930s, the courts sometimes became involved in adjudicating disputes over fees, but they shied away from imposing their judgments about specific treatments on the public. Such was not the case for Tyrell Dueck. In the 1930s, the provincial government was drawn into the controversy over alternative cancer care, but, like the courts, officials refrained from proscribing alternative medicine. By the 1990s, however, the state had made it much more difficult to gain access to unconventional cancer treatments. In the case of Essiac, for example, the federal government permitted use of the herbal treatment on compassionate grounds, for cancer sufferers who had run the gamut of conventional therapies without success. But the road to Caisse's therapy was littered with obstacles, including gaining the support of a physician and negotiating the labyrinthine application process. As one journalist concluded in 1989, "If you have been diagnosed as having cancer and you want to try Renee [sic] Caisse's herbal treatment, Essiac, you'll need to persevere if you wish to obtain it through approved channels."[67]

The history of cancer in Ontario thus casts doubt on assumptions or arguments that conventional medical practitioners enjoyed a "golden age" in the decades before World War II. According to John Burnham, "For half a century, they [doctors] were relatively free from public censure or actual interference in clinical and professional activities, and they enjoyed great public and personal admiration."[68] Clearly, in the 1920s and 1930s, the authority of the medical profession and the support of the state was far more circumscribed—at least with respect to cancer care—than Burnham's comments suggest. Moreover, the ostensible loss of freedom and status among physicians in the 1960s and 1970s was not as far-reaching or enduring— again with respect to cancer care—as we have been led to believe by Burnham and others. In these decades, the state was much more likely to side with the medical profession in matters of health and healing, and to resist public pressure, than it had been half a century earlier. If doctors ever enjoyed a "golden age"—and the idea itself begs for analysis—it appears to have reached full flower in the aftermath of the Second World War rather than the First.

SCIENCE AND THE SHADOW OF IDEOLOGY IN THE AMERICAN HEALTH FOODS MOVEMENT, 1930S–1960S

Michael Ackerman

WHEN TEXAS PHYSICIAN Joe D. Nichols declared that "America is a sick nation" in a promotional brochure for Natural Foods Associates (NFA), the statement must have struck most of his colleagues as mighty odd. For Nichols did not offer this bleak view of public health in the nineteenth or early twentieth century, when infant mortality was high and frequent outbreaks of infectious disease took a heavy toll of lives; instead, he wrote it in the 1950s, a time when Americans were living longer, and were said to be healthier, than ever before. In stark contrast to contemporary medical authorities, Nichols believed that rising rates of heart disease, cancer, and other chronic diseases were signs of a progressive deterioration of the nation's health. Nichols also disagreed with the vast majority of physicians in contending that a significant amount of illness in the country was caused by the consumption of nutritionally impoverished processed foods. As president of the NFA, Nichols announced his group's determination to "save America from poor food grown on poor soil."[1]

Nichols was not the first physician, and NFA was not the first organization, to undertake this task. As early as the 1930s a number of doctors and dentists throughout the country had come to believe that a significant amount of the ill health that Americans suffered was the result of eating too many processed foods deficient in vitamins and minerals. In 1936 a group of southern California dentists sought to stem the tide of diet-induced physical degeneration by establishing the American Academy of Applied Nutrition (AAAN) to educate health practitioners in "the science and art of nutrition." During the 1940s and 1950s the health claims made by members of the AAAN and NFA earned a popular following, thanks to dispensers of dietary advice, such as author Adelle Davis, magazine publisher J. I. Rodale, and radio broadcaster Carlton Fredericks, and perhaps most of all to purveyors of dietary supplements, who urged Americans to consume these products to compensate for deficiencies in the nation's foods. Because of the centrality of the "health foods" store in promoting these ideas, this popular crusade to improve America's eating habits has sometimes been called the health foods movement.[2]

The physicians and dentists who founded the health foods movement in the years just before World War II had developed a keen interest in the new science of vitamins and minerals at a time when the majority of American doctors (other than pediatricians) saw little practical value in the discoveries of nutrition researchers. As the stated purpose of the AAAN indicates, the founders of the movement saw themselves as conduits of information between the nutrition laboratory and the medical and dental professions. Yet their bleak appraisals of the public health and the nutritional quality of the food supply were quite different from the views held by most nutritionists and physicians, who came to perceive the movement as little more than a vehicle through which charlatans and quacks could foist useless products on a gullible public. As a result, in the early 1950s the Food and Drug Administration launched an attack against the movement, accusing it of distorting the findings of nutrition science, and "spreading the false doctrine that our staple foods are debased and deficient . . . [and] that all our diseases . . . are due to malnutrition."[3]

Yet even the movement's critics acknowledged the sincerity of the majority of health foodists, who had no financial stake in the supplement industry. Furthermore, it is clear that most health foodists believed that their nutritional claims had been substantiated by scientific research. This article will attempt to reconcile these conflicting assessments of the scientific legitimacy of the health foods movement from its origins in the 1930s through the mid-1960s. It will show how health foodists found in nutrition science meaningful explanations for the continued prevalence of illness despite all that modern medicine had accomplished. Yet it will also show how doubts and fears about modernity—and about modern food production methods in particular—cast an ideological shadow on their interpretations of this science, leading them to form extreme conclusions about the extent of malnutrition in the country and to offer unorthodox dietary advice.[4]

SCIENTIFIC BACKGROUND OF THE HEALTH FOODS MOVEMENT

The roots of the health foods movement go back to the 1910s, when researchers found that deficiencies of hitherto unknown organic substances occurring in very small amounts in foods—designated "vitamins"—produced serious illness in both animals and humans. One such disease was beriberi, an incapacitating and often fatal illness, which was rampant in East Asia at the time. Investigators traced this disease, which is caused by a deficiency of thiamine, to the consumption of a highly milled form of rice that had been introduced into the region in the late nineteenth century. This discovery was quickly followed by others that showed that various methods of processing food severely impaired the vitamin and mineral content of many commonly consumed items, and that this impairment had potentially disastrous health consequences. Before long, a number of nutritionists suspected that many illnesses prevalent in the United States and Europe could be attributed in part to the consumption of too much white flour and other highly refined foods. Throughout the interwar period several of them publicly questioned the generally held assumption that recent "advances" in food production methods were beneficial to humankind. "We have been trying an experiment in human nutrition on a nation-wide scale, with a dietary which is of a kind which no people in history ever tried to live upon before," mused Johns Hopkins University professor of biochemistry Elmer V. McCollum, America's best-known nutrition scientist. Because of this concern, from World War I on nutritionists regularly advised Americans to eat more fresh, natural foods, and fewer highly processed ones.[5]

Initially, nutritionists' concerns about the nutritional quality of the American diet had little impact on the medical profession. Most American physicians believed that vitamin deficiencies were rare among the nation's adult population, since there were so few identifiable cases of deficiency disease in the country (with the exception of pellagra in the South). In the latter half of the 1930s, however, this complacency was shattered. The development of synthetic vitamins and other clinical tools in that decade enabled researchers for the first time to identify and treat the early stages of deficiency disease. One of these researchers, American physician Tom D. Spies, found that many extremely common ailments—including gastrointestinal disturbances, irritability, forgetfulness, and fatigue—were in fact symptoms produced by minor, subclinical deficiencies of vitamins. (Spies coined the term *subclinical* to describe these deficiencies, because doctors had trouble diagnosing them correctly due to the nonspecificity of their symptoms.) The work of Spies and other pioneers in the field of clinical nutrition led to speculation that vitamin deficiencies were widespread in the United States. In the meantime, enough information about human nutritional needs had been amassed to enable authorities to formulate the first sets of quantitative vitamin and mineral requirements. Using these values as a yardstick, several groups of researchers conducted food consumption surveys to evaluate the adequacy of the American diet. The most extensive study, conducted by the U.S. Department of Agriculture, reported in 1939 that one-third of the nation's families had diets classified as "poor," while just one-fourth had diets that could be considered "good."[6]

With the country mobilizing for war in 1940, the discovery that millions of Americans were malnourished caused health officials to worry that the nation's ability to defend itself was in jeopardy. This fear received apparent confirmation when Brigadier General Lewis B. Hershey, deputy director of the Selective Service System, announced in early 1941 that 20 percent of the first one million men drafted had been rejected as unfit for duty, and that "perhaps one-third of the rejections were due either directly or indirectly to nutritional deficiencies." In response, the Roosevelt administration organized a federally coordinated nutrition program. While the program was essentially a vast educational campaign to teach Americans how to eat better, it did sponsor more direct methods to eradicate nutritional deficiencies, including the provision of vitamin supplements to industrial workers. Most notably, it endorsed the production and use of a new type of white flour enriched with three vitamins and one mineral—thiamine, riboflavin, niacin, and iron—which had been removed from wheat in the course of milling, and which health officials believed were in short supply in the American diet.[7]

There was one other scientific development that had a tremendous influence on the health foods movement. In the early years of the twentieth century agricultural scientists discovered that the mineral content of crops was greatly influenced by the mineral content of the soil in which they were grown, and that pasture-fed animals in various regions of the world where the soil was deficient in calcium, phosphorus, and other minerals suffered greatly from nutritional disease. At first American nutritionists believed that mineral deficiencies in the soil had little direct impact on human health, but in the 1930s they found evidence of malnutrition among people living in mineral-poor regions of the country who could only afford to eat locally grown foods. During these same years, the ravages of the Dust Bowl raised alarms about the state of the nation's soil. As a result, when nutritionists and public health officials determined that millions of Americans were suffering minor deficiencies of vitamins and minerals at the end of the decade, they expressed the fear that declining soil fertility posed a threat to public health. Although they mostly worried about the effects of impoverished soil on the health of the isolated rural poor, they sometimes maintained that mineral deficiencies in the soil made a small contribution to the wider problem of malnutrition in the country.[8]

PRINCIPAL CLAIMS OF THE HEALTH FOODS MOVEMENT

Because the health foods movement emerged at the very moment when American health authorities were most concerned about the consumption of vitamin and mineral-deficient foods, there was little, if any, antagonism between the two groups during the early years of the movement. The establishment of the World War II nutrition program pleased the movement's founders, who, like nutritionists, warned that malnutrition undermined the ability of Americans to defend their country on the battlefield, in the factory, and in the home.[9] Meanwhile, a number of nutritionists advocated the use of natural "health foods," such as brewer's yeast and wheat germ, to augment the nutritional content of the diet, and at least one well-known nutrition scientist told the burgeoning health foods industry that it could render a great public service by educating consumers on the value of vitamins.[10]

The harmony of views between these two groups did not last long. After the war health authorities gradually grew less concerned about the problem of nutritional deficiencies, as economic prosperity, changes in the food supply, and the enrichment of flour all contributed to a marked improvement in the diet of millions of Americans and a drastic reduction in the incidence of deficiency disease. At the same time, several nutrition experts began to suspect that that the standards used to evaluate the adequacy of the diet in the 1930s and early 1940s had been too high.[11] Postwar health foodists, in contrast, continued to maintain that millions of Americans were being crippled by nutritionally inadequate diets. In support of this contention they pointed to the rising percentage of young men rejected for the draft and to the comparatively poor performance of American children on physical fitness tests in the 1950s.[12]

Dissenting from the cultural consensus of the postwar era, health foodists expressed only lukewarm admiration for recent achievements in medicine. While American doctors were being celebrated for the large increase in life expectancy that had occurred during the first half of the twentieth century, health foodists accurately pointed out that almost all of this increase had resulted from the prevention and treatment of infectious diseases, and that the medical profession had accomplished very little in regard to the chronic diseases, which had now become the nation's leading killers and disablers. They rejected the claim made by most health officials that Americans were healthier than ever and that cancer, heart disease, arthritis, and the other chronic illnesses generally associated with old age were on the increase simply because people were living longer. Furthermore, they maintained that chronic disease was afflicting not just the elderly but millions of middle-aged Americans as well. The doctors of the health foods movement constantly lamented the fact that too many of their patients were forced to restrict their activities long before they reached the end of their productive years. "More ominous still," physician W. Coda Martin asserted, "the incidence of degenerative disease is creeping ever deeper into our life span, affecting progressively larger numbers of young people and even children."[13]

At a time when the larger medical community admitted knowing relatively little about the cause of most chronic diseases, health foodists confidently asserted that these diseases were the result of years of improper eating. "More often than not," wrote radical social critic James Rorty in collaboration with New York physician Philip Norman, "the early onset of the degenerative diseases in men and women of fifty and sixty represents the explosion of a physiological time bomb planted early and assiduously built up by a lifetime of malnutrition." As proof, health foodists cited numerous studies scattered throughout the medical literature that found a relationship between nutritional deficiencies and various chronic illnesses. Epidemiological data also served to substantiate the link between malnutrition and chronic disease. Rorty and Norman argued that extreme variations in the incidence rates of cancer and heart disease throughout the world indicated that these diseases were caused by environmental factors, most likely by diet.[14]

Health foodists believed that the destruction of vitamins and minerals that took place during the processing of foods made it very difficult for all Americans to secure a nutritious diet, and they therefore recommended that the consumption of processed foods be avoided almost entirely. "No food is safe," declared health food entrepreneur and nonpracticing dentist Royal Lee, "unless it is fresh enough to have retained most of its perishable vitamins . . . [and] it has incurred no processing that would remove or impair its vitamin and mineral content." Many health foodists even recommended that people drink certified raw milk instead of pasteurized milk, because pasteurization destroyed some of the vitamins found in milk. As for foods enriched with synthetic vitamins and minerals, some health foodists initially expressed lukewarm support for these products, because they were nutritionally superior to the foods that they were intended to replace in the diet. Eventually, however, all health foodists came to view enriched foods as nutritionally inadequate and potentially harmful. "Sticking back in a paltry three synthetically made drugstore vitamins of the known eight to ten of the B-complex alone, is not going to make a hoot of difference about the needed minerals removed from white flour and other processed cereals that load down the American breakfast, lunch and supper tables—to say nothing of the still missing vitamins," Pennsylvania dentist Fred D. Miller maintained.[15]

The founders of the health foods movement opposed the use of synthetic vitamin and mineral preparations to compensate for the shortcomings of the American diet, for they believed that people would deprive themselves of the wide array of nutrients present in natural foods. They also suspected that dietary supplements constructed by man rather than by nature might contain unhealthful amounts and combinations of nutrients, leading to possible nutritional imbalances or toxic reactions. Popularizers such as Adelle Davis, however, recommended the daily consumption of natural dietary supplements—including wheat germ, brewer's yeast, cod liver oil, and desiccated liver powder—that contained unusually large amounts of vitamins or minerals in relation to their caloric value, since they believed that it was extremely difficult, if not impossible, to construct a nutritionally adequate diet from the ordinary items in the nation's food supply. Yet the physicians and dentists who founded the movement never emphasized the nutritional significance of dietary supplements, for they always maintained that eating dairy products, fruits and vegetables, and whole-grain foods was the key to good health. Moreover, unlike nineteenth-century natural food advocates, who embraced vegetarianism, mid-twentieth-century health foodists advised Americans to eat meat, especially organ meats such as liver, which were esteemed by contemporary nutritionists for their high vitamin and mineral content.[16]

Above all, health foodists urged consumers to seek out foods that were grown on highly fertile soil. Despite the relative insignificance of the soil-nutrition relationship in the minds of most nutritionists, health foodists developed a tremendous interest in the subject, thanks largely to the efforts of two men. Between 1940 and the late 1950s allergist Jonathan Forman, editor of the *Ohio State Medical Journal*, helped organize an annual conference on soil and health under the auspices of the popular conservation group Friends of the Land. During these same years Pulitzer prize–winning novelist Louis Bromfield, the organization's vice president and chief financial backer, discussed the soil-nutrition relationship in a number of books and articles devoted to agricultural matters. Having spent most of the interwar period in France, Bromfield had returned to his native Ohio in 1938 to fulfill a lifelong desire to become a farmer, determined to prove that even the poorest land could be made productive by following the practices of scientific agriculture and soil conservation.[17]

Alarmed by conservationists' warnings that soil erosion jeopardized the country's future, health foodists believed that impoverished soil was a major contributor to the nation's malnutrition problem. Some of them maintained that soil fertility was the single most important factor affecting health in the United States, but even those who acknowledged otherwise worried about the condition of the nation's soil. Bromfield, for example, agreed with nutritional authorities that most Americans had little difficulty consuming an adequate amount of minerals, since their foods were grown and raised on a variety of soils, but he still feared that the country might suffer the fate of other great civilizations that collapsed because they had failed to protect their soil. He contended, in fact, that the process of decline had already begun, alleging that many poor residents living on the impoverished soil of the rural South and border states had lost the mental and physical capacity to work productively due to malnutrition.[18]

Finally, some health foodists embraced an unorthodox approach to agriculture, known as "organic farming," which had developed independently in the 1920s and 1930s from the ideas of controversial British agricultural scientist Albert Howard and Austrian occult philosopher Rudolf Steiner. According to these two men and their followers, crops grown with the aid of natural, organic fertilizers were nutritionally superior to those grown with commercially produced fertilizers. Proponents of this claim maintained that humus—the dark, odorless mass of decaying organic matter that is the primary source of plant nutrients in the natural world—contained nutritionally valuable substances not present in commercial fertilizers, which were mainly composed of inorganic compounds of nitrogen, phosphorus, and potassium. In addition, many of them argued that commercial fertilizers caused harm to the soil and ultimately to the plants that grew in it. They therefore urged farmers to stop using commercial fertilizers and to work instead on increasing the humus content of their soil by applying composts of vegetable and animal wastes. Some health foodists, however, did not accept the proposition that commercial fertilizers should never be used to improve soil fertility. Bromfield, who was greatly influenced by Howard's teachings and was just as appreciative of humus as he, nevertheless believed that it was usually necessary to apply inorganic fertilizers to the soil as a practical matter. The movement even contained a small group of "mineralizers," who recommended that the soil be fertilized "by means of a shotgun prescription of all the major and trace elements—somewhere around thirty then known."[19]

HEALTH FOODIST IDEOLOGY

Except for organic farming, all the major health and dietary claims made by health foodists were inspired by the discoveries and pronouncements of mainstream nutrition researchers. Yet health foodists interpreted this information through an ideological filter that led them to form conclusions about public health that differed from those reached by the nation's nutritional authorities. The fundamental premise of health foodist ideology was the conviction that the natural environment is healthful to humans and that disease is largely the result of human interference with natural processes. Health foodists with a religious orientation maintained that good health is a God-given birthright and that sickness is a sign that humans had violated divine laws. More secular-minded individuals used insights from the sciences to argue that good health is humankind's natural condition. Jonathan Forman, for example, combined ecology and Darwinism to contend that disease occurs whenever an organism fails to adapt to man-made disruptions to its environment.[20]

On the specific matter of nutrition, health foodists believed that the foods that God or nature provides contain everything that humans need to avoid illness and thrive. They therefore felt that any alteration to a natural food imposes a potential health risk. They objected to the consumption of processed foods, for they worried that some valuable nutritional element might be destroyed while the foods were being processed. "The study of human nutrition has not yet reached the point where we can state definitely the use to which the body puts *every* element in food, but that does not mean that an ingredient whose usefulness is still unknown must be valueless and can be removed from food with impunity," Coda Martin wrote. "On the contrary, if present research points toward any generality at all, it is that every element occurring naturally in food has some role in our bodily functions." Health foodists were even more troubled by the concoction of "artificial" foods—whether they be vitamin preparations, foods fortified with synthetic vitamins, or infant formulas—since they believed, as Philip Norman did, that the "*component elements in natural foods have been assembled and proportioned by natural synthetic processes subservient to immutable and inexorable factors which are, for the most part, incomprehensible to man*" (italics his). The millers received the most criticism in this regard for adding just four vitamins and minerals to "devitalized" white flour and then marketing this product as a nutritionally adequate substitute for whole-wheat flour. "Are Communists who deny God any more irreverent than men whose egos make them believe they share God's power to bring the dead to life?" Fred Miller asked rhetorically.[21]

Despite their belief that modern food production methods were harmful to human health, health foodists did not reject all new technologies. What they disliked were technologies that substituted for natural processes or those that significantly modified the products of nature. They therefore rejected any food processing method, such as flour milling or sugar refining, that altered the nutritional composition of natural foods. Frozen foods, however, usually received their endorsement, because freezing was a natural process that preserved the nutrients in food. In general, health foodists were fond of any technology that made natural foods cheaper, easier to produce, or more available to consumers, so long as it did not impair the nutritional quality of the product.[22]

Health foodists also embraced agricultural technologies that (in the words of organic farming advocate Ehrenfried Pfeiffer) "work[ed] with Nature and not against it." Although they opposed the use of heavy machinery, they heartily endorsed equipment that increased farm productivity without harming the soil. What distinguished a good technology from a bad technology was not always clear-cut, however, and health foodists had mixed feelings about innovative ways of growing and raising food. Louis Bromfield speculated that aquaculture would someday supply the world with lots of high-protein food, but he did not think that hydroponics would ever do much good, in part because of "doubts concerning the full nutrition value of plants grown outside the range of the natural process taking place in living soil." Jonathan Forman, meanwhile, condemned the development of certain high-yield plant hybrids. "Nature cannot be hijacked by bandit horticulturists—those who introduce new plants or new strains of plants capable of old-time growth in soils depleted of their vital substances," he wrote. Such plants, he claimed (citing the views of controversial University of Missouri soil scientist William Albrecht), contained less protein and minerals and more carbohydrates than traditional crop varieties.[23]

One consequence of technology that troubled all health foodists was the growing presence of synthetic chemicals in food, which they suspected caused serious long-term damage to human health. In fact, by the end of the 1950s the chemicals-in-food issue rivaled the nutritional-quality issue as the foremost concern of the movement. Health foodists were particularly troubled by the widespread spraying of DDT—which they sought to halt—more than a decade before Rachel Carson alerted the public to the possible dangers of this insecticide in her 1962 classic *Silent Spring*. Furthermore, health foodists maintained that most chemicals being used in the production of food were completely unnecessary. Bromfield, for example, testified before Congress in 1951 that the use of pesticides could be significantly diminished and perhaps eliminated altogether if farmers properly maintained the fertility of their soil.[24]

The most controversial chemical technology that health foodists opposed was the addition of fluoride compounds to public water supplies to reduce tooth decay. The leaders of both major health food organizations, the AAAN and the NFA, took the position that water fluoridation was neither safe nor effective, and a violation of individual rights. Yet not all health foodists started out as opponents. Because fluorine is a mineral, and because health foodists highly valued mineral-rich foods, some of them initially viewed the proposal to fluoridate water as a beneficial public health measure. But just as most American physicians and dentists started jumping on the fluoridation bandwagon after 1950, almost every health foodist who had supported fluoridation jumped off. Rather than viewing fluorine as a nutrient, they began to see it as a drug intended to treat an easily preventable disease. "If only our laws and customs could move faster toward making it illegal to remove valuable nutrients from the foods our bodies need daily for building sound bodies from head to toe, rather than making it legal to add toxic substances to what we must take into our bodies daily," declared Fred Miller, "I am sure we would move more rapidly toward the goal of [the pro-fluoridationists] . . . whose aim I do not doubt is to give children better teeth and do no one any harm." Furthermore, even though some health foodists acknowledged the hygienic value of fluorine, they opposed fluoridation, because they distrusted humans' ability to manipulate what nature provided. In contrast, they maintained that naturally fluoridated water was safe, because it contained other substances, including calcium, that supposedly counteracted the toxic effects of fluorine.[25]

Many health foodists blamed the misuse of technology on a market-driven economic system, which had propelled farmers to plunder the soil and food manufacturers to sell devitalized products. Health foodists were especially critical of corporate capitalism, for they believed that big business placed its own interests ahead of the public welfare. They frequently alleged that the makers of nutritionally deficient foods used their money and influence to win acceptance for their products from nutritionists, health authorities, and government officials. Fred Miller charged that the flour enrichment program was a scheme by the milling industry to maintain a market for a product that every nutritionist in the country had come to realize was a detriment to good health. The most comprehensive indictment of the food industry came from James Rorty and Philip Norman, who argued that advertising was chiefly responsible for persuading Americans to choose foods that were bad for their health (and pocketbooks), and who called for a massive expansion of the consumer cooperative movement in order to reorient the nation's food system so that it served the needs of consumers instead of industry. They also endorsed the idea of national health insurance to assist Americans with limited resources, and they proposed that a new food stamp program be established, whereby the government would sell poor families coupons redeemable for nutritious foods at just a fraction of their cost.[26]

The progressive prescriptions offered by Rorty and Norman were quite atypical of the health foods movement. In fact, extreme conservatives found certain aspects of health food ideology especially congenial to their political views. Jonathan Forman, for example, believed that nutritional improvement along the lines laid down by the health foods movement could halt the nation's drift toward the "despotism and slavery" of the welfare state and possible revolution. "Hungry, undernourished people are . . . the real menace to our republic," Forman declared. "Through their apathy, their ignorance, their lack of intelligence, their stunted social judgment, their sexual immaturity and their emotional instability, they are an easy prey for psychopathic compatriots among the professions, politicians, and labor leaders." Several health foodists, including Forman, commented that nutritional improvement would undercut political efforts to have the government build hospitals and provide universal access to health care, since Americans would suffer fewer illnesses if they were well fed. "Better medical facilities and a wider distribution of doctors and dentists will never overcome the fundamental causes of our disgraceful sickness and death rate," Forman wrote. "It is th[e] prevention of sickness largely through proper eating and not a social revolution that we should seek."[27]

Health foodists of all persuasions endorsed education as a means of solving the nation's malnutrition problem. Conservatives preferred this approach, because it required no coercive action by the state. Once consumers had been taught to desire nutritious foods, the food industry would be compelled by market forces, not the government, to give them what they wanted. Several health foodists recognized, however, that even health-conscious consumers needed to have information about what they were buying, so they proposed legislation to establish a grading system for food based on nutritional quality and to require manufacturers to list the nutrient content of their products on the label.[28]

Other health foodists wanted the government to take much stronger action to improve the nation's health than the enactment of mandatory food labeling. They felt that the educational process, while valuable, was too slow and ineffective to effect the necessary dietary changes in a timely manner, especially when the food industry was using its vast marketing apparatus to maintain the nutritional status quo. They therefore called for laws to prohibit the sale of the two most nutritionally worthless foods: white flour and white sugar. "We are entering into the final stage of a battle that will find either our health standards destroyed, or the devitalized food manufacturer destroyed (the latter by legislation, the former by malnutrition)," Royal Lee predicted, advocating legislation.[29]

Despite the appeal of health foods ideology to radicals like Rorty and conservatives like Forman, the movement cannot be located on the traditional left-to-right political spectrum. If any generalization can be made, health foodists tended to reject mainstream politics, since none of the major parties addressed the issues that health foodists were deeply concerned about. In contrast, the one political cause that all health foodists supported was the conservation movement. Convinced that good health could not be attained if the natural world that humans depended upon for sustenance was sick, health foodists became spokespeople for environmental protection. Because they felt it imperative that farmers produce crops of only the highest nutritional value, they called on the nation's farmers to preserve and restore the fertility of their soil by applying fertilizers and following the conservation practices recommended by the U. S. Soil Conservation Service. In a more radical

vein, advocates of organic farming and some middle-of-the-roaders, such as Jonathan Forman, criticized cash-crop agriculture for being especially destructive of the soil, and they
urged a return to mixed farming. Long before ecology became widely popular in the 1960s,
health foodists drew upon the teachings of the young science to support their contention
that man-made disruptions of the environment had undesirable consequences. Ehrenfried
Pfeiffer, for example, used the concept of energy equilibrium to promote his method of organic farming for its sustainability.[30]

Besides conservation, there was one semi-political movement with which health foodists
had close ties. This movement, referred to either as decentralism or distributism, was
formed in the mid-1930s by a diverse group of conservative social critics, who called for the
widespread distribution of property, the decentralization of industry and government, and
the dispersal of the urban population. Decentralists offered a political, economic, moral,
and aesthetic critique of modern urban industrial society. They abhorred the rise of big
business and concentration of wealth and power, which (they maintained) deprived most
Americans of true political and economic freedom, but they equally disapproved of the alternatives that had arisen—socialism, fascism, the welfare state—all of which depended
upon a huge, centralized government. They also deplored the effects of industrialism and
urbanization on the lives of workers and consumers. They considered factory work to be
unpleasant and unhygienic, and they charged that mass-produced goods were poor in quality, adulterated, overly expensive, and often unnecessary. They hated the ugliness of cities
and the toll that living there took on the physical and mental health of their inhabitants.
They were not, however, critical of every technological advance brought by industrialization, for they believed that certain technologies, especially electricity and the automobile,
could actually abet the decentralization of the economy and the population and make rural
life less burdensome. Decentralists believed that life on the farm was not only healthier than
life in the city, but more spiritually and emotionally satisfying, because it brought family
members closer together and fulfilled people's need to work with their hands and have contact with nature. The dissatisfaction with modern society and the appreciation of nature
that marked decentralist philosophy made it appealing to health foodists, and some leading
health foodists, including Bromfield, Forman, and Pfeiffer, promoted the decentralist cause.
Conversely, some decentralists—most notably homesteading advocate Ralph Borsodi—
embraced the teachings of the health foods movement.[31]

Decentralism had a very short heyday. The successful expansion of federal authority
during World War II undermined much of the case for decentralization. Moreover, the return of prosperity ended the likelihood that the movement would ever attract much of a
mass following. Nevertheless, the anti-modernist sentiments that fueled decentralism
lived on long after the war within the growing health foods movement.

SCIENTIFIC CONTROVERSY AND THE SHADOW OF IDEOLOGY
Compared with the rest of the public, health foodists were highly informed on the latest
scientific developments in medicine and nutrition, but their anti-modernist views shaped
the way they interpreted this information. Troubled by anything that impaired the nutritional content of foods, no matter how insignificant, health foodists concluded that the
food supply was so deficient that all Americans, regardless of class, had great difficulty
securing a healthful diet, and that much of the population was malnourished as a result.
In contrast, most nutritionists maintained that Americans could easily obtain adequate

nutrition if they chose their foods wisely, and that the chief obstacles to proper food selection were nutritional ignorance and a limited food budget. They thus believed that the
poor were much more likely to eat poorly than the middle and upper classes, who could afford a healthful diet if they knew which foods to purchase and desired to buy them. Furthermore, they never opposed the consumption of all processed foods, such as pasteurized
milk or canned foods, which retained a large percentage of their natural nutritional content. Some nutritionists even tolerated the consumption of a certain amount of vitamin
and mineral-poor foods, so long as the rest of the diet was nutritionally adequate. Finally,
most nutritionists paid no heed to the soil–nutrition issue after World War II, since they
never felt that the impact of mineral-poor soil on food quality was very great, even when
they were most concerned about nutritional deficiencies during the war.[32]

This difference of opinion on the extent of malnutrition stemmed in large part from how
each group felt about the nation's quasi-official set of quantitative nutritional requirements,
the Recommended Dietary Allowances (RDA), which were established by the National Research Council (NRC) in 1941 and then revised every five years or so thereafter. Nutritional
authorities considered the RDAs to be the best yardstick for measuring the adequacy of the
American diet. Health foodists, in contrast, generally ignored the issue of quantity when
they discussed nutrition, although it is clear that they felt that the RDAs were too low. Author Adelle Davis advised readers that it was almost impossible for anyone to consume too
much of any vitamin, and the more the better (except for vitamin D, which was known to be
toxic when consumed in large amounts). Both Davis and vitamin pitchman Carlton Fredericks established their own sets of requirements, which were as much as four times greater
than the RDAs. With standards so high, it was indeed quite difficult for people to obtain adequate nutrition without supplementing their diet with extra vitamins and minerals.[33]

The rejection of the RDAs for much higher values was not entirely unjustified. Prior
to World War II and to a greater extent thereafter researchers discovered numerous stress
factors—physical exertion, exposure to toxic substances, and certain disease conditions—
that increased an individual's nutritional requirements. They also learned that dietary imbalances could interfere with the utilization of nutrients. Partly to compensate for these
situations, the NRC set the RDA for each nutrient by taking the amount it determined was
sufficient to keep the *average* person in good health and adding a margin of safety to it. Nutritionists generally found this approach satisfactory, since the RDAs were designed for use
in planning diets for population groups, not for use with individuals.[34] Health foodists,
however, assumed that the various conditions that heightened nutritional needs were quite
common, and thus they felt that standards based on an average person's requirements were
much too low. They found support for this position in the work of controversial University
of Texas biochemist Roger J. Williams, who argued that nutritional needs of individuals
varied widely because of genetic differences, and encouraged consumers to purchase vitamin and mineral supplements to meet their needs.[35]

Health foodists had one other scientific justification for their belief that the RDAs were
much too low. Between the late 1910s and the 1930s two of the country's most renowned nutrition researchers, Elmer McCollum and Columbia University professor of chemistry Henry
C. Sherman, determined that a diet previously deemed to be adequate because it enabled rats
to grow and reproduce could be made even more nutritious by up to a fourfold increase in its
content of vitamins, minerals, and high-quality proteins. They found that rats fed such a diet
grew more quickly, acted more vigorously, had larger litters, had fewer infections, aged more

slowly, and lived longer than rats that ate the so-called adequate diet. Both men publicly stated that these experiments proved that humans too could grow faster and remain active and youthful longer if they consumed a vitamin and mineral-rich diet. While nutritional authorities embraced the teachings of McCollum and Sherman in principle, the NRC was reluctant to apply the results of animal-based experiments in formulating the RDAs, relying instead on more conservative values derived from research on humans. Health foodists, meanwhile, were totally convinced of the benefits of what McCollum and Sherman referred to as "optimal nutrition." "In the future," Jonathan Forman opined, "Medical Science promises to those individuals who will take advantage of the new knowledge of nutrition, a greater stature, a better physique, increased resistance to infections, comparative freedom from disease, the insertion of ten additional years into the active mid-span of their lives, an increased vigor and vitality at all age levels, the postponement of the usual signs of senility until the very end, better morale, a happier disposition and a higher level [of] cultural attainment."[36]

Besides the controversy surrounding the RDAs, the other major disagreement between health foodists and the nation's health authorities revolved around the former's contention that heart disease, cancer, and other illnesses of old age were the result of dietary deficiencies. Although researchers produced some evidence that nutrition played a role in chronic disease—including vitamin therapy pioneer Tom Spies, who maintained that all disease was chemical and could be corrected by chemical and nutritional means—the medical community as a whole refused to accept the claim that nutritional deficiencies caused these illnesses without conclusive evidence from controlled clinical studies. Health foodists, however, had no trouble finding reports in the medical literature to support their claim. Ever since it was discovered that a lack of vitamins could produce disease, researchers had studied almost every major disease of undetermined cause to ascertain if it was caused by nutritional deficiencies. Positive results were obtained on numerous occasions, and reports of these investigations could be found scattered throughout the medical literature. Few of these studies stood the test of time, and some had quite limited significance, but their presence in reputable journals gave health foodists reason to believe that their views on chronic disease had scientific legitimacy, despite being rejected by most medical authorities.[37]

CONCLUSION

Despite their differences of opinion with nutritional authorities, there was a certain scientific plausibility to the arguments of health foodists. Given the lack of knowledge about the etiologies of most chronic diseases and the statistical evidence showing that the incidence of these diseases varied in countries with different dietary patterns, it was not unreasonable to speculate that nutritional factors were somehow involved in their causation. Health foodists could also make a good case that the vitamin and mineral content of the typical American diet was less than optimal because of the uncertainties surrounding individual nutritional requirements and the spectacular results of the animal-feeding experiments conducted by McCollum and Sherman. Much of the legitimacy of their claims derived from the fact that health foodists could always find some medical article or controversial scientist to back them up. It is not entirely surprising, then, that in the past two decades researchers have produced considerable, albeit controversial, evidence to support the hypothesis that vitamins and other constituents in food help prevent a number of chronic illnesses, including cancer and heart disease. Furthermore, the discovery of potential benefits from large intakes of vitamins has led authorities to replace the RDAs with a more complex set of nutritional requirements known as the Dietary Reference Intakes. Health foodists were also correct in predicting that scientists would discover previously unappreciated beneficial substances in whole grains not present in enriched grain products.[38]

While health foodists looked to science for their information on diet and health, their deep dissatisfaction with urban-industrial society determined how they interpreted this information. Their concerns about the effects of modern food production methods and their bleak view of the current state of health were predicated on their belief that the natural world was healthful to humankind and that the tremendous environmental changes wrought by industrialization threatened the population's well-being. The idea of "civilization as risk" was not new; as far back as the early nineteenth century allegations had been made that the artificiality of urban life was responsible for various physical and mental ills. Ever since that time, sizable groups of Americans have continued to question whether modern social and economic arrangements are beneficial. In the mid-twentieth century anti-modernist sentiments fueled the two causes allied to the health foods movement: the decentralist and popular conservation movements. In the late 1960s a new generation of Americans began to express concerns about the destructive impact of modern technology. These young people quickly discovered their kinship with the health foods movement, and they swelled its ranks.[39]

However prescient health foodists may have been regarding the relationship between nutrition and chronic disease, their views on food and health were determined less by scientific reasonableness than by how well a particular idea accorded with their anti-modernist commitments. Some of their claims, such as the notion that the soil is the most important determinant of a food's nutritional value and that naturally fluoridated water is safer than artificially fluoridated water, far exceeded the bounds of scientific credibility. Ideological purity led them to reject pasteurized milk and enriched bread, even though these foods provided obvious health benefits. Health foodists (Rorty and Norman excepted) also ignored the fact that modern food processing has made nutritious foods available to those who in the past did not have access to them or could not afford them. Generally speaking, the health foods movement was blind to the unique nutritional problems of the poor. In fact, the supposition that most illness is caused by bad eating made the movement appealing to political conservatives, who believed that health was a personal responsibility and not an issue for governmental involvement. Finally, however one may feel about its ideological perspective, as a practical matter, the main thing that movement has had to offer is the recommendation that people go out and buy relatively expensive health foods and dietary supplements—products of mostly doubtful value, except, of course, to those who have earned a living from their promotion and sale.

INTERSECTIONS: ALLOPATHIC MEDICINE MEETS ALTERNATIVE MEDICINE

"VOODOO DEATH"

Fantasy, Excitement, and the Untenable Boundaries of Biomedical Science

Otniel E. Dror

Hoodoo, or Voodoo, as pronounced by the whites, is burning with a flame in America, with all the intensity of a suppressed religion. It has its thousands of secret adherents.[1]

Zora Neale Hurston, Mules and Men, *1935*

Voodoo. . . . Nobody knows it, everybody uses it as a paradigm of backwardness and confusion. And yet Voodoo has a firm though still not sufficiently understood material basis, and a study of its manifestations can be used to enrich, and perhaps even to revise, our knowledge of physiology.[2]

Paul K. Feyerabend, Against Method, *1975*

In 1942 Walter B. Cannon, head of the Department of Physiology at Harvard Medical School, published his now-famous essay " 'Voodoo' Death." In this study, Cannon elucidated the mechanisms responsible for the detrimental physiological effects of "magic" spells or "voodoo" rituals in "primitive" societies. Cannon's essay, which appeared in the *American Anthropologist,* soon became a staple of anthropological studies on magic-induced death.[3] Pioneering anthropologist Claude Lévi-Strauss, for example, had expressed a common view in 1958, when he argued that Cannon's 1942 " 'Voodoo' Death" essay had provided the physiological rationale for "the efficacy of certain magical practices" to cause death in normal and healthy individuals. Lévi-Strauss's own study "The Sorcerer and His Magic" depended in important ways on Cannon's physiology of voodoo death and the scientific legitimacy that Cannon's article bestowed on the study of death through voodoo ritual.[4]

The subject of voodoo death engaged and negotiated several important late-nineteenth- and early-twentieth-century concerns that lay at the boundaries between mainstream and fringe, alternative and orthodox, and subversive and normative. Questions relating to the relationships between science and the occult, knowledge and emotions, colonial and indigenous people, and—particularly in the United States—black and white Americans, as well as between women and men, were all implicated in Cannon's " 'Voodoo'

Death" study. Although Cannon was oblivious to important aspects of these engagements and was unaware on a personal level of the work that his essay performed in these contexts, his study continued to evoke and destabilize some of these boundaries well into the post–Second World War period.

In this chapter, I situate Cannon's " 'Voodoo' Death" essay within these different contexts. I provide an expansively interpretive, rather than exhaustive, account of his essay. I begin with an examination of the voodoo contexts of Cannon's work and the problems and negotiations that Cannon and his correspondents faced in attempting to transform the fantasy of voodoo death into a legitimate object of knowledge. I study the status of the mechanism for subjugating voodoo death: emotional "excitement," and its fringe and problematic position in the ecology of medical knowledges of the first half of the twentieth century. Then I examine the new and fascinating laboratory model that Cannon proposed in explaining voodoo death—the decerebrate cat. This laboratory model of voodoo death resolved the unregistered cultural dilemmas that Cannon and modern biomedicine faced in tackling voodoo death. Ultimately, the study of voodoo death forced fringe and counter-cultural discourses into the center of the biomedical sciences during a period in which these issues were supposedly already resolved.

On a broader front, I also wish to contribute to the literature on the political dimensions of modern knowledge by presenting a model in which biomedicine fails in its endeavors to completely subjugate alien forms of knowledge, yet unwittingly legitimates these untamed disorders. Voodoo ritual signified a presence of the "primitive" and disruptive in the midst of modern Western society and excited the popular, literary, ethnographic, and medical imagination. Despite the fact that Cannon was only partly successful in his attempts to incorporate voodoo into modern biomedicine, postwar biomedicine "discovered" that voodoo-like phenomena were ubiquitous in modern Western experience. The radical shift from earlier attempts to distance and distinguish between Western and "primitive," to the post–World War Two "discovery" that the primitive is ubiquitous in Western societies signifies and reflects the broader transmutations that Western knowledge underwent during the cultural and political upheavals of the post–World War Two period.

FANTASIZING VOODOO: ONTOLOGIZING FANTASY

Nobody knows for sure how many thousands in America are warmed by the fire of hoodoo, because the worship is bound in secrecy. . . . That is why these voodoo ritualistic orgies of Broadway and popular fiction are so laughable. The profound silence of the initiated remains what it is. Hoodoo is not drum beating and dancing. There are no moon-worshippers among the Negroes in America.[5]

Zora Neale Hurston, Mules and Men, *1935*

Cannon published his scientific analysis of voodoo death after long and protracted deliberations. Though his essay appeared in print only in 1942, Cannon's personal papers reveal that he had struggled with voodoo death over a period of seven years prior to its publication. From 1934, Cannon developed an expansive network of correspondents with whom he engaged in a massive fact-collecting project relating to "voodoo death" or "magic." Particularly during the years 1934–1935—and unbeknownst to his readers, as well as to later commentators—Cannon, the quintessential laboratory man, corresponded, like a nine-teenth-century Victorian naturalist, with numerous physicians and several anthropologists.[6] By 1935, he had already collected all the required ethnographic data and had formulated the physiological model of voodoo death, which he would publish only in 1942.

When Cannon embarked on his voodoo death venture in 1934, his sole objective was to gather reports of

> what might be called "voodoo death." By this I mean the casting of a fatal spell on a person by a king or priest or voodoo doctor exerting an influence among savage and superstitious people, with the result that the person who is credulous and terrorized by the spell is said to die. I am searching for authentic cases of this type.[7]

The diverse reports of his interlocutors testified to the difficulties entailed in defining voodoo death as a legitimate object of scientific knowledge. Some of Cannon's correspondents refused to support his physiological model or even the very reality of voodoo death. Though they agreed with Cannon's contention that death followed upon "bone pointing," they offered competing interpretations, which subverted Cannon's enterprise. "Poisoning," "wasting away," "acute hysteria," "suggestion," or "sub-acute hysteria" were some of the proffered alternative explanations and paradigms for voodoo death.[8]

J. B. Cleland, professor of pathology at the University of Adelaide, for example, explained that "most of the deaths resulting from bone pointing in Australian natives took, however, apparently weeks or months to eventuate—that is, when an individual knows that a bone has been pointed at him and thinks that the effects cannot be counteracted he just seems gradually to lose interest in life and die, I presume, from asthenia."[9] Or as others argued, natives often attributed occult reasons for what the biomedical autopsy revealed to be endemic diseases, such as tuberculosis or malaria.[10] Moreover, even when the autopsy "failed to reveal any etiology for the death," supporting Cannon's thesis of death by fear, "the condition is too slow in progress to be explicable on the basis you suggest."[11]

R. P. Parsons, one of Cannon's correspondents and a lieutenant commander (Medical Corps) in the United States Naval Hospital, San Diego, had spent three years in Haiti and had no personal knowledge of any "real authentic cases" of voodoo death. At autopsy, he explained to Cannon, he always found a physical basis for death: "Deaths by poison . . . may explain many of the deaths attributed to psychic causes through the various methods of sorcery," he asserted.[12] G. W. Harley also believed that death following a spell was due to concealed "chemical poisons."[13]

Several correspondents were even more critical. They not only challenged Cannon's mechanism and model for voodoo death, but defined his object of knowledge—voodoo death—as a figment of the American imagination. Since the American occupation of Haiti (1915), voodoo had overtaken the American popular mind. Kent C. Melhorn, a captain in the United States Fleet (Canal Zone), had served in Santo Domingo and Haiti, "the assignment . . . quelling revolutions": "At no time," he noted in his letter to Cannon, "did I witness or hear of an authentic death caused by the casting of a fatal spell. Many fanciful tales have been published," but these just wanted to create a "best seller."[14]

M. E. Higgins, of the U.S. Naval Hospital, New York, was even more disparaging. Since the U.S. occupation of Haiti, the question of voodoo had "been given wide publicity" with numerous books and magazine articles. This subject, Higgins continued, had an "exceedingly popular appeal . . . and writers have not failed to take advantage of it."[15] One "Captain Craig[e]" had even given a radio talk on the subject of voodoo in the context of a National Geographic broadcast.[16]

Dr. Leslie Tarlton, of Nairobi, British East Africa, expressed well the semantic field of significations that voodoo death evoked in some of Cannon's correspondents: "Poison, autosuggestion, mesmerism, or whatever you please results in fatalities here," she wrote to Cannon.[17] Lurid Voodoo stories, Hollywood-produced cinematic representations of voodoo horrors, and popular magazines created a Western fantasy of voodoo or hoodoo.[18] "Ever since the time of Uncle Remus," Franz Boas observed in his introduction to Zora Neale Hurston's 1935 *Mules and Men*, "Negro Folk-Lore has exerted a strong attraction upon the imagination of the American public. Negro tales, songs and sayings without end, as well as descriptions of Negro magic and voodoo, have appeared."[19]

For many of Cannon's correspondents, voodoo death or magic owed its existence to the credulous nature and enthusiasm of the American public. Cannon's project was an attempt to physiologize an American fantasy and to transform a figment of the imagination into an object of knowledge inside the laboratory. Westerners who believed in the reality of voodoo death were no less credulous than those indigenous people whose "primitive" belief structure was responsible for the gesture that kills, according to Cannon's model.

Other physicians, however, supported Cannon, providing the justification and fodder for Cannon's publication, at least in Cannon's eyes. S. de la Rue, for example, reported that most of the doctors serving in West Indian and Central American countries were "pretty well convinced that killing by suggestion is possible."[20] Ralph Linton, editor of *The American Anthropologist*, wrote to Cannon in 1941 to tell him that after reading Cannon's essay he was convinced of the authenticity of such reported deaths, and had had at least one firsthand experience: A native who said that he had seen a long-tailed spirit and that he was going to die "lay down and died in forty-eight hours."[21]

These physicians and anthropologists substantiated the authenticity of voodoo-death-like occurrences, though they did not distinguish among voodoo death, "bone pointing," "enchanted" spears, "sorcery," "magic," and the like. These observers provided a catalogue of case studies in which rapid death followed a curse.[22]

AN INVISIBLE-VISIBLE SUBVERSION[23]

The difficulties that Cannon's correspondents raised for his project of ontologizing voodoo death—by challenging the very reality of his object of study—were absent from Cannon's published article. Also conspicuously absent was the very mention of voodoo's presence in the United States. To all intent, voodoo was an exotic and foreign practice. Yet it festered at home and, indeed, on the same American shores as Cannon's highbrow Harvard Medical School.

Cannon was not unaware of this proximity. His correspondents had, in fact, explicitly alluded to the voodoo invasion of America and to its *locus classicus*—New Orleans. As one of his interlocutors wrote in 1934, a Dr. Dyer of New Orleans had reported "death among negroes undoubtedly caused by superstitions fear-threats of Voodoo 'Doctors.'"[24]

In contrast to Cannon's disavowal of the American brand of voodoo, other researchers did recognize its ubiquitous presence in Afro-American culture. Franz Boas, Zora Neale Hurston, Newbell Niles Puckett, and Harry Middleton Hyatt, for example, either engaged in or were aware of ethnographic research on voodoo or hoodoo in the United States. Harry Middleton Hyatt's four-year odyssey (1936–1940) across the Southeast and his massive collection of interviews exemplified the omnipresence of hoodoo in many Afro-American communities.[25] Hyatt's ethnographic tour of the United States was itself indebted to the earlier work of Hurston and Puckett.[26]

By the time of Cannon's publication, the voodoo presence in the United States had also been formally recognized, exoticized, and canonized as part of the Federal Writers' Project of the 1930s. The *New Orleans City Guide* emphasized and exaggerated the voodoo presence in describing the local Spiritual churches of New Orleans—and their long history, which extended back to the nineteenth century.[27]

Cannon's disavowal of an entrenched American voodoo presence and his insistence on the alien and "primitive" elements of voodoo expressed wider anxieties concerning the relationships between science and "magic," masculine and feminine, and orthodox and alternative beliefs and knowledge. Establishing "sorcery" and voodoo as legitimate objects of knowledge demanded that Cannon and his cohort avoid the local, popular, and suspect representations of American-produced voodoo in sustaining the clear demarcations between institutionalized science and its others. Beyond this, Cannon and his cohort also had to confront the subversive cultural significances of voodoo and its explicit and contentious historical relationships with Christianity.

Voodoo ritual was a particularly disruptive cultural praxis. It not only presented a lurid and cannibalistic image in the popular imagination, but—on a much more profound level—also served as a vehicle for Afro-American women's empowerment. Voodoo was a culturally subversive and transgressive practice that challenged Western boundaries and hierarchies between male and female and between primitive (African) and modern (Western).

As several recent authors have argued in studying voodoo history in the American and Haitian contexts, voodoo ritual embodied subversive, liberating, and empowering motifs for enslaved, disenfranchised, and disempowered blacks—particularly women—in Haiti and the United States. It functioned, as Rachel Stein has argued in her suggestive analysis of Zora Neale Hurston's *Tell My Horse* and *Their Eyes Were Watching God*, "like Donna Haraway's cyborg"—breaching "assumed boundaries (of race and gender) and thus became a powerful means of indigenous Afro-Caribbean resistance to colonial strictures." By refusing the Western religious "distinctions between spiritual and carnal, and view[ing] sexuality as sacred, to be worshipped as the divine source and ultimate mystery of life," Haitian voodoo inverted a basic hierarchical structure of Western tradition.[28]

In the United States, hoodoo—the American type of Vodun—was also a "source of female empowerment," as Cheryl Wall has argued in her analysis of Hurston's writings. Through hoodoo, Afro-American women not only controlled their interior lives, but also participated as spiritual equals with men and subverted man-made hierarchies. Moreover, and before abolition, hoodoo challenged the omnipotent power of whites by representing a realm in which "slaves could act with more knowledge and authority than their masters." These functions of hoodoo continued into the early decades of the twentieth century.[29]

Voodoo was also represented as a corruption of Christian practices. The adoption of and mutual exchange with Christian symbols and practices, common to Afro-American belief, was perceived as a distortion of "pure" Christianity. As Yvonne Chireau has argued, "unauthorized claims to supernatural empowerment presented a challenge to one of the primary assumptions of the Christian worldview: the singular, uncontested sovereignty of

God's power and will. According to official Protestant thought and doctrine, magic and occultism occupied the realm of heresy and heathenism."[30] The Christian establishment resisted the particular syncretism of African-American belief.

Cannon and his correspondents did not register these culturally subversive significations of voodoo in their epistolary exchange. Yet through their narratives of voodoo death, they nevertheless introduced their own disruptions of modern biomedicine. As Seward Hiltner, executive secretary of the Federal Council of the Churches of Christ in America, wrote to Cannon after reading Cannon's prepublished voodoo death manuscript in 1941:

> Naturally we have a special interest in the "other side of the coin." With the facts and hypothesis which you present, do we not now have some basis for understanding what may occur during "sudden" cures? Though this could be only an hypothesis at present, there is some evidence of such cures at least of tubercular lesions and of similar disorders.

Might it not be possible, Hiltner suggested, that "fear had aided in producing the condition in the first place; that a change in personality had taken place relieving the fear . . . and thus permitting the healing forces of the body to work. . . . This would not suggest the complete connections, but I wonder if it might lead us further along." Could Cannon send him reprints so that "the 50 members of our Commission might be sure to see the article"?[31]

Hiltner's appropriation of Cannon's work on voodoo implicitly threatened Cannon's project and, paradoxically, challenged the distinction between voodoo and Christianity. By juxtaposing Christian health with voodoo death, Hiltner mobilized Cannon's laboratory for his own "fringe" project of substantiating the real effects of Christian healing. The subversive implications of this parallelism between the healing powers of Western Christian belief and the pathologizing effects of "primitive" voodoo ritual were lost on Hiltner and Cannon, though Cannon's reply did not commit his work on voodoo to the Christian healing process. "Perhaps sometime in the future," he wrote to Hiltner, "physiologists will be able to learn how . . . [the subtler influences] may operate" on "illness or restoring health." Voodoo death was an extreme phenomenon that did not function according to the logic of Christian healing, Cannon maintained. Cannon's laboratory was ready to take on and authenticate voodoo death, but it was unwilling to support alternative modes of Western healing.[32]

Other correspondents contributed to the destabilizing effects of voodoo by implicitly challenging modern biomedicine's gregarious ability to swallow up competing systems of belief. These correspondents agreed with and participated in Cannon's depiction of the primitiveness of non-Western voodoo death societies. Yet, even while supporting Cannon, they contributed from their local experiences narratives that often subverted biomedicine, just as it stood poised to retranscribe primitive belief into its own models, practices, and classifications.

As some physicians argued, it was true that local inhabitants were duped into dying by a word or a gesture. Yet biomedicine had failed in its attempts to cure these patients. As these physicians observed, often the victims of spells were cured only by adopting local practices and by literally tricking them out of their deathbeds. As Leslie Tarlton wrote to Cannon, "Where science was apparently failing, I effected a complete and rapid cure, by the simple method of persuading the boy that Dr. Burkitt [the attending physician] was a bigger Witch Doctor than the spell caster!" Tarlton showed the boy a "scar over my liver: informed him that I had formerly had 'a snake in my stomach': that Dr. Burkitt had therefore killed me: cut me open and removed the snake: and brought me to life again! . . . within a very short time the boy was as fit as ever."[33]

This typical report depicted not only the credulous culture of the natives in Nairobi, British East Africa, but also the deficiencies of Western biomedicine. The natives were naive and primitive, but at least in some cases their culture-specific ailments could not be cured by Western medicine. Primitiveness and otherness were sometimes so extreme that modern biomedicine failed to retranscribe and appropriate these bodies and ailments into its own models and therapies. The limits of modern biomedicine were thus implicitly sketched and identified by these failures to cure, the abandonment of the biomedical model and its prerogative over the sick body, and finally by employing a local remedy, even if a caricatured one.

Cannon's project was, ultimately, an attempt to subsume a very great variety of these types of very different, fantastic, and local reports under one all-encompassing and new classification—"voodoo death"—in order to incorporate these variegated deaths into bio-medicine's nomenclature. Voodoo death was, according to Cannon's new terminology, a state of intense emotional "excitement."

THE POLITICS OF EMOTIONS

The interpretation of voodoo death as a state of emotional excitement drew on several decades of laboratory and clinical research on the emotions. More importantly, and not coincidentally, in arguing for his emotion model Cannon mobilized what had already become a powerful vehicle for opposing alternative medical cosmologies. Emotion was one of medical orthodoxy's most important concepts for defining and negotiating its relationship with alternative modes of healing and with its own history, particularly beginning in the late nineteenth century.

Throughout the nineteenth century, various forms of resistance to and disempowerment of alternative knowledge or knowledge makers were conspicuously present, as the ecology of knowledge had not yet assumed its more familiar and modern configuration. Debates over "fringe" phenomena, such as mesmerism, spiritualism, or psychical research, were still part of public discourse, because authority, as Alison Winter has argued, had not as yet shifted from the public sphere to a cohort of experts. Early- and mid-Victorian negotiations around "fringe" sciences were, in fact, instrumental for the late Victorian consolidation of the malleable scientific, medical, and intellectual cultures of the early Victorian period.[34]

In the medical realm, orthodox physicians vied with a multitude of alternative approaches and cosmologies for authority. They not only established the American Medical Association in the context of these contestations, but also developed new concepts and new rhetorical strategies in rationalizing away the apparent successes of alternative systems: the emphasis on the body's natural healing powers, the promulgation of the notion of "self-limiting" diseases, and the formulation of a theory of placebo—all were mechanisms that explained alternative knowledge claims in terms of orthodox theory.[35]

Fundamental questions regarding what constituted scientific knowledge, who could make knowledge claims, and how to maintain authority over knowledge claims continued into the early twentieth century, in spite of the fact that physicians developed "scientific medicine."[36] Particularly relevant to our discussion on emotions and fringe knowledge was the development of various psychosomatic approaches in American medicine. During the early twentieth century psychosomatically oriented physicians were fascinated by the emotions and the occult.[37] These physicians attempted to enlist the apparent success of alternative cosmologies for their own medical system. They were engaged in a Cannon-like, precarious, and dual process of rejection and assimilation: they rejected the ontology of occult medicine, but incorporated its practices and its history into their own corpus.

These physicians often found themselves the target of lay correspondence that explicitly positioned them within the camp of spiritual healers. One of the correspondents of the prominent Cornell psychosomatic clinician Harold G. Wolff expressed a general lay understanding of psychosomatic medicine, praising the doctors for "catching up" with those of us who have been "years ahead of the medical men." She had been interested, she wrote to Wolff, in the study of health through "right thinking" for thirty years.[38] Other lay correspondents perceived psychosomatically oriented physicians as natural allies in their quest for and interest in various forms of bodily "energy."[39]

The central mechanism that allowed psychosomatic clinicians to mediate between orthodoxy and the occult was emotion. Emotion explained millennia of apparent premodern medical successes, naturalized the power of the occult, and marshaled these naturalized powers—in the form of emotion—for orthodox medicine. "[P]re-scientific" practices, Harold G. Wolff explained to his students in 1938, were all unrecognized mobilizations of the power of emotions. Or as Franz Alexander, head of the Chicago Institute for Psychoanalysis, wrote in the opening editorial to the first issue of the *Journal of Psychosomatic Medicine*, psychosomatic medicine was "nothing but a revival of old prescientific views in a new and scientific form."[40] Other prominent emotion-focused clinicians, such as Helen Flunders Dunbar, Stewart Wolf, and George Draper, were also interested in emotion, the occult, and alternative practices of "healing."

The mobilization of emotion, however, was a two-edged sword. Emotion was a culturally negative and suspect phenomenon. It was allied to marginal or oppositional social and cultural movements, and it smacked of the popular and of the superstitious. Its appropriation by mainstream biomedicine entailed various anxieties and a tenuous renegotiation of emotion.[41]

One particularly negative and visible cultural sphere, which was associated with emotion, was the feminine. The feminine, in its turn, was associated from the nineteenth century with oppositional and alternative political movements and systems of knowledge. From the early nineteenth century—and in the context of the contestations between orthodox and alternative medicine—American orthodox physicians were represented as masculine, while alternative or oppositional forms of knowledge and praxis were feminized. While orthodox physicians adopted heroic practices, such as bloodletting or purging, homeopathic physicians promulgated gentle and nonintrusive types of interactions. As Naomi Rogers and Martin Pernick have argued, this mildness "was part of the reason homeopathy had become the preferred medicine for many women and children. By mid-century a number of families began to select different systems of medicine for different family members and different kinds of diseases."[42]

In sheer numbers, alternative medical systems were also feminized. They accepted women into their ranks far more readily than orthodox medicine and appealed to women because of their "less rigid sense of gender and class division."[43] Moreover, during the late nineteenth century, charismatic women led several alternative medical movements—

Christian Scientists, Seventh-Day Adventists, and the International Church of the Foursquare Gospel.[44]

These links between women, oppositional movements, and alternative and popular cosmologies were also visible in other spheres. As Judith R. Walkowitz has argued, medical men "caricatured spiritualists as crazy women and feminized men engaged in superstitious, popular, and fraudulent practices."[45] These divisions between mystical women and scientific men were well expressed in the writings of one of the prominent founding members of the Society for Psychical Research, William James.[46] As Cynthia Schrager has argued, William James sought "to overcome what he saw as the unfortunate antipathy between the 'scientific-academic mind' and the 'feminine-mystical mind.'" His project was framed not as another attempt to appropriate and subjugate the mystical by the scientific, but as a mutual accommodation.[47]

These associations between emotion, women, the feminine, and oppositional knowledge ultimately congealed in the particular late-nineteenth-century political constellation that grouped alternative medicine together with the animal protection and anti-vivisection movements, the anti-vaccinationists, and women.[48] Thus, to the consternation of physiologists and physicians, the most powerful tool for subjugating alternative knowledge—emotion—held a leading and visible position in feminized, oppositional, and alternative political and medical discourses.

DEATH BY EXCITEMENTS

Cannon navigated these dangerous waters by circumventing nineteenth- and early-twentieth-century modes of subjugating alternative knowledge. In confronting voodoo death, he avoided nineteenth-century terms, such as *hysteria, suggestion, faith, hope, mind-body* interactions, and so forth. His physiological model of voodoo death eliminated these Victorian terms and replaced them with *excitement.*

From Cannon's perspective, the final common pathway for the devastating effects of a variety of different cultural practices on the body was "excitement." Cannon had already proposed his death-by-excitement mechanism during the mid-1930s. "Some years ago," he wrote to numerous correspondents,

> I found that after removal of the cerebral cortex the exhibition of emotional excitement which thereupon appears will result in death in approximately three hours. This is in the cat. The death is not explained by hemorrhage or any other feature which I could find. Recently one of my students [Norman Freeman] learned that great excitement causes a progressive reduction of blood volume until the shock-like state develops, which results in death. It has occurred to me that the death from the casting of a "spell" might be of this character.[49]

Eight years later, in his published essay, Cannon was more specific, defining voodoo death as a state of excessive activation of the sympathico-adrenal system—an extreme alarm reaction of the body. The excessive activation of the sympathetic system led to an escape of fluids from the blood vessels, producing shock and death. A "persistent and profound emotional state," Cannon concluded, "may induce a disastrous fall of blood pressure, ending in death."[50]

Cannon modeled the physiological mechanisms that led to voodoo-induced death in the decerebrate or decorticate cat.[51] This model laboratory organism was an animal from which the cortex or cerebrum—the location of the higher functions of the brain—had been removed surgically. Cannon and his cohort of physicians and physiologists paradoxically chose an animal that literally had no higher brain functions in order to simulate the effects of the highest functions of the brain—a culturally specific belief system—on the body.

Harold G. Wolff's 1938 lecture notes in physiology for first-year medical students reveal a strikingly similar solution to the same tensions. Wolff attempted to naturalize the focus on the occult and to bring the mystical and spiritual into the category of scientific curricula. As his notes indicate, it had been difficult to "talk about such things in scientific circles without blush"—before the laboratory had demystified the mystical.[52]

In an interesting and revealing twist, Wolff structured his thoughts in 1938 much as Cannon did in his essay four years later. He followed the same logic, but presented the argument in the inverse order: Wolff began his lecture with a description of laboratory experiments on the decerebrate dog and concluded with a discussion of the relevance of these laboratory experiments for the mystical and spiritual in human beings. Cannon's article began with voodoo death and culminated with the decorticate cat as the model that explained how sorcery and magic lead to death.

The selection of a brainless cat as the most appropriate model for the physiology of human belief exemplifies the way in which modern biomedicine coped with a medically and culturally subversive phenomenon, though these coping mechanisms were not acknowledged or even intentionally conceived by their inventors. The choice of the decorticate cat clearly marked the boundaries between the biomedicalized variant of voodoo death and various fringe, suspect, or alternative knowledge systems. The decorticate cat served as an ideal model precisely because it had no spirit, no culture, no faith, no hope, and no real—experienced—emotions. The cat presented an ideal model because it functioned almost like a machine and represented a radical break from alternative, fringe, and occult modes of modeling human organisms and societies.

CONCLUSION

In 1941, Cannon wrote to W. Lloyd Warner of the Department of Anthropology at the University of Chicago, "The article which I was preparing then on 'Voodoo Death' I have not published because I wanted to obtain further observations regarding a possible physiological explanation of the phenomenon."[53] Yet Cannon had already been familiar with all the relevant and necessary facts during the mid-1930s. In 1934, he proposed the same physiological mechanism that he would publish, almost to a word, in 1942.

Perhaps Cannon felt reassured when his former student Norman Freeman told him in 1939 of his own publication on emotions. In his forthcoming chapter on shock—to appear in William D. Stroud's edited volume *The Diagnosis and Treatment of Cardiovascular Disease* (1941), Freeman intended to present a case of fear leading to shock. Freeman had attached a copy of the chapter to his letter.[54] Be that as it may, we may never know why Cannon delayed the publication of his essay for close to seven years, and what changed his mind at that moment in time.

The debates concerning the reality of voodoo death did not abate during the postwar period, in spite of Cannon's essay. Some anthropologists persevered in maintaining that voodoo death was a fabrication of the Western imagination, while others retorted with their own proof of its reality. Cannon's object of knowledge was still a contested entity, shifting between its status as a reality of some cultures and its status as a fantasy of American popular culture, Hollywood and Broadway industries, and academic scholarship. According to this latter reading, Cannon demystified and physiologized a Western fantasy that was fabricated by an implicit collusion between academics, screenwriters, and popularizers.[55]

The subversive implications of voodoo death also continued during the postwar period, as evidenced by the spate of letters that appeared in the *British Medical Journal* in 1965. The debate about whether "voodoo," "fortune-tellers," or being "scared to death" implied, in some instances, extrasensory perception, extreme fear, or a state of "hopelessness" was again visible in the medical press.[56]

More important for my argument is the observation that voodoo's blackness, its American habitation, its popular register, its Christian associations, and its subversive significations were never mentioned in Cannon's published essay. Cannon, as we have seen, fashioned voodoo death into a characteristic phenomenon of "primitive" societies, granting a similar status only to presurgical patients or soldiers during war. His disavowal of the "primitive" and subversive, in spite of their manifest presence, was his contribution to the cultural work of Western biomedicine in its attempt to delineate not only between orthodox and alternative medicines, but also between Western and non-Western societies. Voodoo was, to borrow Mary Douglas' term, modern biomedicine's pollution.[57]

Postwar authors took a radically different stance. Instead of relegating voodoo death to the exotic, they universalized voodoo death, ultimately transforming it into one of the distinct characteristics of modern life—sudden death resulting from the acute stress of modernization.[58] The voodoo experience was now discovered in a variety of acute medical emergencies that were observed in everyday Western lives.

I would suggest that Voodoo's continued presence exemplifies what Peter Stallybrass, Allon White, and Chris Rojek have described as the "fundamental rule . . . that what is excluded at the overt level of identity-formation is productive of new objects of desire." The persistence of haunting and alluring voodoo-like images in medical texts can be interpreted as an expression of the "secret" fascination of "respectable society . . . with bodies and minds which were not 'respectable' and 'self-disciplined.' "[59] The scientific study of voodoo death epitomizes the productivity and the contributions of the persistent return of the 'repressed' to the development of the modern life sciences.

The postwar engagement with the repressed—transformed from its earlier identification with the "primitive" to its new identity as the emblem of modern Western "stress"—captures one aspect of the dramatic transformation that occurred during the postwar period. If Western identity had been structured along the dyad "primitive"-"civilized," then during the postwar period the transformed politics of the "primitive" had destabilized the very essence and meaning of its otherness. The primitive now resided in and was emblematic of that very process that previously had distinguished between it and the West—modern civilization.

WESTERN MEDICINE AND NAVAJO HEALING
Conflict and Compromise

Wade Davies

INSIDE HIS SIX-SIDED HOGAN in Winslow, Arizona, Jones Benally treated patients in the traditional Navajo healing ways. Like many other Navajo traditional healers (or "medicine men"), he crystal-gazed to discover the causes for their illnesses, and he tended to their symptoms using joint and muscle manipulation and the occasional herbal remedy. Sometimes Benally said traditional prayers over his patients, and he occasionally conducted minor ceremonies. Like all Navajo healers, Benally knew that his healing abilities were limited, and in certain cases he referred patients to a medicine man who could conduct some of the more complex healing ceremonies.[1]

What Benally did for his patients in Winslow during the 1990s differed little from what other Navajo traditional healers had been doing for Navajo (Diné) patients on the reservation for centuries. What was unusual about Benally's case was that his hogan (the traditional Navajo dwelling) sat on the grounds of a United States Indian Health Service (IHS) hospital. The federal government paid Benally to tend to patients referred to him by the hospital's physicians. The idea of Western medical practitioners and Navajo traditional healers working together would have struck most Navajos and non-Navajos as absurd one hundred years earlier, but it made sense to Benally, the IHS physicians, and their patients.

Benally's arrangement with the IHS reflected an ongoing process of cross-cultural accommodation between practitioners of Western medicine and Navajo healing. That accommodation required the eventual cooperation of non-Navajo medical providers such as the IHS, but Diné demands and efforts initiated and drove the process. Through adaptation, compromise, and cultural perseverance, Navajos in the twentieth century found ways to seek the health benefits of Western medicine and traditional Diné healing in combination. In large part, the Navajos were open to multiple healing ways because they had great needs. They, like other American Indians, faced high rates of infectious disease, alcoholism, infant mortality, and accidental deaths. Navajos also wished to determine their own medical future as a key component of their quest for greater political, social, and cultural autonomy.

Many different actors helped make it possible for Western medicine and Navajo healing to coexist and cooperate on the Navajo Nation. Patients did much to initiate the cross-cultural process, because many of them chose to seek care both in hogans and in hospitals. Navajo healers found ways to compromise with non-Navajo caregivers and also led efforts to pre-serve traditional healing ways that modern trends threatened. These healers thus ensured that the incorporation of Western medicine into Navajo lives could be done with as little harm as possible to the traditional ways. Although many non-Navajo physicians, nurses, government officials, and missionaries attempted to overwhelm and eliminate Navajo healing practices, others aided the cross-cultural process. And Navajos in tribal government played vital roles as well once they recognized the desires of many of their constituents. By encouraging the extension of federal medical services and actively participating in the delivery of Western medicine, the tribal government helped make the use of multiple healing forms a more tangible option for Navajo patients.

Before discussing how these healing ways related to each other and to Navajo patients, it is necessary to explain how they differ. While both Western and Navajo medical traditions are incredibly complex and encompass varieties of styles and beliefs, it is useful here to understand one basic way in which they contrast. Western medicine tends to focus on treating specific ailments and bodily organs, while Navajo healing is holistic, focusing on the individual's spiritual and physical relationship with his or her environment. Unlike Western medicine, traditional healing cannot be divorced from spirituality or any other aspect of life. In Navajo tradition, good health is related to *hózhó,* which is defined in part as "beauty," "harmony," and "balance." The purpose of the traditional healing ceremonies is to restore that state of harmony if some action or event disrupts it, such as taboo transgression or contact with the dead.[2]

Navajo healers, like Western physicians, must go through years of training, and even then, an individual healer can never learn more than a fraction of all the healing ceremonies. The ceremonies (or "sings") must be performed in exact detail and must be treated respectfully because they are handed down to the Navajos by their deities, the Holy People. The words and symbols used in the sings have powers and if misused can bring disharmony and sickness. The ceremonies are necessary to truly cure the patient, but Navajo traditional healing allows patients to accept medical practices that temporarily relieve physical symptoms, even if those practices are alien to Navajo culture. Many Navajos eventually came to acknowledge Western medicine's power to relieve symptoms and therefore began to view it as a possible supplement to traditional healing. Other agents of change in the twentieth century, including mass culture, Christian missionaries, and the wage economy, threatened the Navajo healing ways. Navajo acceptance of Western medicine, however, did not overshadow traditional healing, because the two forms of healing served different functions.

Although the potential always existed for Navajos to incorporate Western medicine as a supplement to traditional healing, this did not initially happen. Few Navajos were willing to consult Anglo physicians in the late nineteenth and early twentieth centuries, and few healers or Western physicians were willing to coexist, much less cooperate with one another.

American physicians around the turn of the century were part of a profession in search of social, economic, and political power, and few had any interest in regarding a Navajo medicine man as a colleague. The first physicians to serve the Navajos came either as government employees or as missionaries belonging to the Presbyterian Church, the Christian Reformed Church, or other Protestant denominations. Both government and nongovernment physicians attempted to eclipse Navajo healing with Western medicine. They came to the Navajos at a time when federal and church policies were aimed at assimilating

American Indians into American society and Christianizing them. As the protectors of tradition, the healers seemed to stand in the way of those goals.[3]

The physicians' cultural arrogance antagonized the Navajo patients and healers, and that negativism overshadowed any potential benefits their medical services may have offered. Navajo healers were aware of such attitudes and had little reason to approach the physicians. A famous singer, Manuelito Begay, remembered those early relations:

> When the doctors and hospitals were first established among us, the doctors thought they were the only ones who knew how to apply medicine to the patients. The Navajo people were not recognized at all and, in that connection, we thought the same way, we could not agree as to whose treatment should be recognized.[4]

Most Navajo healers and patients rejected Western medicine before the 1920s, not just because of cultural tensions, but because it offered limited medical benefit. Physicians on the reservation, especially those appointed by the U.S. government, were poorly trained and often had low morale. A trip to a reservation physician often required painful treatments with few positive results. Medical doctors could set broken bones and distribute pain relievers, but Navajos were not overly anxious to go under their knives. Many Navajos viewed hospitals as places of suffering and death rather than of healing.[5]

Until the 1930s few Navajos could gain access to Western medicine even if they wished to. The Navajos first made significant contact with physicians in 1864, when the military provided medical services to Navajos confined on a reservation at Bosque Redondo in eastern New Mexico. Even in close quarters with the U.S. Army and living in miserable conditions, most Navajos avoided Western medical services. After 1868, when the Navajos were allowed to return to a reservation on a portion of their homeland in northern Arizona and New Mexico, Anglo physicians could find few patients other than children attending boarding schools.[6]

During the early part of the twentieth century, the federal government hired only one physician at a time to serve a reservation area as large as the state of West Virginia. These men came to the Navajos through the Bureau of Indian Affairs (BIA), an agency that supervised almost every government program on the reservation. Handling duties from education to livestock management, the BIA devoted only limited attention to Indian health care.[7]

Despite the general inaccessibility of Western medicine and the antagonistic relationship that originally existed between practitioners of Western medicine and Navajo healing, some individual Navajos and non-Navajos eventually saw the potential for the combined use of the two forms of healing. A few physicians understood that cultural arrogance would bring them little success in finding willing Diné patients. Some, like Dr. Clarence Salsbury, found that positive relations with local traditional healers could help them gain the trust of Navajo communities. Shortly after Dr. Salsbury began serving Navajos around Ganado, Arizona, in 1927, a little girl died of an embolism while on his operating table. He had spent three days convincing the girl's parents to let him do surgery, so he had little margin for error. As soon as other reluctant Navajo patients heard about his failure, they all deserted the small hospital. Salsbury feared for his safety when an angry crowd formed outside, but an unlikely savior came to his aid. A Diné healer named Red Point calmed the crowd and pointed out that he and other healers had also lost patients in the past. Although Salsbury still believed that Navajos should discard their traditional practices, he learned a valuable lesson from this episode. Soon after Red Point's intervention on his behalf, Salsbury took photographs of other healers who had come to his hospital for treatment, and he passed the images around as an endorsement. Navajo patients soon overwhelmed the small facility.[8]

The 1930s brought significant changes to the relationship between Western medicine and Navajo healing. Navajo patients found more reasons to use Western medicine as sulfa drugs and other medical innovations began to offer real medical benefits. Increased federal funding during the New Deal also made medical services more accessible for Navajos. Furthermore, BIA commissioner John Collier worked to establish a more culturally sensitive approach to government medical care for Native Americans. Unlike his predecessors, Collier did not believe that Native American traditions had to be sacrificed in the name of modernization.

In the later years of the New Deal, Commissioner Collier hired noted psychiatrists and anthropologists to study Navajo culture in the hope that their work might help BIA medical workers breach cultural barriers. In the early 1940s, Alexander and Dorothea Leighton and Clyde Kluckhohn published works about Navajo culture. In a report, the Leightons explained their basic philosophy regarding Navajo health care:

> If our medicine is to help and not harm the Navajo, we must avoid clean sweeps. We must get them to accept and use our pertinent, practical knowledge without undermining their faith. That faith must grow and adjust also, but it must not be ruthlessly attacked simply because it offers some obstacles to medicine. Instead, white medicine should be expressed to the Navajos in terms of their own culture, in ways that fit into their understanding of the world and their scale of values.[9]

It is difficult to gauge the effect Collier's attitudes and the Leightons' work had on relations among physicians, Navajo healers, and patients, but there were signs of an improving relationship between physicians and healers in the postwar era, perhaps a result of the influence of these studies. After World War II, some younger physicians on the reservation were more open to Navajo traditional beliefs and practices than had been their predecessors, in part because they had different educational experiences than had their predecessors. They understood and took advantage of the fact that patients were more likely to accept medical care if physicians respected their desire to have healing ceremonies before or after going to a hospital.[10]

When these physicians, and also nurses, were willing to cooperate with traditional healers, healers often reciprocated. In 1954, for example, Manuelito Begay and other healers met with a group of government physicians and established an informal referral policy for Navajo children. Begay explained the terms of this agreement to the Navajo Tribal Council. "If you bring a child to the hospital and they cannot do it any good with their medicine," said Begay, "they will have the child returned for our treatment, if we make no progress with our medicine, then we return the child to the hospital."[11]

Many physicians and healers came to respect each other's abilities even if they did not accept the beliefs underlying the various healing ways. Western medical practitioners were more likely than in earlier years to see some value in traditional healing, even if they could explain it only in psychotherapeutic terms. In return, many healers acknowledged that

Western medicine offered some real benefits, but they usually did not accept physicians' explanations about disease. As Sam Yazzie indicated, traditional healers tended to categorize their power as different from, but complementary to, Western medicine's power:

> I have great respect for white doctors; there are things they can do that we cannot. For example, they can remove an appendix, they can take out a gall bladder, or treat a urinary tract infection ... There are certain sicknesses that a doctor can never cure that we can—lizard illness, for example—or an illness that comes from one of those small green worms you sometimes find on an ear of corn. Sickness might last over a long time and it might be a lingering illness. No white doctor can cure an illness of that type, only a medicine man can cure such patients ... In any situation when a patient isn't getting better then I, or any other medicine man who knows his business, should allow the patient to go to the hospital and have his x-rays and other treatment there. Then he can come back and have the rest of the sing in the hogan.[12]

Of course, some physicians and nurses in the mid-twentieth century remained hostile to Navajo traditional healing, but the tools and opportunities were now there for those who wished to find ways to bridge the cultural divide between them and their patients.

As the BIA gradually became a more culturally sensitive health care provider during the 1930s, it also expanded the scope and improved the quality of its services, but World War II brought economic strains and political pressures that eventually ended its medical role. In an attempt to pull back from federal obligations to American Indians, a conservative Congress tried to reduce the BIA's activities. The government transferred Indian health care responsibilities to the Public Health Service (which then created the Indian Health Service) in hopes that the agency, with its greater medical expertise, could bring Indian health statistics to parity with national averages. It would then be more acceptable politically for the United States government to terminate its special health care obligations to American Indians. The IHS took over the BIA's medical duties for the Navajos in 1955. Ironically, instead of reducing federal involvement with Navajo health care, the HIS, under President Kennedy's and Johnson's administrations in the 1960s, expanded reservation health care services dramatically. The HIS approached Navajo health care with a relatively effective comprehensive system that combined clinical care with sanitation services, nutrition services, public health nursing, and health education.

The availability and medical effectiveness of government medical care thus increased in the last half of the twentieth century, and Navajo patients responded by utilizing Western medicine in even greater numbers. This increased utilization did not, however, reflect a Diné rejection of their traditional ways. Instead, there is strong evidence in the late twentieth century that the majority of Navajos accepted both Western medicine and Navajo healing. A survey in 1978 showed that about three in four Navajos used both forms of healing. To say that many Navajos accepted Western medicine, however, is not to say that they were always pleased with the quality of care they received in government hospitals. Administrative blunders, funding problems, arrogance or indifference on the part of some employees, and cultural misunderstandings continually plagued the relationship between the IHS and the Navajo community. A high employee turnover rate also meant that few IHS physicians or nurses remained on the Navajo Nation long enough to form bonds with their patients or with traditional healers.[13]

Nevertheless, the IHS showed greater respect for Navajo traditional healing and traditional beliefs than had the BIA or other medical providers in the past. The IHS did not make a strong push to educate its employees about traditional healing, but administrators encouraged physicians and nurses to accommodate traditional healers and patients who wished to consult them. After the 1980s, the IHS also kept Navajo concerns in mind when constructing new facilities. Government hospitals were built with their doors facing east, like the doors on traditional hogans, and some of the facilities were equipped with special rooms that healers could use to treat patients.[14]

As the IHS's role in delivering health care to the Navajo reservation grew in the postwar era, missionary medical programs declined. Faced with the increasing cost and complexity of health care delivery, the churches began to reconsider medical care's role in the missionary process. Those services had been conceived as a means to aid the spread of Christianity, but they now hindered the mission programs with administrative hassles and funding woes. Perhaps ironically, the missionaries, who had been most vehement about the need to wipe out traditional healing and Navajo culture, may have done more than the government to aid the tribe in its quest to control its health care options. As the Presbyterians, Christian Reformed Church, and other missionaries pulled out of the health care business on the reservation, they turned their facilities over to local Navajo communities. Running their own medical facilities proved challenging but gave those communities greater control over the relationship between Western medicine and traditional ways. The community efforts also served as successful models for the tribe as a whole, as it considered taking greater control over the delivery of Western medicine for the Nation.[15]

As the twentieth century progressed, the Navajo Nation had become more dependent on Western medical services. In recognition of this fact, the tribal government became more and more involved with medical issues. Tribal leaders worked throughout the century to make Western medicine more accessible for the whole reservation and more sensitive to Navajo concerns. There were a variety of ways that the tribal government stayed involved in reservation health care. The Tribal Council played a role in Western medicine by awarding scholarships to Navajos interested in pursuing medical careers and by funding its own medical programs. The tribe also advised and criticized the BIA and IHS and helped facilitate communication between doctors and patients. From time to time, the tribal government also acted to preserve and protect the ceremonial ways. They did not want to simply exchange one form of healing for another. Instead, the hope was to expand the healing options for the people, giving them better access to effective Western medical services while preserving the traditional ways that were so intertwined with their culture and identity.

To a significant degree, the BIA and IHS encouraged the tribal government to become more involved with health care. A working relationship between the BIA and Tribal Council on health issues began in the 1920s when agency officials tried to win tribal cooperation in anti-trachoma and anti-tuberculosis efforts. Throughout the 1920s, BIA representatives reported on their medical activity and asked tribal leaders to encourage Navajos suffering from those diseases to seek help. Council members, such as chairman Chee Dodge, listened thoughtfully and voiced their own opinions, demonstrating that they cared deeply about health issues and wanted to see a larger medical presence on the reservation. This early participation eventually led to the tribe's creation of a Health Committee within the council in 1938.[16]

More direct tribal action in Western medicine followed the Second World War, in part because of a sudden decrease in federal health care services during the conflict. BIA medical care became scarce at a time when Navajo patients were utilizing hospitals and clinics in growing numbers. Wartime funding cuts for reservation health care programs were a cause of great concern for tribal leaders. Chee Dodge and his son, Thomas Dodge, then the chairman, led the protest. During a meeting in 1943, Thomas Dodge introduced a petition complaining that sick Navajos were being turned away from government hospitals and urging that those facilities be maintained. His father, Chee Dodge, stood before the council three years later and expressed his disappointment in what had happened to the government medical program he had helped convince his constituents to accept. The hospitals at Fort Defiance, Arizona, and Crownpoint, New Mexico, were the only two federal medical facilities he considered worth patronizing. "There are some other hospitals on the reservation," Dodge said, "but they have been neglected for so long that they have become like discarded rags."[17]

That same year, Chee Dodge and other tribal leaders went to Washington to voice their concerns to the House Committee on Indian Affairs and to encourage them to appropriate sorely needed funds for health care. They explained how Navajo people had to travel as many as one hundred miles over poor roads to reach the nearest medical services. "We, like yourselves have sickness and pain," said the Navajo delegates. "We are only asking what you would want for yourselves; good medical aid to relieve our suffering. Good medical service would enable us physically to be of greater service to our nation."[18]

Tribal activity in health care continued to increase in the postwar years. At midcentury, another Dodge stepped to the forefront: Annie, the youngest of Chee Dodge's four children, born in 1910 near Sawmill, Arizona. She grew up with concerns for health, education, and leadership. As a boarding school student in Fort Defiance, Arizona, she witnessed influenza and trachoma epidemics firsthand and always remembered what those diseases had done to her friends. Annie Dodge came away from her school experiences with a strong commitment to education and a deep concern about her people's health. In her thirties and now married, Annie Dodge Wauneka had a close relationship with her father, who served as tribal chairman from 1944 to 1947. From him, she learned that understanding both the Navajo and non-Indian worlds would help her become an effective tribal leader. In 1951, Annie Dodge Wauneka earned a seat on the Tribal Council and soon thereafter became chairperson of the Health Committee.[19]

Wauneka, along with Paul Jones and other tribal leaders, worked diligently to turn the Health Committee into a well-informed and influential body. The committee served as an effective mediator among Western medical providers, the Tribal Council, and Navajo patients because it fostered simple, straightforward communication. Wauneka had learned well from her father the power and necessity of communication and instilled that principle in the Health Committee. "The Navajo haven't been deliberately resistant to modern health methods," she explained. "It's just that they didn't understand, and you've got to throw yourself into explaining things. That wasn't done enough in the past, in the health field."[20]

Supplementing her words with action, Wauneka made annual visits to the three hundred or more Navajo patients then being treated for tuberculosis in off-reservation sanatoriums. What they needed most of all, she discovered, was for someone to listen to their concerns and speak to them clearly. Without action on the part of tribal leaders, these patients felt confused, scared, and alone, prompting many to avoid seeking treatment or to leave the sanitoriums. She reported back to the council that Navajo patients often deserted the medical facilities prematurely because they did not understand how long it took for the treatments to work. They assumed that a cure would take only a few days, and no one had told them otherwise, at least not until Annie Wauneka sat down with them. Needless to say, council members and physicians were impressed that, after her visits, patients no longer left the sanatoriums.[21]

Other Navajo politicians, such as Taylor McKenzie and Peterson Zah, would follow in later decades as proponents for more accessible, higher-quality, and more culturally sensitive Western medicine. Referring to itself as the Navajo Nation, as an expression of its desire for greater political and cultural autonomy, the tribe, through its government, became increasingly active in health care from 1960 to 2000. The tribe spent more and more of its limited funds to offer its own Western medical services. It also created tribal government agencies, such as the Navajo Division of Health, that acted in advisory roles to the IHS, as had the Health Committee. But these agencies did more than had the Health Committee. They also administered a growing number of tribe-sponsored health care services, including health education, scholarship, nutrition, HIV/AIDS, and alcohol and substance abuse programs.[22]

As the century drew to a close, the Navajo Nation considered taking an even greater step in its effort to promote and shape the delivery of Western medicine. By taking advantage of contracting arrangements with the IHS, first made possible through the Indian Self-Determination and Education Assistance Act of 1975, the tribe could take over the administration of some or all of the IHS hospitals and clinics on the reservation. Although other tribes used contracting to take over the administration of IHS hospitals on their reservations, the Navajos hesitated in this regard. Because the IHS medical network on the reservation had grown so large, and because Navajo patients were so reliant on IHS services, some tribal leaders worried about the potentially devastating consequences of contracting. Despite federal assurances, many feared, based on past experiences, that contracting was a veiled attempt by the U.S. government to withdraw from its health care responsibilities to the reservation. Other tribal leaders voiced the concerns of Navajo IHS workers who worried about possible changes in employee benefits resulting from a transfer of responsibilities. But many agreed that the opportunity such a move would give the tribe to determine its medical future compelled them to accept the risks. Which path the tribe would choose remained to be seen as the century ended.[23]

When considering all of the groups who aided the Navajo Nation in improving Western medicine while preserving the traditional ways, it is also important to discuss Diné medical workers. Navajo medical doctors and nurses introduced a different cultural perspective to Western medicine. Although many Navajos viewed the BIA and IHS as alien presences on the reservation, Navajo physicians, nurses, and administrators made those agencies more responsive to their patients. Navajo women and men served as government nurses from the early decades of the twentieth century. Navajo physicians were slower to arrive, but they became key players in the process of cross-cultural accommodation in the last three decades of the century. For instance, Dr. Lori Arviso Alvord served her Navajo patients as more than a skilled surgeon. She showed a strong commitment to her traditional culture and language and even had healing ceremonies conducted on her behalf. Even while practicing Western medicine, Dr. Arviso Alvord felt the strong influence of Navajo traditions on her life and could empathize with patients who felt the same way.[24]

Many Navajos thus did a great deal to encourage and shape the delivery of Western medicine as a supplement to Navajo healing, but the greater challenge proved to be preserving the traditional ways. No matter how effective and culturally sensitive Western medicine became, it could not fill the healing and spiritual void that would be left if Navajo medicine disappeared. By the 1960s, many Navajos believed that the traditional healing ways would not survive. It is difficult to quantify the number of traditional healers who served the Navajo Nation after World War II or the number of ceremonies they knew. But many Navajo elders judged ceremonialism to be in decline, and there is every reason for scholars to agree with that assessment. As the population continued to grow rapidly, the number of young people learning the traditional ways clearly decreased. Traditional healing nonetheless endured through times of dramatic change in the Navajo Nation. Navajos continued to value the old ways and to demand sings, and some of those who were most worried about the decline took action to preserve the ceremonies.

Traditional healers, older Navajos, and other observers in the mid- to late twentieth century commonly referred to a declining number of singers and a loss of respect for traditional ways. "I have been acquainted with several medicine men who have recently died who were not able to teach ceremonies they knew to their grandchildren or anyone else," said Yazzie Begay, a Navajo educator. "Today their sacred instruments sit unused." For Begay and others, this situation endangered more than Navajo health. "The Navajo ceremonial system has given our lives meaning, our personalities dignity, and has been the reason our people and land have increased," said Begay. "We believe that, if the harmony and beauty that are part of the Navajo way are lost through the deaths of medicine men, then we as people are lost and have no future."[25]

Interviews conducted by the University of New Mexico and Navajo Community College in the 1960s and early 1970s provide some sense of how older Navajos explained the decline of traditional healing. The Navajo respondents generally did not attribute the loss of traditional healing practices to Western medicine's influence on Diné society. Only a few of the Navajos even spoke of Western medicine in the same context with traditional healing. The ceremonies were not in direct competition with the IHS or any other Western medical providers, and respondents were more likely to view Christianity, economics, education, and broad contact with the non-Navajo world as the real threats.[26]

Navajo elders, including traditional healers, were most worried about how modern society had affected the young people responsible for carrying on the traditional ways. Younger people relied on wage work and went away to school more than in the past, and this absence made it difficult for them to find the time and money to commit themselves to years of apprenticeship with a traditional healer. Under the traditional livestock-herding economy families could support a young person while he or she studied to become a singer, but the wage economy, which became more prevalent in the mid- to late twentieth century, made it more challenging to do so. Some healers in the 1960s also believed that people returning from school off the reservation did not want to become singers because they had not been sufficiently exposed to traditional culture. Many of these students also came back to the reservation unable to speak Diné, and this made it difficult for them to follow the traditional ways.[27]

Modern technology also appeared to distract younger Navajos. Tape recorders and radios filled up their leisure time and steered them away from the traditional teachings. Such concerns were particularly serious because Navajo elders had to pass on essential ceremonial information orally, and they required attentive audiences. Deescheeny Nez Tracy, for one, considered Diné youths disrespectful and unfocused, and he lamented that they were headed down the wrong path:

In the homes the refrigerators are full of pop and Kool Aid. Our children sit in front of the TV and consume gallons of pop into all hours of the nights. When morning comes they want to sleep until noon. That is life to them. We seldom hear about a person running at dawn yelling at the top of his voice, or the screams that come from taking an ice-cold plunge or rolling in the snow. We hear only the screaming of the radios and stereo players. Who is to blame? The white man made the inventions.[28]

John Dick did not blame just the young people or non-Indian influence. Dick believed that the elders themselves had failed to instill the proper values in the children and did not work hard enough to pass on the traditional stories and ceremonies. "Our elders should have continued to tell their stories," he said, "then our religion would have been made stronger and we still would have enough medicine men to serve our people where they are needed." According to Dick, the children were also to blame for failing to be attentive when the elders did speak to them. "Such talks bug them," said Dick, "and they do not listen."[29]

Many of those Diné who worried about what the future held for Navajo healing took action to preserve the traditional ways. Some healers, such as Hosteen Klah and Frank Mitchell, were willing to share their knowledge with outsiders and allowed themselves to be recorded, believing that this would preserve the prayers and chants for posterity. "Gathering all of the information that is vital and keeping it on records or tapes, or printing it in books, can be our Bible, like the white man has," said Deescheeny Nez Tracy. Others were cautious about doing so, because revealing such information, especially at the wrong times, could bring about illness or other harm.[30]

Although the Tribal Council did little to directly promote traditional healing, Navajo-controlled education played a key role in protecting and preserving the culture. During the 1960s, the tribal government and local communities focused energy on taking control of education by administering their own schools, free from BIA influence. By the end of the 1960s, the effort had led to the establishment of Navajo Community College in 1968 and a variety of community schools, such as Rough Rock Demonstration School in 1966. These new institutions made Navajo history and culture official components of their curriculum and provided a possible support base for initiatives focused on training new healers. Robert Roessel, an educator from Arizona State University who helped establish both institutions, took a personal interest in traditional healing. In 1967, Roessel and others at the Rough Rock Demonstration School, in conjunction with some traditional healers, decided to establish a training program for singers.[31]

Rough Rock found funding for what became known as the Navajo Mental Health Program through a grant from the Public Health Service's National Institute of Mental Health. It seemed natural for funding to come through an agency related to mental health. Psychiatrists had normally been more interested in Navajo healing than other medical doctors because they considered it to be psychotherapeutic.[32]

Under the direction of John Dick and Frank Harvey, the Navajo Mental Health Program selected six healers to receive stipends through the Rough Rock Demonstration School to teach twelve apprentices. The school also supported the apprentices with a smaller stipend to help them through the long program. Actual instruction went on outside the classroom, often in the healers' homes, just as it had traditionally. The IHS agreed to take part in the program by dispatching physicians every other Monday for discussion sessions with the healers and apprentices. At those meetings, healers and physicians shared information about their practices and agreed to formalize procedures for referrals. Physicians gave lectures on these occasions during which they explained the use of X rays and other medical technology and answered questions from the healers and apprentices, and the Diné participants responded positively to what the physicians told them.[33]

Although the program had institutional roots, the Rough Rock staff emphasized the need for training to follow the traditional pattern. Apprentices were not rushed through the learning process but were allowed to go at a pace they and their teachers set. This meant that the first group did not finish until after 1970, but it ensured that the new singers were fully prepared to carry on the ceremonies. The healers taught their apprentices the complex chants and prayers, a process non-Navajo observers compared to learning how to recite a Wagnerian opera or the New Testament from memory. Apprentices also learned the use of herbs, sand paintings, and other ceremonial items.[34]

Just as the tribe organized official bodies to supervise the development of Western medicine in the Navajo Nation, many traditional healers believed that modern times required modern methods to promote Navajo healing. In 1978, about fifty traditional healers came together in a group called the Medicine Men's Association (MMA), which committed itself to "develop new health care systems which combine the healing arts and skills of trained Navajo healers and medicine men in conjunction with practitioners of western medical science, and thereby improve the health and well-being of the Navajo people." Referred to as the Navajo healers' equivalent of the American Medical Association, the MMA sought to encourage and regulate traditional healing. It considered establishing certification standards for healers to combat the contamination of the ceremonies by alcohol and improper contact. The MMA also hoped that certification procedures would persuade private companies on and near the reservation to include traditional ceremonies as part of their employee health benefits. The organization's activities included working with the IHS to help design new hospitals, successfully prompting the tribal government to pass a resolution protecting ceremonial objects, and offering healing services to prison inmates in New Mexico.[35]

Some Navajo healers disapproved of the MMA, showing that while many or most Diné believed that the traditional ways had to be preserved, they did not agree on how to do so. Opposing traditional healers argued that the MMA's structure and methods, such as the use of certifications and bylaws, were based on non-Navajo organizational models. Opponents also feared that the organization would reduce healers' individual freedom, and that its proposal to certify singers was "ridiculous" and might be a means to prevent non-MMA singers from practicing. The MMA persevered despite its critics, but many Navajo healers remained outside the group.[36]

The tribal government and MMA took even more direct action to preserve traditional healing during the 1990s. Together, they began in 1997 to plan for a tribe-sponsored apprentice healer program to replace the Navajo Mental Health Program, which had ceased to operate in the early 1980s. The apprentice program planned to train two groups of healers during a given year, paying a $400-per-month stipend to students and $500 to teachers. The Navajo Medicine Man Apprenticeship Program, as it was designated, began recruiting students in 1999.[37]

Through such efforts, it seemed that the Navajo Nation would retain the benefits of traditional healing. Irvin Tso served as a testament to such optimism. In 1984, at the age of fifteen, Tso became the youngest Navajo healer. "When I saw my first ceremony, with the chanting, prayers, and sand painting, it drew me in so much that I knew immediately that this is what I wanted to be," Tso later explained. His struggle to attain that goal exemplified the obstacles young Navajos faced in balancing their desire to become healers with modern demands, and the strong discipline some of them demonstrated. "I would go to school, come back and do homework until nine P.M. or ten P.M.," said Tso. "My uncle, Norris Nez, who was teaching me, would come over and we would go over the chants and prayers until one A.M. or three A.M. Then I would go to sleep and get up at seven A.M. to get ready for school."[38]

The Navajo desire to draw from the benefits of different healing ways did not just extend to Western medicine and traditional Navajo healing. Other healing ways also became available to the Navajos as the twentieth century progressed, including the Native American Church (NAC). Probably introduced to the reservation during the 1930s, the NAC involves the use of peyote in spiritual ceremonies that can be directed toward healing. Because the NAC originated among non-Navajo American Indians, and because some Navajos saw its spiritual nature as a threat to traditional ceremonialism, its practitioners faced criticism from many Navajos in addition to non-Navajo missionaries. Although made illegal by the tribal government in 1940, the NAC continued to draw more Navajo members throughout the twentieth century, prompting the tribal government to overturn the laws and support its growth after 1960.

At century's end, the NAC stood alongside Western medicine and Navajo healing as one of the many medical options available to the Navajo Nation. Using those, and sometimes other, forms of healing in conjunction with one another, Navajos in the twentieth century were able to draw upon multiple sources of power to combat the serious medical challenges confronting them. At the same time, by promoting and protecting those multiple healing ways, the Navajo Nation demonstrated its ability to control its own destiny.

CONTESTING THE COLD WAR
MEDICAL MONOPOLY

SISTER KENNY GOES TO WASHINGTON

Polio, Populism, and Medical Politics in Postwar America

Naomi Rogers

IN MAY 1948 Sister Elizabeth Kenny went to Washington, D.C., to speak as an expert witness before the House Committee on Interstate and Foreign Commerce. Wearing a corsage and plumed hat, the white-haired Australian nurse praised a proposed National Medical Research Foundation that would study polio as well as cancer and other "degenerative" diseases. "Mobilization of forces and pooling of knowledge concerning this disease are imperative," Kenny told the committee, which was investigating whether the government should fund and direct medical research. Although Kenny admitted she had been advised "not to interfere in any way with American politics," she nonetheless was certain that "the Federal government, by appropriation, should support both . . . clinical and scientific research" and "should undertake to see that every avenue is explored to wipe out this disease."[1]

Why was Kenny, a lowly foreign nurse, invited to debate postwar science policy? And why was she taken so seriously? True, she was a prominent figure in 1940s America, featured in newsreels and magazines. Her unorthodox polio therapy enabled crippled children to walk again and promised hope for a disease that was the focus of intense public interest and fear. The hope was enhanced by the ambiguity of her title, "Sister," a British Commonwealth term for head nurse, but with religious connotations for many Americans. Parents, doctors, nurses, and physical therapists flocked to her research and teaching institute in Minneapolis and watched her dismiss the standard use of braces and splinting, treat paralysis with muscle therapy and heated blanket strips ("hot packs"), and explain her new concept of polio as a skin and muscle disease.

It was as a healer and medical celebrity that Kenny was welcomed to Congress in 1948. But, I will argue, it was most of all as a medical populist who transformed the Washington hearings into a platform to attack organized medicine, especially the policies of the nation's largest polio philanthropy, the National Foundation for Infantile Paralysis. The National Foundation, Kenny complained, used its power as a polio monopoly to deny her scientific respect. Indeed, officials were organizing an international conference on polio to be held in July, but Kenny had heard that "my appearance at this meeting would mean that they would have to close the door in my face."[2] A new government agency directed by her supporters, she was sure, could challenge the National Foundation's power and ensure the

United States, in an era of global tensions, an international reputation for providing American children with the best care and most modern knowledge of the disease.

The National Foundation for Infantile Paralysis was without a doubt America's polio establishment. One of the country's most powerful disease philanthropies, but without an endowment like the Carnegie and Rockefeller Foundations, the National Foundation relied on public funds raised through its sophisticated March of Dimes campaigns. It used this money to help the families of polio victims pay for hospital care and rehabilitation, as well as to train health professionals and to support scientists at universities around the country as they pursued laboratory and clinical research. To avoid contentious professional debates over diverse medical practices, the National Foundation had developed careful policies: it agreed to pay for any treatment recommended by a physician, and in order to cope with the many inventors of polio "cures," it funded only researchers recommended by its scientific committees, which were staffed by the nation's clinical and scientific elite.

From its founding in 1938 the National Foundation had been directed by Wall Street lawyer Basil O'Connor, President Franklin Roosevelt's former law partner. A highly centralized organization, the National Foundation's local chapters were led by prominent businessmen and society women and coordinated by a national office in New York City. Although Roosevelt's death in April 1945 left the National Foundation without a political patron in the White House, O'Connor, a Democrat whose brother was a former New York congressman, had strong ties to America's social and scientific elite, especially the conservative leadership of the American Medical Association (AMA) through his friendship with Morris Fishbein. Fishbein, the AMA's powerful secretary and editor of the *Journal of the American Medical Association (JAMA)*, was a fervent public critic of socialized and alternative medicine and disliked any government incursion into medicine, whether for research or patient care; his ideology underlay the politics of the National Foundation as well.[3]

Kenny's appearance before the House committee reflected a wider public suspicion of the National Foundation as an elitist medical monopoly, "a sort of medical closed shop, run for the benefit of certain doctors and certain politicians, perhaps more than for the benefit of the patients," as Marion Bennett, a Republican congressman from Missouri, explained during the 1948 hearings.[4] Its ties to the AMA further consolidated the public view that it was just part of the medical establishment whose leaders had defeated national and state health insurance programs and attacked any critics of mainstream medicine as quacks exploiting the lay public. Against opponents such as Kenny the National Foundation had to defend its control of polio research funding in terms of democratic, responsive health care management and to convince Congress and the public that corporate philanthropy should retain a respected place in the unsettled world of health policy.[5]

Telling the story of the battle between Elizabeth Kenny and the National Foundation allows us a new, rather unexpected look at the ways medical populism shaped postwar science policy. Populism in medicine is difficult to analyze and even harder to categorize. Since the 1970s historians have tended to link medical populists with consumer advocates, environmentalists, and health care reformers, as well as to proponents of alternative medical therapies. My study seeks to trace a particular type of medical populism, as represented by Sister Kenny and her allies in the late 1940s: challenging orthodox medicine's claim to authority, yet demanding access to medical science so that the people's health could be protected through scientific research. We need to understand these opponents of established medicine on their own terms. Yet a focus on such critics of medical orthodoxy has the added benefit of complicating the accepted picture of postwar America as the era of organized medicine's Golden Age, when public respect for white coats and medical science was unrivaled and doctors on film, radio, and television were always the good guys.[6]

The stream of populism that Elizabeth Kenny drew on was composed of elements from both the left and the right. These dissidents were against the medical establishment but for government regulation, feared elitism and corporate conspiracy but idealized the tools and products of science. The people's health was threatened, according to Kenny and her supporters, by narrow-minded medical professionals unwilling to consider ideas promoted by anyone outside mainstream medical institutions. Yet truth could be gained not only by the work of orthodox scientists, but when scientific tools—laboratory and clinical research—became resources available to all. Indeed, Kenny's defense of science was the most distinctive and modern-sounding aspect of her version of medical populism.

The struggles between Kenny and the National Foundation played out publicly at the 1948 hearings were not just over whether and how the government should fund polio research. They were part of a wider battle over the direction and authority of research policy, over whether Congress should mandate lay representatives on the boards of its new research agencies who could provide alternative views to the scientific and medical establishments. In this essay, I will first examine interactions between science politics and medical populism in Washington, then Elizabeth Kenny's distinctive style of populist expertise and her challenge to polio orthodoxy, and finally the fight between Kenny and the National Foundation inside and outside Congress, with its implications for the shaping of American medical research. My story ends in 1949 with the deposing of two of the main players: Kenny herself and AMA secretary Morris Fishbein.

Listening to Elizabeth Kenny in Washington blasting medical elitism and parochial, inaccurate science helps to amplify the debate—largely neglected by historians of medicine and science—among politicians, philanthropic officials, the public, and even a few scientists in postwar America over the relationship between research and democracy. In the process, Kenny becomes only one of many voices challenging a scientific elite for cultural authority.

RESEARCH, POPULISM, AND THE GOLDEN AGE OF AMERICAN MEDICINE

From the followers of botanical reformer Samuel Thomson in the 1820s who merged Jacksonian democracy with attacks on medical elitism to the anti-vivisectionists in the 1910s who targeted the scientific enterprise as endangering both humans and animals, medical populism throughout American history has meant different things at different times. Populists with diverse views have consistently attacked professional monopoly and its claims to special knowledge and truth, but they have been least unified over two crucial issues: the proper role of government and the explanatory power of science. Nineteenth-century homeopaths lobbied for state licensing laws that would recognize their professional standing against those of osteopaths, chiropractors, and Christian Scientists; anti-vaccinationists feared government health officials would deny citizens civil liberties and infect the public with poison in the name of disease prevention. The authority of science, similarly, was sometimes embraced, sometimes resisted. In the early twentieth century homeopaths set up laboratories and proudly claimed bacteriological research as homeopathic; anti-vaccinationists saw all researchers as "experimenters" and turned to the emotive evidence of photographs and testimonials to demonstrate the harmful effects of vaccines.[7] Lumping together all such critics as quacks and cultists, organized medicine fought them through its growing influence in state legislatures, the courts, and the media.[8]

When AMA officials spoke of medical freedom in the 1940s, they meant freedom from government oversight. But during the 1930s talk of medical freedom had been most often employed by alternative medicine promoters and entrepreneurs as they battled the AMA and the Food and Drug Administration. Discoverers of anti-cancer tonics and rejuvenating operations, naturopaths, chiropractors and others on the margins of the medical profession developed an ideology of political populism that drew on the public sympathy for outsiders fighting elitism. At times these struggles entered the political arena. John R. Brinkley, a Kansas "goat gland" doctor with his own radio station, ran as a populist independent for governor in 1930 and 1932, calling for free school textbooks, children's health clubs, pensions for the elderly and blind, and government clinics for the poor. Michigan inventor William F. Koch and his evangelical supporters turned to the vocabulary of orthodox science when they set up their Christian Medical Research League to study Koch's cancer elixir. These men attracted political support from right-wing populist groups including the American Fascist Party as part of a broader program suspicious of the secrecy and power of the AMA and its suppression of the "people's" medicine.[9]

This strand of medical populism suffused the postwar debate over science research policy. Elizabeth Kenny was a newcomer to American politics, but her claim that as an outsider she deserved scientific respectability and needed to be defended against Big Medicine and Big Science (as represented by the AMA and the National Foundation), which dismissed her as a "quack," had deep political resonance.

The achievements of the Manhattan Project had led the public to believe that disease, like war, could be fought and won through collaborative, government-led agencies, despite a lingering faith in of the Thomas Edison–type lone inventor. The prospect of massive government investment into research on disease, beyond the individualistic efforts of the private Rockefeller Institute and Mayo Clinic, grabbed the public imagination. But there was no consensus on how the government should ensure a fair distribution of national resources to enable the public access to preventive public health work, medical care, and medical technology. Indeed, until the expansion of the National Institutes of Health in the 1950s and 1960s, most medical research remained diffuse and unregulated, reflecting parochial interests. Researchers relied on funds donated by myriad private organizations, large and small, often known as "foundations," frequently single-disease charities that funded patient care and only a little relevant research.[10] After the war this patchwork system of research funding seemed old-fashioned and inefficient, but what model should replace it was less clear.

Although American scientists argued that research funding should be based on a "best science" model, politicians in postwar America recognized a competing popular appeal for a "geographic" model, a kind of science democracy where government research money was distributed state by state, available not just for elite health providers and academic physicians but for "ordinary" investigators. In what one historian has called the "highly pluralist postwar system of medical research" Congress divided over whether the development of such research should be left in the hands of universities, private research institutes, and philanthropies or be made part of the highly volatile debate on the government's role in directing the organization of health care.[11] This nascent research populism fit well with the growing anti-Communist, anti-intellectual right-wing populist movement that feared the liberal, eastern establishment and its decadent bureaucracy. Not only elite scientists resisted any kind of states rights science policy but so did leaders of organized medicine, such as Morris Fishbein, representing an older right-wing conservatism, where every government intervention was a step on the path toward Communist dictatorship. Indeed, until the mid-1960s the AMA also opposed Social Security coverage for physicians, expansion of the Veterans Administration, federal loans for medical students, and, most vehemently, government health insurance.[12]

So the question of whether or not populist-defined democratic principles could apply to scientific research necessarily invited a contentious battle. An early attempt to forge such scientific populism came in 1945 when Harry Hoxsey, who had set up his own National Cancer Research Institute in Taylorsville, Illinois, traveled to Washington, D.C. Accompanied by three congressmen, Hoxsey went to the National Cancer Institute to ask for federal investigation of his anti-cancer powder. William Langer, a maverick New Deal–Republican Senator from North Dakota, defended him in Congress.[13] Langer, who mistrusted big government, Communists, and Jews, also extended his distinctive Plains populism to embrace Sister Kenny. The federal government, Langer proposed, should establish a national polio clinic, and to ensure democratic control, its board would be made up not of physicians but of "persons who have had infantile paralysis and have been treated for such disease in accordance with the methods discovered and practiced by Sister Elizabeth Kenny."[14]

It was to gain government-sponsored research resources, not a health clinic, that Elizabeth Kenny had come to Washington in the midst of a raucous debate over the National Science Foundation (NSF). In August 1947 President Truman had vetoed a NSF bill giving outside scientists significant control, explaining that it would "vest the determination of vital national policies . . . in a group of individuals who would essentially be private citizens . . . [and] would be divorced from control by the people to an extent that implies a distinct lack of faith in the democratic process."[15] Immersed in postwar politics, the NSF became a powerful symbol of the changing relationship between government and the research community. Scientists feared rigid government bureaucrats; federal officials distrusted ivory-tower researchers; politicians wanted research that would lead to innovative technologies as dramatic as penicillin and the atomic bomb; and the public sought fair, democratic, and representative science research policy. Historians have traced these dynamics in the struggle to control domestic atomic energy, but they were also a crucial element in shaping federally funded scientific and medical research. Privately Truman told science advisor Vannevar Bush that a science foundation run by a board of scientists outside government would become "simply a log-rolling affair to make grants to things that its members were interested in."[16] As the NSF bill was reintroduced in 1948, a provocative study in *Science* reinforced Truman's doubt that scientists could be relied on to put the public's interest ahead of loyalty to their own institution or subdiscipline. The study, quoted during the NSF congressional hearings, found that almost three-quarters of the research funds distributed by the scientific advisory boards of ten private philanthropies—including the National Foundation—went to researchers at elite northeastern universities.[17]

The defeat of the NSF bill in June 1948, only weeks after Kenny's appearance in Washington, was no coincidence. The bill floundered again over the issue of governance but also over the highly charged inclusion of medical research commissions, including the special commission on polio.[18] Debated while Republicans still controlled Congress and Truman was beginning his presidential election campaign, the 1948 NSF bill passed the Senate but was held up in the House Rules Committee long enough to miss being put on the House calendar, so it could not be voted on before Congress adjourned that session.[19] Behind the scenes the National Foundation made sure that any version of the NSF bill that included polio research would fail, assuring Congress that such a provision was part of a " 'Communistic,' un-American . . . scheme."[20] Thus it was the National Foundation's struggle to control polio research that helped to kill NSF legislation in 1948. It was not until May 1950, after the Democrats regained control of Congress, that Truman finally signed a watered-down version of the NSF bill, with a director appointed by the president but sharing power with a part-time private board made up of academic and industrial scientists. And there was no polio commission.[21] By this time government-funded medical research was clearly shifting to the NIH empire, and Surgeon General Leonard Scheele was calling for bids for a new building at Bethesda to house research facilities for the recently approved National Institute of Mental Health, National Heart Institute, and National Institute of Dental Research.[22] In the legislative battle between Kenny and the National Foundation, Kenny was unable to muster support for a government research agency that targeted polio, much less for her distinctive theory of the disease, and the National Foundation was able to make sure no National Polio Institute was ever established. But the 1948 hearings did help legitimate the mixing of populism into the politics of science research.

KENNY: POPULIST EXPERT

Elizabeth Kenny's path from unknown nurse in the Australian bush to medical celebrity had become a familiar tale by the late 1940s, retold in family magazines, her autobiography, and a 1946 Hollywood movie starring Rosalind Russell.[23] Born in rural Australia in 1880, the daughter of an Irish Catholic immigrant farmer, Kenny had developed her polio treatment while working as a nurse in the isolated bush. Following the ambiguous advice of a local physician in 1911 to "treat the symptoms" of a patient with polio, Kenny found she could heal paralyzed arms and legs by wrapping them in heated blankets (later known as hot packs) and using muscle therapy as early as possible. These methods, she came to realize, challenged the usual polio care of long-term immobilization through splints and braces. Despite resistance from physicians, she was able to set up government-funded clinics in the mid-1930s with the support of patients' families, a few local health officials, and politicians from the Australian Labour Party.[24]

Kenny's autobiography, published by an American press in 1943, presented herself as a female medical populist, challenging stereotypical gender roles and embracing the rough-and-tumble world. Rejecting Victorian delicacy, the young Kenny rode horses and "loved the wind and the rain, the sunshine and the earth-rocking thunderstorms." Confident, canny, and with a sense of compassion, she tried to help local hungry children by trading their fathers' crops, work that made her unpopular in the local farming towns, for "I had stooped to do a thing no woman would think of doing. I was not refined, I was not *nice*." Feeling "strangely apart and alone," Kenny imagined herself as a missionary in India, and she initially trained as a nurse with that in mind.[25] This yen for danger and for self-sacrifice never left her. As a nurse on Australia army troop ships treating injured and paralyzed soldiers during the Great War, she claimed, "I spent more time on dark ships in danger zones than any other woman in the world." After Brisbane's medical elite greeted her polio method with "looks of obvious disgust" and "jeering laughter" her supporters urged her to leave Australia and go to the United States. She agreed reluctantly, for she was "comfortably settled in my own establishment," but concluded that "whatever that Power is that guides our destinies, it had a different plan for me, and I felt obliged to follow it."[26] The appeal of the United States for a woman with an unorthodox medical method was, she made clear, its openness and lack of hierarchy. "The American doctor, in my opinion," she told her American readers, "possesses a combination of conservatism and that other quality which has put the United States in the forefront in almost every department of science—that is, an eagerness to know what it is really all about."[27]

Despite her claims to naiveté and egalitarianism, Kenny demonstrated from the outset her keen understanding of the nation's medical politics. Armed with letters of introduction from Australian politicians and health officials, Kenny went first to the New York City headquarters of the National Foundation and then to the AMA's headquarters in Chicago. Basil O'Connor politely explained the National Foundation's policy of offering grants only to individuals at institutions approved by the medical advisory board, while Morris Fishbein and a Chicago orthopedist rebuffed her as yet another quack with a polio cure. Kenny's third stop was the Mayo Clinic, where orthopedist Melvin Henderson tactfully pointed out that Minneapolis had far more polio cases than Rochester and sent her there.[28] Minneapolis became her base for the next nine years, and she skillfully gained local political, financial, and medical allies, including the city's mayors (Republican Marvin Kline and his successor, Democrat Hubert Humphrey), as well as a number of physicians at the University of Minnesota's Medical School.[29] John Pohl, an orthopedic surgeon who directed the Infantile Paralysis Clinic at the city hospital, and his colleagues Miland Knapp and Wallace Cole published glowing accounts of the "Kenny method" in *JAMA*, followed by cautious but positive editorials from Morris Fishbein himself.[30] In 1941 Pohl invited Kenny to offer a training course for doctors and nurses at the medical school, receiving funding from the National Foundation. And when Pohl and Kenny collaborated in 1943 on a textbook, *The Kenny Concept of Infantile Paralysis and How to Treat It*, Basil O'Connor agreed to write the preface, where he commented that although "in medicine it is not well to believe the eye alone," nonetheless "those who work in the laboratories with problems in histopathology, anatomy, and physiology claim that the major concept is reasonable and rational."[31]

Such limited achievements within a single medical institution were not sufficient for Kenny. In December 1942 she left the medical school, set up her own institute, and, after the National Foundation refused to fund her institute as a research site, established her own fund-raising Kenny Foundation to compete with the National Foundation. By 1945 most polio courses around the country, whether sponsored by the Kenny Foundation or the National Foundation, taught health providers how to administer hot packs, relieve spasm, and reeducate muscles. A few states had freestanding Kenny clinics, and many—perhaps most—hospitals treating polio patients across the country used some version of the Kenny method. As Kenny traveled around the country from epidemic to epidemic, she began denigrating the orthodox polio establishment and identifying her work as its antithesis and the only safe and effective means of treating polio paralysis. She demanded that hospitals hire therapists professionally trained—at her institute—to apply her method. Neglecting therapy, she recognized, meant neglecting the human clinical picture, patients' pain and despair. As the confident title of her 1943 autobiography *And They Shall Walk* promised, Kenny's method would do what other therapies had not: heal those polio had crippled.

But Kenny did more than point out the need for improved therapy. She created and articulated the notion of a polio orthodoxy as a way of showing her work to be a revolutionary path out of medical deadends. Standard polio therapies—splinting and surgery—became symbols of a old and harmful clinical program compared to her modern healing method and polio theory. In her film "The Kenny Concept of Infantile Paralysis," which she showed the congressional committee, the narrator praised the "newer science" based on the "advanced concept."[32] In posters and pamphlets produced by the Kenny Foundation young children walked into the arms of their delighted mothers. The National Foundation's posters, by comparison, had children in wheelchairs, often in braces, awkwardly getting to their feet.[33]

Widespread dissatisfaction with prevailing polio methods made Kenny's attack on orthodox therapy all the more convincing. Standard polio care could be isolating and depressing for child and family. After being kept for weeks in the infectious disease ward of their local hospital, children deemed noncontagious would be, depending on the extent of their paralysis and their family's resources, sent back to their families or to a crippled children's home, where they were frequently immobilized in splints, sometimes in a double-brace frame, for many months. This therapy was designed to keep muscles in their "correct" positions, but it often left growing children with deformities that no amount of surgery could heal.[34] In 1942 one science reporter suggested that "even many leading orthopedic surgeons are dissatisfied with the prevailing methods and have felt it was time to break away."[35]

Physical therapy for polio patients was applied intermittently, backed by little institutional or professional support. Few hospitals or crippled children's homes in the 1930s and 1940s employed more than a few physical therapists, and rehabilitation was largely considered women's work, often done by mothers at home. The AMA had its Council on Physical Medicine, and most medical schools had a single chair in the field, but physical or rehabilitation medicine did not gain a national professional standing until Howard Rusk's work with disabled World War II veterans in the 1950s.[36] As a result, before Kenny politicized polio therapy, there were few serious studies of polio aftercare, and its development was left to individual doctors, nurses, and physical therapists. Further, most scientific research centered around investigating characteristics of the polio virus grown in laboratory animals in hopes of developing a vaccine.

Many doctors, especially specialists in pediatrics and physical medicine, were impressed when they saw patients overcoming what they had thought were unyielding deformities; nurses and physical therapists also appreciated the significant easing of patients' pain through the use of hot packs. Awed by Kenny's charismatic fervor when they met her in person, a few even said she had "healing hands."[37] Her confident challenge to medical orthodoxy attracted a few labor unions, such as the Niagara Falls local of the CIO's United Chemical Workers, and progressive medical groups, including University of Illinois medical students who were members of the Association of Internes and Medical Students.[38] But other health professionals were alienated by Kenny's arrogant self-confidence, her abrasive teaching style, and her clear disdain for those who, as she characterized them in her 1943 autobiography, "eyes have they but they see not."[39]

Even more provocative was Kenny's claim that her theory undermined the standard understanding of the way the polio virus traveled through the body. The "classical picture . . . as taught in medical schools," she explained, was polio as "a virus disease attacking the central nervous system and damaging or destroying the motor neurons . . . deformities were caused through muscle imbalance or strong normal muscles pulling against the flaccid or paralyzed ones."[40] According to Kenny, muscles were not paralyzed but in "spasm," alienated from their corresponding nerves, and could regain normal motion (be "reeducated") through the use of hot packs and careful muscle therapies. Doctors were unable to heal because they did not understand the "true symptoms" of polio and therefore treated the "wrong" disease. This point was highlighted in a scene in the 1946 *Sister Kenny* film where Kenny's orthopedic opponent tells her that "these are not scientific terms."[41]

The orthodox polio theory Kenny castigated was a fair representation. Most virologists in the 1930s and 1940s, such as Simon Flexner at New York's Rockefeller Institute for Medical Research, considered polio a disease of the nervous system and argued that the polio virus grew primarily in neurological tissue.[42] The National Foundation popularized this concept in its pamphlets, training programs, and health education work. An exhibit on polio sponsored by the National Foundation at Chicago's Museum of Science and Industry in the summer of 1948, for example, showed "a life-sized transparent man with a simplified nervous structure, showing the muscles affected when poliomyelitis attacks certain areas in the brain and spinal cord."[43]

Although the medical establishment never accepted Kenny as a scientific theorist, she was effective in stigmatizing immobilization and splinting, and even her critics acknowledged that she had transformed stagnating polio therapeutics.[44] More rarely acknowledged (outside Kenny's own camp) was her influence on orthodox polio theory. This was already a field in turmoil, as Yale virologist Dorothy Horstmann admitted in 1948: "In spite of all the information collected by many investigators in many lands, we still cannot say why poliomyelitis suddenly became epidemic almost sixty years ago, why it is increasing rather than decreasing like other infectious diseases, why it is a summer disease with a preference for certain lands, how it is spread or how it may be prevented."[45] Simon Flexner, the earlier view's most fervent proponent, died in 1948, and a new generation of virologists began to consistently find the virus in blood and in non-neurological tissue, thus increasingly undermining the picture of polio as primarily a disease of the nervous system. In 1949 John Enders' team at the Boston Children's Hospital published their innovative demonstration of the way the polio virus (and therefore a vaccine) could be grown in safe, non-neurological tissue and won the Boston group a Nobel prize in 1954, just as Jonas Salk's polio vaccine was being tested in trials organized and funded by the National Foundation.[46]

Until 1949, however, talk of a safe vaccine was only talk. Aware of the intellectual turmoil faced by polio researchers, Kenny referred to little of this work explicitly, although she did tell Congress at the hearings that there would be no vaccine possible until the scientific community accepted her concept of the disease.[47]

Throughout her life Kenny tried to balance her role as a medical celebrity (having cocktails with Rosalind Russell and her Hollywood friends), as the people's healer (attacking medical trusts and elitists, rescuing patients from disability and from orthopedic surgery), and as a scientific innovator and medical administrator directing a research and teaching institute. These somewhat contradictory elements of her public persona had come to serve her well. In a 1945 Gallup poll 52 percent of Americans had "heard or read about" Kenny and the Kenny method. And in a 1947 poll of the ten most admired living people in the world, the only women ranked were Eleanor Roosevelt (sixth) and Sister Kenny (ninth).[48]

Being a populist expert, though, was tricky. Elizabeth Kenny yearned to be welcomed as a scientific discoverer, invited to speak at conferences, have her work quoted in medical journals, and see her concept become the basis for scientific investigation. But she directed an institute named after herself and promoted a method and theory, both with her name; it all sounded uncomfortably like a patent medicine hawker. Her use of publicity—her technical films, her interviews in local newspapers and national magazines such as *Reader's Digest* and the *Saturday Evening Post*—was as extensive as the National Foundation's but lacked the patina of the latter's elite medical contacts.[49] When Kenny came to Washington in 1948 her audience was already familiar with her story. But by this time Kenny was struggling not just for legitimacy (on her own terms) but also for her legacy. Even as medical texts and public health bulletins on polio came to reject splinting in favor of hot packs and muscle training, they often left out Kenny herself, and physicians were mixing elements of her method with their own therapies. While traveling around the country during the previous summer's polio epidemics, Hart Van Riper, the National Foundation's medical director, remarked at the 1948 hearings that he had seen "orthodox" care supplanted everywhere by Kenny's method, but, he added, "in many places this kind of treatment was not *called* 'the Kenny treatment,' since in minor ways it was modified by the physicians ordering it."[50]

Not only was the Kenny method no longer new, but its promise to heal, its stark comparison to harmful previous therapies, had only briefly captured public attention. A healing nurse could not trump the popular fascination with the scientist in white, the drama of the laboratory, and the magical products possible from research. By the late 1940s National Foundation posters featured not only a walking child but also a scientist holding a test tube.[51] Thus the prominent University of Cincinnati virologist Albert Sabin told the local medical society of Akron, Ohio, in June 1948 that "the Kenny treatment is a waste of energy, effort and money. It fills the hospitals with extra nurses and creates an unnecessary bedlam there." The money, said Sabin, "could be better used for rehabilitation of the few crippled by the disease, and for further research." Its widespread use was "part of a wave of hysteria," he concluded, and "what is good about the Kenny treatment is not new. What is new about it is not good."[52] Crippled children and hot packs were not as exciting or modern-sounding as the promise of a polio vaccine, and the Australian nurse's claim to theoretical discovery came to be easily dismissed.

RESEARCH, PUBLIC RELATIONS, AND THE NATIONAL FOUNDATION

For some time, National Foundation officials had recognized that the public support for science populism threatened their organization. They were therefore delighted to use the 1948 hearings to contest the claim that Elizabeth Kenny's disparagement proved a undemocratic use of public funds. Nor was this the first time the National Foundation had felt the need to defend itself this way. "An organization built upon the most democratic principles," the National Foundation was not just "a few men in a New York office, nor a group of scientists and medical leaders constituting the Medical Advisory Committees," a 1942 publicity pamphlet had firmly asserted. "It is a force of the people themselves, expressed in work and money."[53] While Kenny's characterization of the National Foundation at the 1948 hearings as part of organized medicine was clearly an effective rhetorical strategy, it was also not a great exaggeration. Over the previous decade the National Foundation had come to play a significant if somewhat hidden role in shaping American medical politics. Led since its founding by Basil O'Connor, it had moved away from its early Democratic affiliations and closer to the Republican Party, the political affiliation of most American physicians in the 1940s and 1950s.[54] Like many leading medical administrators, O'Connor, a wealthy Wall Street lawyer, believed in free-market medicine, and he placed the National Foundation firmly behind his faith.

Scientific research and health care were crucial parts of national politics between 1945 and 1950. Not surprisingly, many witnesses at congressional hearings framed the debates on research policy within a broader program by liberal Truman Democrats to centralize and restructure American health care.[55] The AMA had testified fiercely against government health insurance but maintained a careful neutrality on medical research and the NSF.[56] Not so the National Foundation. The 1948 hearings gave it a chance to speak as the nation's expert on polio policy and explain the danger of too much government interference in medical and scientific affairs. Of course, the National Foundation did not want to portray itself as unreasonably antagonistic to any government research funding. Officials claimed that they did "not want to corner the market" and thoughtfully pointed to the "crying need for research" in other fields such as multiple sclerosis and cerebral palsy.[57] Besides, one official told the congressional committee frankly, the funding of polio research had been a crucial part of public fund-raising since the National Foundation's founding. The "interest and hope" of the thousands of "men and women [who] work at the grass-roots level . . . is our research program," and if the National Foundation's research program were "taken over by the Government . . . we believe our greatest appeal for public support will be removed."[58]

The fear that government research could lead to socialized medicine was most starkly laid out by former New York Democratic congressman John O'Connor, Basil's brother and a National Foundation representative. Even if the proposed NSF would be only a "government research bureau," John O'Connor argued at the hearings, "we believe, [it] is the proverbial camel getting its nose under the tent and from that time on you have the whole animal, and the whole carcass, right in the center of the ring. You have got the Government taking care of the personal diseases of our people, a completely totalitarian idea that never was intended in America."[59] In an elitist appeal to his fellow lawyers in Congress, he asked them to imagine their own families threatened by the disease. In 1947, John O'Connor's son, just after graduating from Harvard Medical School, had developed polio, and, John O'Connor added, "I appreciated then, and I submit to you gentlemen that I did not want then, and I do not want now any Government representative, whether he is a scientist or a doctor, treating me or my people under such circumstances. I want to get the best private treatment. And this proposed research by the Government is bound to develop by the Government taking over completely."[60] Philanthropic groups such as the National Foundation, executive director Joe Savage reiterated at the hearings, were large enough to pursue scientific research but also efficient and democratic. With more than twenty-seven hundred county chapters run by around thirty thousand volunteers, our polio program, he declared, was "the greatest research campaign ever carried out against a single disease by the voluntary effort of a free people."[61]

Basil O'Connor relied on his friend Morris Fishbein to promote the National Foundation's interests in his public role as editor of *JAMA* and, behind the scenes, as private censor. Fishbein, an impressive writer and editor, had long shaped the medical content of magazine articles and scripts for movies and radio shows, and the National Foundation often sent him copy to edit.[62] After Minnesota physicians Cole and Knapp's first *JAMA* article on the Kenny method appeared in 1941, for example, the editor of *American Weekly* told journalist Robert Potter to write a story on Sister Kenny. Potter wrote to the National Foundation, promising to "cooperate fully," and O'Connor sent his manuscript to Fishbein, who made sure Potter's published article changed "amazing" to "remarkable," altered "only correct way" to "preferable way," and deleted a section that quoted John Pohl calling previous polio therapy "criminal."[63] During the congressional debates in 1948, at O'Connor's prompting, Fishbein's editorials in *JAMA* declared that the NSF bill should omit "any and all special commissions for specific diseases."[64]

By the late 1940s, however, both Fishbein's influence in the AMA and his wider popularity were waning. His caustic rejection of any kind of prepaid group practice (even organized by physicians themselves) had alienated patients as well as many doctors trying to give the public alternatives to the attractive health insurance proposals being offered in Congress and by governors such as California's Earl Warren.[65] During the war the AMA, represented by Fishbein and a local medical society in Washington, D.C., had suffered a public humiliation when it lost an antitrust suit before the Supreme Court brought by the Justice Department. The AMA's embrace of right-wing groups such as the National Physicians Committee drew it closer to the Republican Party. When the AMA initiated a fierce campaign against Truman's health insurance plan and any Democrats who might support it, Truman's Justice Department in 1947 began another antitrust investigation of the AMA.[66]

Throughout the congressional debates of the 1940s liberal reformers castigated Fishbein's AMA policies and proposed instead an expansive role for government in health care and scientific research. Not only did liberal and left-wing physicians groups such as the Physicians' Committee for the Improvement of Medical Care (founded in 1937) and the Physicians Forum (founded in 1941) voice these populist arguments, but so did other progressive organizations such as the Progressive Citizens of America and the American Veterans Committee, whose spokesmen assailed *JAMA* as a journal that "damns other points of view without presenting them," creating a "shockingly prejudiced" medical profession, and warned that government health agencies should be "placed in the hands of administrators responsible to the public, and not in the control of a private doctors' association."[67] Although the intense anti-Communism of the Cold War helped to isolate and defeat these groups, such moments were, nonetheless, the beginning of the end of organized medicine's Golden Age.[68]

The state of polio science, moreover, weakened the National Foundation's claim to stand proudly as America's polio expert. Researchers funded for a decade, critics pointed out, had not found a cure; perhaps the government could do better. A Pittsburgh surgeon, outraged that *JAMA* would not publish an article on the efficacy of a controversial polio curare treatment, asked Fishbein privately: "How can the A.M.A. justify the refusal to publish this article when they and the National Foundation, despite the millions of dollars collected, have to date little or nothing to offer the profession, patients, or the public?"[69] The association between the AMA leadership and the National Foundation had worked well in the interwar years, but with such postwar critiques the benefits were unraveling.

KENNY AND CONGRESS

As a witness at hearings ostensibly about three unimportant medical research agencies but in fact to gather support for the House committee's position in favor of including special disease commissions in the proposed NSF, Elizabeth Kenny sought to benefit from the shaken reputation of the AMA. Linking the National Foundation to Morris Fishbein, she recognized these complicated medical politics and was able to tell her story of discrimination in terms that fit well with the current congressional climate. Republicans, who had gained control of both the House and Senate in 1946, found supporting Kenny—an underdog battling a medical trust—made good politics and good press. "For the better part of two hours she belabored [the] National Foundation for Infantile Paralysis, to an obbligato [*sic*] of photographers' bulb-flashes," one reporter commented, "[and spoke] to a sympathetic committee, present in numbers which have not been equalled this year at any Congressional hearing on health or medical legislation."[70] In the midst of this public scrutiny, Republican Congressman Joseph O'Hara of Minnesota described relations among Sister Kenny, the National Foundation, and "some of the doctors" as a "civil war."[71] New Jersey Republican Charles A. Wolverton, chair of the House committee, was especially sympathetic, and, reiterating many of Kenny's own arguments, pointedly questioned National Foundation officials about their refusal to fund her work.[72]

Truman had vetoed the 1947 NSF bill, claiming that it did not provide sufficient democratic representation. Framing her struggles similarly, Kenny made her work a symbol of medical populism. An especially powerful way Kenny sought to draw in her congressional audience was to demonstrate her trust in the abilities of lay observers to judge evidence put before their own eyes. At the hearings she screened one of the technical films produced at her institute that she had just shown the previous summer in Europe. Such "documentary evidence," she said in introducing the film, could only be rejected through neglect, ignorance, or prejudice.[73]

Kenny made her exclusion from the upcoming International Conference a central issue during the hearings, arguing that Congress had the power to force the National Foundation to invite her as a scientific participant.[74] She confidently phrased her claims in terms of the new global health politics of the late 1940s. In Geneva that summer the first assembly of the World Health Organization would meet, and then in September the second international meeting of the World Medical Association. In 1947 Kenny had traveled through both Western and Eastern Europe, and she made much of her familiarity with these countries, the international character of the upcoming conference, and the global significance of her work. She had, she explained, already discussed with Columbia University professor Claus Jungeblut the possibility of setting up an International Science Council and a parallel conference, and "several outstanding scientists have already expressed their willingness to take part in such a procedure."[75]

Her participation in the National Foundation's conference, she believed, would give "the Federal Government" an opportunity to present to "governments of all countries . . . through the medium of the Elizabeth Kenny Foundation, this link in the golden chain of friendship." Turning this argument into a threat, she warned that friends could become enemies. "Your Government can present to the peoples of the world a gift that may, in no small measure, cement the much desired friendships. However, if this gift is withheld or covered up with subterfuge and inaccurate statements, it is possible that a bitterness will enter the hearts of the people when the truth finally becomes known." And she knew whom to blame: "I consider that the National Foundation is perpetrating a grave injustice on the people of this country by assuming this attitude which, to me, is not American."[76] The Cold War implications of the politics of medical openness were persuasive. If the

International Conference could carry "governmental implication . . . to the people of this country and other countries," Massachusetts Republican John Heselton reflected, the committee should "inquire as to what further consideration has been given to the [Kenny] Institute's request, and as to whether or not . . . there has been a run-around or a pigeon holing of this very reasonable request to participate in developing all the facts."[77]

One of the most provocative moments in the case against the National Foundation's polio monopoly was the appearance of a scientist Kenny had long claimed as an ally. Claus W. Jungeblut, a German professor of bacteriology at Columbia University, had been working with the polio virus for the previous two decades. His work had not been funded by the National Foundation, he explained at the hearings, because he focused on mice rather than primates. His research, in other words, although orthodox, was out of the mainstream compared to other polio virologists favored by the National Foundation's research council.[78] Nor was he the only scientist in this position: "[T]here is a considerable number of people who have either refused to go with the regimentation of research by the National Foundation, or otherwise have been pushed out by them."[79] A government agency, he believed, would be more likely to be fair and disinterested, or at least it could be organized with "devices that make this sort of thing impossible."[80]

Jungeblut's presentation of himself as a struggling outsider recalled the image of the scientific discoverer popularized by Hollywood in *The Story of Louis Pasteur* (1936), *Dr. Ehrlich's Magic Bullet* (1940), and *Sister Kenny* (1946), as well as in science journalist Paul de Kruif's *Microbe Hunters* (1926), *Men against Death* (1932), and *The Fight for Life* (1938). In Cold War terms, the creative individualist could also be compared to the sterility of Communist group thinking, satirized the following year in George Orwell's novel *1984*.[81] The characterization by Jungeblut and Kenny of a dangerously autocratic National Foundation convinced some members of the House committee. "Too often the medical profession is too orthodox, and unwilling to recognize the individual who is traveling along a path that is different from what is recognized by orthodox medicine," Wolverton told Jungeblut sympathetically "yet . . . so many of our great inventions have come about in a most unexpected way, through the vision or the thought of some individual who was thinking differently than others thought, and it is to encourage that individual thought that the committee has in mind in the preparation of much of this legislation."[82] Minnesota Republican Joseph O'Hara went further by arguing that a lack of professional training should not necessarily undermine scientific respectability: "[O]ftentimes the layman contributes something in the way of science to something in the way of relief that too often we might be inclined to be a little jealous of or overlook it. I do think . . . we must recognize the importance of everything in the way of science, and everything that can be contributed to any one problem should be recognized."[83] Kenny did not tell the committee, however, that Jungeblut had already informed her privately that he thought a separate conference funded by the Kenny Foundation was a bad idea, fearing that few of his fellow scientists would be willing to proclaim such "open rebellion against the National Foundation." "The course I have chosen for myself—not without considerable mental anguish—is to continue my experimental work," he had admitted to her, "and hope that with further diffusion of knowledge the objective facts will eventually be accepted."[84]

Hart Van Riper, the National Foundation's most articulate defender at the hearings, believed the facts were on the establishment's side. Although he also criticized Jungeblut's science, the bulk of Van Riper's testimony was in response to Kenny. Praising her "very valuable contribution," which had led to a widely used method, Van Riper tried to deflect Kenny's attacks, arguing, "There is no controversy between Miss Kenny and the National Foundation, because the National Foundation does not prescribe treatment." (The National Foundation had for some years a policy of referring to Kenny as "Miss" rather than "Sister.")[85] Characterizing Kenny as unfit to participate in the July conference or indeed in any serious scientific meeting, Van Riper dismissed her claim to scientific innovation. Kenny's treatment, he explained, was not new; years ago, physicians in Baltimore and in Boston were "not placing patients in plaster casts" but "were using early physical therapy and some forms of heat."[86] Like Sabin, Van Riper found what was "new" about Kenny not good. Stubbornly, she refused to acknowledge her ignorance of the pathology of the disease. "Miss Kenny is not a physician," physician Van Riper explained, and "has made statements that certain things do not exist which, in the laboratory animal we can reproduce," and "unfortunately Miss Kenny feels that unless you accept her concept of the cause, you cannot accept her treatment."[87] That is, Kenny refused to separate her technical work—as healer and therapist—from her theoretical insights; she was not content to be lauded only as a nurse.

Van Riper identified the two most glaring weaknesses in Kenny's claims to scientific respectability: her reluctance to abide by the conservative etiquette of the scientific establishment—exemplified by her speaking so brashly to the press of her "contribution"—and her inability to recognize the kinds of evidence professionals regarded as authoritative. (The balance between respectable popular acclaim and unprofessional celebrity-seeking was indeed a tricky one: in the 1950s Jonas Salk was denied membership in the elite National Academy of Sciences, partly on the grounds that he had too eagerly accepted a role as polio hero.)[88] Although Kenny spoke often of her desire to obtain scientific confirmation of her theories through clinical and laboratory studies, in her statements to the press and in her formal reports she relied heavily on personal testimonials, evidence she described as "reports of unbiased medical men and the findings of science."[89] Such testimonials had been commonly used to convince the public, in Kenny's youth, of the worth of a new medical technique or a patent medicine. Throughout her career she relied on such "unbiased" statements to counter journalists' efforts to denigrate her words as untrustworthy and simply those of a nurse. Thus she wrote in frustration to a supporter in 1943, "[T]he poor presentation made to the public by the lay press would dwindle into insignificance if I made a leaflet of the signed statements of medical men of unquestionable ability and many of international repute and distributed this leaflet."[90] But such a leaflet would not impress the scientists on the International Polio Conference's organizing committee, which dismissed testimonials as "a restatement of Sister Kenny's contribution to the field of poliomyelitis" and requested instead "some concrete scientific evidence and not merely statements that are based on personal opinion."[91]

Van Riper carefully did not call Kenny a quack. He could have mocked those who claimed her as an ally: anti-vivisectionists, for example, who saw her work with patients as undermining any need for "monkey research" by National Foundation grantees. In fact the National Foundation worked closely with the recently established National Society for Medical Research, the preeminent defender of animal experimentation in research, and helped edit drafts of any scripts for its radio show, *Research Report*, that discussed polio. A 1948 puff piece in the *Saturday Evening Post* mocked anti-vivisectionists who believed that polio epidemics were due to "polluting the blood stream of little ones with some filthy vaccine or toxin" and warned that any attack on animal research "menaces the life and health of every person in this country" and put "the future of medical research . . . in the shadow of serious danger."[92] Van Riper's reluctance to attack Kenny more sharply reflected her national popularity, her shrewd use of the press, and the fact that, in the 1940s and '50s, anti-vivisectionists remained a potent political force in some states, protesting dog pound laws and other legislation in order to restrict the use of animals as potential research subjects. And although Morris Fishbein continued his own unrelenting attack on all alternative practitioners, osteopaths, especially in California, had substantial public support— as the California Medical Association recognized.[93]

Kenny often used the term *quack* in the telling of her story. "At first, I was called a quack, a charlatan, and worse, year after year, in Australia, England and the United States," she told readers of the *American Weekly* in 1944, "by men who simply refused to believe that a nurse from 'the bush' could devise a treatment which succeeded where they had failed."[94] She recognized that her work appealed to anti-vivisectionists and to other anti-orthodox critics.[95] But in public she did not acknowledge such alliances, and even in private letters she was very circumspect in her comments. At the 1948 hearings she explained that she had long ago promised the surgeon who had been her mentor in Australia "that I would keep with the duly qualified medical practitioner until he saw the light," for "I know that if I did veer out a little from the straight and narrow path, that the duly qualified medical practitioners would have nothing to do with me."[96]

After appearing before Congress Kenny received many letters from men and women seeking a clearer stand on her criticism of orthodox medicine. She instructed her staff to write form letters putting them off. In July 1948, for example, Mrs. Virgil Dicke of Goodhue, Minnesota, wrote to Kenny to ask "what stand you take on vaccination and inoculations as the medical doctors recommend . . . [for] I have heard and read so many desperate results of it." One of her daughters would soon be ready for school, and "our entire community is for it and we stand alone in our belief." "In your wonderful work of fighting polio you have proven that natural methods in its treatment have far exceeded surgery," Dicke noted, urging Kenny, "with your world-wide reputation," to "convince many that vaccination is harmful instead of beneficial."[97] Ignoring the content of the query, which was clearly about smallpox (vaccination was required by many municipalities before children could attend public school) rather than polio (which had no vaccine), Kenny's secretary replied that "it would be impossible for Sister Kenny to give any advice as to the efficacy of vaccination as she has nothing to do with [that] phase of the disease and leaves that entirely up to the medical world. . . . we regret that we cannot answer your letter more explicitly."[98] Kenny was unwilling to turn her version of medical populism into a sustained attack on orthodox medical science.

Wolverton concluded Kenny's final day of testimony with sympathetic words, reflecting the distinctive kind of research populism Kenny was promoting. At the hearings the day before, he had told Surgeon General Leonard Scheele that "I am very strongly of the opinion that all of the knowledge that is necessary in the proper functioning of research and research foundations is not reposed in doctors, with all due respect to doctors. I have the highest respect for them. But nevertheless it would seem to me that . . . much can be gained by the presence on these councils of lay members."[99] To Kenny, Wolverton expressed "our very great appreciation for your attendance here today . . . The difficulties that you have had to face demonstrate that you have a spirit which cannot be crushed," concluding, "You are doing a great service for humanity. You are entitled to the respect and the support of all who are in position to give it to you."[100] A few weeks later, wealthy lobbyist Mary Lasker was appointed the first lay member of the new National Heart Institute's advisory council, a reminder that lay representation did not mean class diversity, and "public" could easily be interpreted to mean "patron."[101]

AFTER THE HEARINGS: POLIO, POPULISM, AND THE COLD WAR

Elizabeth Kenny's supporters used her presence in Washington and her reception at the hearings to prove the obstinacy and prejudice of the medical establishment. Sister Kenny had been "prevented from presenting the results of her polio research" to Congress "because of pressure from the National Foundation for Infantile Paralysis, members of Congress and/or the medical profession," the editor of the *San Fernando Sun* incorrectly told readers in October 1948. The editor therefore sent "open letters" to his local congressman, to Basil O'Connor, and to Sister Kenny herself, arguing that "any information which might throw light on poliomyelitis should immediately be investigated by the proper authority. . . . if any group, official, unofficial, charitable, social, medical or any other sort, actively works to prevent such information from being made known or even investigated, we believe the people ought to know."[102] Congressman Harry R. Sheppard corrected the editor's story, describing the hearing as "courteous"; Joe Savage wrote a careful and defensive reply; and Kenny sent an eight-page letter defending Congress and attacking the National Foundation.[103]

The *San Fernando Sun* story was, the editor acknowledged, "prompted by the recent organization of the Citizen's Polio Research League in the San Fernando Valley."[104] This league had begun to circulate petitions asking Congress "to pass legislation and provide Federal Funds and Control for Extensive Research on Poliomyelitis," implying that only government-directed research into polio could be fair and unbiased. "The millions being spent in private research are only peanuts compared with what could be obtained by direct federal action," founder Sonja Betts told reporters.[105] The implications of this populist ideology were not lost on National Foundation officials. In a private phone conversation in December 1948, recorded and transcribed by a National Foundation secretary, Hart Van Riper told Edgar J. Huenkens, the medical director of the Kenny Institute, that he was sure this new league was "Kenny Foundation No. 2" and the result of Kenny's resentment at the shifting power relations at the Kenny Institute and her own foundation.[106]

On the defensive, the National Foundation turned the First International Poliomyelitis Conference into a public relations project. Held at New York's Waldorf-Astoria, amid banquets, films, and exhibits, the conference program was filled with Kenny's work— although her labors often went unnamed. This conference inaugurated a series of international polio meetings sponsored by the National Foundation, held every three years until 1962, with Morris Fishbein assisting with the publication of the proceedings.[107] Making polio research an international issue showed the American public as well as Congress that National Foundation policies went beyond parochial medical politics. Indeed, the word *international* was a coded Cold War term, indicating American allegiances with other "free" nations. These conferences, Yale epidemiologist John Paul later reflected, "set both the stage and the American standard for a global type of representation that had not existed before, and was especially welcome [by researchers] in the immediate post–World War II period." But, he added, they were "conducted in a lavish manner, and it was obvious that they could not have been put on without the unique financial backing of the NFIP." This "spectacle of medical science being closely allied to fund-raising and fund-spending techniques," Paul believed, caused "the raising of eyebrows" by both American and European scientists.[108]

In a pointed response to the film Kenny had shown Congress, a new medical film called *Nursing Care of Poliomyelitis* was presented publicly for the first time at the international conference. Produced by the University of Illinois's Division of Services for Crippled Children with a $12,000 grant from the National Foundation, it was four reels, sixteen minutes long, and in sound and color. Kenny's methods appeared throughout, without her name, and once again in a modified version. Thus, the first reel, "The Acute Stage," showed the use of footboards and hot packs (both Kenny Institute hallmarks); the second reel, "Treatment of Spasm," demonstrated "details of administering hot packs" but also showed how to use baths as a substitute; the third reel dealt with the respirator (although Kenny claimed that her method usually made the iron lung unnecessary); and the fourth, on the convalescent stage, showed ways of applying splints "to prevent deformity," and various muscle tests (which Kenny despised). A *JAMA* reviewer thought the film was likely to be useful in training physicians, third- and fourth-year medical students, nurses, and physical therapists, "who may not always appreciate how elaborate the procedure must be if the patient is to have the best possible care and [be] spared unnecessary suffering."[109]

Kenny's appearance at the 1948 hearings did not gain her access to the international conference as a scientific participant. But she was issued a press card by the American Newspaper Guild and attended as a reporter for the North American Newspaper Alliance. Dependent on participants on the floor to raise her questions, Kenny was largely ignored, but she was able to speak in at least three general press conferences amid the country's leading science writers and medical reporters. "During those conferences, Miss Kenny attempted to voice her pseudo-scientific facts to the press," National Foundation publicist Roland Berg reported in a note to the chair of the Los Angeles chapter, "but the press was not at all impressed and reported nothing of her claims."[110] Not long after the international conference, a local branch of the Citizens' Polio Research League met at the recently opened Kenny clinic in the Jersey City Medical Center, where Kenny complained that she had been "thwarted and frustrated while at the conference . . . [u]nable to answer questions, given no recognition, and had to sit with press representatives." Foreign delegates, she told league members, "were disappointed at the treatment given her at the conference."[111]

As Van Riper shrewdly recognized, even in her own institute Kenny was being pushed to the side and pressured to resign. Never easy to work with, she was also showing her age and the beginnings of Parkinson's disease. After returning to the institute after her trip to Europe in the summer of 1947, she "had the painful experience to learn that the documentary film which I had so much trouble with the translating of the film into six different languages, had been cast aside, there wasn't even a single copy in evidence for teaching purposes."[112] In 1949 Kenny did formally retire and was replaced by pediatrician Edgar Huenkens, who had headed Minneapolis's Emergency Polio Committee in 1947. Her populist legacy and its political saliency lingered, however. "Your inestimable work will always be revered in the hearts and minds of the American people," Indiana Democratic congressman Thurman C. Crook, in typical fashion, wrote to her, "and crippled children will rise to walk again and speak reverently of your love and good deeds done for them. Despite the efforts of the Medical Profession to discredit your invaluable discovery, I, for one, highly appreciate what you have done for suffering humanity."[113]

That same year Morris Fishbein was attacked on the floor of the AMA's House of Delegates by California delegates resentful at his unrelenting opposition to affiliation with osteopaths and to group practice. His relationship with the National Physicians Committee, a right-wing medical lobby that had allied itself openly with pro-Nazi extremists, left him even more vulnerable, and he was deposed as general secretary and *JAMA* editor.[114] Basil O'Connor, Fishbein later recalled, "was apparently fuming with anger" when he learned of the coup.[115] It was the end of an era for America's organized profession.

After their dethroning, both Elizabeth Kenny and Morris Fishbein became lobbyists, writers, and consultants. Kenny continued to travel between Australia, where she had retired, Europe, and North America in the final three years of her life. In 1950 she was a guest on the television show *Meet the Press,* as a kind of polio expert emeritus, and that year Congress passed special legislation allowing her "unrestricted entry," a lifetime visa-free passage across U.S. borders.[116] After Kenny's death, in 1952, the Kenny Institute remained a leader in what was now termed rehabilitation medicine, and Marvin Kline named her "The Most Unforgettable Character I've Ever Met" in *Reader's Digest.*[117] But by the early 1960s, as the fear of polio receded with the use of the Salk and Sabin vaccines and the National Foundation reoriented itself to birth defects, Kenny herself, just as she had feared, faded from medical and popular memory.

CONCLUSION

Elizabeth Kenny did not go to Washington as a maverick nurse with a crazy idea. She was invited to speak as a polio expert, a scientific discoverer, and the director of an internationally recognized polio institute. With practiced poise and fluency, Kenny described the anger she felt, on behalf of the American people, at the ways organized medicine had neglected and—at the same time—appropriated her work.

Why was Kenny taken so seriously? Certainly her claim to scientific discovery did not sway the organizers of the First International Poliomyelitis Conference. But it certainly enhanced her celebrity status. "In all my experience on this committee," chairman Charles Wolverton told Kenny on her second day at the hearings, "you have had more photographers interested in taking your picture than any witness we have ever had before the committee." "I am afraid I do not make a very pretty one," Kenny replied with unconvincing modesty.[118] A few months after the international conference, Gallup pollsters asked the American public: "What woman, living today in our part of the world, that you have heard or read about do you admire most?" The top three women listed were first Eleanor Roosevelt, then Madame Chiang Kai-shek, and third Sister Kenny.[119]

Kenny's reputation, Morris Fishbein concluded, was the result of the public's fear of polio and journalists' love of romanticizing the lay discoverer. Some years after Kenny's death, he felt it necessary to spend many pages in his *Autobiography* refighting Elizabeth Kenny. "Like many another historical figure in the history of medicine, and indeed the history of the world, Sister Kenny did the right thing for the wrong reasons," Fishbein wrote. "She knew nothing really of anatomy, physiology, pathology, or any other of the basic sciences on which scientific medicine rests, she was confronted with an emergency, and she tried what she thought would help, and it did, but she never knew why it helped."[120] To Fishbein, Kenny's celebrity reputation in the 1940s was a typical example of how "most of the press liked to portray, another unprofessional investigator and discoverer being denied and overwhelmed by medical authority." The American public fell for Kenny "because of the publicity and attention given to her" and because "the psychological effects of those so burdened with emotion were such as to make further controlled evaluation of her techniques difficult if not impossible."[121]

Despite Fishbein's efforts to marginalize and trivialize her work and her legacy, what Kenny had to say was neither ignorant nor serendipitous. As Kenny recognized, American medical populism had deep popular and political roots. And in the 1940s her advice about the structure of federal research policy effectively resonated with a broader, populist suspicion of medical elitism. A number of congressmen and members of the public shared her sense that lay men and women should play a role directing medical policy (including scientific research) to ensure fairness and objectivity. In the 1940s and 1950s, the expansion of government investment in medicine and science provided a new platform for the articulation of populist critiques of professional elitism and monopoly, phrased in the Cold War language of democracy and freedom. In the politicized debate over the governance of the NSF the presumed objectivity of scientific professionals was subsumed (even briefly) by a populist concern for democratic responsiveness that would lead to research oriented around the people's health. Liberal reformers such as those in the Physicians Forum hoped government-directed research could become part of a larger extension of federal responsibility for medical care; opponents in the AMA and at research universities feared not only socialized medicine but socialized research, and imagined the Truman administration bringing Communistic collectivism to the doctor's office and the scientist's laboratory.

National Foundation officials went to Washington not just to defend themselves against Kenny's attacks but to keep "their disease" out of Washington. Although they recognized that federal funding for medical research had wide public and political support, research for organizations such as the National Foundation was too important a part of public relations to give up or even share with a government agency, much less ordinary scientists who might discover a cure without the imprimatur of the National Foundation's publicity department. Officials resisted being tarred as elitist by arguing that they distributed the public's funds fairly, responsibly, and democratically. And while still protesting against government incursion into polio work, the National Foundation, aware of the popularity of Kenny and her populist critique, tempered its criticism of her.

To be sure, Kenny, Congress, the AMA, and the National Foundation all agreed that modern scientific research was the best way to fight polio. However, populists such as Kenny and her supporters demanded science be linked to medical freedom, which in Kenny's case meant freeing her patients from braces and crutches and from the crippling effects of elitist orthodoxy. It is important to recognize that for Kenny, twentieth-century science was a resource, not a threat, and she confidently demanded the right to the vocabulary and technology of the laboratory. Access to laboratory science, however, was blocked by the monopoly of the National Foundation and its partner, the AMA. Only the government, responding to popular outrage, could ensure a true democracy of science. Kenny's claims for scientific respect and her portrayal as an isolated outsider attracted a public suspicious of corporate elitism. Perhaps medical freedom could be ensured by government fiat, opening the doors of hospitals and laboratories so that the resources of medical science would, at last, be available to all.

THE LUNATIC FRINGE STRIKES BACK

Conservative Opposition to the Alaska Mental Health Bill of 1956

Michelle M. Nickerson

If you respect your flag and love your Maker
And pray that He will guide you to do right
And do not let the first high-sounding faker
Convince you white is black and black is white . . .
If you stand up and say you love Old Glory
And show you're an American with guts
Baby, you'd better get yourself a lawyer
For "Mental Health" is out to prove YOU'RE NUTS . . . !

—Anna Mary Cann, Minute Women of the U.S.A.,
California Bulletin, February 1956

The political left has long criticized the nation's health care establishment for serving its own interests, disempowering its patients, and ignoring the needs of America's poorest citizens. Recently, the controls exerted over health care by insurance and pharmaceutical companies have motivated the Democratic Party to reassert its historical position as the champion of individual medical rights. Democrats are taking the lead in Medicare reform, a patient's right to sue insurance companies, and better prescription drug benefits for the elderly. As the Santa Cruz "pot giveaway," held in September 2002 in support of medicinal marijuana use, reminds us, there are also countercultural roots to leftist anti-authoritarianism worth noting.[1] The liberal political atmosphere of the 1960s inspired resistance to medical experts and experimentation with alternative medicine. Vegetarianism, herbal remedies, yoga, and holistic health practices have gained wide acceptance in the United States, but the hippie generation played no small role in establishing their popularity.

Looking back forty-five years to the first decade of the Cold War, however, shows us how resistance to medical authority can also emerge out of deeply conservative beliefs and political movements. In the 1950s and early 1960s, professional psychiatry came under fire from right-wing anti-communists. As the mental health field gained stature in the medical community and received unprecedented amounts of government funding, McCarthyite conservatives charged that more sinister forces were at work behind it all. Starting with a coalition of anti-communist study clubs in Los Angeles, activists from the West Coast to Dallas to Washington, D.C., launched a campaign to stop the passage of mental health legislation. They called psychiatric professionals "head shrinkers" and "brain tinkerers" and accused them of using their medical expertise to advance a left-wing political agenda.[2]

A seemingly innocuous piece of legislation, the Alaska Mental Health Bill of 1956, touched off this political movement. Written to enable the territory of Alaska to hospitalize its own mentally ill residents, the 1956 bill appropriated land and money to fund psychiatric facilities and programs. Protests led by grassroots anti-communist organizations erupted after the House of Representatives unanimously approved the bill in January. Shortly after the House vote, Mrs. Leigh F. Burkeland of Burbank, California, unleashed a wave of protest when she published an article in Orange County's Santa Ana *Register* called "Now—Siberia, U.S.A."[3] "Based on close study of the bill," Burkeland warned, "it is entirely within the realm of possibility that we may be establishing in Alaska our own version of the Siberian slave camps."[4] The bill's alleged danger lay in the dubious circumstances under which authorities could commit so-called mentally ill persons. Any police officer or health care professional, according to Burkeland, had the power to incarcerate individuals he or she deemed psychologically unfit. In the eyes of its opponents, the Alaska Mental Health Bill provided both the physical structures and the legal mechanisms for a Soviet-style police state in America. The bill signaled a "trend toward the centralization of Government," proclaimed Robert Williams of Orange County, who also appeared in Washington that week to expose, in his words, "boobytraps" that hide in "thick padded bills."[5]

Congress and political observers were taken aback by the "Siberia, U.S.A." furor. The bill should have pleased critics of big government; after all, it legislated a decentralization of power. Territorial representative Bob Barlett crafted the measure himself to give Alaskans control over the mental health care of their own patients. The bill also *divested* the federal government of one million acres of Alaska lands, authorizing the territorial government to lease those holdings for payment of construction, maintenance, and service costs. Local control and self-sufficiency were the heart and soul of the Alaska Mental Health Bill. Why, then, did the measure concern anti-communist activists? How did it come to mean big government and dictatorship? The solitary historical investigation of the Alaska Mental Health Bill, published in 1980, characterizes the episode as a "lunatic fringe" outburst—a typical McCarthy-era moment replete with PTA parents whispering to each other about late-night arrests.[6] Contemporary accounts were equally dismissive. In June 1956 *The Reporter*, a magazine based in New York and dedicated to fighting McCarthyism, chided anti-communist study groups in California for "sniff[ing] through the forty-three-page Alaska bill like bloodhounds."[7] Even the conservative *National Review* accused the mental health bill opponents of "touching off the biggest panic since Orson Welles landed his Martian invaders almost twenty years ago."[8]

Dramatic flourishes aside, "hysteria," "panic," and "paranoia" serve as grossly inadequate explanations of why the controversy erupted in the first place. They simply do not elucidate why legions of intelligent, politically aware Americans all over the country became so alarmed by this particular piece of legislation. "Siberia, U.S.A." was not an isolated incident. The protests of 1956 were part of a larger, sustained conservative anti-communist movement to thwart mental health reforms and initiatives. Opponents saw "Red" in the Alaska Mental Health Bill not because they were crazy, but because new developments in psychology—political and professional—put them on the defensive. The bill evoked massive conservative opposition that demands investigation, for a core set of very real issues united opponents of mental health into a formidable political group. From a conservative perspective deeply suspicious of state power, mental health was a Trojan horse—a tool of the left, wielding influence under the shroud of medical authority and exerting power with the muscle of federal dollars. I argue that the "Siberia, U.S.A." affair had as much to do with the mental health field's postwar growth spurt, professional psychology's forays into social and political reform, and liberal academic critiques of right-wing "paranoia" as it did with overblown fears of domestic communism. Mental health embodied everything that was wrong with the liberal welfare state for two reasons: first, psychology was beginning to appear more ideological (i.e., liberal) than medical, and second, high-profile intellectuals were exploiting psychological theory to try to eviscerate the American right. This essay, then, explores why so many Americans saw the mental health establishment as a communist threat and illustrates the ways in which they attempted to combat that threat.

THE ANTI-COMMUNIST MOVEMENT

Congressmen were clearly shocked by the torrent of protest mail that came across their desks regarding the Alaska Mental Health Bill 1956, but they should not have been. The "Siberia, U.S.A." uproar was hardly spontaneous. Despite Joseph McCarthy's fall from grace in 1954, a postwar conservative movement was brewing in the 1950s, with mental health issues serving as no small impetus. Mrs. Leigh F. Burkeland, author of "Siberia, U.S.A.," was a major player in the vibrant grassroots conservative community taking shape in Los Angeles at the time.[9] She belonged to two active patriotic organizations, American Public Relations Forum (APRF) and Minute Women of the U.S.A., Inc. Through these organizations, Burkeland was also connected to other conservative activists around the country. Phone chains and newsletters linked American Public Relations Forum to groups such as the Philadelphia-based American Flag Committee. Both organizations monitored domestic communism and mobilized swift, decisive action when necessary, as they did with the Alaska bill. Sharing a deep mistrust of the federal government and intense feelings of patriotism, these grassroots organizations conducted their own research and cultivated their own news organs, believing that liberals mainly controlled politics and the national media.

In the postwar era of "consensus," when political stability and social tranquility were high on the list of national goals, Dwight Eisenhower's "new Republicanism" reigned as a popular, right-of-center conservatism. The president prudently referred to himself as middle-of-the-road and kept a safe but polite distance from the McCarthyite and Robert Taft–led right wing of his party. From the perspective of conservatives ready for an end to liberalism in every way, shape, or form, Eisenhower was a tremendous disappointment. He not only failed to dismantle the New Deal welfare state but jeopardized the nation's sovereignty as well, supporting U.S. involvement in NATO and the United Nations. Although Eisenhower himself opposed civil rights measures, he appointed Chief Justice Earl Warren, whose court boldly hastened desegregation nationally with the *Brown vs. Board of Education* decision. Even Martin Luther King Jr. voted for Eisenhower in 1956.[10]

Not all Americans felt secure in the calmer ideological waters of the 1950s. Many conservatives favored more aggressive anti-communist measures; some even accused Eisenhower of abetting communism. Barry Goldwater charged his administration with succumbing to the "siren songs of socialism."[11] Joseph McCarthy did not ignite the postwar Red scare by himself, and after he crashed and burned McCarthy supporters kept the anti-communist movement alive.

Though conservative discontent took on a range of expressions around the country, from overt white supremacy to strident anti-communism to libertarianism, the federal bureaucracy served as a common target. In southern California, where the burgeoning military-industrial complex fueled the economy, a pro-defense, free-enterprise, limited-government brand of conservatism flourished. Civil rights reforms ignited right-wing opposition in California but most often provoked an anti-statist, anti-communist response. For example, opponents of school integration generally avoided racist language by instead attacking the federal government for interfering with local decision making. The Alaska Mental Health Bill imbroglio was a direct outgrowth of this conservative worldview taking shape in postwar California.

Los Angeles housewives were at the forefront of the anti-mental-health movement. "We are wives and mother who are vitally interested in what is happening in our country," announced Stephanie Williams when she founded American Public Relations Forum in 1952.[12] Indeed, the conservative movement thrived largely because of the gendered patterns of political work that women and men adopted out of the routines of their daily lives. Men tended to put themselves forward as office holders, fund-raisers, and spokesmen. Many important conservative newsletters, radio programs, and organizations were attached to the names of influential men: the *Dan Smoot Report,* the *Williams Intelligence Summary,* the *Manion Forum,* Fred Schwarz's School of Anti-Communism. Women, on the other hand, oversaw a large portion of the grassroots organizing going on beneath the radar. They made use of their flexible schedules and community contacts. As Marie Koenig, a former officer in American Public Relations, explained, "Men don't have time to be . . . doing the things that we women do . . . to sit and write letters . . . when they get home at night they don't want to run around to meetings."[13] Contrary to the image of the apolitical 1950s housewife, the women of APRF, Minute Women of the U.S.A., and numerous organizations like them embraced political work as an extension of their household and community duties. Exceptions to this gendered division of labor abounded. Still, only the intense legislative study that women's groups specialized in made it possible for conservatives to uncover the Alaska Mental Health Bill. They researched communist influences in mental health legislation because they believed that political biases drove the latest developments in psychology.

FROM MENTAL ILLNESS TO MENTAL HEALTH

In the 1950s, "mental health" was a relatively new expression, describing an up- and-coming medical field and social-medical movement, both of which were spun out of the latest theories and methods driving the study of psychology in America. More than any other factor, World War II prompted the change in focus from "mental illness" to "mental health" and expanded the reliance on psychological and medical expertise in the United States. The armed services taught fighting men that it was acceptable to ask for help with psychological and emotional problems. Then, as veterans returned to the United States, they and their families sought assistance with the very difficult transition to peacetime.[14] When vets called upon the federal government to subsidize therapy, Congress quickly discovered that treating mental illness was an expensive proposition. As it turned out, though, psychological professionals were well positioned to help the government meet these demands in the late 1940s, for the military had employed them in droves during the war to screen recruits, boost morale, and treat mental illness. "As a result of our experience in the Army," declared William Menninger, one of the most influential wartime psychiatrists, "it is vividly apparent that psychiatry can and must play a much more important role in the solution of health problems of the civilian."[15]

Menninger and others advocated "preventive," community-based initiatives as the most cost-effective solution to these health problems. Mental health programs, they argued, would reduce the need for institutions, medicine, and other expenses associated with the treatment of mental illness.[16] The National Mental Health Act (NMHA), passed in 1946, signaled the widespread acceptance of this view. The legislation directed federal funding toward research, training, and grants for facilities and established the National Institute of Mental Health (NIMH).[17] Mental health programs then proliferated quickly. Too much so, argued conservative critics. From their perspective, mental health "experts" were unwelcome fixtures of the liberal welfare state, expanding their jurisdiction (and the federal government's) into race relations, housing, education, and employment. Mental health advocates also coaxed tax dollars out of federal coffers and provoked an unnecessary flurry of legislative activity. Worse yet, they seemed to be abusing their medical authority for the advancement of a liberal political agenda.

Conservative activists had plenty of real evidence to support their contentions that liberalism was intimately intertwined with the mental health movement and social psychiatry. The ravages of war and the atrocities of the Holocaust inspired social scientists to apply psychology to solving the problem of racism. In 1950 Theodor Adorno, Else Frenkel-Brunswik, Daniel Levinson, and R. Nevitt published *The Authoritarian Personality*, the final product of many years' research into the psychological mechanisms of anti-Semitism and race prejudice.[18] Funded mostly by Jewish organizations, the studies that constituted *The Authoritarian Personality* aimed to understand Hitler's rise to power and the overall growth of small-*f* fascism. Adorno's major contribution was his personality types— patterns of behavior that characterized racially prejudiced people. "The crank," for example, was one of Adorno's feminine prototypes, a category that included "organized war mothers" whose "continuous repression of the id" manifested "frustration in the widest sense of the term."[19]

As American psychology progressed into the 1950s, American researchers applied Adorno's models to their own theories about race thought in the United States. In 1956, Los Angeles psychiatrist Isidore Ziferstein published the article "Race Prejudice and Mental Health," which investigated racism as "a social and psychological disease . . . a symptom of a disordered society and of a disordered individual." Ziferstein's study pursued an explicitly social-political mission. "Every day that segregation continues," he wrote, "our children's feeling and thinking are contaminated with the germs of this profoundly anti-democratic and anti-human 'fact of life.'" [20] Borrowing from Adorno, Ziferstein sketched personality traits exhibited by prejudiced people in America:

> He [the "prejudiced individual"] is full of fears and distrust. . . . He suffers from an inability to love. . . . He is afraid of feeling, and is therefore out of touch with his inner self. . . . The self hate and the repressed hate of the powerful authority produce strong destructive drives which may at times result in delinquent behavior.[21]

Racism, in other words, was wholly antithetical to mental health. Ziferstein's work might seem bold, but by 1956 his theories were almost commonplace in his profession. The fateful *Brown vs. Board of Education* decision is a case in point. When the Supreme Court ruled that school desegregation was unconstitutional, they not only footnoted the latest social scientific scholarship on race by Kenneth Clark, Gordon Allport, and Gunnar Myrdal, but based their verdict on the psychological damage suffered by black schoolchildren. "Whatever may have been the extent of psychological knowledge at the time of *Plessy v. Ferguson*," the opinion read, "this finding is amply supported by modern authority."[22] *Brown* put the rule of law behind cutting-edge race theory.

Mental health policy evoked a conservative backlash also because many highly acclaimed social scientists and psychologists shared an internationalist—indeed, actively anti-nationalist—vision for how psychology could foster world peace and further the goals of the United Nations. The World Federation of Mental Health teamed up with the World Health Organization and the United Nations in what appeared to conservatives to have the makings of a global conspiracy. Especially alarming to conservatives was a 1948 pamphlet called *Mental Health and World Citizenship*, prepared by the International Congress on Mental Health (ICMH), an organization that included the prominent American social scientist Margaret Mead. "Principles of mental health cannot be successfully furthered in any society," read the pamphlet, "unless there is progressive acceptance of the concept of world citizenship. World citizenship can be widely extended among all peoples through the applications of the principles of mental health."[23] Nationalism, the ICMH implied, was a social affliction that mental health measures might help eradicate:

> Such intervention will meet with many and grave obstacles. One obstacle to the growth of a world community is the partial or distorted picture of the outside world inculcated through a nationalist or ideological bias, through the "stereotypes" of thought and feeling.[24]

The progressive undercurrent driving mental health research and policy, and the federal government's willingness to enforce its latest findings, seemed downright heavy-handed to Americans who did not accept the most fashionable academic ideas about race, prejudice, and nationalism. And scholarly work being written about McCarthyism gave conservatives further reason to mistrust mental health experts. In 1954, the nation's most celebrated historian, Richard Hofstadter, borrowed the term "pseudo-conservative" from Theodor Adorno and constructed a "social-psychological" profile of right-wing extremists. Conspiracy theorists, McCarthy supporters, United Nations antagonists, the Ku Klux Klan, "patriotic groups," and "the old lady . . . in the DAR [Daughters of the American Revolution]" all occupied this capacious category. Pseudo-conservatism was a personality type, clarified Hofstadter, not to be confused with classical conservatism, a legitimate political tradition embodied by the Eisenhower administration. "More than ordinarily incoherent about politics," he explained, pseudo-conservatives acted out of "dense and massive irrationality." Hofstadter's study, which grew into the famous work on "paranoid style" a few years later, became one of the most widely regarded critiques of the American far right for decades to come.[25]

No wonder Hofstadter's name came up more than once in the Alaska Mental Health Bill hearings. For among those who fit his criteria, Hofstadter's annihilation of the right, coupled with the internationalist ambitions of social scientists and the liberal overtones of mental health policy, meant politicized ideology, not scientific psychology. Who had the authority to define normalcy? And under what definitions of abnormalcy could people be institutionalized? These questions preyed on conservative minds, and from their vantage point the Alaska Mental Health Bill looked like the ultimate tool of totalitarian control. Despite the efforts of some groups, such as the Minute Women, to make the Alaska bill protest seem spontaneous, though, opposition did not simply rise out of the conservative electorate. The campaign was well organized. In fact, an anti-mental-health movement had been building up to the "Siberia, U.S.A." controversy for more than a year.

THE INSTIGATORS OF THE ANTI-MENTAL-HEALTH MOVEMENT
American Public Relations Forum and Minute Women of the U.S.A., Inc. commenced their study of mental health legislation in the early part of 1955. Both groups had already been active for a few years. Some of their membership overlapped, and their headquarters were close to each other—APRF's in Burbank and the Minute Women's in Edendale. Catholic women, with Williams as their head, founded APRF in 1952 and started meeting in Immaculate Conception Hall, a space that belonged to the Los Angeles Catholic Archdiocese. Minute Women of the U.S.A. was a national organization with a very active California chapter. In 1952 the organization boasted fifty thousand members in forty-seven states. The Minute Women were mostly white, middle- and upper-class, between the ages of thirty and sixty, with school-age or grown children. Although the national leadership identified the California chapter as one of its strongest, its membership numbers are unknown because the Minute Women were deliberately cryptic. Suzanne Stevenson, the founder, instructed members to act as individual citizens and never reveal their Minute Woman status.[26] She reasoned that political action was more effective when it looked unorganized—hence the anonymously penned Santa Ana *Register* article "Siberia, U.S.A." Even when Burkeland revealed herself as the mysterious writer to the subcommittee in Washington, she never identified as a Minute Woman. "I represent myself," she told them.[27] American Public Relations Forum was far less secretive. By 1955 its membership had expanded to one hundred or more and met one Friday each month at the Hollywood Club in La Brea. After opening with the Apostles' Creed at ten-thirty, the women met for two educational sessions, one in the morning and one in the afternoon. Sometimes members presented their own research, but oftentimes outside speakers—former communists, spies, or United Nations supporters—would tell their stories of redemption. Both the Minute Women of California and American Public Relations Forum published monthly newsletters, as well as emergency bulletins when necessary.

The latest developments in mental health inspired both groups to make themselves experts in the political affairs of professional psychology.[28] Marie Koenig, APRF's public relations coordinator, began subscribing to professional journals, clipping newspaper articles, and ordering pamphlets from the National Institute of Mental Health. A Catholic herself, Koenig did not appreciate the blatantly anti-religious message she encountered in some of the literature. One pamphlet she read, *Mental Hygiene in the Nursery Schools,* published by the United Nations Educational, Scientific and Cultural Organization (UNESCO), implied that Catholic nuns posed a psychological threat to schoolchildren. It went so far as to state:

> The question of selection and guidance of intending nursery school teachers is of the essence of the whole problem of the mental hygiene of young children. Where women in the teaching

service are sexually inhibited or are debarred from marriage, neuroses are common, with disastrous results for the children in school.[29]

With medical authorities unabashedly diagnosing religious traditions as neuroses, the Minute Women and APRF began to question how mental health was being defined. They researched dictionary entries on psychological terms and familiarized themselves with the latest academic scholarship. According to one Minute Women bulletin, Webster's defined a "psychopathic personality" as one marked by "abnormal sensitiveness to spiritual phenomena . . . characterized by extreme susceptibility to religious emotion, conscientious doubts and fears." "What individual has not," asked the Minute Woman writer, "been subject to a greater or lesser degree to some of the above symptoms?"[30] The same bulletin quoted a recent article in the *Annals of the American Academy of Political and Social Science* that praised the mental heath movement for making ideas such as original sin, corporal punishment, and men's superiority over women "unfashionable."[31] The bulletin highlighted this work to show that "acceptance of the mental hygiene beliefs" corresponded precisely to the "discard of Christian ethics."[32]

In the postwar era, mental health professionals increasingly filled social niches once occupied by churches and extended families. "The Mental Health movement has set out," argued the same Minute Women bulletin, "to destroy the structure of Christianity."[33] From guidance counselors to newspaper columnists to Dr. Spock, medical and psychological experts were everywhere, dispensing advice on how to raise children, save marriages, and relax.[34] It did not require a conspiratorial mind to observe this. "Every magazine with few exceptions for April and May," reported American Public Relations Forum in 1955, has "carried articles and stories on the mentally ill."[35] The Minute Women pointed out that amid the vast array of self-help literature, including *So You Think It's Love* and *What You Should Know about Parenthood,* available for twenty-five cents, were "Overcoming Prejudice" and "ABC's of Scapegoating."[36] At what point, they wanted to know, did medicine stop and political indoctrination begin?

In March 1955 it was time to stop studying and take action. The California Assembly was considering three bills dealing with community mental health services. Bill 1158, a funding measure, would have allocated an additional $233,000 to the Department of Mental Hygiene for salaries, equipment, and services. Bill 1159 laid out provisions for local governments to receive assistance from the state for mental health programs. Bill 3300, the most dangerous, altered the commitment procedures for mentally ill persons.[37] "Are You Mentally Ill?" asked a headline in the Montrose *Ledger.* "The new laws would make it possible for the state to legally pick you up . . . whisk you away . . . and hold you in a mental institution against you will without the 'formality' of a court appearance."[38] Two months later, the Freedom Club, a Los Angeles patriotic organization, circulated *Your Freedom May Be at Stake!* a letter from Dr. Lewis A. Alesen, L.A. County Hospital's chief of staff, to Governor Goodwin Knight. "Assembly Bills 1158, 1159 and 3300," wrote Alesen, "constitute in my opinion an insidious but nevertheless most serious threat to the fundamentals upon which our system of representative government rests."[39]

American Public Relations Forum was ready to move. Its bulletins urged members to write immediately and often:

This [May bulletin] could very well be our last. . . . Before another one is due freedom of speech may be a thing of the past. Whether it is the last one or not, it will certainly be the most important. See that you read every word of it and do not let the sun go down without taking action on the information.[40]

Stephanie Williams had her day in Sacramento, speaking for an hour before the Senate committee. "She brought out every weak point in the bill," reported the June APRF bulletin, "and was able to swing one vote against it"—enough to send it back to the Rules Committee, where it was shelved for two years. We cannot be sure, but the evidence definitely suggests that Williams and her cohorts had a great deal of influence on the senators' decision. An article published in the *American Journal of Psychiatry* eight years later credits American Public Relations Forum with defeating the bill and inciting the "first significant public denunciation against the mental health movement."[41]

But this was just the beginning. As Williams was preparing her testimony against the Community Mental Health Services Act, legislators in Washington were preparing H.R. 6376, the Alaska Mental Health Bill. As far as Alaska representative Bob Bartlett was concerned, it was the end. He was eager to bring the forty-six-year battle for psychiatric care in Alaska to a close.[42] Bartlett thought this was finally it because this time, the Territory and Insular Affairs Subcommittee had conducted an investigation that shocked and disturbed them. When the subcommittee traveled to Portland, Oregon's Morningside Hospital, where Alaskans received psychiatric treatment, they discovered that most patients arrived without any clinical records or diagnosis reports. Morningside admitted them without any transcripts of their commitment procedures. Hospital personnel reported that the Alaska commissioner who actually committed patients knew very little about the individual cases when they contacted him. The House of Representatives agreed that this neglect and mismanagement could no longer be tolerated and approved the Alaska Mental Health Bill unanimously in January 1956. Ironically, though, outrage over institutionalization procedures, the bill's catalyst, would soon work against it.

THE ALASKA BILL CONTROVERSY

Quietly and in the most sinister manner the heavily financed pressure groups which comprise the people backing mental health legislation were able to get much of it passed before unsuspecting Americans even knew such legislation had been devised. Wording of the bills, admittedly loosely written by the authors of the legislation, could apply to all Americans, especially those who have been active against the New Dealers and their schemes to make this country into a member of a world government and reduce us to slavery.

—*American Public Relations Forum*, Bulletin, *January 1956*

The Alaska Mental Health Bill read simply: "The purpose of this act is to transfer from the Federal Government to the Territory of Alaska basic responsibility and authority for the hospitalization, care, and treatment of the mentally ill of Alaska."[43] Alaskan jurisdiction over their own mental health affairs seemed like an honorable goal, argued opponents, but several provisions of the bill posed grave risks. First, section 103 specified that "an individual may be admitted for care and treatment in a hospital upon written application by an interested party, by a health or welfare officer, by the Governor [of Alaska], or by the head of any institution."[44] "Interested party," according to the bill's definition, meant legal guardian, spouse, parent, adult children, close relative, or "interested, responsible adult friend."[45] That last category could mean anybody. Second, section 101 defined mental illness as a "psychiatric or other disease which substantially impairs [one's] mental health."[46] The "other disease" component of this definition was ambiguous; it might be flexed to include troublesome political behavior. Third, section 118 authorized the governor of Alaska to "enter into a reciprocal agreement with any State providing for the prompt transfer . . . of residents of such State or Alaska who are mentally ill."[47] Might this provision authorize the shipment of political dissidents to Alaska? Lastly, section 202 granted the territory "one million acres from the public lands of the United States in Alaska . . . to lease and make conditional sales of such selected lands." Despite the expressed intent of this land alloca-tion, and despite the long history of states selling federal lands to pay for government insti-tutions such as schools, those one million acres looked frighteningly like a gulag. All of these possibilities contained in one bill were too much to ignore; the clues were all there.

In December 1955 American Public Relations Forum printed an announcement about a very important bill, H.R. 6376, "one that tops all of them." "We could not help remember-ing that Siberia is very near Alaska and since it is obvious no one needs such a large land grant, we were wondering if it could be an American Siberia." The bulletin writers were fully aware of the stated purpose of the bill but reminded readers what "modernizing pro-cedures [including] commitment" really meant. "This provision takes away all of the rights of the American citizen to ask for a jury trial and protect him[self] from being railroaded to an asylum by a greedy relative or 'friend' or, as the Alaska bill states, 'an interested party.' "[48] After the January House vote, the opposition really started to move. California groups took the lead, but conservative writers, radio broadcasters, and grassroots organizers from Ohio to Texas to New Jersey sprang into action. By March, rumors were circulating in Washington that senators had received more correspondence relating to the Alaska Mental Health Bill than to the 1941 Lend-Lease Act.[49]

On March 3, the Catholic weekly *Brooklyn Tablet* published "Not for Alaskans Alone," warning that the proposed hospital "could be for any one of us."[50] The American Flag Committee, a national patriotic organization based in Philadelphia, rallied its members to "get behind the American Public Relations Forum," praising its heroic victory in Sacra-mento and stressing the urgency of the Alaska bill fight.[51] The Dallas-based conservative guru Dan Smoot devoted an entire March issue of the *Dan Smoot Report* to mental health.[52] "What, after all, is normal?" he asked. "Does it mean conformity with generally accepted attitudes, acceptance of generally held opinions?" "There is only one way for a psychiatrist to tell whether or not you are crazy," Smoot argued; "he finds out how closely your thinking resembles that of everyone else."[53] Orange County's *Williams Intelligence Summary*, which boasted nine thousand subscribers nationwide in 1956, warned that the bill was "full of dangerous loopholes."[54] "Sooner or later," predicted editor Robert Williams, "a health or welfare worker will have to beat down a door, break into a home with drawn guns and perhaps shoot somebody or get shot."[55] The Chicago-based Associa-tion of American Physicians and Surgeons (AAPS), an anti-socialized-medicine organiza-tion that claimed ten thousand members, attacked the bill repeatedly in its bulletins: "It's impossible to describe all [its] horrendous provisions."[56]

Meanwhile, the Senate subcommittee had to deal with the barrage of protest mail. The Public Affairs Luncheon Club of Dallas and Houston's Texas Women for Constitutional Government urged a speedy defeat of the bill.[57] "Remember," warned the Houston women, "the frightful experimentation with human beings an their extermination in Germany under Hitler *was legal.* They had seen to it that the necessary laws were enacted first."[58] Some letters called for investigation of the sponsors themselves. The Keep America Committee of Los Angeles suggested that the bill was proposed by a "conspiratorial gang" that ought to be "investigated, impeached, or at least removed from office" for treason. Philadelphia's American Flag Commuittee suggested that instead of passing the bill, the Senate committee ought to investigate "the Department that introduced it."[59]

The subcommittee also had to face opponents who came to protest in person. Stephanie Williams, one of the first, did her best to connect the dots for the congressmen. She was concerned about line 17 of the bill: "The term 'mentally ill individual' means an individual having a psychiatric or other disease," she pointed out. "I was most concerned in finding out who is going to define that."[60] Following Williams, Burkeland asked, "Is an 'other disease' that which is described by Professor Richard Hofstadter, of Columbia University, in his . . . attack on the 'pseudoconservative revolt'?"[61] Continuing along these lines, Mrs. Ernest W. Howard, of the Women's Patriotic Conference on National Defense, testified on behalf of the three million women in eighteen separate patriotic groups that constituted her organization. She echoed Burkeland's concerns about Hofstadter and dared to inform the subcommittee that she and her members were better equipped than Congress to read legislation. "Those of us who have been in the study and research work of the United Nations," she declared, "we feel that we are experts in this . . . you as Senators with all the many commitments and the many requirements, are not able to go into all these things."[62] The hearings grew especially tense, though, when Camden, New Jersey's John Kaspar took his turn in front of the committee. "I think it is important to realize," argued Kaspar, known for his work as a White Citizens' Council organizer in Tennessee, "that almost one hundred percent of all psychiatric therapy is Jewish and that about eighty percent of psychiatrists are Jewish."[63] Kaspar argued that Jews were nationalists of another country. And he did not appreciate their attempts to "usurp American nationality."[64]

John Kaspar's anti-Semitism was too much to bear. "I do not think," Senator Alan Bible told Kaspar, "the committee will be particularly concerned with this trend of your dissertation. I think we have some very fine Jewish people."[65] At one point Senator George Malone threw up his hands and asked, "When did it become so complex and so controversial? All we want to do is to take care of anyone who is mentally incompetent in a way that he might be dangerous to himself or others . . . but when did it become necessary to include so many controversial and apparently extraneous provisions?"[66] Bob Bartlett expressed the collective shock and outrage of the bill's proponents when he declared, "I am completely at a loss in attempting to fathom the reasons why certain individuals and certain groups have now started a letter-writing campaign . . . to defeat the act. I am sure that if the letter writers would consult the facts, they would join with all others not only in hoping this act would become law but in working for its speedy passage and approval."[67] As we know, however, the opponents of the Alaska bill consulted facts; they had filing cabinets full of facts.

With just a few minor changes, the Alaska Mental Health Bill passed that summer. Political commentators emphasized the inevitability of the outcome. The *Reporter* announced that, "no longer hampered by sensationalized opposition, the Senate passed the Alaska Mental Health bill without dissent after a ten-minute debate."[68] "In the end," wrote historian Clause-M. Naske in 1980, "reason prevailed."[69]

The aftermath of the Alaska Mental Health Bill suggests a different narrative, though. This so-called outburst repeated itself often enough that it can hardly even be called an outburst. The conservatism that showed itself in the Alaska bill controversy did not calm down, but snowballed into the Goldwater era. Mental health advocates won the day in

1956, but "Siberia, U.S.A." was a formative movement in the nascent conservatism then taking shape.

MENTAL HEALTH AND THE RISING RIGHT

Our American team has a big job to do, particularly in building citizens who do not need frequent servicing by some psychiatrist, a mental hospital or a prison. We need a deeper spirituality. We need to get our citizens to stand on their own two feet, with a sense of responsibility and personal independence. Our society needs a new posture of self discipline and character. This would be real mental health.

—*Cleon Skousen, "Law Enforcement Looks at Mental Health,"* Law and Order, *1962*

The Alaska Mental Health Bill came as the first of several setbacks for the anti-mental-health movement. The California bill regarding community mental health services re-appeared in 1957 and won passage the second time around. Attempts to dismantle the mental health regime met with continued failure after that. But as many conservatives such as the anti-communist speaker Cleon Skousen learned, the fight against mental health could be better carried out on other grounds. Skousen acknowledged in his newsletter, *Law and Order*, that crime, delinquency, and insanity were indeed mental illnesses and that "mental health has received the all-out support of presidents, governors, business leaders and civic groups" for good reasons. The solutions to these social problems, however, were not to be found in professional psychiatry. "There is a job for parents to do which is not being done adequately," he wrote, "a job for schools, the churches, the police and the courts which can be done far better." Skousen wrote this commentary in 1962, when the conservative movement was picking up steam. The John Birch Society, a national grassroots anti-communist organization with a strong foothold in southern California, often relied upon anti-mental-health rhetoric to prove the existence of a global communist conspiracy. "The Communists," according to a 1965 issue of its magazine, "in a very considerable number of states . . . have induced the legislatures to enact 'mental health' laws to facilitate the incarceration of troublesome Americans."[70] A 1966 study of the John Birch Society, sponsored by the Anti-Defamation League, even points to the 1956 Alaska Mental Health Bill "salvo" as a prelude to the "radical right" fomentation of the 1960s.[71] The 1964 Republican nominee for president, Senator Barry Goldwater, invoked the evils of "mental health" to explain why liberalism had weakened the moral fortitude of the nation. Rebuking the quintessential liberal who "frowns on the policeman and fawns on the social psychologist," Goldwater equated disrespect for the law, parents, and, for that matter, God, with misplaced faith in mental health experts and social welfare programs. Championing law and order, school prayer, and the free enterprise system, he vowed to redeem the nation out of "thirty years of an unhealthy social climate."[72]

Although the "mental health racket" remained a common feature of far right rhetoric in the 1960s, the Alaska bill controversy and its aftermath continued to escape the notice of historians. To some extent, this is due to the failure of contemporary political observers and pundits to take the anti-mental-health movement seriously in the first place. The political grievances represented by opposition to "mental health," including mistrust of government and medical authorities and lamentation over the declining role of families and churches in the development of the child, attracted scant attention. Mental health experts, for their part, continued to diagnose right-wing ideology as if it were a disease. In 1960, three psychiatrists published an article in the *American Journal of Orthopsychiatry* that studied the Alaska Mental Health Bill opposition and other incidents of "scientific conservatism" as "popular anxieties" aroused by "irrational and unconscious source[s]."[73] The essay invoked Adorno's personality types to make its case. "Often these people [scientific conservatives] come from homes in which rigid, repressive and authoritarian patterns have dominated their early developmental years, with consequent patterns of deeply repressed hostility, dependent and libidinal strivings."[74]

Richard Hofstadter similarly used the analysis he had developed in the 1950s to dismiss the views of Goldwater supporters. The "mental heat" of pseudo-conservatism, he wrote, was still at work in the 1960s.[75] Goldwater himself, wrote Hofstadter, "live[d] psychologically half in the world of our routine politics and half in the curious intellectual underworld of the pseudo-conservatives."[76] For this reason, that ultra-conservatism stood apart from routine politics, Goldwater "zealots" would not be able to govern the electorate even if they won power. They were too "ecstatic" and too interested in party domination, concluded Hofstadter, to handle the great American task of consensus building:

> The art of consensus politics, in our system, has to be practiced not only in coping with the opposition party but internally, in dealing with one's partisans and allies. . . . Our politics has thus put a strong premium on the practical rather than the ideological bent of mind, on the techniques of negotiation and compromise rather than the assertion of divisive ideas and passions.[77]

However, as Hofstadter was formulating his theories about the ultra-conservative passions handicapping the right, Ronald Reagan was on his way to becoming governor of California. Anti-liberal and anti-intellectual to the core, Reagan won the 1966 gubernatorial election by wholeheartedly embracing the ultra-conservative wing of the Republican Party, although he evaded the extremist mantle himself. Reagan assailed Berkeley's "beatniks and malcontents" and decried the liberal welfare state ("Big Brother") but never joined the John Birch Society, openly admired Franklin Roosevelt, and refused to let opponents brand him a racial bigot.[78] Not only did Reagan artfully negotiate the conservative movement and "routine politics," but he became a master, the "Great Communicator." He won the U.S. presidency in 1980 and ushered in a new conservative era nationwide. Almost in defiance of Richard Hofstadter, Reagan rode to the White House on the back of the Cold War conservative movement and dared to become one of the most popular presidents in U.S. history.

As it turns out, then, the Alaska Mental Health Bill controversy was not such an historical aberration after all. "Siberia, U.S.A." was off the mark in its assessment of the Alaska Mental Health Bill, but it was not a paranoiac fantasy. When opponents of the bill cried communism, they challenged a whole set of political and social conditions that were very real. Psychologists and social scientists *were* pathologizing certain kinds of political thought. Indeed, they were classifying racism and nationalism as diseases. Scholars and politicians were, moreover, using these psychological theories to publicly question the sanity of right-wing conservatives. While the term *paranoia* may be politically useful at times, its power to explain is severely limited. As the Alaska Mental Health Bill controversy shows, social and historical circumstances led people to see the world in conspiratorial terms.[79] And despite their marginalization from mainstream politics, mental health opponents did not disappear; their activism folded into a larger grassroots movement that eventually found leadership in Barry Goldwater and power in Ronald Reagan. They demonstrate that conservatives, as well as liberals, have formulated powerful anti-authoritarian critiques of organized medicine that remained alive in politics even as their own movement faded.

The example of the Alaska Mental Health Bill controversy shows us that by studying opposition to the medical establishment, historians can gain deeper insight into the diversity of voices that have influenced larger political movements. In this case, we see a thoroughly underexamined contingent of the conservative movement, one that offers a more nuanced and bottom-up perspective of the right-wing ascendancy—housewife activists. Women honed in on mental health legislation because they believed that it threatened their spheres of influence, namely, their homes, families, children, public schools, and communities. In other words, it was precisely the psycho-medical and social dimensions of the Alaska Mental Health Bill that drew them out into the political realm. The attacks made against the housewives by the conservative *National Review* remind us, moreover, that conservatism was not a monolithic political movement and that women did not simply toe the conservative line. The California activists set their own priorities and willingly subjected themselves to ridicule from conservative intellectuals and leaders. They suggest that, for periods such as the 1950s, when gender politics were far less prominent than in other historical moments, movements centered on medical and health issues might have valuable potential for finding examples of female political activity.

"NOT A SO-CALLED DEMOCRACY"

Anti-Fluoridationists and the Fight over Drinking Water

Gretchen Ann Reilly

"IF WE ARE GOING TO COMPEL PEOPLE to do anything they may not want to do," Dr. George Swendiman, an anti-fluoridation dentist, asked in 1951, "why not compel them to refrain from consuming candy, cakes, cookies, and soft drinks? Why not prohibit, by suitable laws, the manufacture of refined sugar, refined flour, and similar devitaminized atrocities?"[1] For advocates of an all-natural healthy diet and alternative medicine, the introduction of fluoridation as a public health measure was more than just another example of the wrongheadedness of modern medicine. Unlike processed foods or even dehumanizing and ineffective medical treatments, the addition of fluoride to public water supplies was not a matter of personal choice. When a community began fluoridating its water supply, anyone who objected to it would have to find an alternative water source or consume what anti-fluoridationists considered a dangerous and useless poison. Certainly, many anti-fluoridationists had coherent ideas about healing and alternative medicine. Yet it was the *compulsory* nature of such water treatment that was always at the heart of their concerns, and therefore politics was always at the center of their attention.

Beginning in the 1950s, public health and dental professionals attempted to begin fluoridation in communities across America, most often through lobbying of local governments and the water boards that managed community water supplies, but occasionally through referenda in communities that required public approval for the decision. They believed fluoridation to be a scientifically and medically sound public health measure that would improve people's lives by eliminating expensive, painful, and disfiguring dental cavities. When anti-fluoridationists began their campaign of opposition, pro-fluoridationists were completely surprised. Indeed, the ability of anti-fluoridationists to convince local governments, water boards, and the voting public to reject such a promising health measure blindsided the pro-fluoridationists. At first pro-fluoridationists comforted themselves with the hope that "the ridiculous charges would eventually prove self-defeating, that the public would soon awaken, and that the fluoridation issue would be settled, quietly and sanely, in the best traditions of . . . American democracy."[2] But this did not happen: opposition to fluoridation did not die down. Some communities that had previously embraced fluoridation rejected it; other communities faced annual challenges. Many more communities

never enacted fluoridation, because after ugly public campaigns led by anti-fluoridationists, voters or elected officials rejected the measure.

Pro-fluoridationists long struggled to understand their opponents, to explain why anti-
fluoridationists rejected the advice of experts, and to respond to the opposition's political
attacks on fluoridation. The anti-fluoridation movement, though, has proved difficult to
understand or counteract. Springing up at the very moment fluoridation was first being
embraced by the medical community, the anti-fluoridation movement, while being focused on the issue of coercion, was actually a changing coalition of groups that objected
to fluoridation for a wide range of reasons. Nor were anti-fluoridationists mere local irri-
tants; they challenged the measure on the national political stage as well. And despite the
fact that no major political party embraced their cause, anti-fluoridationists repeatedly associated their movement with national political and social issues and related it to America's broader political traditions in a way that fluoridation's supporters found difficult to
counteract.

Pro-fluoridationists always labeled their opponents "the lunatic fringe." They characterized the anti-fluoridationists as rabid conservatives, health nuts, anti-social agitators,
and "little old ladies in sneakers." But can a movement that has managed for over fifty years
to fight to a standstill a public health measure backed by federal, state, and local governments and much of the medical and scientific community truly be dismissed as a fringe
movement? The movement's repeated success in voting booths nationwide instead suggests there may be more to this movement than pro-fluoridationists—or latter-day scholars—ever were or have been willing to admit.

ORIGINS OF THE MOVEMENT

Originally, the United States Public Health Service (USPHS) began to study fluoride in
drinking water after the early 1930s discovery that too much fluoride in drinking water led
to brown stains or mottling of the teeth. The USPHS wanted to develop an index that related the severity of mottling to the fluoride content of drinking water so that communities could judge whether the level of fluoride in their water supply was safe. Research
scientists experimenting with fluoride discovered in the late 1930s that fluoride not only
mottled teeth, but also appeared to prevent tooth decay. Epidemiological studies of communities with naturally fluoridated water conducted by the USPHS confirmed these
observations, and in the latter half of the 1940s, the USPHS and a few state health organizations began fluoridating several communities' water supplies on an experimental basis
to determine the mineral's effectiveness and safety. A group of outspoken dentists in Wisconsin, convinced that communities that had been drinking naturally fluoridated water
for centuries were proof enough that the measure was safe, pressured the USPHS and various dental and medical organizations, such as the American Dental Association (ADA)
and the American Medical Association (AMA), to publicly endorse and encourage fluoridation. When these organizations resisted their efforts, the Wisconsin dentists began actively promoting fluoridation on their own. They traveled throughout Wisconsin, urging
communities to begin fluoridating their water supplies.[3]

Their efforts met with great success: by 1949, 85 percent of the urban population of
Wisconsin drank fluoridated water.[4] Only in Madison, Wisconsin, had there been any real
public opposition, and that had been easily overcome; in most communities, there was little resistance to the measure. That changed in 1950, though, when the proponents of fluo-

ridation attempted to convince the community of Stevens Point, Wisconsin, to fluoridate their water. Opposition to the measure arose quickly there, led by a group of men who defeated fluoridation soundly by arguing that the measure was being forced on the community by "outsiders."

The opposition group did not stop their attack on fluoridation once they had defeated it within their own community. They began writing letters against fluoridation to municipal officials and private citizens throughout the state. In Wisconsin communities considering the measure, the group paid for newspaper ads objecting to fluoridation. When in 1950 the USPHS and ADA publicly endorsed it and dentists and public health reformers nationwide began lobbying for fluoridation in their communities, a loose network of anti-fluoridationists developed around the Stevens Point group.[5]

The decentralized nature of public water supplies meant that fluoridation had to be fought locally, encouraging anti-fluoridation organizations to be, primarily, small groups. Yet the national network that formed to support these groups ensured that these campaigns were remarkably consistent over time and space by distributing educational materials and information regarding tactics and strategy. One anti-fluoridation flyer, found in a collection amassed by a Wisconsin anti-fluoridationist, had notations on it indicating that it had been reprinted by anti-fluoridation groups in Seattle, Washington; Lakeland, Florida; and Washington, D.C. The flyer consisted of an anti-fluoridation editorial from a Richmond, Virginia newspaper, as well as a letter from a French Canadian anti-fluoridationist.[6] National organizations in the network offered self-published books and bulk quantities of flyers and brochures for sale to local anti-fluoridation groups. They also provided the names and addresses of other national organizations fighting fluoridation. In one case, a flyer announced that donations to the organization would be used to distribute anti-fluoridation flyers for free in communities where the issue was being debated.[7] Other nationally prominent anti-fluoridationists offered their services as lecturers or debaters for a modest fee.

Despite the coordination between anti-fluoridationists scattered throughout the country, the anti-fluoridation movement was never a single unified force. It was always a coalition of groups and individuals who fought against fluoridation for a wide range of reasons. Opponents of fluoridation included medical and dental professionals, research scientists, alternative health practitioners, heath food enthusiasts, Christian Scientists, conservatives, and occasionally environmentalists. Each group had its own objections to fluoridation.

Medical and scientific objections to fluoridation sprang from the idea that fluoride was a dangerous poison. Some mainstream medical and dental professionals, such as Dr. George L. Waldbott of Michigan and Dr. Frederick Exner of Washington, and alternative health professionals, such as homeopathic doctors and chiropractors, claimed that fluoridation caused heart disease, cancer, kidney damage, birth defects, and other ailments. Scientists also argued that not enough testing of fluoridation had been done; they based this charge on the fact that the USPHS had endorsed fluoridation before its own clinical trials of fluoridation had been completed. Other scientists, such as Dr. John Yiamouyiannis and Dr. Dean Burk, stated that enough research had been done on fluoridation to prove that it was either dangerous or ineffective, or both. They challenged the idea of delivering either a safe or sufficient dose of fluoride through drinking water, arguing instead that children could be given fluoride more easily and safely through tablets, drops, fluoridated bottled water, or milk. Lastly, some medical and scientific professionals argued that fluoridation only delayed dental decay, or that fluoride had the undesirable side effect of staining teeth brown.[8]

Dr. George L. Waldbott, a Michigan allergist, was a typical medical opponent to fluoridation. He fought against fluoridation from the 1950s until his death in 1982. In his book, *A Struggle With Titans: Forces behind Fluoridation*, he described how he was a mainstream doctor who accepted most conventional medical views until his own research into the issue and experiences with patients allergic to fluoride convinced him that the medical establishment was wrong about fluoridation. To establish his mainstream credentials, he went so far as to note that he had volunteered to administer polio vaccine at his local public school, even though many anti-fluoridationists also objected to vaccinations, in particular the polio vaccine. As a prominent anti-fluoridationist, he lent support to local anti-fluoridation campaigns nationwide, wrote numerous books and articles on the subject, and testified in public hearings and court cases against fluoridation in the United States and abroad. With his encouragement, his wife founded and initially edited the *National Fluoridation News*, the longest-surviving and largest anti-fluoridation periodical.[9]

Pro-fluoridationists dismissed medical and scientific opponents as a fringe group composed of individuals either meddling in issues outside their area of expertise or with questionable backgrounds and nefarious motives. Anti-fluoridationists, in turn, insisted that the medical and dental professions were filled with opponents to fluoridation, but because a pro-fluoridation minority controlled the professional organizations and institutions, the anti-fluoridation majority was effectively silenced. Stories of how anti-fluoridation doctors and dentists were censored, harassed, or excluded from professional organizations, and of how anti-fluoridation researchers were unable to win grant money to support their research or were unable to publish their research in professional journals, appeared regularly in anti-fluoridation publications such as Dr. Leo Spira's book *The Drama of Fluorine: Arch Enemy of Mankind*. Spira described in his book how individuals in the medical profession worked to stop his research into how both fluoride and aluminum cookware were poisoning people. Not only did he claim that pro-fluoridationists prevented him from getting grant money or publishing his findings, he also charged that research institutions, under pressure from the pro-fluoridationists, refused to give him laboratory space to conduct his work. Those stories themselves became evidence that pro-fluoridationists were wrong. If pro-fluoridationists were so sure they were right, opponents asked, why did they attempt to suppress debate over the issue within the professional and scientific communities?[10]

Alternative health practitioners, such as homeopathic doctors, osteopaths, and chiropractors, were particularly vocal in their opposition to fluoridation. According to pro-fluoridationists, these groups fought against fluoridation in retaliation for the mainstream medical profession's attack on the legitimacy of their professions. Most chiropractors and osteopaths stressed how opposition to fluoridation fit in with their belief in the benefits of a diet of unrefined natural foods. They stressed that fluoride was a manufactured chemical unnaturally added to pure drinking water, or that fluoride allowed people to eat more refined sugar and processed foods and still avoid tooth decay.[11]

Individuals without professional medical or scientific backgrounds, such as health food enthusiasts and environmentalists, also used the same kind of arguments. Anti-fluoridation books directed at the general public often talked about the complex medical and scientific theories of why fluoride was dangerous, and pamphlets provided bibliographical references to anti-fluoridation scientific publications and studies.[12] This reflected the deeply held anti-fluoridationist view that, despite the complex issues involved, the average American could understand fluoridation. Dr. Exner, in a speech, complained: "I resent the implication that the government, or the P.T.A., or the Junior Chamber of Commerce, loves your children more than you do; or that these people are so much smarter than you are that you can't be educated to give your children what is good for them, and these self-appointed wise men must take over."[13] Not only was the issue something the average American could understand, but anti-fluoridationists believed that the public should insist on knowing all the facts, rather than relying on anyone—either for or against fluoridation—telling them how to vote. Later in that same speech, Exner explained: "I am often asked why you should believe me in preference to the great government experts. The answer is that if you are wise, you won't believe what anyone says simply because of who said it. . . . The best way to be sure you are right is to investigate for yourself, as I have done."[14] In contrast, pro-fluoridationists always worried that the scientific and medical evidence that supported fluoridation was too complex for most people to grasp. One pro-fluoridationist bemoaned: "The average citizen does not have the educational background to sort out claim and counter-claim or to judge which 'authorities' to believe. . . . The sheer bulk of the controversy is itself likely to arouse doubt in the minds of most voters."[15]

Because of these different views, pro-fluoridationists in general believed that administrators or elected officials, advised by public health experts, were best able to decide the issue of fluoridation, but those opposed to fluoridation believed the people should be allowed to decide the issue through referenda. Anti-fluoridationists were confident that if they could fully inform voters about the dangers of fluoridation, they would win these popular votes. As Dr. Exner noted: "I have no fears as to the capacity of the voters to make an intelligent decision on fluoridation when they are given the facts."[16] Pro-fluoridationists, in contrast, saw full public debate over the issue as only confusing and frightening voters, leading ultimately to the defeat of fluoridation at the polls. Warned one pro-fluoridationist: "Overwhelmed by volumes of pseudoscientific information . . . the confused citizenry is unsuccessful in its attempts to collate the claims and counterclaims. The voters therefore tend to be swayed by the advice of whichever group most successfully earns their trust during the campaign."[17]

Just as health enthusiasts and alternative health practitioners were attracted to the movement, organizations that supported these views often spoke out against fluoridation. The American Association for Medico-Physical Research, the National Health Federation (NHF), the Citizens Medical Reference Bureau, and the Lee Foundation for Nutritional Research were not originally anti-fluoridation organizations, but their views on medicine and health meshed nicely with anti-fluoridation medical and scientific arguments. The American Association for Medico-Physical Research was originally concerned with defending alternative cancer treatments, such as "oxygen therapy," but embraced anti-fluoridationism because it believed the federal government had no right to dictate an individual's medical treatment, either by forcing someone to drink fluoridated water or by barring someone from receiving an unconventional cancer treatment. The Citizens Medical Reference Bureau also objected to government intervention in the medical field through such measures as compulsory vaccination and the regulation of cancer treatments. The NHF, founded by Fred J. Hart, a California farmer, rancher, and businessman, worked for an end to government intervention in the medical field, such as the Food and Drug Administration's efforts to suppress alternative cancer treatments such as laetrile, and to regulate vitamins and nutritional supplements. The federation also categorized fluoridation as an example of excessive government intervention in an individual's health. The Lee Foundation for Nutritional Research, whose stated mission was to investigate and disseminate information about nutrition, sold anti-fluoridation books and pamphlets because it associated healthy food with healthy drinking water.[18]

In contrast to anti-fluoridationists who objected to fluoridation for medical or scientific reasons, those attracted to the movement for religious reasons were probably the smallest part of the movement. Christian Scientists, Jehovah's Witnesses, and Seventh-Day Adventists were most likely to disapprove of fluoridation because of their religion, based on the premise that fluoridation was a medication. If fluoridation was defined as medicine, drinking fluoridated water could be considered a sin for these individuals because their religions forbid the use of medication. They claimed that government-imposed fluoridation violated their First and Fourteenth Amendment rights to practice their religion.[19]

Throughout the 1950s and 1960s, anti-fluoridationists, without success, challenged fluoridation in state and federal courts using the argument that the health measure was unconstitutional. Typically the courts ruled that fluoridation was not medicine, since fluoride naturally occurred in some water supplies, or that fluoridation did not infringe on anyone's religious beliefs or their freedom to practice their beliefs because alternatives to public drinking water were available. Still, anti-fluoridationists continued to imply that fluoridation would eventually be found unconstitutional. They claimed that the Supreme Court had never ruled it constitutional. This was true, but only because the Supreme Court had always declined to consider any anti-fluoridation cases.[20]

The other large category of anti-fluoridation objections were philosophical, and these were primarily put forth by political conservatives. Conservative anti-fluoridationists contended that fluoridation was an infringement of individual liberties because whenever a community began fluoridation, individuals who objected to fluorides were forced to ingest it. Whether voters or government officials chose to begin fluoridation was irrelevant to these anti-fluoridationists. Regardless of how fluoridation was implemented, there would always be a minority that was losing control over its bodies.[21]

Conservative anti-fluoridationists also saw fluoridation as only one example of a growing threat to American liberties. They warned that America was slowly becoming socialist or totalitarian, as the federal government was gradually taking over control of the individual's life. Fluoridation was socialized medicine because government tax revenues would pay for medicine and the machinery to distribute it through public water supplies. It was totalitarian because the government was dictating to individuals how they would live their lives. Explained an anti-fluoridationist in the preface of William R. Cox's book *Hello, Test Animals . . . Chinchillas or You and Your Grandchildren?*, "Totalitarian government is not confined to forcing everyone to vote for the same dictator, or go to the same church. It involves also the elimination of liberty to choose your food and drink, choose your remedy for disease, choose your own poison drug in which you may have confidence."[22] Many anti-fluoridationists warned that fluoridation was only the beginning: "Already there is serious talk of inserting birth-control drugs in public water supplies, and growing whispers of a happier and more manageable society if so-called behavioral drugs are mass-applied."[23] This was, according to these anti-fluoridationists, why the USPHS and local health departments were so eager to enact fluoridation, so that the stage would be set for more ambitious programs.[24]

A subgroup existed among the conservatives who objected to fluoridation: those who believed that fluoridation was an actual communist plot to destroy America. For them, the possibility that fluoridation would lead to communism was not a philosophical abstraction or something that would occur as America gradually abandoned its traditional values and freedoms, as other conservative anti-fluoridationists claimed; fluoridation was actually a weapon being used by communists to attempt to kill literally millions of Americans. These anti-fluoridationists stressed the poisonous nature of fluoride, arguing either that long-term consumption would kill or sicken Americans, making the country vulnerable to an invasion by the Soviet Union, or that communist agents would use fluoride equipment installed at water treatment plants to give a sudden lethal dose to the American population, killing off millions before the Soviet Union seized control of the country. One Michigan anti-fluoridationist described how strategically significant cities, such as Sault Ste. Marie, might fall through fluoridation:

[P]erhaps not more than 6 to 10 of their agents could quietly move into the water plant at the Soo [Sault Ste. Marie] . . . finish off the unsuspecting operators and . . . introduce lethal amounts of this stuff into the water. It has no odor, nor color and without suspecting it by taste either, within a few hours a large proportion of the population would be corpses leaving all the facilities of the city with its store of supplies intact. The Locks would be in their hands.[25]

Others believed that long-term exposure to fluoride would cause mental weakness, sterility, or cancer, any of which would make Americans unable to raise an army capable of repulsing a Soviet invasion.[26]

Communist-conspiracy anti-fluoridationists were not only laypersons caught up in the hysteria of the McCarthy era. Some of them also objected to fluoridation for medical reasons but used the communist conspiracy to explain why something so dangerous as fluoride was being promoted as a health measure. Dr. Charles Betts, a dentist from Ohio, was one such anti-fluoridationist. As president of the Anti-Cancer Club of America, he had promoted the idea that food cooked in aluminum cookware caused cancer. He also spoke out publicly against vaccination and pasteurization.[27] Betts argued that fluoridation was being promoted by the aluminum industry, which was inadvertently doing the communists' dirty work. He noted that fluoridation was "better THAN USING THE ATOM BOMB *because* the atom bomb has to be made, has to be transported to the place it is to be set off while POISONOUS FLUORINE has been placed right beside the water supplies by the Americans themselves ready to be dumped into the water mains whenever a Communist desires!"[28]

Dr. Betts was not the only medical or scientific anti-fluoridationist to believe in the communist conspiracy theory. Dr. E. H. Bronner, a research chemist, wrote extensively in the 1950s about the role of the communists in promoting fluoridation. On flyers offering his services as a public speaker against fluoridation, he claimed to be Albert Einstein's cousin and to have escaped from a Soviet concentration camp where his wife had died. The validity of these claims is uncertain; pro-fluoridationists charged that he had been confined in an Illinois mental institution. Possibly because of pro-fluoridationist efforts to discredit Bronner with these allegations, he was active in the anti-fluoridation movement only in the early 1950s.[29]

Within the broader movement, communist-conspiracy anti-fluoridationists were actually prominent primarily only in the 1950s, during the height of the McCarthy era. By the early 1960s, their presence in the movement was fading. Reflecting the inclusive nature of the anti-fluoridation movement, communist-conspiracy fluoride opponents found acceptance among more mainstream anti-fluoridationists, even those who rejected their fears. For example, the Lee Foundation for Nutritional Research, although mainly concerned with medical and scientific objections to fluoridation, reprinted and sold materials warning about a communist fluoridation conspiracy.[30] *American Capsule News*, a newsletter that generally argued that fluoridation was the result of business and government corruption, noted a possible link to communism:

> The USPublic [*sic*] Health Service has been corrupted by the Aluminum Trust. . . . The Soviet General Staff is very happy about it. Anytime they get ready to strike, and their 5th column takes over, there are tons and tons of this poison "standing by" municipal and military water systems ready to be poured in within 15 minutes.[31]

American Capsule News believed that fluoridation was a conspiracy between corporate America and the federal government to make a profit off the disposal of a toxic manufacturing waste product, but the periodical was willing to concede that communists might also be able to take advantage of the program. This stance was typical of how other anti-fluoridationists regarded the communist-conspiracy arguments: they held to their own fears about fluoridation but were willing to accept that there might also be a communist conspiracy.

Despite this acceptance and occasional use of communist-conspiracy anti-fluoridationists' ideas, many fluoride opponents were aware that the communist-conspiracy argument often undermined their cause. Pro-fluoridationists used the communist-conspiracy argument as evidence that all anti-fluoridationists were crackpots. Dr. Exner, speaking at an anti-fluoridation convention in the early 1960s, stated:

> A good example [of a bad argument against fluoridation] is the frequently heard argument that fluoridation is a communist plot. In the first place, it is not. . . .
>
> It is true that the communists are for it. *The Daily Worker* has promoted it, which should be proof enough. Communists will jump on any band wagon that furthers their ends; but fluoridation is not their band wagon and never was. They merely climbed on board.
>
> But the important thing is that most people are not prepared to believe that fluoridation is a communist plot, and if you say it is, you are successfully ridiculed by the promoters. It is being done, effectively, every day . . . some of the people on our side are the fluoridators' "fifth column."[32]

Interestingly, although Exner does not believe in the communist-conspiracy argument, he did not denounce those anti-fluoridationists who believed it, except to point out that they were a liability for the movement. Indeed, mainstream anti-fluoridationists never argued publicly that those believing in the communist conspiracy should be ostracized by the movement, or ridiculed them as pro-fluoridationists did.

Over time, though, mainstream anti-fluoridationists did distance themselves from the argument in much the way Dr. Exner did. As the extreme fears of the McCarthy era faded away, the communist-conspiracy argument exposed the movement to public ridicule. By the mid-1960s, the belief that fluoridation was a communist plot had become even more associated in the public mind with irrational fear and paranoia. The most well-known example of this was the movie *Dr. Strangelove: Or How I Learned to Stop Worrying and Love the Bomb* (1964), in which a character initiated a nuclear war because of his fear of fluoridation. But other less memorable movies of the 1960s, such as *In Like Flint* (1967), used the fear of fluoridation to indicate that a character was insane.

In addition to the communists, possible conspirators involved in the promotion of fluoridation included the aluminum industry, the sugar industry, corporate America in general, and the federal government. For anti-fluoridationists, the history of fluoridation provided substantial support for these conspiracy theories. When fluoridation was first studied, the USPHS had been part of the Federal Security Administration, whose director, Oscar Ewing, had previously been an attorney for the Aluminum Corporation of America (ALCOA), which produced fluoride compounds as a by-product of aluminum manufacturing. According to anti-fluoridationists, Ewing spearheaded the promotion of fluoridation in order to solve the problem of how the aluminum industry could dispose of a dangerous waste product.[33]

Another group of anti-fluoridationists believed that other large corporations manufacturing products such as bricks and glass were behind the promotion of fluoridation, because they also were having difficulty disposing of the fluoride compounds created by the manufacturing of their products. Gladys Caldwell, in her book *Fluoridation and Truth Decay,* insisted: "No, I don't think fluoridation is a Communist plot; it is Industry's scheme to camouflage their deadliest pollutant, with government officials and Madison Avenue advertisers beating the drums."[34] Still others blamed the sugar industry or the food industry in general, which wanted a way to prevent tooth decay without limiting people's consumption of refined sugars and processed foods. James Rorty, in the introduction to *The American Fluoridation Experiment,* noted: "Among the earliest advocates of the program [promoting fluoridation] was the Sugar Research Foundation, which is the research and propaganda arm of the sugar-refining industry. The Foundation had been giving generous support to *ad hoc* investigations to show that America's 100-pound-per-capita annual consumption of sugar was not excessive."[35] The federal government itself might be part of the conspiracy, either as a patsy of business interests or as an organization dominated by power-hungry bureaucrats trying to expand federal power at the expense of civil liberties. And belief in one conspiracy theory did not necessarily rule out acceptance of other conspirators: as in the case of *American Capsule News,* anti-fluoridationists could reconcile different theories by suggesting that various groups were working together or exploiting each other's actions.

ANTI-FLUORIDATIONISTS ON THE NATIONAL POLITICAL STAGE
Several factors worked to discourage national action against fluoridation: the local nature of public water supplies, the lack of interest in the issue within the major political parties, and the federal government's role in promoting fluoridation. Despite this, anti-fluoridationists did very much attempt to interject the fluoridation issue into national politics. These efforts included bringing the issue before Congress and calling to task presidential administrations for their support of fluoridation, as well as seeking to relate fluoridation to other national political issues.

When the issue of fluoridation first came before Congress, anti-fluoridationists suf-fered a serious defeat: in June 1951, Congress passed a bill to fluoridate the water supply of the District of Columbia. Within a few months, though, the bill's sponsor, Republican representative A. L. Miller of Nebraska, who had been a practicing physician and state health official before becoming a congressman, changed his mind about fluoridation, claiming he had been misled by the USPHS.[36] Miller convinced the House Select Committee to Investigate the Use of Chemicals in Foods and Cosmetics, led by Democratic Representative James J. Delaney of New York, to hold hearings on fluoridation for seven days in March 1952. The hearings were limited in scope, focusing solely on the safety and effectiveness of fluoridation and hearing testimony from only scientific and medical witnesses. The opposition stressed the inadequacy of scientific knowledge of fluoride and recommended that more research be done before the wide promotion of fluoridation. Proponents, mostly from various national organizations that had endorsed fluoridation, insisted that there was adequate evidence to justify the widespread promotion of fluoridation.[37]

Representative Miller had hoped that the Delaney hearings would call attention to the experimental nature of fluoridation and convince Congress to reverse its position on fluoridation for the District of Columbia, but in May 1952, Congress appropriated the funds needed to begin fluoridating the capital's water supply. The Delaney committee's final report, released in July 1952, also was a disappointment for Miller and the anti-fluoridationists. The report noted that none of the opposition had completely opposed fluoridation and concluded that, based on both the positive and negative scientific opinions, a wait-and-see policy should be adopted. Lastly, it recommended against federal legislation on the issue, arguing that local communities could best settle the issue.[38]

Anti-fluoridationists were undeterred by the Delaney committee's recommendation, and they continued to push for national anti-fluoridation legislation. In May 1954, Minnesota anti-fluoridationists convinced their representative, Democrat Roy W. Wier, to sponsor a sweeping anti-fluoridation bill.[39] It not only would have barred the federal government from promoting fluoridation and fluoridating federal facilities, such as military bases, but also would have barred state and local government from fluoridating their water supplies, even if authorized by a referendum. The hearings on the bill were held by the House Committee on Interstate and Foreign Commerce, chaired by Republican representative Charles A. Wolverton of New Jersey, in late May 1954.[40]

Unlike the Delaney committee, the Wolverton committee heard testimony regarding philosophical and moral objections to fluoridation, and the opposition completely rejected fluoridation, rather than advocating more research before its adoption. Witnesses included not only dentists, doctors, and researchers, but lay individuals, including religious objectors and communist-conspiracy anti-fluoridationists. Once again, pro-fluoridationists from organizations such as the USPHS, ADA, and AMA spoke out in favor of fluoridation. Ultimately the Wolverton committee was unconvinced by the anti-fluoridationists' testimony and the bill died in committee.[41]

Even though the Delaney and Wolverton hearings did not produce anti-fluoridation legislation, they were a strategic victory for the opponents of fluoride. Anti-fluoridationists were able to quote the negative testimony from these hearings in their letters to editors, pamphlets, and flyers without mentioning the results of those hearings, suggesting to the uninformed that fluoridation was a questionable practice. Both hearings provided scientific quotes arguing that not enough research had been done on fluoridation, or questioning the USPHS's judgment regarding the dangers of fluoride. The transcripts of the Wolverton hearings in particular became a reference book with materials supporting a wide range of anti-fluoridation arguments. In addition to testimony presented at the hearings, the transcripts contained letters and petitions from individuals and groups who did not attend the hearings, giving the impression that most of the witnesses before the committee opposed fluoridation. And to many anti-fluoridationists, the accusations of a conspiracy behind the promotion of fluoridation gained a measure of legitimacy by being aired before a congressional committee.[42]

Fluoride opponents were not deterred by these early setbacks in Congress. They continued to push for national anti-fluoridation legislation. The major political parties were indifferent to the fluoridation issue, but anti-fluoridationists found that through lobbying, they could win over individual politicians, such as Representative Miller, who were willing to sponsor bills or amendments.

Letter-writing campaigns were one example of how anti-fluoridationists across the country lobbied Congress. Representative Wier testified before the Wolverton committee that "during my 6 years here [in Congress] . . . I have received more mail and communications and material for the bill now before you than on any other subject or issue pending in the Congress during those 6 years."[43] One campaign in 1956 was typical: anti-fluoridationists attempted to get legislation passed that would bar the USPHS from using federal funds to promote fluoridation. The sponsors of the campaign were politically astute. They warned participants that "this plan . . . should not become known to proponents . . . (to head off counter measures)" and advised participants to "use scientific rather than emotional appeal, only facts, not opinions; avoid offensive terms (rat poison); refrain from name-calling, these hurt our cause; reference to communism is not recommended because at this time it will prejudice Congressmen."[44] Aware that pro-fluoridationists stereotyped their opponents as crackpots and fanatics, the sponsors of this campaign clearly wanted to avoid confirming this image.

Anti-fluoridationist groups also introduced legislation at the state level. In 1953, the Connecticut, Massachusetts, and California legislatures defeated bills prohibiting fluoridation. The Wisconsin legislature voted against an anti-fluoridation bill in 1955; that same year, similar bills died in committee in Virginia. In many states, anti-fluoridationists introduced bills regularly: anti-fluoridationists submitted 70 bills to the Massachusetts legislature between 1969 and 1978.[45] In Illinois and New Hampshire in this same period, anti-fluoridationists did not try to ban fluoridation outright but instead attempted to pass laws requiring a referendum before a community could enact fluoridation. Anti-fluoridationists favored these laws because, more often than not, communities rejected fluoridation in referenda.[46]

Statistical data justified this attitude: between 1977 and 1979, fluoridation was defeated on average in four out of five elections.[47] Laws requiring a referendum before the adoption of fluoridation in a community hindered fluoridation. Those laws made it impossible for pro-fluoridationists to enact fluoridation quietly by lobbying city governments and water boards. Winning a fluoridation referendum almost always required a sophisticated and time-consuming public campaign, and even such a campaign did not guarantee that fluoridation would win. So too, when anti-fluoridationists lost a referendum, they often did not give up. They would begin lobbying for another referendum on the issue, requiring pro-fluoridationists to continue their campaign promoting fluoridation in order to maintain public support for the measure.[48]

Maine, New Hampshire, Delaware, Nevada, and Utah, five states that between 1957 and 1976 enacted laws requiring a referendum, were also the least fluoridated states in America in 1979. From 1958 to 1968, Massachusetts also had such a law. At the time of the law's repeal, only 7 percent of Massachusetts' population drank fluoridated water, but by 1978, without the law, over 50 percent of the population had fluoridated water.[49]

In the 1970s, anti-fluoridationists took advantage of a new tool: the statewide referendum. In 1976, anti-fluoridationists were able to get statewide initiatives to prohibit fluoridation in Oregon and Washington on the ballot, and in Utah a statewide initiative to require a referendum before a community could fluoridate. Of the three states, only Utah passed its initiative, but this was just the beginning of a renewed effort to fight fluoridation at the state level that included pushing for a statewide ban in Pennsylvania and weakening Minnesota's mandatory fluoridation law.[50] Also in the 1970s, even when they did lose a referendum, anti-fluoridationists worked to stop fluoridation by attempting, with mixed success, to block local and state appropriation measures to pay for fluoridation.[51]

Compared to their lobbying of Congress and state legislators, anti-fluoridationists made almost no effort to convince presidential candidates that fluoridation was wrong. While individuals sometimes wrote presidents and presidential candidates about fluoridation, the lack of organized lobbying reflected the general belief among anti-fluoridationists that presidents were completely dominated by the pro-fluoridationists in the USPHS. Instead of trying to convince presidents that fluoridation was wrong, anti-fluoridationists viewed presidents as adversaries, holding them responsible for the policies of hostile federal agencies. Anti-fluoridationists were especially critical of how presidents' positions on fluoridation appeared to contradict values these presidents had publicly embraced. This can be seen especially in the case of Presidents Dwight D. Eisenhower and James E. Carter.

In the case of Eisenhower, anti-fluoridationists were particularly disappointed with his acceptance of fluoridation because initially they had expected he might change the federal government's policy on fluoridation. Upon his election, they were led to believe he would support their movement because he had spoken out against government bureaucracy and intervention, especially in health matters, and in favor of individualism and freedom, all ideas that antis were fighting for. Much to their disappointment, Eisenhower not only continued Truman's policies toward fluoridation, but also publicly endorsed fluoridation and was quoted in fluoridation promotional materials.[52]

Anti-fluoridationists dismissed the significance of Eisenhower's endorsement of fluoridation by saying that he had not studied the matter himself, but was just doing what his advisors told him to do. Anti-fluoridationists also minimized the significance of Eisenhower's position on fluoridation by quoting him in their literature as if he actually supported the anti-fluoridation movement. They used quotes from speeches given by Eisenhower warning about the dangers of socialized medicine, in particular a speech he gave at the 1953 AMA national convention. Eisenhower had been attacking proposals for national health insurance, but anti-fluoridationists used his statements as if Eisenhower had included fluoridation in his critique.[53]

Anti-fluoridationists criticized Presidents Kennedy, Johnson, Nixon, and Ford less often, but when they attacked these presidents for their policies, it was also over the perceived conflict between presidential rhetoric and actions. For example, anti-fluoridationists believed early on in his administration that Richard M. Nixon might end the promotion of fluoridation because of comments in his first State of the Union address regarding water pollution.[54] In that case, fluoride opponents defined fluoridation as a form of water pollution, but the Nixon administration did not.

Anti-fluoridationists also misinterpreted President Carter's comments on human rights as favorable to their cause. When the opposite proved true, they bitterly denounced Carter. An article in the *National Fluoridation News* complained: "Apparently President Carter's Human Rights program is nothing but political rhetoric. He proposes to force all Americans to drink medicated water contrary to their medical, health, religious, moral and ethical beliefs."[55] The article's author then predicted that his position might cost him votes in the next election: "If the President pursues his present political path of alienating large blocs of voters such as farmers, blacks, and now all those who vote against fluoridation, he could very well be a one-term president."[56] Other anti-fluoridationists echoed the idea that they could make a difference in the voting booth, despite a complete lack of evidence that they had an impact on presidential politics. Nor were there any organized efforts among anti-fluoridationists to influence presidential elections. For example, they issued no call to vote against President Gerald Ford, even though, of all presidents, he was the most obviously pro-fluoridationist. He came from an area in Michigan that had been among the first places to adopt fluoridation, and his voting record had always been pro-fluoridation. Most damning of all, he had testified in favor of fluoridation as early as at the Wolverton hearings.[57]

What is more striking about the quote suggesting Carter's fluoridation stance would cost him votes is how the author equated anti-fluoridationists with other interest groups, such as farmers and blacks. Anti-fluoridationists never believed that they were a fringe group, as the pro-fluoridationists always insisted. With good reason, anti-fluoridationists interpreted their successes in defeating fluoridation in referendum after referendum as proof of widespread support for their views. Dr. Exner noted, "As to our being a minority. Actually, and with rare exceptions, whenever the people have been permitted to vote on fluoridation they have voted it down, usually by overwhelming majorities."[58] In contrast, pro-fluoridationists always explained the defeat of fluoridation at the ballot box as evidence of voter ignorance, confusion, or fear, or as a result of low voter turnout.[59] One pro-fluoridationist vocalized the frustration of pro-fluoridationists everywhere: "It is shocking but true that many people, even after they listen to professional advice—carefully, competently and intelligently given—blithely ignore it in favour of what they have been told and frightened into by someone with no professional background whatsoever."[60] These divergent interpretations of referenda are the basis for pro-fluoridationists' view of their opponents as a fringe movement and anti-fluoridationists' self-image as a popular mainstream movement.

In terms of presidential politics, anti-fluoridationists were ultimately nothing more than spectators and commentators, but their views on the presidents reveal a movement that saw itself as part of the American political scene and as an active participant in contemporary politics. In addition to their efforts to lobby Congress or challenge presidential policies, anti-fluoridationists sought to fit themselves into the mainstream of American politics by relating their movement to other political issues of the time.

Anti-fluoridationists were especially successful at connecting fluoridation with the larger battles being waged in America in the 1940s, 1950s, and 1960s over a national health insurance program. The medical establishment resisted both the Truman administration's plan for universal compulsory health insurance in the late 1940s and President Eisenhower's moderate efforts to expand access to health insurance. Medical and dental associations, such as the AMA and ADA, launched a $1.5 million campaign to defeat these plans by labeling them "socialized medicine," "communistic," and the first step toward the complete socialization of American society.[61] Successful at first, the medical establishment gradually lost the battle against health insurance legislation. Truman, Eisenhower, and Kennedy's plans were successfully resisted, but Lyndon Johnson, after his 1964 election victory, had the political clout to push through Medicare and Medicaid in spite of AMA efforts to stop it.[62]

As a result of the medical establishment's fight against health insurance legislation, the concept of socialized medicine was publicly debated for nearly twenty years, providing anti-fluoridationists with a vocabulary with which to express their objections to fluoridation. The term "socialized medicine" could accommodate a wide range of objections to fluoridation. To those opposed, fluoridation was socialized medicine because fluoride was being used as a medication when it was added to drinking water, meaning that the government was assuming the role of doctor by prescribing medicine for an entire population. Other anti-fluoridationists claimed fluoridation was socialized medicine because public funds were being used to pay for the medication and the system used to deliver it. Explained one anti-fluoridationist:

> When [a] mechanism is installed for feeding fluorides into the drinking-water, the taxpayer foots the bill. There you have "SOCIALIZED MEDICINE" as certainly as you have it in Socialist Britain or in Communist Russia. Fluorides are crammed down the throats of the people against their wills. They are taxed for "medication."[63]

Others labeled it "socialized" because of its compulsory nature; whenever fluoridation was enacted, everyone was compelled to drink it. One anti-fluoridationist dentist complained:

> As a professional group, we [dentists] have hitherto opposed socialistic practice in all its forms. . . . Have we not denounced every effort that would compel the layman to accept volume dentistry and to submit to the service of a dentist whom he may not choose? . . . Yet now we are sponsoring a program that will necessarily compel everyone from infant to grandfather to drink fluoridated water whether he wants it or not, whether it jeopardizes his life or not.[64]

Besides offering a vocabulary, the medical and dental professions' fight against national health legislation provided anti-fluoridationists with an enemy about which the public was already sensitized. Anti-fluoridationists directly related one issue to the other: "Those same political bosses [officials in the USPHS] are hell-bent for Socialized Medicine and since they couldn't foist it upon the public through legislation, now they're sneaking it in via the back door in the form of fluoridation."[65] The medical establishment's public relations campaign had already familiarized the American public with the specter of excessive government intervention, and the anti-fluoridationists were riding on the medical establishment's coattails by associating the evil of national health insurance with the evil of fluoridation.

Although the accusation that fluoridation was socialized medicine was reflective of the broader debate in America about the role of the federal government in medicine, the term put a name on a specific fear that was always at the heart of the anti-fluoridation move-ment. In 1966, one anti-fluoridationist wrote in a letter to the editor of the *National Fluo-ridation News*: "The latest plan of the United States Public Health Service to compel fluoridation . . . reveals it for just what it is—compulsory mass medication that destroys our most precious human right, protected by our Constitution, to choose what we shall put into our systems."[66] The fear of losing personal control and freedom had always been present in the movement and actually outlasted the use of the term "socialized medicine." In the 1970s and 1980s, that fear, renamed "compulsory mass medication," could be seen in warnings in anti-fluoridation literature that fluoridation "deprived all consumers of pub-lic water of their right to choose what medical advice and medication they will accept or reject for themselves and their children."[67] Even as the terminology changed, then, the fear of government intrusion has remained a constant theme in the movement.

In contrast to the issue of socialized medicine, anti-fluoridationists' efforts to associate themselves with the civil rights movement were a failure. Anti-fluoridationists in the 1960s sought to attract supporters of civil rights to their movement by linking the issue of mi-nority rights with freedom from fluoridation:

> Recent pressures for establishment and maintenance of the sanctity of civil liberties with regard to certain minority groups stand out in incongruous contrast to the apparent deliber-ate repudiation of civil liberties in the case of fluoridation.
>
> We are asked, or told, that we should surrender our basic right to refuse to take a drug so that those children under 8, who may benefit, can avail themselves of it. Depriving anyone of this basic right is unjustifiable.[68]

Another anti-fluoridationist asked in a 1968 article in the *National Fluoridation News*: "Why, at the very moment that we are so concerned with the 'dignity of man' and the civil rights of minorities, do we seem to be forgetting, in our zeal for health, that the ultimate minority is the individual?"[69] Despite these attempts to define fluoridation as a civil rights issue, anti-fluoridationists did not win support from the civil rights movement for their cause.

Attempts to equate opposition to fluoridation with demands for minority rights might appear exploitive, but they were not. Anti-fluoridationists truly believed that their cause should be part of the civil rights movement. They had often used the term "civil rights" in their discourse. Typical of this was the letter an anti-fluoridationists wrote in 1958 to the *New York Times*: "To me, it is an invasion of my civil rights to have *anything* put into my water supply."[70] Anti-fluoridationists genuinely could not understand why organizations and prominent individuals in the civil rights movement did not support their cause. In a letter to the editor of the *National Fluoridation News*, one person wrote: "I call upon the ACLU [American Civil Liberties Union] . . . to reconsider its decision [not to support the anti-fluoridation movement] and to join the anti-fluoridation forces. I feel that the right to choose one's own medication should be defended."[71] New York City mayor Robert Wagner Jr. actively supported the fluoridation of the city water supply in the 1960s. In reference to his support of the civil rights movement, an anti-fluoridationist asked in a letter to the edi-tor of the *New York Times*: "Now that Mayor Wagner has concurred fully in the fight for civil rights, what about the right of all citizens to decide what they shall or shall not ingest?"[72]

Anti-fluoridationists also tried during the 1960s and 1970s to relate their movement to the consumer movement, in part because they had already embraced much of that movement's rhetoric. As early as the 1950s, the anti-fluoridationists related their crusade to the Progressive-era food safety legislation and the efforts then to fight adulterated foods and drinks. In particular, they claimed as their hero Dr. Harvey W. Wiley, head of the Department of Agriculture's Division of Chemistry from 1883 to 1912, who had focused on food safety issues and worked for the passage of the Pure Food and Drug Act.[73] "My attitude is simply that of many other citizens who feel as did Dr. Harvey W. Wiley, that it is a bad practice to permit the adulteration of any food or drink with poisons in any amount whatever, regardless of the smallness or assumed insignificance of the amount," an anti-fluoridationist wrote in 1951.[74] Anti-fluoridationists sympathized not only with Wiley's struggle to improve the food Americans ate, but also with the fact that Wiley was forced out of his job in 1912 because of political pressure placed on the federal government by business interests. His experience supported their own belief that business interests were behind the federal government's promotion of fluoridation.[75]

In the 1960s and 1970s, a number of exposés, such as Rachel Carson's *Silent Spring*, reinvigorated the consumer movement in America. Anti-fluoridationists tapped into this new spirit by beginning to define fluoridation in terms of the consumer issues of fraud and misuse of tax funds. Gladys Caldwell, in the introduction to her book *Fluoridation and Truth Decay*, called fluoridation the "most disastrous and costly consumer fraud of this polluted century."[76] Anti-fluoridationists insisted that the issue should concern everyone, even people in communities without fluoridation, because pro-fluoridationists were using federal tax dollars to promote fluoridation. Pro-fluoridationists were "soaking the U.S. taxpayers with artificially fluoridated water."[77]

Like civil rights supporters, consumer advocates disappointed anti-fluoridationists with their lack of support for the cause. One anti-fluoridationist wondered in a letter to the *National Fluoridation News* in 1971 why senators who supported strong consumer protection legislation also supported federal funding for community fluoridation programs: "how can anyone who supports legislation to protect the health and lives of consumers, simultaneously support legislation which promotes further pollution of nature's elements whether they be air, water or vegetation?"[78] Not only did some consumer advocates support fluoridation, a few consumer groups actually attacked anti-fluoridationists. Consumers Union published a two-part series supporting fluoridation and critical of the anti-fluoridation movement in its magazine, *Consumer Reports*, in 1978. The Lehigh Valley Committee against Health Fraud classed anti-fluoridationists with occult healers, fad diets, and healing cults in its 1980 book *The Health Robbers*. Through the publication of books such as *The Health Robbers* and *The Tooth Robbers*, a collection of pro-fluoridation articles, the Lehigh Valley Committee against Health Fraud attacked faith healers, vitamin sellers, and the promoters of alternative cancer treatments such as laetrile. Anti-fluoridationists were unique among those the committee attacked because they were not selling anything.[79]

The exception to the general apathy or hostility of the consumer movement was Ralph Nader. Nader did not actively fight against fluoridation, but throughout the 1970s he questioned publicly the cost-effectiveness and environmental impact of fluoridation and criticized pro-fluoridationists for their hostility toward debate on the issue. Anti-fluoridation publications, such as the *National Fluoridation News*, eagerly reported Nader's accusation that fluoridated toothpaste ads exaggerated the benefits of their use. Nader was an isolated case, though, and even he never did more than publicly question the practice.[80]

ANTI-FLUORIDATIONISTS AND THE AMERICAN POLITICAL TRADITION
Beyond relating their movement to contemporary political and social issues, the anti-fluoridationists also pointedly defined themselves within the American political tradition. They angrily rejected the "lunatic fringe" stereotype that pro-fluoridationists had successfully created. Anti-fluoridationists evoked such icons of American culture as the Constitution, the Bill of Rights, and the Founding Fathers. They insisted that they were fighting for core American values such as freedom, democracy, and liberty and couched their arguments in terms typical of American politics, such as "un-American" and "tyranny."

The American Revolution and the founding of the nation were a particularly important theme in anti-fluoridationist literature. An announcement of the Wolverton hearings in a health organization's bulletin, for example, called on "Minute Men of Medical Freedom" to register their support for the bill.[81] Anti-fluoridationists not only compared themselves to those who had helped found the nation, but also drew inspiration and encouragement from the past. A prominent anti-fluoridationist in the 1970s, Gladys Caldwell, wrote in her book *Fluoridation and Truth Decay:* "George Washington did not cross the Delaware on that blustery Christmas night in 1776 to found a country whose presidents would permit pillorying of scientists and doctors for telling the unpolluted truth two centuries later."[82] An anti-fluoridationist at the Wolverton hearings evoked America's past as setting a precedent for the rejection of fluoridation: "At the risk of their lives, their fortunes, and their sacred honor, our fathers fought and died to establish in this country—not a so-called democracy that would allow any majority vote to tyrannize a helpless minority—but a Republic, with a Constitution."[83] Implicit in these quotes is the idea that fluoridation and the behavior of pro-fluoridationists were un-American and not consistent with the values that had led to the nation's founding.

Of all American values, democracy was perhaps the most important to anti-fluoridationists. According to them, their opponents' efforts to enact fluoridation without a referendum threatened the nation's democratic tradition. Anti-fluoridationists warned that pro-fluoridationists were setting a dangerous precedent by pushing for the adoption of fluoridation through administrative measures. The *National Health Federation Bulletin* reprinted an editorial from a California newspaper that challenged the pro-fluoridationists' reasons for avoiding referenda:

> [If] the people of the East Bay [San Francisco area] are adjudged so stupid that they cannot be trusted to pass on the matter of fluoridation—as they did three years ago when they rejected it—then, as any fool can plainly see, there will soon be other matters on which they are not intelligent enough to decide also. . . . If the mass of the citizenry . . . cannot be trusted to vote on fluoridation, why should they be considered intelligent enough to vote for their choice of officials who might get us into war or bring us a dangerous peace?[84]

As with most aspects of the movement, there were those who went to the extreme. A few anti-fluoridationists rejected even democratic measures as a legitimate way to settle the question. Fluoridation of public water supplies, regardless of whether people voted on it or an administrative body enacted it, could never be acceptable because some members of society would always be forced to consume fluoride against their will. One anti-fluoridationists wrote to the editor of the *New York Times* in 1974, responding to another anti-fluoridationist's letter: "Although I agree ... that compulsory fluoridation ... is an abrogation of civil rights, I do not agree that the matter should be resolved by public referendum because I do not believe that my neighbors, any more than my government, should decide whether I drink fluoridated water."[85] Other anti-fluoridationists denied that a majority vote in favor of fluoridation was an example of democracy:

> Many people seem to feel that if a majority can be persuaded to vote in favor of doing something, it is in line with democracy for that something to be done. This is a gross misconception of the nature of democracy, which is primarily concerned with the rights of people as human beings, and not with the dominance of the majority. A majority vote which violates ethical or moral principles or deprives individuals of rights they should be free to enjoy, is not democracy, it is tyranny.[86]

Most anti-fluoridationists did not share this view; they argued instead that when they lost referenda, it was because they were unable to properly inform the voters, or the anti-fluoridationists themselves ran a poor campaign.[87]

For those opposed to it fluoridation was not just a threat to American traditions, it was "un-American" and "alien." Anti-fluoridationists characterized pro-fluoridationists as "this alien influence."[88] Anti-fluoridationsts defined their own cause as patriotic and noble: "As loyal Americans, it becomes our duty to courageously defend and preserve, always, our traditional American heritage of individual freedom!"[89] Dr. Waldbott described the typical anti-fluoridationists as "the cream of this nation's citizenry. They are self-sacrificing, intelligent, independent in their thinking, able to distinguish truth from fiction, willing to stand up and be counted. . . . The ranks of opponents include people from every walk of life, of every creed, color, economic and intellectual status. Outstanding Catholics, Jews, Negroes, Italians, Poles are among the leaders opposed to fluoridation, who have actively helped to spread the truth."[90] The defensive tone in anti-fluoridationists descriptions of themselves was a response to pro-fluoridationists' characterization of the opposition.

For anti-fluoridationists, defining themselves as good Americans and their opponents as "un-American" was not just a way to win over supporters. They needed to give legitimacy to their movement in order to counter the negative labels given to them by pro-fluoridationists. By emphasizing how their movement was consistent with American values and traditions, anti-fluoridationists were directly refuting the idea that they were crackpots and charlatans. Yet despite these efforts, and their regular victories in referenda, anti-fluoridationists were never able to shake the label of "lunatic fringe."

CONCLUSION

Pro-fluoridationists were not the only ones baffled by the longevity and the success of the anti-fluoridation movement. Starting in the 1960s, fluoridation came under the scrutiny of social scientists. They studied nearly every aspect of fluoridation campaigns, from voting patterns to the effects of the media on voters and correlations between type of local government and referendum outcomes. All of these studies made no startling discoveries. Initial studies suggested that those who voted no in fluoridation referenda were most likely to be older, with middle- or lower-class occupations, low incomes, and no children under the age of twelve. Others found a link between education and support for fluoridation: college-educated voters were more likely to vote for fluoridation, but oddly, those with less than an eighth-grade education also favored fluoridation. Studies noted these correlations but could not explain the link between education and fluoridation. Efforts to associate fluoridation with specific political and social attitudes also failed to find distinctive attitudes associated with any particular group. Many studies concluded what pro-fluoridationists already knew: the average voter who rejected fluoridation did so not because of a strong belief in the opposition's charges, but because of vague doubts raised during the campaign.[91]

After studying fluoridation campaigns, sociologists came up with numerous explanations for the reaction to fluoridation. Early researchers proposed that opposition to fluoridation stemmed from anti-scientific attitudes, but most later researchers rejected this as too simplistic. Other researchers suggested that opposition to fluoridation reflected feelings of alienation in society. According to these researchers, anti-fluoridationists' anti-authority attitudes and arguments appealed to those on the social and political margins.[92] Later studies presented evidence that conflicted with this view.[93] Ultimately, social scientists were unable to satisfactorily explain who anti-fluoridationists were and why they were so successful. Pro-fluoridationists had hoped that by knowing why anti-fluoridationists won, they would be able to develop more effective methods of countering them. The failure to explain the movement forced pro-fluoridationists to rely on the difficult and often unsuccessful campaign tactics and education programs they had traditionally used to promote fluoridation.

What pro-fluoridationists and researchers studying the anti-fluoridation movement failed to realize is that the very nature of the anti-fluoridation movement made labels irrelevant. The movement was not made up of one type of person or one group with one set of values. It was a coalition of groups and individuals with a wide range of arguments. That anti-fluoridationists were able to defeat fluoridation time and again was not because they frightened or confused voters, but because their many different objections resonated with a wide range of voters.

Pro-fluoridationists tried to vilify their opponents, but in a sense anti-fluoridationists are an excellent example of good American citizens. Social commentators and politicians have bemoaned the decline in participation in politics in the twentieth century, noting not only the decline in voter participation, but also a growing apathy in society toward the political process. Anti-fluoridationists bucked this trend. They believed in expressing an opinion publicly, in using the political process to communicate with the broader society. They were not a lunatic fringe, quite simply because they—accurately—did not see themselves as outside society. They saw themselves as belonging within and valuing American society and its political traditions.

Judging the anti-fluoridationists and their place in American history is not easy. Reading years of pro and anti propaganda has made someone like me, who does not have a technical background in science or medicine, less sure about who is right or wrong than when I first started. Few individuals have the technical knowledge to evaluate anti-fluoridationist or pro-fluoridationist scientific studies or the other side's critiques of those studies. From my own personal experience, I have nothing but favorable things to say about fluoridation—

I come from a community where the water was fluoridated and I have reached adulthood without a single cavity. However, I am left-handed (which some anti-fluoridationists said could be caused by fluoridation), and I did need braces (some claimed fluoride caused children's teeth to grow in crooked). I brush with fluoridated toothpaste, but when I lived in an area with fluoridated drinking water, I never used the fluoride mouth rinse my dentist would offer me when I got my teeth cleaned. I object to some of the anti-fluoridationists' tactics, but as a post-Watergate, *X-Files*-watching member of Generation X, I am sympathetic to their skepticism of the federal government and "experts" and to their demands for personal control of their bodies. I find something admirable in their passion and willingness to fight— especially early anti-fluoridationists, who used mimeograph machines and typewriters to produce many of their newsletters and flyers. Today, with the Internet and widespread access to technologically sophisticated copying machines and publishing software, it is easy to object and complain. Those early anti-fluoridationists really had to work to get their message out. And the themes of their movement, that individuals should take responsibility for their health and that control over one's body is an important personal freedom, are important lessons that more Americans need to take to heart. On the other hand, many of the pro-fluoridationists were extremely earnest and made valid arguments about the "needs of the many outweighing the will of the few," the impossibility of science ever proving 100 percent that something is safe or effective, the importance of public health, and the responsibility of society to take care of its young. I object to some of the pro-fluoridationists' attitudes toward their opponents, but I also understand how the pro-fluoridationists felt threatened by the anti-fluoridationists and often ambushed by them. In the end, perhaps the value of the anti-fluoridation movement comes not from whether they were right or wrong, but from the example they set of how individuals should value their health and take responsibility for it.

CONTEMPORARY PRACTICES/CONTEMPORARY LEGACIES

ENGENDERING ALTERNATIVES

Women's Health Care Choices and Feminist Medical Rebellions

Amy Sue Bix

EVERY DAY, AMERICAN WOMEN MAKE important choices about their health care, whether deciding to take multivitamin pills or agreeing to undergo risky surgical procedures. Individual decisions are influenced by very personal factors, yet in a broader sense, modern medicine has been thoroughly politicized. The persistent popularity of alternative healing, in particular, represents a vehicle through which people dissatisfied with conventional recommendations may seek to empower themselves in a quest for more satisfactory treatment. Individuals' frustrations may combine with (and in turn be reinforced by) the agendas of oppositional political movements. Major social and cultural trends also play a strong role in promoting options outside standard therapy. This article focuses on women's choices of alternative medicine, particularly in respect to the feminist challenge to the mainstream medical system during the late twentieth century.

Starting in the 1960s and through subsequent years, under the maxim of "the personal as political," feminists transformed discussion of women's health from individual problems into a mutual concern and impetus for action. In protesting against what they perceived as the twin disasters of diethylstilbestrol treatment and the Dalkon Shield, and in rejecting condescending treatment by mainstream health systems, feminist medical rebels embraced alternative concepts. Women's health activists explicitly defined holism as superior to allopathic medicine, not only medically, but also politically and socially, in its sensitivity to gender, race, class, and environmental concerns. They cast the struggle for women's medical choice in terms of a political and philosophical quest for fairness and freedom, deliberately inserting their cause into the history of the civil rights struggle, anti-Vietnam protests, and of course the earlier women's rights movement. Advocates rallied women to stand fast, defending their interest in alternative treatments against scorn and criticism from the male-dominated health care establishment.

Such mobilization led to an intensified political confrontationalism, as feminist critics charged the medical establishment with systematic neglect of women's health. Activist individuals and groups prioritized breast cancer as a particular focus of concern, demanding and often winning recognition of their cause at the highest levels of Washington politics and New York/Hollywood/middle American culture. During the 1980s, controversy also erupted over chronic fatigue syndrome; unhappy with doctors' slowness to acknowledge their complaints as a "real" disease, many women turned to holistic practitioners for sympathy and help. In 2002, research highlighting the dangers of hormone replacement therapy encouraged thousands to explore alternative approaches to menopause.

While feminist leaders and publications touted alternative care as a female-friendly, politically correct improvement over crude, impersonal, masculine-oriented allopathic medicine, holistic healers themselves constructed a personal and political appeal to American women. Herbalists blended New Age goddess mythology with talk of restoring "wise women's" legacy, adding an ecofeminist emphasis linking femininity to the earth. Therapeutic touch and energy healing added a rhetoric of women's empathy and intuition. Practitioners commonly promoted themselves by offering testimony, anecdotes of how they had granted long-suffering individuals relief from serious health problems. Such stories served to personalize the appeal of alternative therapy, cultivating the listener's faith through a personalized, emotional touch rather than through cold statistics. From these critics' viewpoint, the nature of scientific "proof" was questionable and also unnecessary, since they considered it self-evident that nature and holism provided inherently better medicine.

By the end of the twentieth century, commercialization and popular culture had come to reinforce these gendered dimensions of alternative medicine and take them mainstream. Popular general-audience periodicals and women's magazines encouraged female readers to explore holistic treatment, with articles offering accessible (if not always thorough) discussion of options. Manufacturers of herbal supplements and aromatherapy products cultivated female customers with great success. Marketing played on imagery of nature and well-being while evoking emotions ranging from self-indulgence to paranoia. More than that, questions of women's health routinely made front-page headlines, especially with reports of research undermining old assumptions and raising troubling doubts about the "right" course of treatment. Women who in the late 1960s would not have agreed with the feminists discussing cervical self-examination and who had shunned any impression of radicalism might in 2003 find themselves questioning institutionalized dictates on the value of hormone replacement therapy in menopause. The personal and political appeal of alternative medicine had become entwined, creating a new individual and collective context for women's health choices.

WOMEN'S HISTORICAL CONNECTIONS TO ALTERNATIVE MEDICINE

Historically, alternative medicine carried special meaning for American women, as both practitioners and patients. Many colonial-era women gained reputations as valued family nurses, community healers, and midwives who acquired expertise by shadowing experienced practitioners. As formal medical training and professionalization expanded in the early nineteenth century, most allopathic colleges either refused to let female students enroll or limited their numbers. With these doors closed, women sought educational opportunities elsewhere. Many "irregular" institutions embraced coeducation as both a practical measure and a philosophical statement. Hundreds of women attended New York's homeopathic Women's Medical College, the eclectic Penn Medical University, and the American Hydropathic Institute. Some entered sectarian schools out of necessity when access to allopathic education was blocked; others were drawn by ideological commitment to nature cures.[1]

Many female (as well as male) patients were also attracted to alternative medicine by belief in its superiority in healing and by its relative accessibility. Allopathic care was commonly characterized by "heroic" measures, such as bloodletting, purging, and blistering. Doctors defined the violent nature of these procedures as proof of their efficacy, dramatically reflecting the struggle to conquer disease and force it out of the body. However, the physical toll exerted could easily arouse fear and mistrust among observers, especially when physicians failed to save patients. Critics in the 1830s and 1840s warned that many people barely escaped with their lives after being "butchered by pill givers" and poisoned with mercury-based calomel. By contrast, Samuel Hahnemann's homeopathic formulas promised gentle handling, a message that carried a specifically gendered appeal for women to use on themselves and on children.[2]

The popularity of irregular therapy in the mid-1800s reflected not only a backlash against extremes of mainstream medicine, but also nineteenth-century political enthusiasms and social causes. Historian James Whorton has argued that in its defense of free choice, its anti-intellectual emphasis on common sense, and provisions for self-treatment, Samuel Thomson's botanic philosophy "was democratic medicine . . . tailored to fit the desires and biases of the newly enfranchised masses" of the Jacksonian age.[3]

In its emphasis on preventive medicine and self-doctoring, along with its claims to improve on the allopathic approach, sectarian medicine appealed to many women in the nineteenth century. Elizabeth Cady Stanton, Susan B. Anthony, Louisa May Alcott, Harriet Beecher Stowe, Catharine Beecher, and Julia Ward Howe, among other notables, favored various irregular treatments. Describing the "clear links between early feminist reforms and sectarian partisanship," historian of medicine Naomi Rogers writes, "Women sectarians became reformers and entrepreneurs, conscious of the power of their sisters as consumers and patients and even as potential fee-paying students. Feminists in nineteenth-century America saw health reform as a significant part of the women's rights movement."[4]

In attacks on allopathic arrogance, irregular medicine enabled women to question the authority of orthodox male physicians. Indirectly, some (though by no means all) irregular systems also challenged allopathic assumptions of female weakness. Such ideas extended far back; following the philosophy of Aristotle, the ancient Greek physician Galen had idealized men as the true and normal type of human, with women as comparatively incomplete and flawed, physically and intellectually. Over the centuries since, superstition and the misogyny of Church authorities helped perpetuate such assumptions about women's inferiority. Many nineteenth-century scientists and doctors defined women's nature in terms of their reproductive system, which was seen as virtually pathological, causing a long list of emotional, mental and bodily complications. Defining menstruation as a particular source of female vulnerability, Boston doctor Edward Clarke warned society in 1874 against letting young women pursue too demanding an education; other Americans would refer to such assumptions in opposing women's suffrage. Such arguments combined with religious authority, etiquette instruction, and legal restrictions to declare women unsuited for the public sphere of politics, business, and intellectual life. The end result was a connection between issues of women's health and women's rights. In experimenting with dress reform, for example, activists such as Stanton linked women's physical ease to their political, social, and mental freedom.[5]

The role of sectarian medicine in highlighting this alternative vision of female capability rather than weakness and passivity appears notably in the history of hydropathy. In dumping cold water on patients or immersing them in icy pools, this water cure would not be associated with pleasant handling but nonetheless attracted a prominent midcentury clientele, including Anthony and Beecher. Modesty dictated that female patients undergoing immersion should be attended by female staff, and thus, for reasons of propriety, hydropathy welcomed women practitioners. More than that, Susan Cayleff has suggested, rather than focusing on female limitations, hydropathy normalized women's reproductive physiology as part of the natural world. Assuming responsibility for their own well-being, female patients temporarily residing at hydropathy centers could concentrate on personal needs, relieved of daily household responsibilities and family pressures. "[W]ater-cure leaders argued that once patients began controlling their physical lives, the entire spectrum of self-determination and choice was within reach," Cayleff writes. Translating this progressive gender vision into tangible concerns, hydropaths denounced tight corseting as unhealthy and oppressive, encouraging female patients to adopt bloomer dress.[6]

Through the late 1800s and early 1900s, American women continued their involvement with alternative medicine as both practitioners and patients. This trend was especially significant in the history of homeopathy, which capitalized heavily on women's interest. The American Institute of Homeopathy (AIH) voted to accept female members in 1869, forty-six years before the American Medical Association would officially change its bylaws to permit women's admission. Female homeopaths served as delegates to AIH annual meetings throughout this period and were chosen to hold local and national offices, including that of AIH vice president, as Anne Kirschmann has documented. Homeopaths valued women's participation as testers of therapies to treat female diseases, in an ongoing effort to improve homeopathic knowledge and thus subdue dissension in the ranks over choice of treatment. More than that, women constituted a clear majority of homeopathic patients, and advocates looked to the continuation and expansion of this female constituency to help their beleaguered cause remain alive into the twentieth century.[7]

FEMINIST POLITICIZATION OF WOMEN'S HEALTH

Over the first half of the twentieth century, Americans' interest in alternative medicine remained active, especially for cancer and other diseases of desperation. The 1960s and early 1970s would bring a new energy to the nineteenth century's connection between non-mainstream medicine and a drive toward political and social reform. Interest in alternative healing burgeoned in association with the modern cries of rebellion, which rejected authority in medicine as in other mainstream institutions. Instead, the counterculture admired primitive shamanism for its exotic mystery, Chinese medicine for its non-Western emphasis on balance, and herbalism for its harmony with nature. While counterculture critics denounced establishment medicine for narrowness of philosophy, the energetic feminist movement added charges of outright abuse of women's well-being.[8]

Although many strands fed into modern politicization of women's health, one signal development originated from a 1969 Boston-area feminist conference featuring discussion of "women and their bodies." Over continued meetings, participants voiced "frustration and anger toward . . . the medical maze," especially toward "doctors who were condescending, paternalist, judgmental, and non-informative." To fill in the communication gaps, some began reviewing medical information for themselves, a process that "exhilarated and energized" them: "starting to take control over that area of our life . . . has released for us . . . a life-changing effect." Women had lived with "ignorance, uncertainty—even, at worst, shame—about our physical selves" for too long, the group decided. "[B]ody education has been liberating for us and may be a starting point for the liberation of many other women. . . . Learning to understand, accept, and be responsible for our physical selves, we . . . can start to use our untapped energies," becoming "more self-confident, more autonomous, stronger, and more whole."[9]

This personal awakening fed a parallel political transformation, these health feminists declared. In wrenching control over their bodies back from the medical establishment, women would gain courage to challenge it. All but roughly 7 percent of American physicians were male, creating a system that fostered devaluation of women. Medical education promoted sexist stereotyping, as in textbooks instructing gynecologists to measure patients' "femininity quotient." Women must reject such patronizing treatment and refuse to be intimidated by physicians' professional status, activists urged. "Remember: . . . the doctor is no longer a god." Rather than staying silent and dependent on physicians, women must become critical health consumers who "feel entitled to more information [and] . . . demand better."[10]

While gender bias in medical institutions insulted women, the complaints ran, it also contributed directly to specific problems. Too many women lacked access to decent sex education and could not obtain birth control without embarrassing inquisitions by "moralistic and punitive" gynecologists. Due to lack of respect for women's bodily autonomy, many hysterectomies performed in the United States were medically unnecessary. Doctors concentrated narrowly "on treatment of the symptom, isolated both from the rest of the mind and body and from the social context of the illness." Calling for health care alternatives, the Boston group concluded, "[W]e feel that a very different model of disease causation should be developed."[11]

Initially, the Boston Women's Health Book Collective shared this assessment of the politics of women's medicine locally, through courses and inexpensively printed material. Published commercially in 1973, *Our Bodies, Ourselves* spawned numerous "Know Your Body" women's self-education courses and within a decade sold more than two million copies nationwide. A 1975 edition employed still sharper language to attack a medical establishment fragmented into minute specialties, "arrested for too long at the level of symptoms and mechanisms and chemical tinkering." Demanding a more integrated perspective, the feminist medical rebels wrote, "Health is more than just the absence of disease."[12]

Since male-dominated medicine appeared unable to offer this balanced approach, the book suggested, women must organize to create positive alternatives. Authors welcomed the recent opening of "grass-roots community clinics formed by local women . . . fed up with the lack of helpful health services for women, and who became radicalized by the hostility of local male doctors." In working outside the medical establishment to provide self-help groups, establish health education centers, run female-friendly clinics, and employ midwives, feminist critics declared, women were recapturing a vital element of history. "[T]he women's health movement . . . [is] deeply conscious of linking up with our lost identity as healers in the distant past."[13]

In this feminist context, personal care became aggressively politicized, and the politics of medicine became intensely personal. Specifically, the Boston Women's Health Book Collective emphasized the importance of feelings as well as facts about women's health. *Our Bodies, Ourselves* contained a wealth of diagrams and details about biology but also quoted women describing their experiences with sex, childbirth, and more. An individual's right to choose on such essential life matters always remained paramount, the book emphasized, and when mainstream medicine made those major events miserable, women should not hesitate to find alternatives. For many women, attacks on modern hypermedicalized, assembly-line childbirth rang particularly true, as critics accused interventionist gynecologists of manipulating the pace of labor, pushing drugs or cesarean sections, or otherwise forcing a woman's stirrup-bound delivery to fit the hospital's and doctors' convenience and prejudices. Feminist health critics of this era encouraged women to regain control over childbirth from the sterile, male-dominated institutionalized childbirth routine by considering midwife attendants, home births, and more unusual labor experiences.[14]

Feminist openness to alternative medicine was particularly noticeable in discussions of contraception, a topic fraught with tension. After scientists had spent decades researching hormones and synthesizing substitutes, the Food and Drug Administration (FDA) approved the manufacture and sale of birth control pills in 1960. Although many women were thrilled to have a relatively reliable, easy-to-use form of contraception (especially in the days before the *Roe v. Wade* abortion ruling), the pill's popularity also brought controversy. Especially in its initial version, before dosages were adjusted, women complained about annoying side effects, including nausea, breakthrough bleeding, water retention, and weight gain. There was also uncertainty about long-term risks, particularly about possible connections between hormones and breast cancer. For those and other reasons, although the feminist health movement encouraged women to embrace and explore their sexuality, uneasiness about the pill remained in many quarters.[15]

The subject of contraception became explosive with the calamitous case of the Dalkon Shield. Around 1970, this new type of intrauterine device (IUD) was being heavily promoted by manufacturer A. H. Robins, which drummed up customers partly by emphasizing warnings about the alleged harms caused by birth control pills. The pharmaceutical company's aggressive advertising promised that the Dalkon Shield was safer than other IUDs and almost 100 percent effective. In truth, as a few scientists already noted, studies behind those claims were incomplete, riddled with fatal methodological flaws, and tainted by conflicts of interest. Nevertheless, FDA rules of the era allowed Robins to put its device on the market. Within two years, doctors began reporting that some Dalkon Shield users developed severe pain and pelvic inflammatory disease, sometimes causing infertility or necessitating hysterectomies. Worse, design of this particular IUD significantly increased the likelihood of infected miscarriages, a complication implicating the Dalkon Shield in at least twenty fatalities. Despite accumulation of such evidence, Robins delayed and obfuscated until pressure finally forced the firm to suspend further U.S. distribution in 1974. Some of the roughly two hundred thousand women injured through Dalkon Shield use subsequently filed suit, but the drawn-out legal process proved futile after Robins filed for bankruptcy.[16]

Amid ongoing uncertainty about the pill and the Dalkon Shield disaster, it should not be surprising that some feminists found alternative choices in contraception intriguing. Noninvasive, nontechnological, and "natural" methods, such as "astrological birth control," carried special appeal. The second edition of *Our Bodies, Ourselves* described this approach as "another level of fertility awareness which might be added to the tools of natural family planning. This method has not been widely tested or proved, but it is a subject of . . . interest to many." The book did not give precise instructions for astrological contraception, but offered bibliographical references and personal contacts for further information.[17]

For details on astrological contraception and other "natural birth control," women of the late 1970s could consult Berkeley's *Holistic Health Handbook*. In an indictment of mainstream medicine, Merilee Kernis condemned both the pill and the IUD for side effects and the risk of death. "[T]hese devices . . . are only primitive jabbings in the dark, and . . . interfere with the delicate balance of the body . . . reflecting the social and political statements of the times: imbalance, obstruction, and eradication. . . . No wonder there are so many angry and disillusioned women." By contrast, Chinese women had relied on safe herbal contraception for centuries, while according to anthropologists, tribes in India and the South Seas had "a fantastic ability . . . to use mind control as a contraceptive . . . just as effective as the current . . . pill . . . [without the] harmful side effects." Western women too could master psychic contraception, using meditation, breath regulation, and yoga to control body conditions, Kernis wrote. As another option, a Czechoslovakian gynecologist had shown how to calculate a woman's fertile cycle in relation to her natal sun and moon position. Women could combine astrological analysis with the rhythm method or self-analysis of their cervical mucus for "at least 98 percent" contraceptive accuracy, the *Holistic Health Handbook* testified. Such "powerful" techniques allowed women to "prevent unwanted pregnancies without relying on potentially dangerous chemical and mechanical devices . . . [by] living in harmony with natural laws which support mindful celebration of sexuality and conscious choices about contraception."[18]

For women who didn't want to study their cervical mucus, create their astrological charts, or do yoga, the *Holistic Health Handbook* endorsed the "well-thought-out system" of "lunaception." For women living in traditional villages or who slept outdoors, ovulation and menstruation eased into synchronization with moon phases, allegedly responding to the same energy in the universe that governed plant growth. Western women could simulate such natural rhythms by sleeping under low-watt lamps at midcycle and in total darkness on other nights, thus regularizing fertility, Kernis wrote. "This creative process . . . raises a woman's consciousness of herself . . . as a functioning whole. . . . [A] woman may become aware of powerful creative feelings three days before she ovulates each month."[19]

Probably for good reason, the feminist movement's flirtation with alternative birth control proved short-lived. In 1992, *The New Our Bodies, Ourselves* contained a single sentence on astrological birth control: "This doesn't work."[20]

Even though the promise of lunaception waned, feminist distrust of the medical and pharmaceutical establishments remained. By the mid-1970s, women already embittered over the Dalkon Shield episode became outraged over another disaster, the prescription of diethylstilbestrol (DES) to more than five million pregnant women from the late 1940s through the 1960s. Researchers promoted it to prevent miscarriage, and manufacturers promised that DES also improved babies' health, although clinical trial results brought both claims into question. In 1971, after observing numerous young women in their twenties with a form of vaginal cancer normally rare before middle age, researchers linked those cases to exposure to DES in utero. For months, the FDA delayed responding to those reports. Later research detailed further long-term harm, extending even two generations down. Daughters and granddaughters of women who took DES might experience increased risk of infertility, ectopic pregnancies, and certain types of cancer; male descendants experienced their own heightened health risks. As such conclusions emerged, many women became furious over the difficulty of getting good information about their medical risks and need for proper follow-up care. In 1974, women in Berkeley, California, created the grassroots organization DES Action, and elsewhere hundreds of women formed similar groups to provide each other with psychological support and tangible advice about medical evaluations. Against criticism from the pharmaceutical industry and many doctors, these women mobilized to raise public awareness and maintain pressure on the medical system. Some traveled to Washington to testify at congressional hearings. In 1975, in the wake of the DES crisis, activists established the National Women's Health Network, institutionalizing the politicization of women's health on a nationwide scale.[21]

During the 1980s, feminist activists widened the attack to suggest that beyond specific catastrophes such as DES and the Dalkon Shield, women's health had been systematically endangered by the mainstream medical establishment. Biology was gendered, with solid evidence of important physiological differences between men and women on conditions such as heart disease. Nevertheless, medical textbooks often tacitly assumed or explicitly stated that men represented the human norm, while researchers frequently conducted major studies or tested new drugs only on all-male samples. Though drug companies and some investigators defended that practice, a growing number of physicians called for increased representation of female subjects in research. Major medical journals featured articles and editorials concerned about, as the *Journal of the American Medical Association* (*JAMA*) put it, "too much extrapolation from data on middle-aged white men." Activists succeeded in bringing their campaign to the consideration of the Congressional Caucus for Women's Issues, whose co-chair, Representative Patricia Schroeder, blamed male policy makers for leaving women's health "at risk." Amid this rising political momentum, in 1990 the NIH established a new Office of Research on Women's Health.[22]

Interest groups such as the Women's Health Action and Mobilization (WHAM!) expanded the case to argue that beyond women's underrepresentation in studies, gender bias extended to systematic inequity in federal health funding. The National Women's Health Network pressured government to rectify past imbalances by immediately enlarging research on female-specific health problems. In 1991, one week after her confirmation as first female director of the NIH, Bernadine Healy announced plans to create a $600 million, fifteen-year Women's Health Initiative (WHI). This commitment made national news, while its sheer magnitude caught the attention of prestigious researchers; plans to enroll 160,000 women in studies made the WHI the largest single clinical trial effort in NIH history.[23]

The amazing momentum of breast cancer activism in the 1980s and 1990s illustrates the transformation of women's health interests into a Washington-savvy lobby wielding substantial clout. Previous generations of victims tended to keep breast cancer secret, considering it a private concern or fearing that the disease reflected badly on them. Politicization of breast cancer offered women a means to stop feeling powerless and to rechannel their frustration into a positive direction. Organizing drew women beyond their individual struggles against an internal enemy (the disease itself) into a broader crusade against outside opponents (the political establishment, the medical system, or both). Operating from the same conviction that had galvanized the 1960s Boston Women's Health Book Collective, activists accused mainstream medicine of systematic bias against women's concerns and, in particular, of ignoring breast cancer even as the disease approached "epidemic" proportion. News commentator Cokie Roberts observed (inaccurately) that women's 44,500 breast cancer deaths in 1991 exceeded the total of American soldiers killed in Vietnam. To redress this injustice, the National Breast Cancer Coalition called on the federal government to increase support for breast cancer research immediately, a demand backed by petition drives, marches, and public-awareness campaigns. Surgeon and activist Susan Love compared the battle for breast cancer funds to past fights over "civil rights and war resistance and the early women's movement."[24]

As activists poured enormous energy into the cause, cover stories in *Newsweek,* the *New York Times Magazine*, and *Ms.* made breast cancer research a high-profile topic and established pink ribbons as a fashionable sign of enlightenment. The activism paid off; by 1995, federal appropriations for breast cancer study rose to $465 million, up from $90 million just five years earlier. Many activists still judged that amount inadequate; the National Breast Cancer Coalition directed supporters to ask President Clinton and Congress to "invest $2.6 billion in quality breast cancer research to find a cause and cure, between now and the Year 2000."[25]

Even as breast cancer organizations won millions for research, many continued accusing mainstream medicine of irresponsibility, of misplaced priorities, of literally playing with women's lives. In particular, activists faulted authorities for not paying more attention to evidence linking breast cancer risk to environmental contamination and nutrition. With a headline asking, "Why Did They Dismiss Dietary Fat?" *Ms.* magazine bemoaned cancellation of a study on whether low-fat diets could lower cancer rates. In this cover article, the head of the National Women's Health Network's Breast Cancer Committee identified a set of villains: the National Cancer Institute (NCI), the American Cancer Society (ACS), the "mostly male" university establishment, clinicians "accustomed to having a virtual monopoly on the breast cancer research pie," and a pharmaceutical industry with a vested interest in profits from high-tech, "highly toxic" cancer treatments. *Ms.* accused this "golden circle of power and money" of denying evidence implicating "endocrine disrupters" in pesticides, industrial pollution, and organochlorines as possible causes of breast cancer. Such sentiments roused real passion; critics who accused the NCI, FDA, and ACS of ignoring pollution's role in breast cancer directly confronted researchers at a 1994 American Association for the Advancement of Science meeting.[26]

Many women with breast cancer hoped that given increased funding, medical experts would eventually discover ways to reduce rates of the disease and perfect a cure, so that their daughters and granddaughters would not experience similar trauma. As thousands of women knew to their cost, surgery, radiation, and chemotherapy were stressful, painful, and not even guaranteed to succeed. A 1996 *Atlantic Monthly* article concluded that today "breast cancer is every bit as incurable" as in the late nineteenth century. Susan Love blamed a heroic-medicine philosophy in which "we [doctors] radiated, we slashed, burned, and poisoned. . . . I think we'll look back on this era and think we were totally crazy that we did these barbaric things." New research, Love suggested, allowed us to see cancer less as an "evil invader" and more as a lapse in the body's normal regulation of cell growth. Given that understanding, "we've got to change the paradigm . . . [to a] much more subtle" approach, working *with* the body to pause or reverse that biological misdirection. Linking the crudeness of conventional medicine to humankind's abuse of the planet, one ecofeminist quoted in *Ms.* denounced chemotherapy and radiation as "natural responses from a society that thinks in terms of chemical warfare and nuclear power."[27]

The 1998 edition of *Our Bodies, Ourselves* emphasized the negative dimensions of conventional cancer treatment, warning about the carcinogenic danger of radiation therapy and cautioning that doctors often exaggerated the benefits of chemotherapy. In contrast, the book offered many positive comments about alternative medicine. A paragraph on the Simonton visualization technique, for example, stated, "Although too new to have long-term survival statistics, this therapy appears to have been a major factor in the recovery of many people with cancer, including some for whom the conventional treatments had failed."[28]

Many breast cancer patients indeed turned to alternative treatments to supplement or substitute for mainstream medicine. The feminist magazine *On the Issues* told the story of one woman whose oncologist dismissed her complaints about post-lumpectomy hardness in her breast. When tests finally showed that cancer had spread through her system, the woman became convinced that "the medical establishment is deliberately withholding cures in order to profit from costly but ineffective treatments like chemotherapy." In addition to taking shark cartilage and numerous other supplements, this woman traveled to Mexico to obtain Hoxsey therapy tonics. She regarded her shopping around as self-defense, saying, "It's naive to believe there's only one way of treating this disease. There's a lot of information out there. It's like buying a couch; you go from store to store . . . . No physician talks straight." In a similar drive to explore alternatives, the celebrity Suzanne Somers made national news in 2001 with her decision to reject chemotherapy and treat her breast cancer by injecting herself daily with a European homeopathic mistletoe compound.[29]

ALTERNATIVE DIRECTIONS FOR WOMEN

Feminists' challenge to medical authority developed during a period when numerous Americans were ready to look beyond conventional health care, especially to treat headaches, back pain, depression, and other chronic problems.. Forcing many experts in mainstream medicine to take notice, a well-regarded study in 1990 suggested that one-third of the adult population, sixty million Americans, had supplemented visits to regular physicians with at least one form of alternative therapy during that year. Even more striking, a 1997 follow-up survey revealed a continued trend; over just seven years, the estimated number of Americans turning to alternative treatments had further risen to eighty-three million, 42 percent of all adults. A clear gender distinction existed: 49 percent of women reported using alternative medicine, versus 38 percent of men. Offering more detail on women's interest in alternative medicine, a 1999 *Newsweek* poll of more than 750 women showed that 43 percent had tried herbal medicine and another 34 percent had considered it. Thirty-three percent had tried chiropractic care and another 28 percent had considered it; 30 percent had tried massage therapy and another 40 percent had considered it. Ten percent had tried acupuncture, and another 32 percent had considered it, while 7 percent had tried biofeedback and another 21 percent had considered it.[30]

Women's interest in homeopathy remained strong; according to some estimates, women constituted a clear majority, roughly two-thirds, of all homeopathy users in the United States. Homeopathic writer Dana Ullman explained that pattern as a logical consequence of mainstream medicine's faults. "Because women tend to seek professional medical care more than men do, they also tend to experience more of its dangers. . . . When women reach the limits of modern medical expertise and experience some of the harsh side effects . . . it is certainly understandable that they seek out alternative health methods." Homeopathy offered a "considerably safer," effective, easy, and more affordable choice of harmonistic holism, Ullman and his colleagues suggested. Homeopaths particularly cautioned pregnant women that most obstetricians prescribed multiple drugs to women before and during labor, and that these substances crossed the placenta into the fetus. Homeopathic medicines promised a less risky way to relieve nausea and other discomforts of pregnancy, as well as to strengthen uterine muscles and shorten labor.[31]

Having attained status as a classic feminist reference, *Our Bodies, Ourselves* expanded coverage of alternative medicine in the 1980s and 1990s, devoting full chapters to "a compelling range" of holistic options. Authors portrayed alternative medicine as particularly suited to women, reflecting traditional knowledge "handed down from mother to daughter"; one firsthand reflection quoted a woman's recollections of her Puerto Rican mother collecting herbs. By listening to mothers and grandmothers, women could preserve that wisdom; by forming female self-help groups, they would build confidence to "withstand the cynicism and doubt you are likely to encounter from those who put all their faith in Western biomedicine." By educating themselves and consulting each other about which practices helped them, women could make themselves smart consumers who would always ask themselves, "Who profits from this mode of healing?" Women should "[e]xplore the politics of the method you want to use," the book advised. In general, holistic philosophy was inherently superior, since "it is an important political act to acknowledge that the interconnection between body, mind, and spirit is fundamental to well-being." Holistic medicine was politically correct, since it paid attention not only to individuals, but also to the community and environment, including problems of pollution and "the hostility we face in the form of racism, sexism, homophobia and so on." In *Our Bodies, Ourselves*, the definition of a good practitioner was one "especially sensitive to the larger political and economic issues that affect women's health."[32]

"[A]lternatives have often helped where the conventional methods of drugs and/or surgery could not," *Our Bodies, Ourselves* declared. Specifically, authors recommended yoga to reduce blood pressure and stress, improve joint movement, and possibly ease asthma and other respiratory difficulties. Touting the "positive healing effect" of imaging, the book instructed, "Relax and let your attention go to the particular body part causing discomfort. . . . Now begin to visualize something happening . . . to make it . . . heal. You might see energy, light or color flowing into it. . . . A powerful image could help you feel better right away." Other sections discussed herbal medicine, meditation, tai chi, massage, chiropractic care, dance and movement therapy, acupuncture, homeopathy, spiritual healing, and therapeutic touch. While the book noted that not everyone responded to every alternative treatment, it only included one firsthand comment speaking of disappointment, a woman for whom acupuncture failed to relieve chronic fatigue syndrome. In other quotations, one woman praised the chiropractor who let her "walk again in comfort" following an accident; a second asserted that a Chinese herbalist made a "tremendous difference" in relieving her menstrual cramps, while a third testified that self-healing visualization almost eliminated her post-cancer-operation pain.[33]

Similarly encouraging words about alternative medicine appeared in the feminist periodical *Ms.* One 1994 piece recommended twenty herbs and other "natural" remedies as "alternatives to prescription and over-the-counter drugs." Articles in 1996 promoted Rolfing,

Feldenkrais body work, therapeutic touch, and high-soy menopause diets. *Ms.* also extended the politics of women's alternative medicine, building health activists into feminist heroines. A profile titled "Info-Power" praised Janice Guthrie, a woman with ovarian cancer who refused to "unquestioningly submit" to radiation therapy. To "help others" enjoy that "empowering" feeling, Guthrie built a business supplying clients facing health care decisions with analyses of their options for mainstream, alternative, and experimental therapy.[34]

To some observers, supporting alternative medicine represented not just a personal health care choice, but a statement condemning the current economic and political order. Ecofeminists argued that inasmuch as pollution created sickness, keeping people well involved caring for the earth, and vice versa. More than that, psychiatrist Judith Orloff asked:

> Could illness, in part, be the body's desperate attempt to reequilibrate itself with a planet fighting to survive? Depression, chronic pain, autoimmune disease, in which the body literally attacks itself, are growing at apocalyptic rates. There's a parallel between our suffering and the relentless assault on the earth, the ravaging of rain forests, underground nuclear testing, pollution of air and oceans. Can we empathically feel our planet's cry? Do our bodies mimic the disease we are inflicting?

Calling for a complete paradigm shift, environmentalists argued that modern society needed more gentleness and balance, traits holistic medicine identified as feminine. Indeed, some warned that "the earth will not be able to heal until women reclaim their power as healers."[35]

For other women, support of alternative medicine blended with New Age beliefs. Redefining women's "curse" as positive, feminist holism insisted that there was more to menstruation than cramps, bloating, and mess. "Rather than feeling attacked and wiped out by their hormones, women can learn how to harness their wild, undomesticated power, riding them to a deeper understanding of their body/mind/spirit. . . . Every month the wildness courses through the female, enriching her blood." Turning Native American anthropology into feminist inspiration, healers told modern women that Indian cultures revered menstruation as a sacred symbol of eternal life-giving forces, women's connection to nature's cycle. During their "'moon time,' an extraordinary interlude when the world of intuition and spirit unveiled its deepest mysteries," tribal women "retreated to the Moon Lodge to rest, reflect, dream, and gather wisdom." Holistic healers urged all women to "celebrate the power of your blood" by relaxing in the moonlight, taking a renewing nighttime swim, keeping a journal of special visions, holding mother-daughter ceremonies, or "whispering to a spider as she spins her web." Herbalists concocted recipes for "lunar tea" for women to drink during their periods. New Agers recommended that women follow Native American traditions of returning blood to the earth by rinsing reusable menstrual pads in the garden. "If you live in a city, perhaps you could give your potted plants a monthly treat!" Such rituals honored women's signature changes, rather than giving into social pressure to hide all signs of bleeding and pretend that menstruation never happened. "Menstrual blood is the water of life . . . feel its energy coursing through you as a river runs . . . [T]hink of your blood as 'moon drops'—gifts from the moon, pulling on your inner tides."[36]

Tales of Native American women's biological wisdom fit into a broader interpretation of the past, which grew from and in turn supported the feminist health movement. While developing a "women and health" class in 1972, writers Barbara Ehrenreich and Deirdre

English collected material for a self-published booklet, *Witches, Midwives, and Nurses*, and a later Feminist Press companion, *Complaints and Disorders: The Sexual Politics of Sickness*. Ehrenreich and English detailed a preindustrial "gynocentric order," in which care of sick people was entrusted to village "wise women" who possessed healing skills and understanding of herbs. Other writers built up a picture of society before male domination as a paradise, an idyllic sisterhood. Nursing specialist Margarete Sandelowski wrote that ages ago, "women provided each other with emotional and physical comfort. . . . Mother-daughter bonds were strong, empathetic, and intimate, and all older women were mothers to younger ones."[37]

According to this feminist history, superstitious paranoia about women's seemingly magical capacity to cure or harm led to their persecution as witches in fifteenth- and sixteenth-century Europe. Thus "the feminine art and knowledge of healing, . . . a positive affirmation of female energy, was expropriated by men" greedy for power and financial reward. In denouncing establishment medicine for stealing women's healing legacy, modern feminism sanctioned alternative medicine as closer to wise women's original knowledge. One practitioner of traditional Chinese medicine urged his mostly female clientele to "travel back into the distant past . . . when the words *feminine* and *healing* were synonymous."[38]

These accounts condemned professionalization and commercialization for changing medicine from women's nurturing art into man's cold science. During these same decades, feminist scholars such as Sandra Harding, Carolyn Merchant, and Evelyn Fox Keller raised a wider challenge to scientific authority itself. Science could never be isolated from its historically male-dominated political and social context, feminist philosophers argued. "Women have been more systematically excluded from doing serious science than from performing any other social activity except, perhaps, frontline warfare," Harding wrote. More than that, the defensive misogynist posture of male scientists had permeated the nature of the discipline; authorities from Sir Francis Bacon to Richard Feynman had invoked metaphors of rape, mistresses, and motherhood in defining the scientific method. "The sexist meanings of scientific activity were evidently crucial resources through which modern science gained cultural acceptance; they remain the resources that contemporary scientists and philosophers use to justify and explain their activities," Harding concluded. "Why should we regard the emergence of modern science as a great advance for humanity when it was achieved only at the cost of a deterioration in social status for half of humanity?" As generations of men maintained control over the scientific enterprise, their research became contaminated by a sexism and racism that belied the ideal of science's sacred objectivity. Harding, Londa Schiebinger, Anne Fausto-Sterling, Emily Martin, Donna Haraway, and many others documented examples of biased research, from anthropologists' obsession with "man the hunter" to reproductive biologists' assumptions about "the passive egg." The most extreme feminist critics denounced science, especially in its partnerships with military research and industry, as ultimately contributing to the oppression of women, minorities, homosexuals, and the underprivileged.[39]

Alternative medicine proponents also sought to pull Western science down from its pedestal. When physicians dismissed energy healing because their research showed no possible mechanism for it to work, holistic healers said that only proved the limitations of "logical" analysis and the parochialism of scientists. Herbalist Rosemary Gladstar advised women to be "openminded to the fact that science can be just as fallible as it can be infallible. If a plant has been found safe and effective for a thousand years of human use, it may be wise to question the validity and applicability of the scientific tests now being used."[40]

Where Cartesian philosophy divided matter and spirit, where Baconian science sought to tame nature, alternative healers claimed to reunite all. According to the 1996 *Harvard Guide to Women's Health,* the holistic model of integrating body, mind, and spirit with each other, society and environment, was "sometimes regarded as a traditionally feminine" philosophy. Healer Jason Elias defined alternative therapy as expressing "archetypically feminine traits of tender care, gentle touch, or massage . . . and the deep-rooted belief that health and happiness cannot be sustained without a reverence for nature." Indeed, Elias traced many of the world's problems to the way that "classically feminine virtues of spiritual nurturance, love of peace and harmony, and sensitivity to the needs of others have been . . . suppressed in a world increasingly enamored of the archetypically masculine ideals of competition, confrontation, and conquest."[41]

As yet another dimension of its appeal to women, alternative medicine often echoed feminist criticism about society's persistent gender discrimination. Healer Andrew Weil sympathized with "superwomen" who "work in male-dominated businesses and professions [and who] get paid less for equivalent work." Even non-career-oriented women or those who hesitated to call themselves feminists might respond to language that resonated with personal concerns. Christiane Northrup promised that her care would address the needs of "[w]omen of my age . . . the 'sandwich' generation, . . . caught between caring for their still-dependent children . . . [and] elderly parents." For these women trying to "meet impossible demands," natural healers particularly recommended meditation to ease stress and headaches. One book advised, "Women's hectic role-switching can wreak havoc with their lives and with their health. . . . Meditation gives women a psychological buffer so that life's hectic pace doesn't knock them out. . . . It allows you to turn inward . . . like taking a vacation once or twice a day."[42]

Such language blended medical concerns with personal-growth psychology. Through alternative healing, advocates promised, women could change stress into renewal, converting traumatic disease into a life-transforming opportunity. "There are possibilities within illness that you may not anticipate" for "profound spiritual initiation," Orloff wrote. "See all health challenges with these eyes and the night sky will be lit up with a million stars. If you don't there will be only darkness. It is your decision. Illness is not failure. Approach it as a student, accept what it has to teach. Ride the dragon. Let your spirit grow strong." To illustrate the moral that "there's a purpose to everything," Orloff used the case of an unhappy administrator whose cancer diagnosis gave her courage to switch to her dream job selling real estate. In another episode, Orloff told a "control freak" lawyer to follow Buddhist principles and "harmonize" with her back pain, rather than fighting it with painkillers. The "mystical alchemy" of meditation and visualization healed this overcommitted woman not only physically but emotionally, teaching her to accept help from friends, slow down, and be "more mindful of beauty. The glistening sunlit boughs of magenta bougainvillea arcing over her front porch don't go unnoticed anymore."[43]

Once a woman resolved to experiment with alternative medicine, she could choose between dozens of therapies. For women with premenstrual syndrome, for example, traditional Chinese medicine recommended ginseng, homeopaths recommended pulsatilla, and herbalists recommended aloe root and a multitude of other preparations. Shiatsu massage and reflexology each called for pressure on ankle points to stimulate the feminine energy or qi. To relieve cramps, energy healers suggested women place magnets on the abdomen to repolarize cells and rebalance the body's positive and negative charges. Advocates of raw-food diets, meditation, light therapy, acupuncture, hydrotherapy, chiropractic care, and therapeutic touch all claimed that their particular discipline carried special power to relieve PMS. Some women might find this multitude of options liberating, while others see it as confusing.

ENERGY HEALING AND THERAPEUTIC TOUCH

Energy healing represented the perfect example of an alternative therapy that evolved into a popular fad among some circles in the late twentieth century. Though healing celebrities Deepak Chopra and Judith Orloff did not target their best-selling books and television shows exclusively to women, their philosophies conveyed a female-oriented appeal. Orloff's writing highlighted concepts of emotion and nurturing, and she emphasized the healing power of intuition, frequently regarded as a female trait. By learning to consult the body's inner signals and sense its energy fields (chakras), she announced, anyone could tap into the "intuitive healing code that contains the blueprints for our health and happiness." People could find "magic" and "miracles" by going beyond the rational mind, letting spirituality guide them into "the realm of genius—where ideas, imagery and dreams ignite, making healing an absolute reality even when science deems it impossible."[44]

Orloff advised patients whose doctors told them to live with chronic disease to ignore such "dangerous, debilitating, untrue" opinions. "There are always options; to find them may require you to become a kind of revolutionary. Dare to go beyond conventional medical wisdom." Orloff recommended honing visualization and meditation skills. "[F]rom listening to the language of starlight . . . illness can often be detected and reversed long before physical signs appear." She provided specific instructions on how to practice "body scanning," by focusing attention inward to localize feelings of energy depletion or tingling in specific organs. One woman who discovered a large mass in her breast turned to meditation before panicking, Orloff wrote, and received a clear image that it wasn't cancerous. "Every cell of her body agreed . . . she was fine. Not long after, her diagnosis was confirmed by ultrasound." Another technique, remote viewing, let users "tune into the past, present, and future, [to] help diagnose illness by picturing the body's organs, predict proper treatment, appraise current therapies—all mandatory when conventional medicine seems unable to find a cure." Finally, Orloff recommended that people analyze their dreams to recover "revelations about illness" and "straightforward health advice" on treatment options. Dreams could even "mend the body" by accessing healing instincts, Orloff wrote, citing the case of her friend who hoped to avoid surgery to remove a painful benign tumor. "That night she dreamed there was a huge syringe next to her bed. Seemingly on its own, the syringe pierced . . . her spine, and extracted a milky fluid. . . . When she awoke she . . . rushed straight to the mirror. The lipoma was gone."[45]

Alternative medicine promoters also encouraged women to explore different types of touch healing, as simple and familiar as a back rub. Professionals claimed that therapeutic massage accelerated removal of bodily toxins, improved circulation, and promoted natural immunity. Practitioners maintained that overstressed women particularly needed not only the physiological benefits of massage, but also its nurturing of mind and spirit. Female patients improved simply by giving themselves time to relax on the massage table, one therapist explained. "You've set aside an uninterruptible hour just for you. That alone is a powerful healing message, which for most women is too often denied."[46]

Energy healers claimed still more powerful effects from touch treatment. Orloff wrote about attending a book club meeting where the hostess broke down in tears from recurring pain. Touching the woman, Orloff "requested energy to flow through me, out my hands." Under her guidance, the other women, "mostly housewives living in privileged Palos Verdes Estates . . . [with] no experience in sending energy," encircled the sufferer "lovingly" to create a vortex that interrupted the attack, giving the woman overnight relief until she could have her gallbladder removed. Though not reserved for women, touch healing carried feminine connotations for both users and practitioners. Popular holistic philosopher Andrew Weil asserted that "women often learn these techniques more readily than men, and all of them are valuable."[47]

Indeed, by century's end, believers in hands-on energy healing had built their ideas into a characteristically female discipline. Therapeutic touch was allegedly invented in the 1970s by a nursing professor at New York University and steadily acquired adherents through special seminars and nursing-school classes teaching the technique. Practitioners often identified themselves as holistic nurses, who sought to define a unique role for themselves as the caring face of an overly technologized health care bureaucracy. Differentiating themselves from other medical professionals, these nurses claimed to look after the whole patient, mind, body, and spirit, in contrast to physicians' fixation on disease. By meditating and projecting compassion, therapeutic touch users asserted, they could manipulate patients' energy fields to promote wellness. Citing one woman who credited therapeutic touch with forestalling her migraines, *Our Bodies, Ourselves* (1998) commented, "Like shamans in 'primitive' societies and religious or faith healers in Western societies, modern psychic healers can mobilize the body's healing forces." Although skeptics sneered and sought to show that claims of energy manipulation had no basis in reality, for many female patients and practitioners alike, touch treatment offered both a personal meaning and a political statement.[48]

HERBS AND AROMATHERAPY: NATURE FOR WOMEN, AND WOMEN'S NATURE

Another gendered alternative medicine gaining popularity in the 1990s was herbalism, which blended feminist interpretations of medical history with New Age and environmental principles. Female practitioners defined the modern "herbal renaissance" as recovering their foremothers' legacy. Herbology teacher Rosemary Gladstar wrote, "For thousands of years women . . . gathered herbs by the waning and waxing of the moon. . . . Through an intuitive communication with the plants, women learned the healing powers of their green allies." Herbalists reverently described the herbs collected by twelfth-century mystic Hildegard von Bingen or reprinted medieval illustrations showing an abbess grinding her own remedies with a mortar and pestle.[49]

Reaching into mythology to claim healing knowledge as innately female, Anne McIntyre proclaimed herbalism the "art of Artemis." As the moon goddess, McIntyre declared, Artemis symbolized "the essential feminine principle" behind women's menstrual cycle and served as "protector of young maidens." As goddess of agriculture, Artemis represented women's customary role as food gatherers, reflecting the belief that "only women could make things grow. as they are under the direct guardianship of the moon." Finally, McIntyre noted, women asked Artemis for protection in labor, honoring her role as fertility goddess in the names of herbs valuable in childbirth, such as *Artemisia absinthium* (wormwood).[50]

Other practitioners linked their field to more ancient mythology, citing the work of anthropologist Marija Gimbutas on Paleolithic "Venus figurines" and that of Joseph Campbell on "goddess societies." In this interpretation, the Great Goddess had created the special feminine healing power of herbs, infusing different aspects into particular plants. One version of this herbal polytheism connected echinacea to the protective warrior strength of Athena, chasteberry to the nurturing love of Demeter, false unicorn root to the life-giving spirit of the Irish figure Danu, and dong quai to the Chinese fertility goddess Chang-O.[51]

Other herbalists declared that the divine spirit of Mother Nature was always ready to help women, providing plants to ease pregnancy, assist in birth, and serve other female biological needs. Reflecting the broader resonance between environmentalism and holistic medicine, some herbalists referred to their work as "ecological healing," connecting women to Mother Earth's profound rhythms of life. As one wrote, plants "offer a system of healing that is gentle, imbued with 'soft power,' and attuned to the feminine spirit . . . Beautiful, strong . . . herbs . . . provide a deep source of nourishment and vitality to the female organs and have an innate ability to heal imbalances that have lodged in these deep, moist places of our female being."[52]

Herbalists such as Susun Weed portrayed plant cures as simultaneously powerful and gentle, free of conventional drugs' noxious side effects while acting more effectively, almost miraculously so. For instance, herbalists cautioned anemic women that taking commercial iron supplements might prove useless or cause digestive trouble. Instead, they promised, countless iron-deficient women had been restored to full energy by taking a "humble weed," yellow dock root. Practitioner Kathi Keville wrote, "Although the way that this herb increases iron remains a mystery, the proof is in the results."[53]

By exploring this centuries-old herbal heritage, advocates promised, women could handle illness in a naturally superior way and find self-fulfillment in the bargain. Western society had led women too much toward masculine priorities of work, competitiveness, and objective rationales, causing feelings of "inner conflict," McIntyre argued. Herbalism helped women recapture their lost feminine spirit, returning to "inner mysteries of creation and nurture."[54]

Women already familiar with herbs such as rosemary from preparing family meals would find it simple to extend such knowledge from cooking to healing, herbalists said. Creating one's own herbal teas, oils, capsules, syrups, tinctures, liniments, salves, and ointments would prove "easier than making cookies and just about as fun." Popularly oriented herbals supplied recipes, illustrated with artistic drawings of plants or gorgeous photographs of flowers. Instructions for a tea to be drunk twice daily to ease breast swelling, for example, specified one teaspoon each of burdock root, mullein leaves, and dandelion root, plus other ingredients. Remedy names played on appeals to female New Age mythology; "Bringing on the Moon Tea" (pennyroyal and peppermint) promised help for amenorrhea, while "Crone Candy" was a sesame butter and royal jelly menopause aid "in honor [of] the wise old woman in each of us."[55]

During the 1980s and 1990s, aromatherapy became trendy in some circles; upscale spas and beauty salons offered massages with scented oils as not only an indulgence, but a valuable health treatment. By 2002, brands such as the Healing Garden marketed aromatherapy to mainstream consumers. Women browsing through the cosmetics department of Target stores could purchase a chamomile "drift away milk bath" as relaxing "zzz theraphy" [*sic*] or a St. John's wort "upbeat bath and shower gel" as stimulating "gingerlily theraphy [*sic*] [to] fill your mind, body, and spirit with positive energy." The company touted "aromachology" as "the study of olfactory powers that measurably improve your physical state and emotional well-being." Fostering the idea of aromatherapy as risk-free, accessible, and enjoyable self-treatment for women, the Healing Garden Web site offered "personalized" product recommendations to help buyers cope with stress, relieve sleeping difficulties, or fit other self-diagnosed emotional or physical needs.[56]

Herbalists promoted aromatherapy as a natural and naturally feminine form of healing, appreciated by anyone who ever relaxed with a cup of peppermint tea, sniffed an orange while cooking, or loved wandering through a fragrant garden. Advocates cited the ease and pleasantness of aromatherapy as its strength, "built on the concept of finding the fragrances . . . appropriate to each person's emotional needs. The simplest way to determine the best healing fragrance for you is to determine which scents you find most appealing."[57] Rather than feeling guilty for enjoying a luxuriously warm, scented bath after a stressful day, women overwhelmed by work and family demands could excuse it as a medical justification to take care of themselves. Aromatherapist Joan Clark declared that this physical and emotional self-healing was especially important for ambitious "business women who may feel the need to put forth lots of male energy and sublimate their essential feminine natures." Women too short on time for soaking could relieve stress or menstrual cramps simply by sniffing essential oils, herbalists promised. They recommended rose oil for alleviating postnatal depression and low libido, peach scent for calming anxiety and fighting narcolepsy, vervain as a nervous system tonic to relieve exhaustion and restore mood balance, and geranium for easing depression and premenstrual syndrome.[58]

To support these claims, herbalists cited numerous cases in which they had helped women dissatisfied with mainstream care. Keville lovingly described how a neighbor reversed her precancerous cervical dysplasia (and thus avoided surgery) by taking sage tea sitz baths, putting castor oil packs on her abdomen, and using calendula-soaked tampons. Herbalists also validated their recommendations as traditional mainstays in Chinese, Native American, and other cultures, telling pregnant Americans that for centuries, European women had trusted raspberry tea to relieve nausea, avert miscarriage, and ease labor. In the modern world, a "woman who takes the time to use herbs will always have a good outcome with her birth," said herbalist Nan Koehler. In devoting daily time and energy to harvesting or purchasing herbal remedies, "the woman reinforces the idea that she's doing everything she can to insure that she will have a healthy baby—a bit of positive thinking."[59]

CHRONIC FATIGUE SYNDROME: FRUSTRATION WITH MAINSTREAM MEDICINE

Alternative medicine appealed to many American women specifically for care of certain diseases, as the history of chronic fatigue syndrome illustrates. In the mid-1980s, a wave of media attention highlighted reports of mysteriously debilitating fatigue from hundreds of people in several Nevada communities. Medical analysis proved elusive; affected people presented with a wide range of symptoms, including malaise, joint and muscle pain, severe headaches, disorientation, cognitive difficulties, neurological abnormalities, sleep disorders, and depression. Given the vagueness of this profile, many doctors doubted whether a specific medical syndrome truly existed. In the absence of clear diagnostic physical tests, some analysts believed that cases stemmed from psychological causes. Skeptics suggested that complaints represented extreme episodes of ordinary exhaustion. This assessment was reinforced by an impression that cases disproportionately hit overstressed go-getters, leading to the nickname "yuppie flu."

The sense that many physicians and medical researchers discounted their misery infuriated Americans facing the mystery illness. Activists estimated the incidence of chronic fatigue immune dysfunction syndrome (CFIDS) as affecting two million to ten million Americans, with women constituting 60 to 80 percent of cases. To many, denial of chronic fatigue reflected the medical establishment's long tendency to dismiss female complaints as hysteria, malingering, or hypochondria. Clinical psychologist and CFIDS patient Katrina Berne wrote, "[D]octors who hadn't known me . . . before CFIDS . . . often treated me like a 'crock,' a neurotic woman . . . who . . . enjoyed being attended to by the medical profession. . . . The illness itself was crazy-making; the insult added by insensitive, disbelieving physicians made the ordeal worse."[60]

Following the feminist slogan of "the personal as political," CFIDS activists interpreted their individual frustrations as a collective challenge. One explained, "I began to understand I was facing another battle in addition to the one raging in my body, a battle I and countless other women had fought before. Like survivors of rape, sexual abuse, or harassment, women were again being told that what we suffered was trivial, or even unreal." In 1988, following persistent pressure from activists, the Centers for Disease Control announced new funding to investigate chronic fatigue. Critics derided the CDC's commitment as ridiculously inadequate, reflecting the medical establishment's structural underfunding of female health issues.[61]

Some observers concluded that the very nature of mainstream medicine made it unhelpful at best, hostile at worst to people with CFIDS. Many complained that they had to visit ten, twenty, or more doctors before finding one willing to take their symptoms seriously. From doctors' perspectives, such office hopping only reinforced perceptions of hypochondria. Activists maintained, however, that the high-tech, crisis-oriented medical establishment had made it impossible for people to find the individualized attention necessary to manage the complexities of chronic sickness. Chronic fatigue sufferers insisted that their problem could be properly diagnosed only by the rare physician who believed in the existence of CFIDS and who dedicated time to listen to patients.

Under this conviction, that regular medicine had failed and even humiliated people with CFIDS, many turned to alternative treatments for hope and understanding. For those who resented being "shuffled among specialists while never being given an opportunity to present the whole picture or to be treated as a whole person," holistic medicine promised to focus on the individual's particular manifestations of symptoms and to balance the whole body, mind, and spirit. For those who had been dismissed by conventional medicine when standard procedures failed to identify any problem, it came as welcome news that homeopaths "do not rely heavily on lab tests to produce diagnoses; labels are not considered important." Some alternative practitioners even blamed allopathic medicine for creating a predisposition for CFIDS, theorizing that overuse of steroids and antibiotics suppressed the immune system and led to extended weakness. Significantly, as evidence of allopathic medicine's failures, critics highlighted previous cases that had most infuriated feminists. Berne wrote, "Any substance powerful enough to affect body chemistry may cause serious side effects or severe complications. Many of today's 'miracle' drugs will be deemed worthless or even harmful in the future. Thalidomide and DES are examples of pharmaceutical products once considered helpful and safe that later produced tragic results."[62]

Different disciplines of natural healing claimed to provide help for CFIDS. Some holistic practitioners advocated examining the subconscious or trying to contact the "inner child." Through imagery, one said, he had diagnosed one woman as continually searching for her parents' approval; "the pain and the grief of not having that love were not only weakening her immune system but keeping her stuck in the unhealthy way she was living." By healing such open wounds, holistic healers promised to restore well-being. Traditional Chinese healers recommended ginseng and blood tonics; other herbalists prescribed echinacea, dong quai, and ma huang. Some CFIDS patients reported gaining renewed energy from acupuncture, while others credited meditation and ayurveda. Through support groups, newsletters, e-mail lists, and Web sites, people with chronic fatigue exchanged information and shared assessments of various treatments, while discussing the political struggle to get recognition of their disease and venting their anger with mainstream medicine.[63]

Patients often felt that chronic fatigue had robbed them of normal existence. The very process of pursuing different treatment options gave some a feeling of reasserting control over their lives. Biomagnetic and Reiki healer Janice Strubbwe Wittenberg, herself a CFIDS patient, defined exploration of alternatives as a necessary component in recovery. "People who have achieved the greatest degree of wellness or . . . live in harmony with these illnesses are those who have taken off on their own path, not waiting for someone to come along who will fix them. There are some . . . going at their own healing using very unusual, subtle measures. Chanting, visualization, energetic healing practices . . . are some." Wittenberg urged readers not to let pain and frustration box them into the role of passive victims. "[B]y saying 'I *am* healing' or 'I *am* in charge,' positive physical states are stimulated that cause the cells to awaken."[64]

By empowering themselves to cope with CFIDS, holistic medicine stressed, patients could achieve "true healing" in the form of "transformation of consciousness . . . a point of departure from the old self." Wittenberg linked chronic fatigue to the tendency of women in particular to serve family and community first. "[R]epressing your true needs—may be . . . the source of much anger and 'dis-ease.'" To heal, women must break behavior patterns and explore new ideas, "discovering who you are underneath all of the rules and expectations . . . to reshape your life into anything you choose."[65] The story of chronic fatigue syndrome thus blends women's personal and political embrace of alternative medicine. When many perceived that regular medicine had contemptuously dismissed them (individually and collectively) as hysterical, alternative medicine accepted the self-diagnosis and welcomed the CFIDS business.

MENOPAUSE: ONGOING CONTROVERSY

The end of the twentieth century and the start of the twenty-first witnessed extended uncertainty over a major question: women, menopause, and medicalization. In 1942, the FDA had approved use of estrogen to mitigate hot flashes and other annoying symptoms; within the decade, brands such as Premarin hit the market. More than that, estrogen therapy promised to fight wrinkles and vaginal dryness, helping postmenopausal women retain their sexuality and resilient skin. Synthetic hormones seemingly offered older women a magic fountain of youth, the gift to remain "feminine forever," as Robert Wilson (a New York gynecologist with connections to hormone manufacturers) promised in his wildly popular 1966 book. As articles in mainstream magazines such as *Look* and *Harper's*

Bazaar echoed Wilson's praise, estrogen sales skyrocketed. Studies in the 1970s linking estrogen to escalated risk of endometrial cancer caused concern, but the addition of progesterone promised to limit the danger.[66]

An important shift came in subsequent years as researchers examined the possibility that women could take hormone replacement therapy (HRT) not just for short periods to fight hot flashes but over a longer term to avert chronic diseases associated with aging. Studies conducted during the 1980s and early 1990s highlighted suggestions that HRT could help lower cholesterol and keep blood vessels healthy, thus fending off heart disease, the major cause of death among postmenopausal women. Manufacturers also touted hormone treatment as a virtual panacea for preventing strokes, osteoporosis, depression, even mental decline and Alzheimer's disease. With approximately forty million women already in menopause and as many as two million joining that population annually, HRT became big business, worth more than $2.5 billion annually by 2001. An estimated 40 percent of American women at menopause began using hormone treatment, although doctors reported that a number chose on their own not to renew their prescriptions after a few years.[67]

Though some researchers claimed impressive results for benefits of hormone therapy, overall medical evidence remained incomplete and ambiguous. In particular, given knowledge that estrogen could fuel the growth of breast cancer, critics worried that years of hormone treatment might create a dangerously cumulative risk. Skeptics such as health activist Sandra Covey emphasized that the worth of hormones in preventing cardiac disease and bone fractures had been "grossly oversold." Reminding women that exercise could also protect bone strength, Covey charged that "drug companies make osteoporosis sound much more common and more severe than it actually is."[68]

Not coincidentally, observers calling for reexamination of menopause treatment placed the issue within a context of baby-boom feminist health politics. As popular women's medicine author Susan Love noted, the same generation that had broadened discussions of sexuality and joined the push to understand "our bodies" during the late 1960s and 1970s had now reached middle age, still ready to challenge old assumptions. Holistic doctor Christiane Northrup hailed politicization of the menopause debate as a continued advance in women's personal and collective self-assertion. At midlife, she wrote, today's women are "no longer invisible and silent, but a force to be reckoned with: educated, vocal, sophisticated in our knowledge of medical science, and determined to take control of our own health. Think about it: forty million women, all undergoing the same sort of circuitry update at the same time. By virtue of our sheer numbers, as well as our social and economic influence, we are powerful—and potentially dangerous to any institution built upon the status quo."[69]

Feminist critics accused pharmaceutical corporations of having turned menopause, a normal part of a woman's life, into an illness ready for corporate exploitation. By defining menopause as a disease, drug companies insidiously defined premenopausal women as a desirable norm, while older women became inherently defective. HRT advertisements showing older women riding bicycles through a park played on American baby boomers' obsession with youth and fear of aging. Love urged women to resist such manipulation. "Obviously, a lot of people are invested in this 'disease' and its treatment. . . . It's unfortunate that corporate profits and media fads should determine anyone's medical treatment. . . . But they do, and just as consumers need to distrust the glittering promises of car companies and perfume manufacturers, they need to question the promises of the pharmaceutical industry."[70]

Love, a breast surgeon herself, warned that physicians had been seduced by pharmaceutical representatives touting the mythology of necessary treatment. "[W]e're often working long hours seeing patients, and we don't always have the time to critically review all of the literature. We're rarely educated on alternatives such as lifestyle changes, supplements, and other approaches to wellness. . . . [I]t does make the *doctors* feel better . . . when they can give you a pill to solve your problems." Prescribing hormone treatment represented the easy solution for doctors without time or incentive to probe individual needs and risk factors.[71]

Contrary to the drug industry's image of menopause as inevitably devastating, Love pointed out, individual women might experience no problems at all or only mild discomfort, for which powerful hormones would be pointless. Consequently, "I would strongly recommend that you look into [alternative approaches] before you try Western drugs. There are fewer dangers, and for the most part equally good effects." As with chronic fatigue, critics of hormone therapy pointed to history as proof of how the "experts" could go wrong. Love asked readers, "Do you really want to take a hormone pill every day for the rest of your life? Hormones are powerful. . . . Are these things safe? . . . Wasn't DES supposed to be a miracle drug?"[72]

Alternative practitioners pointed out that while "the menopause industry" issued identical hormone prescriptions to millions, homeopathic medicine promised women individualized assessment. Advocates also noted that during the decades when American doctors routinely directed menopausal women to HRT, European women felt comfortable relying on herbal treatment. Herbalists promised remedies proven across centuries and cultures, recommending both a traditional Native American agent, black cohosh, and various Chinese herbal formulas to treat hot flashes. Advocates portrayed herbal remedies as so safe that women could self-prescribe. Christiane Northrup wrote, "The wisdom in nature is user-friendly, and you have a lot of it within you already. To tap in to it, just pick the herb, the formula, or the foods that seem to jump out at you and say 'Try me.' Because all of the herbs . . . I've mentioned . . . have virtually no side effects, feel free to experiment."[73]

During the 1990s, herbal healers and dietary supplement companies paralleled the mainstream pharmaceutical establishment in targeting the new generation of menopausal women as potential clients. According to one study, over 20 percent of menopausal women treated hot flashes and other symptoms with herbs or other alternative treatments, while another 25 percent mixed mainstream and complementary therapies. Health food stores and vitamin companies, even groceries and chain drugstores, devoted entire sections to products aimed at menopausal women. Wal-Mart stores attached handy herbal guides to supplement shelves, allowing consumers to look up their category ("women," "mature adults," etc.) and select their own medicine. The black cohosh tablet Remifemin was a strong seller, as were soy products such as Soy Balance, a "Nature's Resource herbal supplement for a more comfortable transition through menopause [which] helps relieve hot flashes [and] night sweats." In advertising and pamphlets distributed in stores, health businesses touted phytoestrogens as "natural" hormone replacement therapy. Alternatives had become accessible; by 2001, sales for over-the-counter menopause-related products reportedly totaled $100 million. Purchases of the most popular choice, black cohosh, had jumped more than threefold since 1998.[74]

Other unconventional healers offered a broader New Age and personal-growth reconceptualization of menopause, citing non-Western beliefs that the end of menstruation lifted women from the physical plane into a higher spiritual resonance. In this interpretation, Native American tribes revered "grandmothers" who used their mystical powers to guard human life, animals, and the earth itself. Naturopathic philosophy interpreted menopause not as a disease, but as a natural "gateway" full of meaning. In traditional Chinese medicine, Nan Lu wrote, menopause reflected an "enormous energy shift." By rebalancing and strengthening internal qi, women could "[e]mbrace the unique and magnificent transition."[75]

Especially for women whose priority for years had been tending babies and young children, holistic medicine advised, menopause represented nature's signal to tend their own needs. Northrup wrote, "As the vision-obscuring veil created by the hormones of reproduction begins to lift, a woman's youthful fire and spirit are often rekindled, together with long-sublimated desires and creative drives." Those who accepted this empowerment could find "emergence of what can only be described as pure joy, the feeling that arises when a woman is truly coming home to herself." Biology might force this message on those women who resisted change. "Bodily symptoms are not just physical in nature; often they contain a message for us about our lives. . . . [W]e attract precisely the illness or problem that best facilitates our access to our inner wisdom." When she herself developed fibroid tumors at age forty-one, Northrup testified, it served as a "wake-up call" to quit her stressful surgical practice and devote more energy to teaching.[76]

Though society marginalized older women and mainstream medicine emphasized their weakness, holistic medicine told women to resist such negative messages and make the second half of their lives even better than the first. One group of natural healers advised, "Perhaps you'll . . . end a meaningless marriage, stop being a slave to your kids, move to an exciting city, or wear flowing purple clothes . . . travel to far-off lands you've always wanted to see."[77]

That vision of menopause as adventure made its way into popular culture, with T-shirts reading, "They're not hot flashes; they're power surges!" In a 1999 *Time* cover story, Barbara Ehrenreich hailed such slogans as part of an emerging "femaleist" consciousness. Uniting in support groups such as the Red Hot Mamas, hundreds of women affirmed their strength and celebrated female biology. Ehrenreich referred to them as "estronauts," the "lawyers and homemakers marking their menopause by throwing a party or climbing Mont Blanc," ready "to feel the delicious tug of the hormonal tides as well as the gleaming challenge of the mountain peaks."[78]

This awakening was political as well as personal, Northrup emphasized. "Like the rising heat in our bodies, our brains also become fired up!" Hormonal changes "give a woman a sharper eye for inequity," an "increasing intolerance for injustice," and "the courage to voice it." With more baby boomer women reaching this enlightenment every year, Northrup declared, the potential multiplied:

> Once we truly become partners with our own spirits at midlife, we not only restore our faith in ourselves, but also become part of a force to be reckoned with. . . . Though the mainstream media has tried to make midlife women all but invisible, . . . [t]here is a critical mass of us . . . beginning to know . . . the power that has always been there but that our mothers and grandmothers were

talked out of. . . . As we flex our economic, mental, and physical muscles . . . the world will change in ways that reflect our inherent women's wisdom.[79]

Northrup remained vague about the exact mechanisms of female empowerment, declining to specify exactly how women would exercise this biologically based politics. Other observers often cited environmentalism as one political characteristic of a new world created in harmony with female wisdom, but holistic health writings generally stopped short of detailed discussion about the precise meaning and implementation of environmental thinking.

Indeed, some marketing of alternative treatments for menopausal difficulties drew on this context of feminist empowerment, praising the growth of women's public presence in the United States. One 2003 advertisement for the Woman's Wellbeing Menopause Relief Supplement headed the page with a declaration in large, bold type, "By 2005, women will be 55% of the workforce, 50% of all business owners, 47% of all stockholders. Take care of yourself! Get Menopause Relief Without the Risks of HRT."[80]

Soon, millions of baby boomer women, along with physicians and other health workers, would revisit questions of how to handle menopause, amidst political controversy and personal agonizing. New medical evidence on risks of hormone therapy would abruptly and radically shift terms of debate. The first shock came in 1998, with a major clinical trial of Prempro, the nation's most popular combination estrogen-progestin pill. The manufacturer, Wyeth-Ayerst Laboratories, had funded research involving more than twenty-seven hundred women, anticipating that favorable results would support claims that Prempro could prevent recurrence of cardiac trouble in postmenopausal women with preexisting heart disease. Ironically, the Heart and Estrogen/Progestin Replacement Study (HERS) revealed that women taking the hormone combination experienced more heart attacks over the first one or two years than those receiving placebo pills. Over a longer period, evidence suggested, Prempro failed to confer any cardiac protection on users, eliminating one justification for prescribing it. Data also linked Prempro with increases in the frequency of blood clots, urinary incontinence, and need for gallbladder surgery. Reversing its previous support for the hypothesis that hormone therapy might improve heart health, the American Heart Association cautioned women with cardiovascular disease against taking Prempro.[81]

An even bigger clamor arose in July 2002, when the federal Women's Health Initiative suddenly canceled its landmark study of Prempro, three years ahead of the scheduled stopping point. Researchers had randomly assigned half of sixteen thousand healthy postmenopausal participants to take hormones, the others placebos. Almost five years into the study, intermediate data showed that the group on Prempro experienced small but statistically significant increases in heart attacks, strokes, and blood clots. Most ominously, WHI evidence clearly associated Prempro with higher rates of breast cancer. Ironically, it appeared that the progesterone added years before to reduce the risk of uterine cancer had escalated breast cancer risk. Independent experts concluded that the apparent benefits of hormone treatment (a limited reduction in hip fractures and slightly smaller risk of colorectal cancer) did not outweigh the adverse effects. Although the WHI tested only Prempro, medical analysts (including the American College of Obstetricians and Gynecologists) warned there was no reason to assume that other formulations would prove more safe or valuable.[82]

Although many questions about the full medical effects of hormone therapy remained unanswered, announcement of these major clinical results provided powerful grounds for concern. Many leading physicians found the results more convincing than earlier studies highlighting the alleged benefits of hormones, where observational data could have been contaminated by selection bias. The HERS and WHI studies did not deny the effectiveness of estrogen as a quality-of-life drug alleviating hot flashes, night sweats, and the resulting insomnia. A number of analysts recommended that women battling such incapacitating symptoms try at least to minimize the length and dosage of hormone use, gradually weaning themselves off medication. However, other researchers cautioned that short-term use might not ensure safety. In-depth examination of WHI evidence seemed to suggest that women who had stopped taking Prempro early faced the same elevated rates of breast cancer as those who continued, a risk that might linger for years.[83]

Protests against overselling of hormone medication led to a backlash against the "forever young" philosophy that had been estrogen's initial selling point. In October 2002, the NIH ruled that the name "menopausal hormone therapy" should be substituted for the term "hormone replacement," which misleadingly implied that the treatment was an innocuous biological mechanism. The theory of permanently recapturing youth by simply filling a deficiency had been a commercialized mirage, critics concluded.[84]

Not surprisingly, Wyeth executives challenged the quality and interpretation of studies targeting their product. Pharmaceutical interests accused critics of overreacting, exaggerating increases in breast cancer risk to the point of making the disease seem inescapable. Nevertheless, reports indicated that Prempro sales dropped more than 40 percent following the damaging revelations.[85]

Although some users chose to continue taking Prempro or switched to other firms' regimens, anti-hormone headlines drew public attention to alternative treatments. The *New York Times, Newsweek,* and *U.S. News and World Report* all highlighted anecdotes about women who experimented with black cohosh extract, soy milk, dong quai, wild yam pills, or red clover until they found relief from hot flashes. Reporters noted that German clinical trials had demonstrated the value of black cohosh but that other studies on herbal therapy's effectiveness and long-term safety were negative, inconclusive, or nonexistent. Moreover, experts cautioned that "natural" substances carried unnatural risks; while red clover conjured up images of flower-filled meadows, that seemingly innocent substance carried blood-thinning chemicals, potentially creating negative interactions in women who combined it with aspirin or anticoagulants.[86]

Clearly, all the answers about menopause treatment were not in yet. The process of weighing competing health risks and benefits was inherently complex and imperfect, to the point where many physicians admitted feeling uncertain how to advise patients. Women reported feeling confused, frustrated, and sometimes amazed and angry that possible harms of estrogen therapy were still being explored sixty years after its introduction. While their mothers might have accepted the promise that swallowing hormone pills would maintain youth and health, women of 2002 had been politicized, and consequently disillusioned, on medical matters. To many, swallowing black cohosh tablets like Europeans or cooking soy-based meals like Asian women suddenly seemed like easier, better alternatives. Literally illustrating the scope of possibilities, *Newsweek* filled a 1999 article titled "The Estrogen Dilemma" with pictures of Premarin tablets, soybeans, red clover, wild yams, and wild yam root capsules. It had become easy for women to discover alterna-tives. Making decisions about them remained more difficult.[87]

CONCLUSION

By 2000, the American press had picked up on women's interest in alternative medicine and described this trend in generally positive terms. It seemed almost mandatory, for example, for popular articles to include photographs of beautiful flowers and magical-looking herbs, of women receiving massages or meditating with hands folded. A January 2003 *Time* cover featured a poised young woman sitting in yoga's lotus position, illustrat-ing "How Your Mind Can Heal Your Body." A December 2002 *Newsweek* cover depicted a lovely woman smiling serenely, with three acupuncture needles stuck into her forehead. Aside from a few quotations from conservative skeptics referring to unconventional medi-cine as "voodoo," the accompanying article, "The Science of Alternative Medicine," praised popular demand for compassionate, personalized integrative medicine as "bringing about a revolution in modern health care."[88]

Women's magazines often recommended alternative therapies as part of articles advis-ing readers on how to take better care of themselves. *Heart and Soul*, a magazine catering to African-American female readers, casually advocated Ayurvedic remedies. *Family Circle* cautioned people with "serious ailments" not to abandon conventional medicine for un-proven treatments, but mostly it spoke favorably about herbs, acupuncture, transcendental meditation, and homeopathy. Its article "The ABCs of Alternative Medicine" concluded with a plug for Tibetan medicine, advising readers to "keep an eye on this lesser-known discipline, which we'll soon be hearing more about."[89]

Celebrities' use of New Age treatments added a glamorous endorsement. Shirley MacLaine testified to the wonders of acupuncture and crystal healing and Britain's Queen Elizabeth reportedly used homeopathy and aromatherapy, while the late Princess Diana allegedly favored acupuncture and energy healing. In 2002, American readers learned that Cherie Blair, wife of Britain's prime minister, not only wore "acupressure earrings" to counteract stress and an anti-radiation "bioelectric shield pendant," but also had report-edly undergone a "rebirthing ceremony." Far from scoffing, the *New York Times* offered supportive statements from other women, who suggested that as a public figure, high-powered lawyer, and mother of four, Blair deserved all the tension relief and nurturing she desired.[90]

Alternative therapy products catering specifically to female consumers had become a substantial niche, especially in the health-food business. The Zoe Foods Flax and Soy Granola Bar billed itself as "good for the overall health . . . energy for the heart and soul," allegedly following a recipe the founder's mother had concocted to ease her menopausal change. On the same shelf, shoppers might find the New You "women's supplement" chocolate-crisp "hormonal balance" bar. The ingredients ("black cohosh, dong quai, red clover, wild yam, 37 herbs, vitamins and minerals") promised "support for hot flashes, PMS, mood, increased energy, breast and bone health," although small type noted that the FDA had not evaluated those claims. Drawing on a rhetoric of empowerment, the label read, "Women can take charge of their health by choosing safe, natural solutions." Playing up emotional connections, each Luna "whole-nutrition bar for women" carried a "per-sonal dedication" from "the women of Luna" to female friends and relatives who "touched us, inspired us," such as a sister who "taught me to . . . be happy with the person I am."

A 2003 *Cathy* cartoon poked fun at the way manufacturers had jumped on the bandwagon of marketing food with gender-specific health claims and at female consumers' apparent eagerness to accept such claims. The strip showed female office workers refusing to let their male boss share their "hormone-balancing 'for women only' soy shake, "energy-boosting 'for women only' mocha blend," or "energy-quieting 'for women only' mint tea." When their female-health-food fixation drove him to take pills promising "extra pain relief for a man-sized headache," the women snarled, "Honestly . . . how self-indulgent can they get?" In truth, marketing often came to overshadow the political roots of women's alternative health foods, and a shopper did not have to be an involved feminist activist in order to toss a Zoe Foods bar into her cart at the checkout stand. Nevertheless, though obscured, the history of feminist medical rebels had helped set the stage. Consumers who purchased Luna bars or soy shakes might not always know the story of the Dalkon Shield or have mastered the latest menopause research, but the feminist, environmentalist, and New Age politics of alternative medicine had nonetheless facilitated that trend.[91]

At its best, female-authored and female-oriented criticism of mainstream medicine and support of alternative approaches had enlarged political, professional, and public awareness of female health issues. Even some mainstream doctors acknowledged that in challenging established medical authority and demanding a response, feminists and other critics had spurred the medical establishment to dedicate new attention and increased funding to women's health matters. As results from the Women's Health Initiative's study of menopausal hormone therapy so vividly demonstrated, there was indeed reason to investigate some old assumptions about women's health and press for answers to unsolved questions. As the feminist medical rebels behind the various editions of *Our Bodies, Ourselves* had intended, an extended focus on female health needs opened avenues of political and social debate for many women, giving them forums to express opinions on topics ranging from air and water pollution to marginalization of the poor and underprivileged. In agitating for specific causes such as research on breast cancer or CFIDS, many activists found a sense of sisterhood, dedication, and sometimes at least partial accomplishment. In rejecting the biological explanations and cultural messages that had attached negative overtones to menstruation and menopause, women could gain confidence and comfort. In pursuing alternative health care, they could enjoy feelings of empowerment and possibility. Especially in an age when many Americans complained about feeling lost, intimidated, or infuriated by hospital and insurance firm bureaucracy, defecting (even occasionally or temporarily) from conventional medicine could seem like freedom, whether embracing one approach or in testing several. Health self-education became important to many women, and to the extent that holistic practitioners directed clients toward more nutritious dietary patterns, exercise, and proper sleep habits, the result could amount to an important gain in well-being. Massage, aromatherapy, meditation, and yoga could provide bodily relaxation and sensory adventures rare for overstressed Americans immersed in a fast-paced, information-intensive world. If nothing else, the placebo effect could provide satisfaction for women who felt sure that homeopathic compounds boosted their energy or that echinacea helped ward off colds. Holistic healing provided a rich promise of personal and environmental balance that millions of women chose to explore as a substitute for or meaningful complement to regular medicine.

At its worst, women enraptured by searching through alternative-medicine options for a magical cure for cancer could find the mirage fatal. Although rhetoric of feminist empowerment and consumer independence sounded positive, selecting medical treatment could not, and should not, be "like buying a couch." Practitioners might encourage people to test-drive various alternative approaches, but it simply was not wise to experiment casually with a treatment mentioned in a popular magazine, described in four sentences in the do-it-yourself guide attached to the herbal product shelves at Wal-Mart, recommended by a friend of a friend, or touted on some Web site possibly full of misinformation. Contrary to the appealing image of "natural" cures as perfectly safe, herbs and food supplements carried definite health risks. Authorities warned, for example, that consumers who took ephedra in search of an easy weight-melting or bodybuilding miracle might develop dangerous, even deadly, side effects. Many Americans assumed wrongly that all supplements appearing on the market and any other product making health claims must have been tested for safety and effectiveness by the Food and Drug Administration, not realizing the absence of strict government oversight in this area. The marketing of herbs, natural foods, and other alternative health products had become just that, *marketing*, often playing more on imagery and consumers' credulity than on sound science. As for the principles and ideology behind feminist health ideology, fervor at times descended into crude critiques of patriarchy and simplistic blanket condemnations of modern medicine. While some alternative healers might indeed offer valuable advice on balanced eating habits and other self-care strategies, such commonsense principles were often mixed with or outweighed by utter mumbo jumbo. Judith Orloff, for instance, encouraged her followers to choose between health practitioners, even before meeting them, by remote viewing, "intuitively focusing on their names [even just a first name] and noticing any images, impressions, or insights that strike you . . . [to] get a good take on your compatibility . . . illuminating a universe of information unattainable by logic alone. . . . Be an empty rice bowl waiting to be filled."[92]

For all the pitfalls inherent in such appeals by alternative practitioners, however, it remained difficult, not to say politically incorrect, to argue with women convinced that alternative medicine had "worked" for them. Celebrities and ordinary women alike testified to their satisfaction with various therapies. Alternative healers of the later twentieth century had evolved a dynamic practical and ideological, individual and collective, appeal to women. Practitioners pledged to satisfy American women by moving beyond regular medicine, exemplified in their readiness to recognize CFIDS as a disease and their refusal to reduce menopause to an illness. While the Boston Women's Health Book Collective's critique of conventional medicine had derived from and reflected the oppositional political culture of the 1960s, the eagerness to explore female-friendly alternatives had spread far beyond radical consciousness-raising groups. As the twenty-first-century debates over menopause clearly revealed, female-oriented alternative practices had become mainstream in their accessibility and public acceptability. In publishing *Our Bodies, Ourselves*, America's feminist medical rebels had articulated a political philosophy promoting consideration of alternative medicine. Over the three decades since, that perspective had merged with New Age beliefs, environmentalism, consumerism, and commercialism, constructing a very specific context for a renewed interest in female-friendly alternative medicine. Feminist medical rebels had made the personal into the political, and in turn, modern alternative medicine had made the political into the personal.

INSIDE-OUT

Holism and History in Toronto's Women's Health Movements

Georgina Feldberg

Before the onset of modern medicine, healing was a traditionally female domain, co-existing with woman's role as mother and nurturer. A fundamental difference between female lay-healers and the male dominated medical profession was in their approach to knowledge. Female lay-healers operated within a network of information sharing and mutual support.

—*Healthsharing*, November 1979

"WCH [Women's College Hospital] gets its day in Court," read a banner headline in August 1997.[1] It was a small victory, but the Friends of Women's College Hospital—an association of loyal physicians, patients, and staff—nonetheless celebrated that Toronto hospital's latest effort to resist a merger with Sunnybrook, the city's veterans hospital. Less than a decade earlier, WCH, Canada's oldest and premier women's facility, had successfully averted a plan to integrate its operations with Toronto General Hospital. On both occasions, the hospital's unique history and its status as an alternative institution where women patients could receive a special kind of care from women physicians formed the foundation of resistance.

The portrayal of a late-twentieth-century hospital as exemplary of an alternative health movement seems inside out. I have chosen this odd turn of phrase deliberately—and I use it here in place of *upside down*, *backward*, or even *absurd*—both to capture WCH's struggles and to position these within debates over the meaning of alternative health care. Since the late 1980s, alternative health and alternative health movements have inspired considerable scholarly analysis and debate. The literature shows no consensus about the meaning of *alternative*, and both scholarly and popular sources use the term in many different ways. Some locate alternative healing within the literature of professions and professional ideologies. Hans Baer, for example, portrays alternative health movements as oppositional to the structures and knowledge base of biomedicine, attractive to a range of peripheral or marginal populations, and coherent in their critique if not their content. Others identify the alternative approaches to medical practice that emerged in late-twentieth-century America in terms of their ideological opposition to biomedicine. For example, Robbie

Davis Floyd and Gloria St. John divide practitioners into holists, who dismiss the practices and beliefs of allopathy and replace them with an integrated form of healing based on the fundamental relationship between mind and body, and humanists, who accept the principles and practices of biomedicine but seek more personal, humanized ways of delivering care. Others, such as Rosalind Coward, adopt an epistemic or Foucauldian approach to the rise of alternative healing that is more cynical. Coward argues that though political action could transform health care, alternative healers do not seek political goals. Rather, she suggests, they are united in a "philosophical opposition to orthodox medicine and attitudes to health" that emphasizes such virtues as nature, healing, and women's special wisdom.[2]

Whether from such scholarly perspectives or the vantage of populist activists, hospitals—homes to and products of the biomedical revolution—represent all that alternative practitioners have come to rebel against. Yet as WCH constructed its history and justified its survival, it made claims to the same battles and goals that motivated other alternative practitioners, as portrayed above. WCH in its early years provided training to those who wanted to be physicians but were denied admission to regular medical institutions. The physicians who trained at WCH and the programs that the hospital developed challenged the scientific status of biomedicine while simultaneously battling for the approval of patients and medical regulatory bodies. Moreover, over the course of a century, WCH affirmed women's special and distinct role as healers. This claim to women's special nature, so central to the struggle to save WCH, resonated with the broader goals and ideologies of the women's health movement (WHM) that emerged in the United States and Canada during the 1960s. As North American women campaigned to transform the substance, organization, and delivery of health care, women's wisdom and ways seemed to offer a powerful counterideology to allopathic medicine. Though few women's health activists would have identified WCH as a comrade in arms, the hospital capitalized on the broader trend and its unique history to forge an alternative based on women's ideals and women's work.

This essay focuses on WCH, as part of the broader Canadian women's health movement, to place women's health in the frame of alternative medicine. I have chosen this "inside-out" struggle to explore the ways in which both women's activism and alternative health have been traditionally situated outside hospitals and medical authority. I have chosen the term *inside-out* carefully, to reflect the political position of standing apart that is so central to alternative health activism and to reflect the debate over whether change can be effected from within or must necessarily come from outside. The focus on WCH also emphasizes the political uses to which history is put and regenders the history of medical alternatives by privileging women over their particular practices and beliefs. From the vantage of WCH and the movement of which it was a part, to be a woman was itself, and by itself, the "alternative." As the title of one best-selling book proclaimed, "All Women are Healers."[3]

SEEKING ALTERNATIVES: WOMEN'S HEALTH MOVEMENTS
IN LATE-TWENTIETH-CENTURY CANADA

Women's College Hospital based its claim to status as a singular, alternative health care provider on its own history and the objectives of a broader women's health movement. Working outside of institutions—indeed, in opposition to institutions—the women who forged the women's health movement of the 1960s and 1970s saw themselves as revolutionary. Highly political and politicized, they critiqued medical dominance, affirmed the authority of women's ways of knowing, empowered women as consumers of medical services, and refuted the authority of science. In their cause, they often invoked history and women's historical work as healers. Physicians, if they figured at all in that past, were usually cast as villains. Hospitals similarly assumed bit parts as bastions of traditional male knowledge and practice. Yet despite an immense political divide, there were many commonalities between the goals and objectives of the WHM and those of WCH, which this section explores by outlining, in depth, the contours of the WHM.

The women's health movement (WHM) that swept North America during the 1960s and 1970s was far from monolithic. It comprised many different women who had diverse goals. Both scholarly and popular opinions often characterize the WHM as a political movement or even a "new social movement."[4] Inspired by the civil rights activism of the 1960s, the consumer protection efforts of Ralph Nader, and an awareness of medical malfeasance and malpractice, U.S. women organized politically for change.[5] They constructed a political critique of medical services, the organization and delivery of which did not adequately meet women's needs. Canadian women confronted a different political landscape in which neither the Vietnam War nor civil rights loomed as large as they did south of the border. Citizens of a welfare state, they had already won such significant battles as coverage for essential medical services, under universal, publicly funded health insurance plans. Yet as Chantalle Maillé observes, "most of the services required for women fall outside this category of required services."[6] For example, birth control and abortion were not covered by public health insurance in the 1960s; midwifery, nutritional, and psychological counseling and assisted reproduction were not covered in the 1980s. Hence, Canadian women joined their southern sisters' challenge to a medical system that women continued to find inadequate, and they marshaled many of the same responses.[7] Over the course of two decades, Canadian women sought legal, political, and social means to transform medical practice and frame alternatives. They promoted self-help, empowerment, and women's special ways of knowing, and they invoked the spirituality and special healing status of women.

In both nations women initially engaged in a concerted drive to reclaim reproduction. Criticized since for their limited and exclusionary scope, women's efforts to promote birth control, legalize abortion, and refeminize birth nonetheless rallied diverse constituencies of North American women around a common cause.[8] As Lesley Biggs suggests, reproduction provided a unifying force. Despite the many differences among them, all women had reproductive systems and hence could claim to know and experience oppression that derived from their physical sex. All women could mobilize politically around the cause of reproduction to fight their shared oppression.[9] Hence, the campaign for reproductive rights allowed for varied personal, public, and legal actions. It came to dominate and shape historical scholarship and activist efforts, and it inspired two distinct feminist alternatives.

On one hand, as the campaign for reproductive rights took shape around efforts to improve access to safe, legal abortion and contraception, it defined an overtly activist and political agenda focused on the limitations of both medicine and law.[10] For example, in 1968, a group of McGill University undergraduates openly linked political change with reproductive rights in their race for student leadership positions. If elected, they promised, they would produce and distribute information on birth control that was illegal at the time. The Montreal Health Press emerged from their victory, and its pioneering *Birth Control Handbook* educated and "sexually liberated" students across North America. As the table of contents for the first edition of the Boston Women's Health Book Collective's *Our Bodies Ourselves: A Book by and for Women* (1971) illustrated, women sought emancipation through their control of reproduction and their creation of new understandings of sexuality, relationships, violence, venereal disease, and menopause. Along with the Boston Women's Health Book Collective, the Montreal Health Press set the agenda for a campaign that combined political action and a critique of established medicine.[11]

The reproductive focus that was so central to the WHM also had another more ethereal or spiritual side, exemplified in efforts to reclaim natural childbirth and reinstate midwifery. Through the 1970s and 1980s, choice in childbirth became a rallying point for diverse constituencies of North American women. While some activists viewed the campaign to legalize midwifery as part of a broader, liberal political campaign to maximize women's health care choices, many others used the campaign to promote midwife births as a spiritual departure from allopathic health care. What Rosalind Coward has described as a shift "from Politics to Mythology" occurred as spiritualism and history became central to debates over midwifery,[12] and in Ontario, as elsewhere, the profession and its public divided along lines of sentiment versus practicality.[13] Alongside the more overtly political efforts to transform medicine and law so that midwifery was legal and acceptable, some women sought ways to recapture women's essential spirit and abilities. They made claim to women's affinity with nature—a special relationship women ascribed to their menstrual cycles and ability to give birth. Women, by virtue of their ability to bear children, were deemed one with the physical world.

History, a symbolic retelling of the rise and fall of woman-dominated healing, became central to this effort, and the telling of this history became a kind of political action. Women's harmony with the earth and its cycles was both rooted and reflected in the practices of goddesses and witches, who had mastered the secrets of the universe and used these to heal. The publication of the classic pamphlet *Witches, Midwives and Nurses* in 1973 had set the stage for scholarship and activism that would reclaim woman's healing role. "Women have always been healers," Barbara Ehrenreich and Deirdre English wrote in what would become a common phrasing:

> They were the unlicensed doctors and anatomists of western history. They were the abortionists, nurses and counsellors, they were pharmacists, cultivating healing herbs and exchanging the secrets of their uses. They were the midwives. . . . For centuries women were doctors without degrees. . . . They were called wise women by the people, witches or charlatans by the authorities. Medicine is part of our heritage as women, our history, our birthright.[14]

Thereafter, the number of works that proclaimed women's distinct ways of healing, and attempted to recapture a history that scientific medicine had erased, proliferated.[15] While some feminists denounced the rise of male-dominated medical obstetrics, others extolled the virtues of a female-dominated birth.[16] To many in this latter group, home births and midwife-attended births, services delivered by women, formed part of a gentle but venerable historical tradition. The experience of birth came to represent what Pamela Klassen has termed a cosmology. It exemplified all that was female and feminine about the natural order, and it offered the promise of an essential and uniquely female health experience.[17]

The myriad women's health collectives that emerged in Boston, Toronto, Vancouver, and other cities across North America mirrored the broader movement as they struggled to balance political action with spiritual change. Among these, Women Healthsharing became the most prominent and influential of the Canadian collectives, and it explicitly and implicitly offered what seemed a dramatic departure from the kind of hospital care that WCH provided.[18] Healthsharing, comprised of women from diverse backgrounds that included nursing, public health, and law, published the first issue of its journal, *Healthsharing*, in 1979. Initially, the Healthsharing Collective received grants from Canada's federal government under program funding to nonprofit agencies. This financial support continued into the 1990s, when the government withdrew funding to grassroots organization. Cast as a matter of fiscal restraint, the demise of the program that funded Healthsharing and similar nonprofit alternatives coincided with a new era of funding for health research. As it withdrew its funding from Healthsharing, the Liberal government announced its new Centres of Excellence for Women's Health Programme, designed to foster collaboration between academic and community researchers. The parallel and coincident events, which shifted funding from grassroots to institutions, captured the inside-out dilemma of women's health activism.

The words and work of the Healthsharing collective, its journal, and its resource guide exemplified the WHM's search for alternatives. A decade of North American successes in promoting women's health inspired the Healthsharing collective to dream of consolidating and building upon Canadian women's health interests. Founded a decade later than the Boston and Montreal collectives, Healthsharing began with the conviction that women's health activism needed to reach beyond reproduction to transform relations with physicians, challenge the scientific basis of allopathic medicine, and recapture women's traditional wisdom and ways of healing. "A feminist critique of the health system," members of the collective wrote in their inaugural essay, "is not addressed solely to issues relating to sexism and gynaecology . . . the repeatedly apparent oppression of women is indicative of the inherent oppression of the whole system. It is the whole system which we, as women, are struggling to change."[19]

Changing "the whole system" could not be achieved without a fundamental transformation of the ways in which medicine was practiced. The pages of *Healthsharing* created a space in which women could share their dissatisfaction with existing medical services and unite their individual and personal experiences to reconfigure health care. Articles in the journal's first issues promoted improvements in existing services for women. Each issue drew readers' attention to new and different sites for service delivery, among these freestanding birthing centers (in which women bore their children in a setting that more closely resembled the home) and sexual assault care centers, which provided women who had been assaulted with more respectful and sensitive treatment. These alternatives changed the physical places in which health care was delivered, with many feminists specifically advocating the relocation of women's health services away from hospitals.

Healthsharing challenged both the sites in which health care was delivered and the means by which it was practiced. Medicine's insensitivity to women's needs became a common theme, and a plea for practitioners who both recognized the physical differences between the sexes and women's desire to be treated differently appeared again and again. "The aspects of allopathic medicine—reliance on laboratory science for diagnosis and cure, dehumanization and specialization—have all been criticized by feminists and other social critics," the collective suggested. "There has been both a demand for changing allopathic medicine and for creating alternatives."[20] A women's health clinic in Montreal, Quebec, the Centre de santé des femmes du Quartier, became the prototype for "changed" allopathic medicine. Instead of the traditional hierarchy of doctor-nurse-patient, the center was run by nurses and nonmedical staff. This clinic claimed to shift the "imbalance of power between a doctor and a 'patient'" by including women in decision making and offering them less intrusive, "woman-oriented care." For many women, simple inclusion in decision making was the key element of woman-centered care, but the center also went beyond this to offer a range of options for services, such as self-administed Pap tests and vaginal examinations, that it believed to be less invasive than standard procedures.[21]

For some contributors to *Healthsharing*, allopathic medicine seemed beyond repair. Hence, the magazine and the women it served also reached outside to consider a range of alternatives, at once "traditional" and revolutionary. An article promoting health care choices outlined some of the ways in which a woman with premenstrual syndrome (PMS) might seek relief. The piece began with a typical critique of the medical approaches and treatments so many women found unsatisfactory. "If she had access to other resources," the author noted, a woman suffering from severe PMS might avoid taking hormonal treatments. Choice, rather than any single modality of care, was the alternative, and the article outlined some of the many options a woman in need might pursue:

> An herbalist could have told her about raspberry leaf or brancha leaf tea and tamari tea. A nutritionist might have recommended that she take dolomite calcium and decrease her intake of caffeine and sugar the week before her period. She could have gone to a masseuse for lower back massage. A women's health group might have put her in touch with a feminist yoga instructor to learn exercises which might relieve menstrual cramping. A different doctor or a nurse-practitioner might have suggested an increase in very ripe bananas or fresh orange juice to help increase potassium levels. A friend might have suggested taking a sauna or having an orgasm to help increase her menstrual flow.[22]

The range of alternatives described here reflected the diverse therapeutic modalities Canadian women turned to in their quest for better care.

Healthsharing educated women about long-standing alternatives to biomedicine, including nutritional healing, naturopathy, herbalism, midwifery, and homeopathy. Articles and advertisements encouraged women to try these varied options and train themselves in new healing practices. The women of *Healthsharing*, like other proponents of alternative care, deemed natural remedies and practices—whatever their source—safer than, and preferable to, the technologies and synthetic pharamaceuticals that allopathy offered. In addition, *Healthsharing* introduced readers to newer alternatives, often spiritually based, such as "healing with the mind's eye" or guided imagery, hypnosis, and techniques for retrieving lost traumatic memories. Part of a range of populist health practices that became common throughout North America during the 1970s and 1980s, these therapies became especially important to the WHM because they rested on the foundational claim that individuals did not need physicians or experts; they could heal themselves.

The WHM's challenge to allopathy thus reflected women's widespread and fundamental belief that remedies and practices traditionally defined as "alternative" were better for women than biomedicine. The movement's challenge also reflected a faith that medical knowledge need not be hierarchical and scientific. Rosalind Coward, in her analysis of the alternative health movement, argues that one of the movement's failings is that "[w]hat could be a political critique of conventional medicine is instead a critique based on a *philosophical* opposition to orthodox medicine and attitudes towards health . . . it is a symbolic activity."[23] The WHM, exemplified by the readers and contributors to *Healthsharing*, engaged in this symbolic activity as they challenged medicine's knowledge base. Alongside political critiques of service delivery, the quest for alternatives took a philosophical turn that invoked women's special talents. Both *Healthsharing* and the WHM repeatedly complained that "knowledge based on personal experience is not validated by medical professionals" and they promoted different ways of knowing about health.[24] Wisdom came from everyday life and shared experience rather than experiments and books. Philosophers and psychologists alike made claim to women's distinctive ways of using intuition and context. Women scientists, Evelyn Fox Keller argued in her pathbreaking book *A Feeling for the Organism*, collected and interpreted evidence differently than men. Girls, Carol Gilligan maintained, learned relationally and through context.[25] The women's health movement applied these theories unevenly in its effort to change practice, but the appeal to women's special wisdom and ways of knowing was almost universal.

A quest for self-knowledge and self-care became fundamental to the WHM as empowerment, education, and knowledge sharing offered ways to claim women's special ways of "knowing" and recapture a tradition of women's healing work. Healthsharing again exemplified this trend. As members of the collective put it, "the first step toward creating an alternative is to communicate, to share with one another and to trust one another."[26] Knowledge sharing, or Healthsharing, provided a way to shift power and authority, especially within medical systems deemed hierarchical and based on hidden knowledge. The commitment to "sharing information" and "communicating" borrowed from a broader trend toward empowerment and self-help that was part of a very particular and American way of combating differences in economic and social power. Just as information would allow American consumers to make good choices, information would enable women to take charge of their health and well-being. Hence, the women's health activists advocated a shift from "patient" to "client."[27]

In addition to contributing to this semantic power struggle, the commitment to sharing information also reflected a desire to create a new, distinct form of health knowledge. "Healthsharing—the concept of sharing health," the members of the collective wrote, "is for us a feminist approach to health and healing. It denotes the caring and sense of community which are the essence of both feminism and healing."[28] Such affirmations of the power of women's wisdom, women's knowledge, and women's healing became central to—indeed, fundamental to—the WHM. Empowerment, self-help, spirituality, and women's special ways of caring for the sick came to form standard components of the women's health care kit because women's wisdom stemmed from experience, the self, and the knowledge of elders who had forged the path. Building on the historical claim laid down by Ehrenreich, English, and others, the women of Healthsharing noted that "Health Care has always been a special concern of women. It is part of our long designated historical role in the community as midwives, herbalists and healers."[29] The Healthsharing collective took this history one step further and identified women's *historical* connection with medicine as the root of the WHM. "[T]he women's health movement," one Canadian activist suggested, "emerged, in the early seventies, as a reflection of [a] special relationship between women and health care."[30] This affirmation of women's special and *historical* relationship with health care became the uniting, alternative force of the WHM.

When viewed through the work and words of Healthsharing, a women's health movement that seems diverse and fractured, with disparate goals and methods, can be seen to be more unified and united. Healthsharing engaged women in a quest for alternatives to allopathic medicine that ranged from an initiative to increase the admission of women to medical schools to the reclaiming of herbal recipes and to magical and spiritual healing. The movement, such as it was, did not propose any one modality for care. It did not embody one philosophical position or affirm one principle of causal relations. It did, however, unite women in a challenge to the knowledge base of medicine, predicated on women's unique and special wisdom. Again, the critique was both political and philosophical. Women, who constituted the majority of health care workers and the largest population of consumers of health care, sought the power to transform the medical services they both provided and used. But the WHM also laid claim to the assertion that women provided a fundamentally different kind of care. They did more than cure; they healed. Hence, the WHM also attempted to transform the care that women received by recapturing a distinctly female form of healing. Historically grounded, this tradition of womanly healing purportedly predated modern scientific medicine. It relied on gentle products of nature, women's connection with the earth and its people, and their ability to learn from experience rather than from books.

The women's health movement's challenge to medicine, and its search for historically grounded, women-centered healing, took place outside of conventional medicine. Affirming women's innate capabilities, based in a special affinity between women and nature that derived from women's reproductive capacities, it nonetheless recognized that women would not heal within the confines of the regular medical system. "Most of our collective members go to women doctors because we find they are more approachable than men, take more time to listen, explain what they are doing," Healthsharing explained. "Are these differences significant enough to expect a dramatic shift in healthcare as women continue to increase their proportion of the medical profession? Unfortunately, we don't think so."[31] The political and philosophical imperatives of the WHM came into conflict as the goal of increasing the representation of women within medicine collided with the belief that medicine was "masculine" and male. Yet despite the WHM's location outside of and in opposition to mainstream biomedicine, affirmations of women's affinity for healing also had a long tradition within the medical system itself. Over the course of half a century, Women's College Hospital repeatedly reminded Canadians that it had played a major role in shaping this alternative tradition.

WOMEN'S WORK FOR WOMEN'S NEEDS: THE HISTORY OF WOMEN AND HEALTH IN TORONTO

The WHM's claims to women's special status as healers resonated powerfully with Women's College Hospital's own history, and in its struggle for survival, WCH built its own historical claim to women's healing on women's behalf. In its effort to maintain independence from other institutions and perpetuate a tradition of caring it viewed as distinct, the hospital created a history—on paper, in art, and on film—that invoked its status as an alternative institution.[32] The articulated characteristics of an alternative—namely, making a place for medical outsiders, giving them the structures within which to practice, allowing them to confront the limitations of biomedicine in their struggle for status, and affirming women's special and distinct role as healers—all formed part of this effort.

Women's College Hospital prided itself on a long history of creating space for medical outcasts. When it sought designation as a national historic site, in the 1990s, it began its history with accounts of Emily Stowe (1831–1893), the grandmother of Canadian medical women. Stowe, a teacher and suffragist, was also the first Canadian women to practice medicine openly. She personified the alternative vision upon which women's health has been built. Born Emily Howard Jennings, to Quakers who had emigrated to Upper Canada from Vermont, Stowe later described herself as a "scientific socialist," and the octagonal house she built with her husband, John Stowe, suggested a predilection for Theosophy. Her mother was a herbal healer, and the young Emily apprenticed with Joseph Lancaster, an eminent homeopath. She then followed a more traditional path into teaching and worked as a teacher and principal until 1865, when she enrolled in Clemence Sophia Lozier's homeopathic New York Medical College for Women. After her graduation in 1867 Stowe returned to Canada, where her practice included homeopathy and herbalism. Stowe's preference for homeopathy figured prominently in the celebrated death of Sarah Lovell, following which Stowe was tried for performing an abortion because the pregnant Lovell died shortly after taking the homeopathic remedy—ostensibly with abortifacent properties—that Stowe had prescribed.[33]

Stowe's preference for homeopathic principles and practice was only one of the challenges she issued to established allopathic medicine; she also fought for the inclusion of women. Having been unable to study medicine in Canada, both because women were unwelcome in medical schools and because there were no homeopathic colleges, Stowe was also denied a license when, as a medical graduate, she later returned to Toronto. After her daughter Ann Augusta decided to follow her mother into the study of medicine, Stowe played a leading role the campaign to open Canadian medical schools to women. From the time she studied in New York, Stowe had advocated strongly for women's medical needs, and particularly for their need to be cared for by a woman physician. Advertisements for her practice, which appeared in *Might's Toronto City Directory*, listed her as a specialist in the diseases of women and children. Stowe spoke openly of women's special capacity to heal and their responsibility as "mother[s] of the race." Yet Stowe was an egalitarian. She did not endorse sex-segregated medical education and practice. First vice president of the Canadian Women's Suffrage Association and a leader of the National Council of Women, she fought to ensure that women would be accepted as equal to men and their work fully recognized.

Though Women's College Hospital claims her among its founders, Stowe actually had no connection to that institution. However, Stowe did play a part in founding Toronto Women's Medical College (1883), which WCH eventually grew from, and the Medical College bore the imprint of Stowe's political commitment to shaping an alternative medicine that included women. With the men and women she worked with, Stowe endeavored to provide opportunities for outcasts—the women whom other, more established medical institutions made unwelcome. The curriculum of TWMC did not conform to or reflect Stowe's preferences for homeopathy, botany, and other nonallopathic medical treatments. Indeed, in the early years, *Annual Calendars* and *College Announcements*—published to recruit students and report on progress—repeatedly reassured applicants and the public that its women students received the same rigorous, scientific training as men. "The College was founded and has been maintained," reports and publicity statements reminded readers, "at great self sacrifice on the part of subscribers and staff, in order to vindicate the principle that the sexes should not be taught medicine together."[34] Women, both Stowe and the college's board maintained, were medical equals of men.

Yet alongside assurances that women would and could be trained in scientific medicine, statements from the college also affirmed women's special, distinct medical talents. The medical college, and the hospital and dispensary it later gave rise to, both created opportunities for aspiring physicians who had no other options *and* allowed women graduates to practice a different kind of medicine. "Recognizing the great importance of the clinical study of Diseases of Women and Children to women students," the *Announcement* for 1891–92 reported, the college had "amplified" the course of instruction to include special practical classes and clinics in obstetrics and gynecology.[35] The decision to emphasise the college's ever-expanding offerings in diseases of women and children played pragmatically on popularly held assumptions about the kind of medicine women physicians might prefer to practice, where, and with whom.

The emphasis placed on instruction in diseases of women and children also reflected a commonly held belief that women, because they became mothers, had inherent, superior abilities to treat their own sex. The conviction that women would practice a different kind of medicine emerged clearly in a second theme of the college's *Announcements*: the goal of preparing graduates to care for the needy through missionary work in Asia, or among the poor who lived closer to home.[36] Efforts to recruit women as medical missionaries built openly on the interconnections between women's reproductive ability and their religious and medical callings. As recent studies of women and medicine remind us, religion, faith, and spirituality played significant and long-standing roles in women's healing work. Most of these recent works situate women healers outside of medicine, in folk and informal traditions, or within the confines of formal religious orders. Yet other formal possibilities existed for late-nineteenth- and early-twentieth-century North American women, and the founders of the Toronto Women's Medical College both recognized and capitalized on these. As British missions to India and West China flourished during the late nineteenth century, Canadian women assumed a central role in the colonial effort. Despite a rapid proliferation of outposts, Canadian missions failed to reach their targets for conversion, and this failure reflected their inability to reach local women who controlled their households. In the mission field, medicine had become an intermediary. Canadian medical missionaries did not charge for their services but instead extracted conversion to Christianity as the price of care. When Asian women resisted the medical interventions of men, sending women into the field offered one ready solution. Under the direction of Lady Dufferin, wife of the governor general, or queen's representative, to first Canada and then India, hospitals for women, staffed by women, opened throughout the Far Eastern colonies.[37]

Offering services for women, by women, was a pragmatic solution that first and foremost bridged a fundamental gender gap and allowed the male missions to achieve goals they could not otherwise attain. However, women physicians also recognized and took advantage of opportunities for work in areas from which they were otherwise excluded. Canadian women's missionary work in India and China was at once emancipatory and co-optive, colonizing and complicit, and as they took on the work, the women physicians echoed the arguments men had made about their special qualifications. Women, they argued, were more spiritual, had a greater affinity for nature, and were able to heal gently. Marshaling these strengths, Canadian-trained women doctors worked to convert their patients simultaneously to Christianity and to "civilized" methods of healing. They spread the gospel of health. Ironically, on foreign soils, Western principles of faith and medicine were the "alternatives." The germ theory, Western hygienic practices, and allopathic medicines replaced and supplanted the traditional, indigenous Ayurvedic and herbal remedies that late-twentieth-century health activists deem "alternative."

Newly graduated women physicians also provided medical missionary services closer to home, where they similarly made the case for the different kind of care women physicians could provide. In 1898 the students of the Women's Medical College opened a dispensary and clinic at one of the city missions. This dispensary and clinic was the forerunner of Women's College Hospital, and over the course of a century, it metamorphosed into the medical facility that exists today.[38] The dispensary and clinic of the Women's Medical College provided relief work to women living in Toronto, and it identified women's special medical needs as its raison d'être. "That there is always in our midst a number of retiring poor ones that would suffer death almost or quite than seek relief at a public dispensary where men attend is an actual fact," the doctors maintained.[39] WCH graduates met the need with medical services adapted to women patients and provided by women physicians. Among those who sought care, readers of the dispensary's annual reports were advised, was a woman from Alberta who had been "suffering in silence for eight years because there was no woman physician whom she could consult."[40] The women doctors met her needs because, in language used as well by the late-twentieth-century alternative health movement, they had an appreciation for the context of women's lives and the many stresses on their health. College graduates attended to medical and social needs. In addition to "receiving medical attention," the dispensary reported, "one patient was given one of our well-filled maternity bags, as she was quite unprepared for the event." A student taught another woman, sick with tuberculosis, how to cope with her disease. The doctors proudly publicized their success in reaching women who were trapped in unfortunate marriages. For example, "[o]ne woman, with a number of growing girls and a very evil husband has found relief for both body and mind in bringing her troubles to the Dispensary."[41]

WCH, as it grew, continued to provide a place for patients and practitioners who were at the fringes of male medicine. While other hospitals excluded women from fellowships and residencies, WCH created opportunities for female medical graduates to complete their training. Thereafter, it employed them in a facility that, until the hospital became part of the University of Toronto in the 1960s, women operated for women. This alone, the hospital maintained, made WCH different. Annual reports repeatedly interwove the stories of a hospital that women physicians founded for their sisters and to which women patients could turn in times of trouble. They reaffirmed both the special capacities of women doctors and the special needs of women patients. Just as the hospital provided training to renegade women doctors, "[h]omeless, sick, elderly women have been cared for when no other Hospital would take them in."[42]

As WCH told of the many ways in which women physicians served their needy patients, it also adopted a narrative of caring. In 1912, the hospital had begun using the motto "Woman's work for women's needs." Soon this was modified to include the phrase "the union of those who love on behalf of those who suffer."[43] The annual report for 1914 celebrated "women's work among women for the amelioration of suffering."[44] Almost foreshadowing the efforts of the twentieth-century WHM, some of their efforts to ameliorate suffering took shape as a plea for the reorganization of medical care. "The need for beds for those who could not pay the public ward rate became a most pressing one," the hospital reports regularly acknowledged.[45] Hence, WCH found ways to enable women who could not otherwise afford to pay the regular hospital rates to receive professional services. Much as this effort was structural and philanthropic, it was also cast as a distinctively female solution. "The hearts of the doctors were frequently much touched by the expressions of relief and thankfulness of timid, suffering women, too poor to go to a doctor's office and too fearful to go to an ordinary dispensary to seek the needed help," the report noted.[46] Hence, in addition to the reconfiguring of payment schemes, WCH also claimed to provide a different kind of care. Sentiment and compassion characterized the work of the women doctors who took on these difficult cases.

The hospital also used history politically, and it deftly and repeatedly invoked its unique history to situate and enshrine women's special wisdom and their sensitivity to other women's needs. In 1915, the hospital moved from its original quarters, in a small house in Toronto's old east end, to grander, though still residential, premises in the city's west end. When the new facility opened, one of the hospital's founders told the story of its origins. "Upon me," she began, "has been conferred the privilege of representing the 'Mother' of this Branch of 'Women's Work for Women's needs.'" Adopting a distinctly spiritual tone, the unidentified orator spoke of the hospital's early days, and the "great diffidence" with which "we metaphorically stepped carefully to the water's edge to try to do our little bit in helping the sick and suffering . . . then we heard the Divine Call as Paul did when the Voice said 'Come into Macedonia and help us.'" She used similar rhetoric to commend Dr. Jennie Gray, a founding staff physician who had been asked to give the address but was unfortunately not present. "It was she who conducted the first Clinic in the beginning of the history of this work, to whom, timid suffering women flocked in such numbers."[47] Over the course of half a century, hospital reports echoed these words and sentiments. These reports reminded patients and patrons alike of the women physician who willingly, even gladly, made sacrifices for the flock that badly needed them. The stories within them celebrated occasions on which the women doctors triumphed, as when, perhaps by coincidence, WCH delivered the hospital's first baby on December 25, 1911—Christmas Day.

CONCLUSION: OFFERING ALTERNATIVES

Throughout (and through) its history Women's College Hospital presented itself as an alternative to dominant medicine and posed both political and philosophical challenges to the standard delivery of medical services. WCH provided a space for those who were unwelcome elsewhere in medicine. It created a place where physicians could practice a different kind of care. The hospital consistently and repeatedly prided itself for allowing women physicians to pursue more empathetic and compassionate healing.

Some of the institution's novelty lay in the creative ways it found to provide nontraditional services. Early in the twentieth century, it offered care to those who could not otherwise afford it. Later, after publicly funded health care became the Canadian norm, it pushed the boundaries of medicare to open and operate clinics that provided "non-insured" services. The Bay Centre for Birth Control (1973)—a street-front clinic—provided counseling and contraception to women of all ages at a time when the provision or dissemination of birth control information and products was barely acceptable legally or socially. The hospital's Brief Psychotherapy Centre (1987) offered women therapy that was alternative in both its duration and its approach. The Regional Women's Health Centre, established in the 1990s, employed a range of nonmedical staff to provide ancillary services. The Center's programs continued the tradition of alternative delivery. Redeploying public monies, they allowed women access to nutritional advice and counseling that would not otherwise be covered under public or private insurance schemes. Those services also took novel approaches. For example, they addressed issues of nutrition in the context of body image. They used peer group support and lay counseling. The center's library made a range of materials available to women in order to enable them to explore varied options for health care and apply information in their decision making. When the Province of Ontario legalized midwifery in the 1990s and allowed midwives to charge the public health insurance plan, WCH was among the first medical institutions to grant midwives hospital privileges.

Hard as it pushed politically, Women's College also forged a philosophical alternative. The hospital formed itself in the image of women, as healers. In the 1950s the hospital had taken the Egyptian symbol of the ankh, which refers to the spirit of life, and interwoven it with the international *H*, for hospital, to create its own symbol. The female virtues implicit in the ankh were displayed increasingly openly as the hospital came under threat. In 1971 the Board of Governors commissioned a statue to "commemorate the dedicated women who have built the hospital into what it is today." Created by the artist Frances Gage, the marble statue, entitled "Woman," stood in the hospital lobby. As *Spirit of Life*, the official "story" of Women's College Hospital produced in 1993 by the Association of Hospital Volunteers, explained:

> The spirit that animates "Woman" emulates a quiet strength, is one woman who could be all women, is wistful yet resolute, is rooted in the past yet with unwavering gaze looks to the present and beyond to the future. It is a remarkable achievement that both recalls history and inspires it.[48]

"Woman," placed as a sentinel in the lobby of a Toronto hospital, thus captured the same sentiments that inspired the women's health movement. "Woman," along with the new hospital motto "To Teach . . . to Heal . . . with Special Care," resonated powerfully with the affirmation of the historical base for women's healing that had unified the women's health movement.

Women's College Hospital's claim to a historically based alternative status was often politically strategic and self-serving. Its invocations of women's superior and distinct styles of healing ensured the hospital's survival in difficult financial times. Nonetheless, strong commonalities exist between this political, economic, historical, and philosophical posturing and the broader efforts of the WHM and other alternative health movements. Yet neither the women's health movement nor most alternative health care practitioners would immediately recognize WCH as a fellow traveler. Working outside of institutions—indeed, in opposition to institutions—the women who forged the women's health movement of the 1960s and 1970s saw themselves as revolutionary. Highly political and politicized, they critiqued medical dominance over women's bodies, affirmed the authority of women's experiences, empowered women as consumers of medical services, and debunked the authority of science. They issued strong appeals to history and to women's historical patterns of healing. They did not, however, celebrate women physicians as part of that past.

Still, the history of women and health in Toronto suggests that the struggle to reform medicine and reclaim women's healing past was at once historical and current, so those who worked outside often shared much with an older generation of women who worked within institutions. Both inside and out, women sought alternatives to the established relationships between physicians and their patients and to standard allopathic modes of treatment. They shared a desire to transform the delivery of traditional services, and they recognized and affirmed the special healing work undertaken by women. Both were alternative in their efforts to challenge standard medical knowledge, use a range of healing modalities that fell outside biomedicine, and highlight women's unique spiritual and physical qualifications for healing.

The struggles that WCH waged against dominant medicine, its positioning of itself as an alternative, and its emphasis on women's special ways of healing consequently issue a twofold challenge to the study of alternative medicine. First, the alternative status of WCH forces us to reflect on the definition of *alternative*. To most scholars of alternative medicine, the site where healing takes place and the kind of care provided take precedence over the practitioner herself. Ayurveda and acupuncture become alternatives whether delivered by indigenously trained practitioners or Western converts. Yet in the case of the women's health movement, the gender of the practitioner became more central than what she practiced, where, or how. So, for example, in the Far Eastern missions, the allopathic medical care that Western women provided was the alternative to the medical norm, even though this usurping of local knowledge can be deemed as colonizing as more recent Western appropriations of indigenous healing.

The intersecting efforts of the WHM and WCH also force us to pay closer attention to the place of gender in the history of alternative healthcare. Women used homeopathy, naturopathy, acupuncture, and a diversity of other widely recognized alternatives to biomedicine. However, the promotion of these varied modalities was not the primary objective of the women's health movement. Historically grounded affirmations of women's wisdom and women's ways became central to the WHM, even though women did not practice or know in any single way. When gendering alternative medicine's past we must consequently probe the meanings of *alternative*. We must ask whether the alternative existed in women's participation in broad challenges to biomedicine or in the women-centered movement that physicians and populists both forged. The efforts of WCH and WHM beg us to ask not what but who is the alternative.

A QUIET MOVEMENT

Orisha and the Healing of People, Spirit, History, and Community

Velana Huntington

The vast power of the priest in the African state is well known; his realm alone—the province of religion and medicine—remained largely unaffected by the plantation system. The Negro priest, therefore, became an important figure on the plantation and found his function as the interpreter of the supernatural, the comforter of the sorrowing, and as the one who expressed . . . the longing and disappointment and resentment of a stolen people.[1]

Between the fifteenth and nineteenth centuries, millions of Africans were transported from kingdoms and countries in West Africa to colonies throughout the Americas. To their involuntarily new cultural and geographical landscapes, many of them brought the healing knowledge and bodily praxis of *orisha* worship. From that point on, the personal and religious became political as those of African ancestry engaged in meaningful forms and practices of cultural and religious resistance against the colonialist powers that held their bodies captive. Embedded in their religious systems were profound medical beliefs along with notions of personhood and the nature of the human body. For Orisha devotees, religion has not been separate from everyday life in the African diaspora, and the human body is seen to exist on multiple levels, as it is at once physical/material, spiritual, emotional, and communal. Thus, both healing and religious practices were and are understood to be holistic.

In this essay, I explore this notion of holistic healing as I discuss Orisha as it is practiced in the urban areas of middle America, primarily Chicago and Milwaukee.[2] Drawing upon several years of on-site and off-site fieldwork among Orisha practitioners, I will first discuss some of the attributes of this Yoruba-based religion. Second, I will discuss the history of the Yoruba movement within the United States during the latter part of the twentieth century. Finally, I will tie together the politics of healing within this contemporary yet ancient religion as it is practiced by priests and other followers in the midwestern United States. As we will see, the personal, political, and spiritual converge in a particular understanding of African-American personhood.

THE ORISHA AND THEIR DEVOTEES

Orisha can best be understood as a complex and hierarchical set of relationships between Olodumare, the *orisha*, human beings, other living things such as animals and plants, and nonliving, natural objects such as rocks and water. All are embedded in spiritual "webs of relationships" in which each exists in direct and intimate relation to the others.[3] Orisha is what I consider a living religion, as it is an everyday, interactive set of beliefs, obligations, sacrifices, prayers, and deeds in the name of Olodumare, the Yoruba creator god, and the deities that serve as messengers to and for Olodumare.[4] No sacrifices are ever made to Olodumare (the embodiment of *ashe*, the creative force that occupies all things and makes all things happen), and priests and practitioners supplicate via the deities that serve as representative liaisons. The lines that are usually drawn between the sacred and secular realms of existence and understanding, are blurred, as the sacred exists in the secular: for example, the *orisha* reside in pots in people's homes or temples in the forms of specific aesthetically styled stones. To many, this would seem baffling. In fact, in Carl Hunt's book on the Yoruba movement in America, one of his respondents stated, "I remember when the initiation rituals were over and we were preparing to leave the Temple and return to America, our Godfather told us to open our pots and see what we had, and there was nothing in them but stones. And I thought, 'Oh my God! You mean I spent $2000 for some stones to take home to my wife'; and there was embarrassment and shock at the same time."[5] But to the initiated, the fact that the sacred energy of the *orisha* is found in the stones is not baffling: when the *orisha* came to earth to make it habitable for human beings, they left their respective essences, their *ashe*, in various objects and places on earth such as stones, trees, water, soil, and animals. These objects and substances are understood to vibrate with the original energies of the *orisha* themselves and are thus given in initiations and used in other ritual moments and procedures. But the *orisha* are more than messengers for Olodumare. They are extensions of Olodumare that are often associated with aspects of nature and culture, and they all have their own distinct personalities, likes, and taboos. For example, Eshu is understood to be the ambiguously characterized guardian of the crossroads, an eternal trickster yet a stringent judge of act and character. Yemonja, on the other hand, is understood to be the kind and cool maternal deity of the ocean, nursing, and midwives, while Ogun embodies male virility, weaponry, and warfare.[6] Thus, devotees can appeal to a particular *orisha* for guidance and assistance with certain personal life and health problems.

The basis of the religion can be summed up, however simplistically, as mutual and respectful exchanges and relationships between people, the *orisha*, and the *egun*, or ancestors, as well as between godparents and godchildren and between members of the more general community. An Orisha devotee cares for and honors, prays and sacrifices to the *orisha* or to their ancestors, and in return his or her wishes for health, peace, and well-being (*alaafia*) will usually be granted. A godparent (*iyalosha*, *babalosha*, or *babalawo*) nurtures and guides her or his godchild through the religion and in everyday life; likewise, a godchild respects and assists her or his godparents with their ritual and varied needs. The religious "family" operates much as a biological or otherwise kin-based family does: optimally, it is at once a "space" and a set of relationships in which people care for and respect each other and in which everyone does his or her part in making those relationships run smoothly.

It is precisely this sense of family and community responsibility that fostered mutual aid societies throughout the Americas. The purpose of these groups, which varied in form and function depending on which country we discuss, was to offer fellowship and social opportunities, to assist the needy, to aid the sick and to bury the dead.[7] Concurrently, they were places for the safe worship of African deities. Thus, *orisha* worship has long been tied to a more holistic notion of well-being, one grounded in the everyday lives and experiences of people. Although *cabildos* and other mutual aid societies have, for the most part, long been driven underground or otherwise dissolved, their legacies of spiritual guidance, economic help, and healing practices have continued to color the ways in which Orisha devotees understand themselves in relation to the spirits, their ancestors, and other people.[8] Writing of her experiences with her godparents in Cuba, Marta Moreno Vega reflects,

> As visitors praised Eugenia's cooking, an undercurrent of social tidbits filled my ears. The woman next to me commented, "I went to claim my ration of chicken this week, and the butcher told me no deliveries had been made." Another commented, "Forget it, there is no meat to be had, not even on the black market." Someone chimed in, "In my section we haven't seen meat for the past four weeks. I have a collection of meat coupons that mean nothing. What is the point of rationing our food, giving us coupons, when there is no food?" Suddenly, a roar of laughter erupted, as everyone added their stories of unsuccessful attempts to find meat. A voice at the end of the corridor shouted out, "*Que viva Shango*; Shango lives! Today we are eating meat thanks to Oba Koso! Praise be to Shango.' "[9]

The above passage describes how a sacrifice and ceremony in the name of Shango feeds both the *orisha* to whom the sacrifice is made as well as the community of practitioners: Shango asks only for the sacrificed animals' *ashe*; the people present enjoy the feast that follows. Likewise, at the *bembes* (or other rituals and celebrations) I have attended, the *orisha* are honored, people are advised and blessed, and everyone savors the dishes of rice, beans, goat, and chicken that are offered. Although there is certainly no meat shortage in the Midwest, the people present appreciate the sacrificial efforts made by the priest hosting the celebration and the chance to get together and mingle over good company and wonderfully prepared food. Congregating and nurturing the community (initiates and non-initiates alike) are important aspects of this religious practice, and are not so tangentially tied into the longer and wider histories of some of these religious communities. In the next section, we see that since the political is by nature communal, for a history of Orisha in the United States addresses, and perhaps heals, wider issues—such as personal and community empowerment—for the people with whom I work.

RECLAIMING THE YORUBA GODS: EMPOWERMENT FROM AFRICA IN THE UNITED STATES

That Yoruba religions are still practiced in many parts of the Western Hemisphere has been discussed as a multisited success in cultural and religious resistance.[10] That is, in order to retain their religious beliefs and practices, people had to actively remember and claim their African heritage and religion. Often cloaking the *orisha* in Catholic imagery, priests and practitioners stood against an onslaught of cultural, racial, and religious oppression. Bush, writing about slave women in the Caribbean, reminds us:

> From the general cultural perspective slave women were prominent in all areas of resistance against the dominant white culture. Obeah, ritual magic and folk medicine, though frequently

despised and derided by whites, were feared and suppressed through laws and punishments. Yet women slaves, undeterred by the often harsh penalties, preserved and defended African cultural and religious traditions of the slave community. This formed the essential basis of the unique Afro-Caribbean culture which developed on the slave plantations.[11]

For the purposes of this essay, however, it is important to note that Yoruba-based beliefs and practices did not survive in any systematic or overtly recognizable form in the United States. With the United States a largely Protestant country, there were few Catholic images behind which to hide the African deities. Instead, drawing upon the knowledge and practice of relocated Cuban *santeros*, *santeras*, and *babalawos*, African Americans were able to re-claim and reinvent a religious and cultural milieu for themselves, one based in a perceived preslavery set of Yoruba traditions and values.[12] I will return to this point later in the essay.

Overt and systematic forms of Orisha worship had, however, been brought to the United States early this century. By the 1930s, a number of Cuban initiates were living and practicing in New York. Around 1938, Katherine Dunham, the renowned dancer and artist, met a number of Cuban priests/drummers and invited them to join the Dunham Company.[13] Other scholars place the initial introduction of Orisha worship around this time as well:

> The Afro-Cuban community in New York was initially created in the 1930's and 1940's by artists and craftsmen. There was also a small number of intellectuals, such as Romolu Lachatanere, an anthropologist who has written extensively about Afro-Cuban religion. Along with other professionals, Lachatanere organized a social club, called Club Cubano Inter-Americano, to bring together Afro-Cubans and other Latin Americans in New York. Members of the leadership came from a senior club in Tampa; indeed, many of the members of the Tampa club were involved in establishing the New York club. Several members of the club practiced Lucumi; indeed, some were powerful priests, and priestesses. As a result, many club sponsored activities served a dual function with the Lucumi religion.[14]

Thus, the seeds of Orisha worship were in the United States in the early part of the twentieth century and were squarely in place when Pancho Mora came to New York and established the first *ile*, or Orisha house, there in the 1940s, although the first known initiations were not performed in this country until much later (1961).[15]

In 1959, on the eve of the Cuban revolution, two African-American men, Walter King and Chris Oliana, traveled to Matanzas, Cuba, to become initiated into the Orisha priest-hoods of Obatala and Aganju, respectively. Although both men had already been initiated in Haitian Vodou, King, now known as Oba Ofuntola Oseijeman Adelabu Adefunmi, in-corporated the first African American temple to both the *loa* and the *orisha*. The visibility of the temple and of Oseijeman's followers angered many in the New York Cuban commu-nity, since they were used to a more closeted, discreet approach to the religion; after all, it was in part the secrecy that kept it alive for hundreds of years, and the open use of Yoruba names and the wearing of Yoruba clothes only served to attract attention to its practice. In 1970, after further initiation in Abeokuta, Nigeria, Oseijeman moved to South Carolina, where he founded the Yoruba-inspired Oyotunji village and where he began in earnest a reorganization of the religion along traditional Nigerian lines, retrieving it and reclaiming it from Santeráia—a religion he held to be African in origin yet tainted with the symbols of European oppression (i.e., Catholic images).[16]

This reclamation of Africa was indeed a guiding factor for Oseijeman, who was involved in the Black Power movements of the 1950s and 1960s. He was the minister of culture for the Republic of New Africa (RNA) and the founder of the African National Independence Party. Oyotunji itself is rooted in Oseijeman's nationalism, as he announced in 1962 that "an African state will exist in America. The foundation of the state will be African, and it will be purely African in culture."[17] At Oyotunji, founded in 1970, Yoruba is spoken; dress includes *bubas, dashikis, geles,* and *filas*; Yoruba and African diaspora history is taught; and polygynous marriages are allowed, per traditional Yoruba custom. A number of Oseijeman's future initiates and contemporaries were also involved with Black cultural and political movements during the 1960s and 1970s, and although the reclamation of *orisha* worship was in fact a spiritual endeavor, many people with whom I work also tell of the political and personal purpose the religion serves as well for African Americans:

> In the 1970s, it probably was political as well as spiritual. It had a lot to do with concepts of self-determination. It had a lot to do with Christianity as oppressive and not developing the human being. You start looking for alternatives. . . . Christianity will not empower me . . . and Orisha is a quiet movement. It's something we do and it's none of your business. And when . . . there's nothing your FBI or CIA can do to discredit it, then it will be a national thing.
>
> —*Obasanmi, Obatala priest*

> I left the RNA [the Republic of New Africa] because they became very militant and I don't believe the gun is the solution for anything, which is why I went into Orisha. I believe in the magic but I don't believe in violence as a tool to educate or change. And some of the revolutionary brothers—they were so angry and I don't blame them—they said violence was the way but I don't believe that ever, ever, ever. Unless it's in self-defense! And not many women do because we birth the babies. Why would we birth 'em to kill 'em?
>
> —*Adegoke, Shango priest*

> I came out of my Ph.D. program feeling ignorant about my people, where we came from, Africa . . . I obtained the highest degree in my field and nobody taught us anything about our culture. And I had this philosophy about what we were like before we were kidnaped and brought here; I wanted to know what we were before all this . . . so I went to the village and ate up all that information.
>
> —*Ifagbemi, Ifa priest*

A common thread that runs through many narratives of people's early interest in the religion is one of a healing redemption from the multifold oppressions that were evident in America during the times when people of color were denied basic human and civil rights under the federal and local governments. At a time when everything Black was seen as negative, the reclamation of a positive Africa served as a theme around which many began to pattern their lives and practices outside of and within the Black Power movement:

> Art, religion, and politics are impressive vectors of a culture. Art describes a culture. Black artists must have an image of what the Black sensibility is in this land. Religion elevates a culture. The Black Man must aspire to Blackness. God is man idealized. The Black Man must idealize himself as Black. . . . Politics gives a social order to the culture, i.e., makes relationships within the

culture definable for the functioning organism. The Black Man must seek Black politics, and ordering of the world that is beneficial to his culture, to his interiorization and judgement of the world. This is strength. And we are hordes.[18]

These early spiritual and political pioneers have made a difference, as people have increasingly come to "find" the *orisha* and to claim them as a spiritual base that informs how they live their lives within the world, and within the still very much Eurocentric United States in particular. John Mason, a renowned Yoruba scholar of Afro-Cuban ancestry and a priest of Obatala, has written:

> From the 1970s until today there has been a worldwide explosion of involvement in Orisha tradition. Three factors have spurred this movement. The first relates to the resurgence, especially in the United States, in the wake of the Civil Rights and Nationalist movements, and in Brazil, of a vocal and open pride in being of African stock and possessing and maintaining the beautiful and valuable cultural heritage of Black Africa.[19]

To be sure, this sense of "healing" African American people, history, and community throughout the Western Hemisphere has been long in coming and has been facilitated by the numerous global communities that have reaffirmed their sense of African heritage through, in this case, religious thought and practice.[20] Even now, as other generations of initiates enter the religion, although they were not born during the 1950s and 1960s Black nationalist and civil rights movements, feelings of cultural and racial pride still inform how they understand the religion that they are participating in. However, tied into these ideals of race and pride are also issues of healing and a different understanding of the world. For example, Oshunwole was being initiated into Oshun when I spoke with her about her process of entering the religion; we had first met four years prior to her initiation. Her narrative of the religion tied the personal to the spiritual as well:

> How did I get into it? That's a good question and I keep askin' myself . . . I keep looking for the patterns but I don't see any because none of my family's really into it. My family's from the South. We were always told stories about hoodoo . . . but I kinda got into Afrocentric culture and I was still practicing Christianity but it never did fulfill me. So I started reading books and the books kinda got my interest and I started looking for someone who was of African descent in this country that was doing it because I didn't want to go through the Spanish system. . . . And I've been in it for [six] years. . . . It's been an experience. It helps. My mother passed over [in 1998] and it makes a difference. I didn't want to fall apart. It keeps my sanity. Because so much of my family is dead and you can look at it and go, "Hmmm. Everybody's *dead*," or you can say, "Everybody's working on the other side. Okay. So I gotta do my part on this side."

From Oshunwole's account, political and racial concerns are perhaps more subtle than with her predecessors, but they are still there. Although less visible, Black Power still has an effect on African Americans today, as its message and methodology changed from "Black is beautiful" to "I am beautiful and I'm black."[21] History, family, and community are part of people's contexts in which they can be understood to exist; they affect how people see and live in the world, regardless of race. Indeed, although the majority of incoming adherents are young and African-American, many others are White, Latino/a, and Asian. For these devotees, I would guess that the religion has perhaps less to do with racial politics and more to do with global spiritual movements and endeavors. Later in the discussion I had with Oshunwole, I asked her how she saw herself in the priesthood. She stated, "Serve the gods an' serve humanity. That's what I want to do. That would be fine. . . . I mean, I just want to serve in the manner that the gods and my ancestors see fit and that's what I'm working toward." Service to others and to the spirits is a primary aspect of the religion, and in the next section, I examine how Orisha priests serve to heal people by understanding them in relation to spirit, nature, and culture.

ALAAFIA: HOLISM AND HEALING

In her article on healing and Haitian Vodou, Karen McCarthy Brown asserts that "healing is the primary business of these religious systems. In fact it is not an overstatement to say that spirituality and healing are synonymous in the Afro-Caribbean."[22] By this, she means that holistic notions of healing permeate the everyday relationships between priests, practitioners, spirits, and clients, and that physical, social, spiritual, and emotional problems are treated within these religions. Joseph Murphy, writing about Santería, echoes this sentiment, since *babalawos* were and are "at once priests, doctors, and counselors" for their communities.[23] Likewise, for Yoruba-derived religions in Brazil, the role of healer, diviner, and priest falls squarely in the *mae* and *pai de santo's* list of responsibilities, while in the United States, Zora Neale Hurston points out that voodoo and hoodoo are the divine healing "powers of Africa" embodied.[24] And in Trinidad, James Houk tells us, the *orisha* are powerful entities that can assist people (usually via the priests) with "sickness, financial problems, court appearances, and a variety of other matters."[25] The Yoruba term *alaafia* embodies this sense of holism.[26] Although the priests and practitioners with whom I work live in urban areas of the midwestern United States, this African concept—along with their concepts of human bodies—guides their understanding of health and healing.

Human beings, in their bodies, are understood to inhabit multiple levels of existence; that is, they are at once spiritual, physical, emotional, mental, communal, and political. When asked about the nature of health and healing in Orisha, Iyalosha Adegoke told me:

> Well, healing would mean a fixing of things, a setting right of things . . . let's see. I don't want to use the term *fixing*. Healing would be setting things right again. In a physical sense, it would be bringing you back to your healthy condition, which would be you would have to be rid of your disease. In a political sense, it would be a settlement that was satisfactory to all parties. In the emotional realm, it would be . . . an emotional healing would be that you could go on and would not be over- come by the hurt or the negative feelings. And mentally, healing would mean that you are sane, you have your decision makin' faculties and your conscious is in order. Okay? So, you know, setting things right. Oh, yeah. Spiritual healing would be setting you back in sync with your guides. You know, your guides, your guides.

Alaafia embodies these different notions of health that the people with whom I work use to guide their religious practices: if one acts well in the world, then health and prosperity will follow. Likewise, if one cares for and attends to the spirit world properly—that is, keeping one's shrines "fresh," sacrificing to the *orisha* and the *egun* (ancestors), and following one's destiny as chosen before Olodumare—health and well-being will likewise come. According to many of my respondents, almost every problem (or good event) ultimately stems from a spiritual source. Although divination may show that certain cases require both spiritual and physical treatments, some problems are deemed to be simply physical in nature. As one respondent put it: "I don't know how to heal a cavity by doin' a chicken!" Priests and practitioners acknowledge that strep throat should be treated with antibiotics and that someone who is having chest pains should chew an aspirin on the way to the local hospital. But the *orisha* can often work adjunctly with (and within) allopathic medicine in order to physically heal people with very real and very frightening illnesses. When I first asked about healing, I was told to talk especially to Iyalosha Adegoke because she had been involved in some of the most dramatic cases in recent memory. According to a number of people and Adegoke herself, she conducted rituals solely for the intention of healing; as a result, one woman's cancer went into full remission and another woman's brain aneurysm all but disappeared from the CAT scans she regularly received.[27] However, many physical ailments are seen as manifestations of spiritual circumstances. In one reading that I witnessed, a client was told that her physical and economic problems were due to the fact that her ancestors had been neglected. She was instructed to make certain sacrifices and conduct, under the priest's tutelage, certain rituals that would begin to mend the relationship between this person and her ancestors, thus affecting her well-being. In this case, the benefit is bidirectional: the client would enjoy the blessings of her ancestors, and her ancestors, known and unknown, would be acknowledged and honored. Acknowledging the ancestors is an important aspect of Orisha in the Western Hemisphere, since so many people were lost to the Middle Passage and to the horrors of slavery. This, then, is one way, via the vehicle of African-based worship, that people can begin to heal their families and their histories: by remembering where one came from in terms of genealogy and race, one can be guided by the wisdom that the ancestors brought with them, ultimately from Africa.

But Orisha is very much a this-world religion and is concerned with the lives people lead while on earth. In this way, it is similar to other so-called slave religions in that it is very much tied to people's economic situations, family structures, access to resources, relationships, and community needs.[28] Priests deal not only with the supernatural aspects of well-being, but with the everyday aspects as well. Several years ago during a phone call I was making to Iyalosha Oshunfemi in Chicago I was intercepted by her answering machine, which told me that I had indeed reached her temple, and where and how I could find assistance in procuring clothing, shelter, food, or other aid for my family should it be needed. This message greeted all who called her, reflecting the intertwining of the spiritual and the secular, as meeting people's immediate, everyday needs is as important as meeting their spiritual ones. Iyalosha Oshunfunmi also echoed this holistic aspect of Orisha when she told me, "People who are not necessarily practitioners [i.e., not in the religion] utilize Orisha priests' services for a number of purposes. Some priests are good herbalists, Orisha tradition notwithstanding. Some clients go for readings and case work to be done; one priest in particular in Cleveland has a reputation of working well both with jail cases and mental illness. . . . Another works well with people with serious illnesses."[29] In instances of working with social and legal problems, as with other types of healing, it must be noted that moral and ethical considerations are primary. If a person is guilty as charged, spiritual work will be done as a protective measure during incarceration; if a person is innocent, then work will be done with the spirits so that the guilty party will be found and that there will be a just and right outcome to a hearing or trial.

All *orisha* are involved with different kinds of healing, and each has a different job with regards to a person's life, or "path." Adegoke delineated some of these as follows:

> Yemonja is primarily responsible for the womb and the reproductive area. She has a lot to do with mucus-producing parts too, so it's not just the womb; it's also sometimes the lungs, sometimes your glandular system and sinus system and the upper respiratory system. She's very much involved with that . . . and venereal diseases. She can cure those and will. Oshun deals with the blood and the sex organs—the vaginal area and the ovaries. Yemonja is more the womb; Oshun deals with the ovaries, the vaginal area, and the blood. Shango deals with the nervous system and the respiratory [system]. Obatala deals with the head, the brain, strokes, all that kinda stuff. Anything to do with the head, ears, eyes, throat, nose . . . Oya deals with injury. She deals with recovery from injury and bruises and physical cuts and things like that. And Ogun deals with male virility, as does Shango. Shango deals with fecundity and impotence, but Ogun does a lot with that too and Ogun is the medicine man. You can go to Ogun for just about anything. Ogun is like the doctor. He has all the knowledge of all the herbs. . . . Olokun deals with the spleen, the liver, the underpinnings . . . the pancreas, the urinary tract, the cleaning organs . . . and then Osanyin is the *orisha* of medicine.

Besides having responsibility for certain parts of the body, the *orisha* rule over other aspects of people's lives as well: Ogun is the patron of bus drivers, metalworkers, and butchers, while Yemonja would be the matron of midwives, nurses, and day care providers. Obatala would be the patron of professors and ambassadors, while Oya would be the matron of CEOs, businesspeople, and stock traders.[30] Thus, if a person is having trouble with family and children, Yemonja could be appealed to for help; if a person is having financial trouble or trouble with business, Oya could be petitioned for guidance. But it is divination, direct contact with the *orisha*, that would divulge the true causes for misfortune and prescriptions for how to deal with those aggravations.

Notions of health and well-being are so conflated with the religion that many priests don't consider themselves healers. They often minimize their role in the religion as direct lines to the spirit world and will often say things like, "I just give advice. Just general information." However they discuss it, though, health and well-being are inextricably tied into their religious notions of how a person relates in the world as she or he moves within (and from) their various contexts of spirit, community, history, and embodiment.

A QUIET MOVEMENT: CONSIDERATIONS OF POLITICS AND HEALING

Far from being the "opium of the people" that Marx described religion as being, Orisha worship in its many forms has had a long history of cultural, racial, and religious struggle that has shaped how the people involved understand the relationship between people on Earth and the spirits and deities in the otherworld as well as how those worlds are understood to interact. From the slaves who originally carried and practiced their religion to and in their unwelcoming new homes to those who have chosen to embrace and engage their histories as the descendants of African slaves, African-based religious reverence has been inextricably linked to the political and the personal, and that is, indeed, healing. These facts of political religiosity have long been documented in the African diaspora, from Haiti, Brazil, and Cuba to the United States.[31] This perspective affects the people involved, as it offers an alternative way of looking at the world, and understanding what "health" or "well-being" means. Healing in Orisha questions the hegemony of European-American control of religious and biological theories. To be sure, the people with whom I work do make an appointment with their physician if they or their children are ill. But they believe, along with many others, that doctors treat only one aspect of a person—the physical. There may be a whole host of other etiologies behind one's headache. As I alluded to earlier, one's relationship with an ancestor may need attending to, or one might need to offer a sacrifice to an *orisha*. Whatever the treatment prescribed, Orisha, as a group of divine relationships, attends to that particular person's lived events and contexts; it addresses a person's problems holistically.

The DuBois quote at the beginning of this essay speaks to the fact that European oppression did not kill all that was African in the minds and bodies of African (and African-American) slaves. This fact speaks to the tenacity of spirit and person with regard to the practice of African-based religions in the Western Hemisphere. It has already been shown that the existence of these religious systems can be understood as resistance to dominant expressions of culture, thought, and power. That they have been nurtured, and reclaimed, exemplifies that the personally religious has always been, and continues to be, political.

GLOSSARY

Aganju—the (male) *orisha* of the volcano; not usually encountered among most of the people I work with.

alaafia—a Yoruba (originally Arabic) word meaning peace, health, and prosperity as well as a holistic sense of well-being.

ashe—a Yoruba term meaning "may it happen"; the divine power to make all things happen.

babalawo—a Yoruba word meaning "father of the secrets"; an Ifa priest.

babalosha, babalorisha—a Yoruba word meaning "father of the *orisha*"; a male Orisha priest.

bembe—a celebration for the *orisha* in which there is drumming, dancing, and singing.

buba—a Yoruba term for a loose blouse.

cabildo—a Cuban mutual aid society; also a place where the African deities were worshiped.

dashiki—a loose, flowing African robe.

egun—a Yoruba term for a group of one's ancestors; also referred to as *iku,* or "the dead."

Eshu—the (male) *orisha* of the crossroads, uncertainty, and magic.

fila—a Yoruba term for a man's cap.

gele—a Yoruba term for a woman's head wrap.

Ifa—the (male) *orisha* of certainty, coolness, and oracular knowledge.

ile—a Yoruba word meaning "house." The term usually refers to the family/line of godparents and godchildren or can refer to an actual place of worship or temple. In this country, people's homes usually serve as their temples, the places where their shrines are kept and worship is conducted.

loa—the pantheon of Haitian Vodou spirits.

mae de santo—a Portuguese term meaning "mother of the saints"; a female Candomble priest.

Oba—a Yoruba title, meaning "king," or chief.

Oba Koso—a praise name for the *orisha* Shango, meaning "the king did not hang."

Obatala—the (male) *orisha* of coolness, creativity, and the sky.

Ogun—the (male) *orisha* of war, weaponry, and metalsmithing.

Olodumare/Olorun—the Yoruba creator god.

Olokun—the (hermaphroditic) *orisha* of the depths of the ocean.

orisha—one of numerous deities in the Yoruba pantheon; they are both messengers to Olodumare as well as divine extensions of Olodumare.

Osanyin—the (male) *orisha* of plants and herbal medicines.

Oshun—the (female) *orisha* of sensuality, beauty, and sweet waters.

Oya—the (female) *orisha* of windstorms, electricity, and thunder.

pai de santo—a Portuguese term meaning "father of the saints"; a male Candomble priest.

santera—a female Santería priest.

santero—a male Santería priest.

Shango—the (male) *orisha* of thunder, lightning, and fire.

yalosha, iyalorisha—a Yoruba word meaning "mother of the *orisha*"; a female Orisha priest.

Yemonja—the (female) *orisha* of the ocean, motherhood, and midwifery.

THE POLITICS AND POETICS OF "MAGAZINE MEDICINE"

New Age Ayurveda in the Print Media

Sita Reddy

THE PRINT LENS

Most accounts of professionalizing Asian healing systems in America over the twentieth century concentrate on their increasing legitimacy as a form of expert knowledge and therapeutic practice, whether within professional centers of authority such as clinics or politico-legal institutions and the courts. This essay shifts the focus to *popular* representations of Asian medicine, arguing that an important part of professionalization for any healing group is the relation with its "publics" or the widespread dissemination of its public legitimacy. In this view, popular discourses beyond professional centers of authority— such as everyday knowledge or media images—play a critical role in the legitimization of expert medical knowledge. I focus specifically on the American *print* mass media, particularly those health and lifestyle magazines that are widely available at newsstands and promote various techniques for improving health in the face of the stressful demands of "modern" living. "Magazine medicine"—Robin Bunton's evocative term for the broad area spanning expert knowledge on the one hand and lay knowledge on the other—offers a particularly instructive view on the politics of alternative healing.[1] As boundaries between expert and lay health discourses become increasingly blurred, especially within alternative medicine, this arena not only highlights new sites of popular health that may have replaced institutional health care practices but also shifts analyses toward the consumption and representation of health rather than its production or practice. What sociologist Peter Conrad calls the "public eye," defined here as media discourse and images available in the public sphere, thus becomes a crucial site within which professional definitions themselves are modified as well as one that health-seeking individuals use to construct meanings of social phenomena.[2]

For over a century, mass-distributed print media in America and Europe have promoted popular alternative techniques for improving health as antidotes to the stresses of modern living. In this essay, I argue that these health and lifestyle magazines constitute part of the continuing tradition of self-help literature for the upward mobility of the twentieth-century American middle classes. Writing about nineteenth-century Europe, Michel Foucault in his 1988 *Technologies of the Self* notes that the rise of public health programs coincident with the project of modernity fostered the perception of health as the responsibility of the state, and thus a citizen's right.[3] Health quickly became institutionalized as a core modern value, if we understand modernity to be the critical mode of relating to the world in which unlimited progress is both possible and desirable. Health also came to embody idealized notions of modernity such as flexibility and control. Following Foucault, we can suggest that twentieth-century magazines, by making these depersonalized self-study health techniques widely available to mass audiences, were crucial in fostering this trend and in transforming popular perceptions of alternative health. Printed ideas, in other words, encouraged the institutionalization of health as a central value of modernity and as a commodity that could be consumed by the masses.

Among this arsenal of health techniques offered in the American print media, Ayurveda—the South Asian medical tradition dating back to the sixth century B.C.E.—merits particular consideration as one of the latest medical imports to be transplanted from the East and then reinvented as a New Age healing technique.[4] In this essay I analyze some examples from American magazines that point to specific ways in which New Age Ayurveda has been represented for consumption. The consumers of Ayurveda as ideology and practice in fact constitute very different audiences, whose receptivity to Ayurveda as a valuable alternative tool for achieving health and countering stress has been determined by specific historical contexts. Yet while both the audiences and the tactics of presentation used to sell Ayurveda are different, underlying all of these representations is a common Orientalist theme dominated by stereotyping dichotomizing tendencies—such as East/West, mind/body, spiritual/material—that has historical antecedents in the late nineteenth century. New Age healing, in other words, is neither new nor all that innovative, drawing as it does on a particular form of American Orientalism that has enjoyed almost continuous popularity during the past hundred years. Viewed in the context of this volume, it is yet another example of how the reinvention and professionalization of a contemporary Asian alternative system is shaped not only by the politics of American *medical* culture and its ideological opposition to biomedicine, but by oppositional millennial heterodox elements of American *religious* culture that have their most recent modern resurgence in the New Age. For these Asian medical transplants, the cultural authority underlying professionalization is neither science (as it was for biomedicine and some heterodox health systems), nor nationalism (as it was in their countries of origin), but metaphysical sources of authority in America.

Yet for all its links with the past, the language of New Age Ayurveda points not just to continuity but also to ruptures and discontinuities from the holistic rhetoric underlying alternative healing. Although the dominant neo-Orientalist stereotypes running through print images of Ayurveda—of East/West, material/spiritual, tradition/modernity—suggest stark opposition, the magazine articles themselves typically suggest a middle ground that avoids a simple trade-off of one side for another, and points to new ways of reconciling these dichotomies in the American healing context. In this essay, I show how printed ideas of Ayurvedic practice, being more widely available to mass audiences, defined this new middle ground and transformed the way Ayurveda was perceived by mass American audiences in ways that are significantly different from clinical therapeutic encounters. By selectively emphasizing New Age disciplines, practices and techniques over its beliefs or doctrines, print images of Ayurveda highlight popular elements of the New Age that privilege the health seeker and shift the locus of authority away from institutions and practitioners toward lay users, practical preventive remedies and self-help regimens. Ironically, these representations have the unintended consequence of attributing health and illness not to structural factors but to individual moral responsibility. Thus in the end, much like the politics of the New Age, which is neither "red nor green," print images of Ayurveda ultimately suggest neither radical transformation nor social change.[5] If the counterculture first coined the slogan the "personal is political," print images of New Age healing—as the spiritual heirs to the counterculture—turn this equation on its head. For Ayurveda in the media, the political is often reduced to the personal, with the patient increasingly designated as the active creator of health even as the realm of alternative healing expands to appropriate new sources of authenticity and tradition.

I follow John B. Thompson and use the term "mass media" to cover those types of organized information that are "available in principle to a plurality of recipients and . . . are significantly biased toward the dissemination of information from a centralized producer to a dispersed audience."[6] My analysis involves a comprehensive survey of Ayurveda in the mass-distributed *print* media from the time it was first mentioned in 1989 to the present, on the premise that this periodical analysis provides a good barometer with which to gauge popular acceptance of Ayurvedic medicine as a credible New Age alternative to biomedicine. The focus here is on newsstand health and lifestyle magazines, which offer a unique perspective on self-help techniques and health practices as avenues of mobility. I choose not to include newspapers in this analysis because their coverage of health news tends to focus much more on the discovery of miracle "cures" rather than preventive practices, conforming more closely to what Stephen Hilgartner and Charles Bosk call a "public arenas" model of limited carrying capacities in which health problems compete for space with other news.[7]

Viewed more broadly in the context of contemporary healing, "magazine medicine" offers a particularly instructive arena for critical social analysis. Given the rapidly increasing marketization, deregulation and dispersal of contemporary American health regimes, magazines take on added significance as popular health sites that replace older institutional health care practices.[8] Sociologists as different on the political spectrum as Niklas Rose and Anthony Giddens agree that as health concerns extend to an infinitely broader focus on "well-being," everyday life becomes saturated with "expert" knowledge, and the boundaries between expert and lay health discourses grow increasingly indistinct.[9] While there has been a tendency in the sociology of health and illness to distinguish between expert and lay knowledge, we should in fact no longer assume any clear boundary between them. "Magazine medicine"—as a site positioned squarely between expert and lay discourses—thus acquires much of its particular significance by serving as a powerful mediator between them. Moreover, as health continues to embody idealized notions of modernity, such as flexibility and control, it also begins to be viewed as a citizen's personal responsibility.[10] Magazines now fill a crucial role as new information brokers, and magazine medicine becomes an important link in what Wendy Farrant and Jill Russell call the "politics of health information."[11] In this view, magazine knowledge is popular health knowledge that extends beyond the professional epicenter of medical authority yet makes judgments about the quality of that knowledge and interprets it for the general reader.

Two premises about contemporary magazines inform this essay. First, to use Clifford Geertz's term, magazines are classic "blurred genres," in that they are characterized by a radical heterogeneity and the refusal of a singe authorial voice.[12] Magazines are also self-consciously temporal, giving them an open, fluid quality that requires them to be read in a less intense manner than books or journals. Given this diversity of forms and the manner in which they are consumed, magazines are unlikely to position a single reader or even an identifiable "type" of reader. Instead, they are more likely to create "subjects" that are fragmentary and dispersed—in this case, a whole range of "heterogeneous healthy selves," among which the reader is left to pick and mix. Joke Hermes, for instance, identifies at least three women's magazine types distinguished through its diverse readers—traditional, feminist, and gossip—each of which reads the same magazines differently. Thus any analysis of Ayurvedic images in health magazines and the print media would have to rely less on locating a single subject than on finding the various meanings of magazines and distinguishing them through a detailed process of reading and identity formation.

A second premise is that magazines—coming to prominence in the age of capitalist mass production—are not only commodities themselves but also important means of health commodification and product promotion.[13] On the one hand, magazines increasingly carry more health-related articles, and health-related consumer cultures thrive linked to a more general privileging of bodily appearance, youthfulness, beauty and the "aestheticisation" of everyday life.[14] On the other hand, they also encourage the rise of a new field of expertise—health education and health communication—that focuses on the ability of campaigns and advertising to promote or diminish healthy behaviors and lifestyles.[15] Health promotion, rather than health per se, thus becomes the focus of many periodicals and self-help magazines.

This is particularly marked in the world of alternative medicine, where the margins between lay and expert knowledge are unusually permeable. Popular tastes in health consumption accompanied by the invasions of corporations into health markets reflect the gradual erosion of professional biomedicine's autonomy and authority. As sociologist Bryan Turner suggests, we may expect a possible collapse between the hierarchical divisions of scientific and alternative medicine much like the distinction between high culture and mass culture in the postmodern period.[16] This broad blurring of lines between specialist and non-specialist knowledge systems—or between what Ludwig Fleck describes as "inner esoteric knowledge at the center of disciplines and outer exotic circles"[17]—reflects the gradual transformation of medical knowledge by the advent of post-industrial society through the communications revolution, cybernetics, the growth of the Internet, and the dominance of the service sector. Popular magazines covering alternative, holistic or New Age remedies are particularly important communicators of new health messages, and play a central role in the flow of health information to a public already increasingly hungry for alternative therapies and self-help regimens.

For scholars studying New Age phenomena or movements, there is an added methodological advantage to focusing on popular *representations* of health rather than health practices. Given the New Age movement's decentralized, amorphous structure, and lack of an overarching national umbrella organization, scholars claim it is best studied not as a movement but through its varied interests, products, or participation in local voluntary organizations.[18] Fieldwork that focuses on actual practices and disparate local groups may thus have limited value as a research tool if the goal is a national-level picture of the New Age movement. In the view of anthropologist David Hess, a better research alternative would be the cultural interpretation of New Age representations as "texts"—for New Agers, what they *say* (and write) and how they say it may not only be central to any sense of a national movement, but *is* what they do. As Hess argues, quoting James Boon, for this ethnographic community "the scribes are the tribes."[19] A textual analysis of Ayurvedic representations would provide a more comprehensive description of the diverse ideological positions within the movement, but it would also richly articulate the symbolic world of popular health beliefs. This may be particularly important for the holistic health and New Age movement, which is not simply a group of people favoring one alternative health care system over the biomedical paradigm, but an ideological community actively pursuing a desired future—whether this future is based on goals that are millennial, nativist or revivalist.[20]

In the late twentieth century, representations of New Age Ayurveda in print may reflect nothing more than the changing politics of ethnicity in the public sphere. As with other Asian alternatives, the popular appeal of Ayurveda rests as much on its challenge to biomedicine as on its ability to heal modernity and the West itself. In other words, it cures as much through medical efficacy as through cultural difference. The irony here is that print images of Ayurveda end up assembling and commodifying this cultural difference at a time when the popular health arena has never been more multicultural. As Asian alternatives flood the diverse American health market, the politics of healing for New Age audiences in search of perfect health often result in a range of unintended consequences: from a subtle shift toward patient responsibility for illness and a tendency to engage in the "healthicization of everyday life."[21]

AYURVEDA IN PRINT: A BRIEF HISTORY

Ayurveda was first introduced to American health and lifestyle magazine readers in 1989 as an exotic alternative to biomedical orthodoxy. Through the next decade, media articles on Ayurveda increased not only in number, peaking in 1996, but also in diversity and depth of coverage, so that by 1999 the term was almost self-explanatory to familiar audiences. As with other aspects of Ayurveda's reinvention in America—such as its therapeutic practice, pharmacy, or institutionalization—representations of Ayurveda in the print media rely heavily on New Age discourses and their syntheses of Eastern religion, human potential psychology, science, shamanism, and all things considered "natural."[22] What may be *unique* to printed ideas of Ayurveda, however, are particular ideological emphases and elements within these New Age discourses that are not emphasized in clinical practice.

Among the most salient is a disproportionate emphasis on a particular form of American Orientalism—the inheritance by the New Age of "selective American appropriations of the Orient."[23] As Andrea Diem and James Lewis powerfully show, this discourse has historical antecedents in nineteenth-century romantic American discoveries of a Hindu golden age.[24] Despite the fact that contemporary print images of Ayurveda in the American media use varied tactics of presentation to make the East more appealing to Western audiences—such as scientific credibility, or holistic legitimacy—the common Orientalist theme running through all of them is dominated by distinctive notions of the "mystic East" that we can trace back to the previous century.

As long ago as 1893, "Indian medicine and religion" first came to the attention of the American public through Swami Vivekananda, whose lectures in the United States, beginning with the World's Columbian Exposition in Chicago in 1893, received widespread attention in the news media.[25] In America, Vivekananda first became known through his appearances at the Parliament of World Religions, part of the 1893 Chicago World's Fair. Vivekananda made several claims about Hinduism and "Indian medicine" that continue to find their way into contemporary print presentations. Because of his Western-style education and background, for instance, Vivekananda first chose to present Hinduism and "Indian medicine" as sciences, comparable to the sciences of the modern West such as astronomy and chemistry. In his publications and public lectures, Vivekananda emphasized Hinduism's fundamental compatibility with science, making every effort to distinguish it from Christianity, which, for various reasons in his view, was not as compatible.[26] The ideological strategy here was to establish Indian science (and yoga) as not merely "traditional" and therefore irrational, but a happy synthesis of the best that East and West could offer.

Even more interestingly, Vivekananda claimed that the American middle classes were the ideal audiences for popular "Indian religion and medicine." Vivekananda, himself a middle-class, university-educated, English speaker, first directed his communications to a similar audience. In an article entitled "East and West," first published in 1901, he states that humans have a duty to keep their bodies healthy, because the body is the only instrument through which complete freedom, or salvation, can be achieved. Attaining this freedom is easier for those in the middle because: "too much wealth or too much poverty is a great impediment to the higher development of the soul. It is from the middle classes that the great ones of the world come. Here the forces are very equally adjusted and balanced."[27]

While the specific nature of the middle-class audiences attracted to Vivekananda's ideas about religion and medicine varied, they were predominantly university-educated, altruistically-minded women from the educated middle to upper rungs of society, many of whom were also interested in a variety of religious, occult and spiritual matters. These women "adopted" Vivekananda and facilitated his later presentations in Chicago, Boston, Los Angeles and New York. At the same time, they impressed the Indian teacher with their social service projects and influenced his re-orientation of philosophy, medicine and yoga not only as a means of self-improvement and personal salvation, but as techniques based on selfless service to the wider community, a way of emancipating the whole world.

There is every reason to believe that both these patterns—Indian medicine as scientific synthesis of East and West, and ideally targeted toward the middle-class audiences—persist in contemporary American print presentations of Ayurveda. Even though later American audiences for Ayurveda were not restricted to the educated middle classes, and came also from non-university-educated classes, the print media suggest that those most involved with Ayurveda continue to be drawn from the upwardly mobile "middle class" that Vivekananda recommended. Broadly defined as those with a high enough socio-economic standard to have time for and interest in activities beyond mere subsistence, but who do not necessarily fit the standard for being extremely wealthy, the middle class is often used as a self-referential category where self-identity, and therefore consumer and cultural habits, do not necessarily reflect purely economic indicators of class.[28] Thus when the readership of magazines is correlated with the issues addressed, Ayurveda in the media appears to serve the same set of essentially middle-class goals and ideologies—either in terms of the quest for a good life, or how to construct healthy selves that embody modernity, flexibility and personal control—all goals clearly associated with the upwardly mobile and their pursuit of "perfect health" and longevity in order to counter the stresses of modernity and life in the "West." Between 1989 and 1999, for instance, magazines as different on the ideological spectrum as *Dissent* and *Yoga Journal* all promoted Ayurveda not just as the Eastern antidote to Western lifestyles, but as the solution and corrective for modernity and the West itself. Ayurveda emerges here not just as reinvented medical system challenging biomedicine but also as a cultural form that cures difference.

Yet a closer look reveals that the "middle class" invoked in Ayurvedic print presentations is far from homogeneous. There is a significant range of differentiation among audiences to remind us that they vary in their receptivity both to middle-class goals of health and to Ayurveda's appeal as the Eastern antidote to modernity. On the surface, this diversity might reflect nothing more than the New Age roots of late twentieth-century Ayurvedic practice. If the New Age can be termed a popular social movement at all, it is one that is neither coherent nor organized, being marked instead by an overwhelming range of educational and occupational backgrounds, significant social divisions and an overwhelming diversity in audiences.[29] Much like the New Age movement itself, New Age Ayurveda in print might represent nothing more than a decentralized, amorphous series of converging tendencies, ideas and groups.

One way of examining this diversity among Ayurvedic audiences is to view them as reflections of various ideological strategies by which Ayurveda is represented in print—in other words, to analyze *how* Ayurveda is represented in order to understand who these consumers are. Read as texts, ideological strategies for promoting Ayurveda provide a comprehensive description of the diverse positions and possible consumers within this movement. In this essay, I argue that differences in these tactics of presentation both reflect and create disparate social audiences for Ayurveda, the relationship being a recursive one of mutual dependence. If nothing else, the range of these media presentations helps to demonstrate that neither alternative health, nor New Age Ayurveda nor even middle-class modernity is a true monolith. In what follows, I draw on Ayurveda's fifteen-year history in the American print media to address this plurality in two ways: chronologically, through a history of the changing language of Orientalism that underlies print presentations of Ayurveda; and synchronically, through a mapping of the diverse ideological strategies by which Ayurveda is promoted in the print media.

THE LANGUAGE OF ORIENTALISM: CHRONOLOGY AND CHANGE

In one of the first popular magazine articles to mention Ayurveda, Deepak Chopra—the earliest protagonist in Ayurveda's popular reinvention—described a dream he had as a seven year old after he heard a lecture by Alexander Fleming on his discovery of penicillin:

> I saw thousands of soldiers fallen on a battlefield, all dead. A kindly European man wearing spectacles and a beard was walking among the bodies, spraying them out of a nozzle with teeming little white dots. And as he sprayed them, the men each got up and walked away. Gradually everyone was sprayed, and not a single body remained. But right in the middle of the field lay a black cobra in a pool of its own blood. Its head was smashed and its neck broken. A small mongoose having vanquished the cobra, leaped around it in fits and jumps. Medicine in the Western scientific mold is all mongoose and no cobra. All that is wise and instinctive has been banished in favor of constant vigilance and mongoose-like hunt for its prey. The cobra represents Ayurveda—a 4000-year-old medical system rooted in Indian mysticism. Its underlying message: Disease, a failure of the flesh, is the culminating step in several stages of breakdown. If the physician can get beneath the physical problem, and heal the psyche that is out of balance, the body or what I call the bodymind can heal itself.[30]

By 1995, this image of Ayurveda as Indian mysticism began to change. While Ayurveda's ancient Indian origins continued to receive mention, they were no longer considered the source of its uniqueness as a curative system. A typical article in *Vegetarian Times* described it as one among many non-Western alternative medical systems that could be successfully updated for contemporary life as part of a new world herbalism:

> Ayurveda, translated as "the knowledge of life" is the traditional medicine of India that was passed down from Brahma 1000 years ago. As we witness a decline in the effectiveness of antibiotics, increasing deaths from cancer and AIDS, and soaring health care costs, many people—rightly or wrongly—are losing faith in conventional medicine. As they become skeptical about wonder drugs, they are interested in learning how to become *wonder people* [emphasis mine]. Ayurveda's herbal-based medicines and herbomineral compounds are uniquely used in both prevention and cure, and have meaningful application in today's society.[31]

Then, at the end of the decade, there was a clear emphasis away from "cure" toward naturalistic prevention, health maintenance, balance, and self-care, and a simultaneous de-emphasis of Ayurveda's Indian origins. An article in *Natural Health* in 1998, for instance, simply described Ayurveda as the "hot new medicine from 1500 B.C.E. whose name in ancient Sanskrit means "The Science of Life (or Longevity)." The same piece continued:

> This month's discussion of natural ingredients begins with a brief review of what is perhaps the world's oldest system of healing, one which has been practiced continuously for about 3000 years and can trace some of its roots as much as 2000 years earlier than that. We refer to Ayurveda, the traditional medicine with cutting edge holistic insights that treats the specific person rather than the specific ailment or symptoms. In this ancient system, physiological differences are due to immutable individual differences, a unique combination of *dosas* (energies), which must be kept in balance via diet, exercise, meditation and massage therapy. Ayurvedic medicine brings the healing power of the ages to today's work-a-day world.[32]

If these three images of Ayurveda drawn at intervals over its ten-year history in the print media suggest a historical narrative, it is that of a gradual change in perceptions of Ayurveda as a science. In 1989 Ayurveda was presented as a system of mind-body healing, whereas in 1995 it was depicted as rational proto-science, and in 1999 as a form of naturalistic holism. As one of the main early proponents of Ayurveda in the United States, Deepak Chopra's own writings reflect this history. In his 1988 autobiography, for instance, Chopra originally invoked Ayurveda as the best alternative healing system, and asserted that "Ayurveda contains the spiritual element that Western scientific medicine jettisoned three hundred years ago."[33] By the time he had written his next book, *Quantum Healing,* in 1991, Chopra considerably downplayed the role of Ayurveda in alternative healing, and maintained only that individuals need to identify their *dosha* or body type before beginning a scientific effort to improve their health.[34] Later, in 1993 when he wrote *Ageless Body, Timeless Mind,* Ayurveda had emerged in his philosophy as neither science nor ancient system, but as a set of dietary procedures, exercises, breathing methods and other techniques for overcoming fatigue and slowing the aging process.[35] For all their differences, however, these images had a single common language running through them—a particular form of "American Orientalism" through which Ayurveda is promoted as the perfect Eastern scientific antidote to the Western stresses of modernity, materialism and monotheism.

As a set of institutional and ideological representations of Asia and Asians in the United States in the twentieth century, this discourse of American Orientalism consists of two separate but related themes: a romantic notion of the "mystic Spiritual East," and a systematic conflation between the classical past and contemporary life in the East.[36] While most scholars agree that the discourse of American Orientalism differs from the earlier European Orientalism of the eighteenth-century post-Enlightenment period, they disagree on the nature of this difference. Critical theorists, such as Lisa Lowe, claim that the two discourses are materially but not rhetorically discontinuous, and have been merely transformed by quite different state apparatuses as well as by different global and national contexts of material conditions.[37] Religious historians, on the other hand, claim that the difference between the two discourses is ideological, and is informed by the culturally distinctive way in which Americans understand Asia and the particular patterns by which they appropriate the Orient. Part of the American romanticist legacy is a historical tendency to view the Orient through stereotypical idealizations, such as the mythical, sensual East with a classically defined golden age, and to then criticize the West in terms of that ideal.[38] Others argue that understandings of the East in twentieth-century America rely not on these Orientalist stereotypes alone but on how Eastern beliefs are appropriated and thoroughly "Americanized." Sydney Ahlstrom, for instance, claims that American manifestations of Eastern thought should not be viewed in terms of their individual uniqueness, or the original core they retain, or even the historical and theological accuracy of their uses in American contexts.[39] Instead, as Robert Ellwood shows, they must be interpreted *collectively*, through the unique historical style in which Americans tend to appropriate all Oriental beliefs. Observing that the harmonial tradition in American thought, dating back at least to Emerson, has profoundly influenced ways in which Americans have understood the East, Ellwood draws a genealogy beginning with the Transcendentalists, moving to the cults of the depression era, and ending with the beatniks and the hippies.[40] This is echoed by religious historian Catherine Albanese, who cautions against addressing twentieth-century Asian beliefs in America as exotic transplants or Eastern imports, arguing that they are instead "direct expressions of an emerging American ethnicity," by which she means they have become critical cultural constituents of American nationalism.[41] As a *popular* discourse, therefore, American Orientalism, and in particular perceptions of India, needs to be examined not only against the particular cultural understandings that make their way into the print media, but also against their historical antecedents in nineteenth-century discoveries of a classical Hindu golden age.

IMAGINING INDIA

The original picture of an idealized India—with a historical golden age located in classical Sanskrit texts—was the product of British East Indian scholar-officials associated with the Asiatic Society in Calcutta in the late eighteenth century.[42] Within India, this essentially scholarly idea of the "true classical India," and its corollary of "the degeneracy of contemporary Indians," was used repressively by British imperialists, iconoclastically by Hindu reformers, and subversively by Indian nationalists.[43] As this idealized image moved across the Atlantic to America, however, it changed in some interesting ways. First, for romantic twentieth-century Americans, this picture of India's *past* became a description of contemporary, *present-day* India. Second, this image began to embody the theme of the "mystic East" that was initially introduced in literary circles and contributed to popular stereotypes of India and the Orient.

I would argue that both these elements of American Orientalism—the mystic East stereotype and the forward movement of a classical golden age—were so resilient in the print media because popular publications were crucially important to its history and spread in the first place, whether these were nineteenth-century literary translations and religious texts aimed at literate Americans, or the publishing activities of twentieth-century Hindu reform organizations that gave them an influence out of proportion to their membership. As Andrea Diem and James Lewis show, the activities of the Calcutta Asiatic Society and its British Orientalist scholars, for example, shaped American print perceptions of India in two ways: directly, through literary texts and indirectly, through Hindu missionary activities and their publications.[44] While the direct influence of the early Orientalist texts on literate Americans began quite early—the first English translation of classical Sanskrit literature by William Jones was published in the US in 1805—it was not until the Transcendentalist movement that interest in Asia truly came into vogue.[45] By the mid-1800s, the scholar-officials had translated some of the more important Hindu religious scriptures into English, and the ideas in these texts directly influenced the Transcendentalists (evident for example in Emerson's "Over-Soul" essay) and the Theosophists (as seen in Madame Blavatsky's early writings). Based on this, the Transcendentalists were first responsible for introducing the "spiritual East/material West" theme into American literary traditions. This aspect of the East/West stereotype—which as Edward Said demonstrated, would later become almost axiomatic in Western thinking about Asia—gradually became one of the defining features of American Orientalism. If eighteenth-century European Orientalism with its imperialist and colonial underpinnings often portrayed the Other as uncivilized, barbaric, infantile, or savage, American Orientalism with its textual, literary base almost always depicted the Indian Other as spiritual and quite often mystical.

It was not until the late nineteenth and early twentieth centuries, however, when Hindu missionaries began to preach in the United States, that this idealized India of the British Orientalists began to be regularly confused in the popular mind with current Hindu practices. The early stages of this confusion are clearly evident in the public lectures of Pratop Chandra Mazumdar, Paramahamsa Yogananda, and perhaps the first well-known representative of Hinduism in the West: Swami Vivekananda. Instead of British Orientalists' "theory of decline" from a glorious classical Hindu golden age, Vivekananda and the others set about the defense of *contemporary* Hindu religious life.[46] Instead of focusing on classical *Vedic* texts or scriptures, they attempted to dispel myths of contemporary Hindus as polygamous, superstitious or mystical. This "forward movement of the Hindu golden age" was popularized by the organizations they established, such as the *Vedanta* Society in New York, which because of their publishing activities were extremely successful in reaching wide audiences. Eventually, this idealized East was to become a central feature of American Orientalist thinking.

NEW AGE ORIENTALISM

Over the course of Ayurveda's decade in the print media, this discourse of American Orientalism remained important, although there was a gradual, perceptible change in the ideology itself. The clearest trend was a shift from a romantic American Orientalism—that emphasized sacred geographies of the East and historical golden ages—to a "New Age Orientalism" that perennialized and pastiched traditions, conflated high and low cultures, and invoked techniques and practices rather than discourses or beliefs.[47] While magazine articles in 1999 continued to rely on Orientalist dichotomies, the actual image of the Orient invoked gradually changed to reflect shifting historical images of the East over the century—from the profoundly spiritual and mystical Indians of Vivekananda's portrayal; to the iconoclastic 1960s counterculturalists who projected onto the East the reverse images of everything they disliked in America; to the eclectic New Agers of the 1980s who included not just the East, but any and every culture or movement that could reflect their own worldview.[48] If in 1989 articles on Ayurveda drew on romantic notions of the mystic East, by the end of the 1990s they were beginning to rely heavily on New Age images of the non-Western Other in which tribes, movements and other groups were characteristically lumped together in the desire for some sort of worldwide legitimation. In other words, while New Age Orientalism is the most recent *inheritor* of the tendency in American romanticism to idealize the East and to critique the West in terms of that ideal, it is also the *source* of new stereotypes of the East.

Some of these new stereotypes that emerge in the ideological shift to New Age Orientalism can be illustrated through particular examples in Ayurveda's print history. For one thing, its specific *Indian* origins are increasingly ignored—even downplayed—in favor of a generic use of ancient traditions with no specific emphasis on place. Thus while early articles on Ayurveda invoke Sanskrit texts for legitimacy or divine Vedic sages as sources of revealed wisdom, by the mid-1990s these stories of transcendent origins in divine authority largely disappear. Against an early reverence for the past expressed in historical golden ages, superior "knowers," and a continuity of genealogies and lineages, later articles tend to appropriate the past through an ahistorical pastiche of multiple discourses of other times and other cultures. In New Age writing, a variety of time periods—from future-oriented cutting-edge science to ancient wisdom of the Mayans, Egyptians or Hindus—come together in a syncretic juxtaposition of erudite and mass cultures, or religious and scientific discourses.[49] Thus if the Orientalism underlying the first Ayurvedic print images relied on Enlightenment worldviews, we can say that the New Age Orientalism of the late 1990s relies on postmodernist views that question Enlightenment values and celebrate or equate all cultures, particularly if they are non-Western.

MAPPING AYURVEDIC CONSUMPTION : A SYNCHRONIC ANALYSIS

Moving to a synchronic attempt to map the cartography of Ayurvedic consumption in the American print media, I suggest that representations of Ayurveda are directed at a handful of distinguishable audience groups. I focus here on five ideological strategies used to promote Ayurveda, and the five potential audience groups that they target. Each of these marks out, in different ways, a middle ground between tradition and modernity, East and West. The first group comprises the educated, liberal environmentalists who follow Thoreau and the Transcendentalists in looking toward the East for an antidote to Western materialism and the stress created by capitalist life. Ayurveda emerges here as a form of metaphysical holism and India as the original source of spiritual answers and metaphysical medicine. The second group of publications targets the non-intellectual American middle class that seeks relief from stress but also needs to be convinced of the virtues of Ayurvedic practice because it sees India as an alien place. Popular "Ayurveda myths" are dispelled using a mixture of scientific credibility and masculine rationality as ideological strategies. In this view, Ayurveda appears as a rational, empirical system that works and appeals to pragmatic audiences who are not necessarily metaphysically inclined. A third group consists of professionals and executives who epitomize capitalist success, and to the segment of the middle class that looks for a middle way marked by success in both "traditional" and "modern" terms. Ayurveda here becomes the means towards a sacred commerce, a distinctly American "prosperity consciousness" in which health leads to capitalist success and good business ethics. Women, both American and South Asian, constitute a fourth group. Ideological strategies aimed at this large segment attempt to invoke the dual role of women as modern agents of change and as repositories of tradition. This dual role underlies a view of Ayurveda as a system of domestic medicine that is reminiscent of South Asian nationalist discourses on feminization in the wake of colonialism.[50] Finally, I consider a fifth group that includes populations traditionally considered "vulnerable" by Ayurveda—such as the elderly and children—who are targeted by what has been called the "marketing of weakness" and the commodification of health tonics.[51] Here Ayurveda emerges as a system of "radical therapy" that is a source of replenishment rather than restraint, strength rather than control, power rather than purification. Interestingly, in the American print media, this group includes ethnic populations—primarily South Asian but also other nonwestern groups—that are considered "naturally vulnerable" to hot, powerful biomedicine. The image of Ayurveda invoked to counteract weakness and the loss of vitality is one of a "Science of life and longevity" that replenishes strength and rebuilds weak bodies. Thus in the context of American and New Age Orientalism, Ayurveda is promoted as a corrective to the imbalances of a diaspora. This theme of alternative medicine for immigrants is common both to American heterodox medical sects of the pre-Flexner era and indigenous medical therapies in South Asia. In the sections that follow, I examine each of these audiences groups through the ideological strategies by which Ayurveda is sold to them.

EASTERN HOLISM

Popular stereotypes of Ayurvedic practitioners and clients link them with left-wing politics, higher education (though perhaps as dropouts from conventional academic pursuits), environmental or social activism, and alternative lifestyles. The Transcendentalists come to mind as role models, and the media often invokes the theme of the influence of India on the Transcendentalists, and of the Transcendentalists on the American reception of Ayurveda and yoga.

As suggested by this stereotype, there is a range of articles on Ayurveda in specialty publications such as *Yoga Journal*, more intellectually targeted liberal publications such as *Harper's* and *Dissent*, and those considered alternative, such as *Utne Reader*, *Vegetarian Times and East West*. Most of these publications tend to assume that Ayurveda and Indian philosophy are known to their audiences as a good thing, even if it is unclear what "using Ayurveda" actually entails. Popular publications aimed at the "ex-hippies" assume a nostalgia for India as the source for self-development, often including an unabashed exoticization of Eastern culture. An article in *East West* exhorts its readers to use Ayurveda and "Go to the source."[52] Another popular newsstand magazine, *New Age*, ran a piece on Ayurveda that distinguished between "western people who understand things with their intellects" and "eastern people for whom the exact reverse is true, namely, their ability to use visual images and feelings."[53]

Not surprisingly, magazines such as *Yoga Journal* can, and do, assume a shorthand with an audience already convinced of the virtues of a closely related Eastern spiritual discipline. This strategy of "Ayurveda as embodiment of the mystic East" broadly targets the more "speculative" adherents of New Age discourse who show a tolerance for mysticism to complement their metaphysics.[54] In all these media articles, the clear use of nonrational spiritual East versus rational West could have come a century ago, indeed even straight from Vivekananda's pen. It is interesting to note, however, that this particular emphasis on the metaphysical appeal of Ayurveda declined in the print media after 1995. The passage of the Dietary Health Supplement and Education Act for the regulation of herbs and food supplements in 1995 could well have been an important factor in shifting popular preferences from Ayurvedic philosophies to Ayurvedic herbs and "psychotechnologies" that can be isolated from them.[55]

The more environmentally inclined liberal middle classes are targeted by publications like the *Utne Reader* that emphasize the "flower power" behind Ayurveda, and associate it with the values of holism, environmentalism, nonviolence, and social service. The tendency in these articles is to inscribe the moral and political commitments of the 1990s onto Ayurveda. While the tone continues to be romantic, the imagery tends to be wildly eclectic. In such images, the East is often less important as the geographical source of Ayurvedic origins than the fact that it represents a locale that is distinctly "non-Western." For instance, three separate articles on Ayurvedic herbal farms and spas tend to freely mix images that evoke ethnobotany (in the Himalayas), saving the rainforest, and The Body Shop, with images of divine sages, *ashrams*, and sacred texts.[56] The "green" subtext seems to suggest that the production or manufacture of these herbs in ecologically sound contexts is even more important than their consumption or the method of their administration. Equally important is the way that these articles refigure Ayurvedic treatments in line with the gentle, nonviolent values of environmentalism. An article in *New Times,* for instance, described Ayurveda as "a haven, an island of gentle breezes and calm sanity in this world of increasing violence, chaos and overmedication."[57] Just as Francis Zimmermann has shown that contemporary Ayurvedic practice in America completely erases the "violence" of traditional Pancakarma therapies—such as evacuations, purges and enemas—that were part of the traditional Ayurvedic armamentarium,[58] so do the print media articles, especially those that appear to target at environmental activists and potential ecologists. These articles describing the new green Ayurveda selectively ignore the so-called evacuative treatments to emphasize the figure of holism that constantly circulates in discourses of alternative healing. These print descriptions of Ayurvedic *Pancakarma* treatments privilege descriptions of spa-type massages over the more violent activities of purging and sweating that were such an integral part of these treatment packages.[59]

When they turn to Ayurvedic diets and nutrition, magazine articles tend to foreground Ayurveda's *Indian* origins. In *Vegetarian Times,* for instance, an article written in 1997 spoke in glowing terms of the Ayurvedic practice of "purifying blood and muscle through fasts and moderate eating as the ancient Indians did."[60] The article describes the virtues of this moral hygiene of restrained living, and indicates that "it keeps the *Indian* mind sharp and vigilant." Gandhi is invoked often in these articles, as is the discourse of "pure foods," asceticism, and wholesome foods such as Graham crackers.[61] Many of these articles appeal to die-hard vegetarians as well as to recent converts, and they do so without appealing to biomedical language for legitimacy. In other articles, designed to draw in both skeptics and New Age aficionados, Ayurvedic diets are presented as less severe and are defined broadly to include assorted Indian food items newly "discovered" as universally good for health. These items, often staples of Indian diets that are consumed daily, are promoted as "Ayurvedic" medicinals ascribed with healing properties thought to transcend cuisines and cultures. For instance, lentil soups, or *dals*, staple features of North Indian diets, acquire in these writings the status of a "protein-rich mana."[62] On the whole, these images of Ayurveda as a system of holistic dietary restraint offer two things to American audiences—on one hand, an authentic source of knowledge from India, and on the other, a system of nutrition for the modern age in which medicines merge seamlessly with herbs, foods and global cuisines.

There is also a small but critical group of articles, written in magazines such as *Gaia* and *re:generation quarterly*, that romanticize holistic Ayurveda as an emblem of local self-reliance in an age of commodification, globalization, and increasing Third World dependency. By invoking themes common to development discourse, such as "appropriate technology," "sustainable social development," and "local self-sufficiency," Ayurveda emerges as a repository of vernacular, indigenous tradition that successfully resists colonial and biomedical domination. To audiences that may not be convinced of Ayurveda's healing properties, but need no convincing of its political symbolism, these articles serve as reminders about the lessons of postcolonial dependency that are often glossed by the more eclectic New Age Orientalism.

Running through all these printed ideas of "Ayurveda as holism" is the classic counter-hegemonic ideology—competing against the "West" by claiming historical primacy—which has been well-described by scholars of South Asian medicine.[63] Western holism is claimed not only as original to India but as the central idea behind ancient Ayurvedic therapeutics. Thus *East West* in 1992 carried a long piece that traced the eastern roots of New World herbalism to the banks of the Ganges in Benares. In a similar vein, an article in *Vegetarian Times* claimed Ayurveda as the "granddaddy of all patient-centered philosophies and wisdoms."[64] Still other articles appeal to a cosmopolitan legitimacy for Ayurvedic knowledge by linking it with global authority that transcends historical or geographical boundaries. Ayurveda is described in one of these articles as "the world's oldest holistic medicine—the only hope for the post-antibiotic era where a search for pathogens may no longer be that important." The text goes on to claim that Ayurveda is the "hot medicine from the 1500s . . . that may be the only hope for the post-antibiotic era."[65]

Viewed collectively, most of these articles rely on a simplified notion of the "mystic East," and of India, that is a legacy of early American Orientalism. Ayurveda here is clearly viewed as a system of holism or dietary restraint that invokes many of these stereotypes. However, while these publications targeting alternative health seekers constitute a fairly large group, they are still only a fraction of the total number of articles on Ayurveda in the print media. An increasing number of articles on Ayurveda are to be found in magazines targeted toward the mainstream middle classes—both the general middle classes without a university education, as well as professionals and executives bound for economic success—which I explore in the pages that follow.

NEW AGE RATIONALITY

The second group of magazines I consider is aimed at a general middle-class audience, not particularly high on either the socioeconomic or educational scale. These articles tend to direct their attention toward dispelling "Ayurveda myths," with wording such as: "The New Ayurveda: No longer the preserve of ex-hippies, this once-mystical discipline promises perfect health and a total body workout."[66] The article uses pastel colors and photos of a woman meditating on a beautiful beach with ocean waves rolling in the background. It gives biomedical backup for its recommendations but goes on to suggest that "perhaps the ultimate attraction is that Ayurveda, which in Sanskrit means science of life, works to increase longevity . . . [it] may be ancient wisdom, but in the 90's, the idea of trying to live a long, fulfilling life seems thoroughly up-to-date." The primary idea behind articles like this is a form of New Age rationality—a mixture of magic and personal control within an essentially mechanistic world-view—that attempts to rescue Ayurveda from being either too esoteric or too elitist.[67] This rationality makes its way into several articles on Ayurveda primarily directed at "the common man" in an effort to make India less alien and Ayurveda less mystical. By taking Ayurveda out of the exclusive hands of the Indophiles, spiritual "seekers" or environmentalists predisposed to holism, these articles attempt to put it in reach of middle-class audiences everywhere. Ayurveda, in their telling, can be practiced for personal control or practical benefit by the global citizen.

Control over nature is one avenue for these rationalist appeals. In one set of articles on Ayurveda, the "whole" natural body is linked to personal responsibility and control. Ayurvedic health is achieved in these images by controlling nature through hard work, not through meditation which is spiritual, or submission to nature, which is seen as passive. Magazines such as *Whole Earth Review* and *Total Health* thus see Ayurveda as part of a mechanistic worldview bent on governing and dominating the natural world. Ayurveda in these images appeals to those who seek not religion but magic—seen as the capacity to alter, transform, and dominate nature, and to pursue what one article calls "the alchemists' dream."[68] Disease itself is thus a kind of unnatural state, a moral failing demonstrating the level of an individual's personal control over his or her life. The all-important factor is the health of the *body*, rather than the mind or spirit, and Ayurveda in many of these articles is seen as the channel par excellence through which the individual can exercise this personal responsibility.

Other magazines such as *Shaman* that target more specialized audiences—in this case ostensibly the new "sensitive" men of the 1990s—also use nature as the ideological draw for Ayurveda but emphasize connections that are "emotional, instinctual." Ayurvedic healing here continues to be aligned with "nature's way," although this natural state is achieved through emotional work, rather than through hard physical work and control. Middle-class audiences targeted by these appeals to "Ayurveda as instinct" appear to be those in search of direct, non-mystical connections to nature. In an article in *Shaman*, for instance, the author claims that the goal of Ayurvedic wellbeing is achieved not through balance or harmony, but "through the *liberating* of natural energies." He then invites readers "to *feel* your way to health through the natural emptying of impurities." This process, which resembles what he calls a primal scream technique, relies on a cathartic expression that releases natural toxins and buildups in the body.[69]

In contrast with the previous example is an article in the magazine *Men's Fitness*, which caters to male audiences that fall somewhere between the new men's movement and traditional bodybuilders. The piece is titled "Urban Renewal" and notes "Ayurveda offers the sort of pretzel logic that makes perfect sense to stressed-out men." The author draws his audience in with the lure of celebrity-speak (Demi Moore and Michael Fox use Ayurveda) and illustrates its points with a heavily tattooed man, sitting on the pavement in an urban back alley. The article cites a number of medical authorities who now endorse Ayurveda, and evaluates the compatibility among Ayurveda, bodywork, and weight training. The macho American version of Ayurveda focuses on what it can do for the body. The subtext is that Ayurveda is a rational pursuit, not an "airy-fairy spiritual" one, and that real men have nothing to fear from the practice of Ayurveda—it might even help with their weight training.

Related to this theme of machismo and masculine rationality is the issue of sexual virility and performance, which, in this age of Viagra, has become a public preoccupation. Indeed, a number of articles on Ayurvedic medications deal specifically with male sexual anxiety, in magazines as different as *Men's Fitness* and *India Abroad*—a political news journal catering to educated middle-class Indian immigrants.[70] Many of these draw on a specific sub-tradition within Ayurveda, known as *Vajikarana* or the science of sexuality and aphrodisiacs, to highlight the explicit use of tonics marketed in America to augment sexual energy. One article, for instance, addressed all those men worried about "sexual loss" and lauded the replenishing properties of saffron, ginseng as well as a new compound called "*Chyawanshakti*" (*shakti* means energy or power), all of which "enhance enjoyment tenfold."[71] Another stream of articles on Ayurvedic "tonics" weave together sexual, mental and economic indices of strength, and describe a more generalized form of power that encompasses sexuality. Advertisements in magazines that range from *Body Builder* to *Utne Reader* offer images of successful businessmen who turn to Ayurvedic tonics for strength in a stressful world. This is a tactic I describe in greater detail in the fifth group I describe.

In a small minority of these articles focused on Ayurveda, sex or sexuality is linked in a complicated semantic network with modernity and the West. While some of these articles vilify biomedicine as the root of all that is evil, even pornographic, still others use the classic counterhegemonic argument often invoked in Ayurvedic circles. In this view, ancient India is said to have already produced whatever new sexual sophistication the West displays—whether these are sexual surrogates, marital aids, virility enhancers, and dietary replenishers—which are then reappropriated and offered as examples of the primacy of Indian tradition and the diversity of Ayurvedic sexual remedies. In perhaps an extreme example of this tactic, a 1997 article in *Trikone*, a magazine for gay South Asians of the diaspora, even makes the argument that Ayurvedic sexual remedies might be particularly compatible with homosexual lifestyles, given the fact that both may have first originated in the "sensual East."[72]

By focusing on Ayurvedic remedies as replenishers of "strength" and sexual vigor, this group of articles highlights a vision of Ayurveda different from the one promoted in the first group. Instead of Ayurveda as a system of holistic restraint or moral hygiene, what is promoted here is Ayurveda as a system of radical therapy, augmentation and replenishment. This latter view is often related, particularly in the print media, to one of the leitmotifs in tropical medicine and in Indian colonial discourse—namely, the debilitating effects of the Hindu vegetarian diet on growth and "development," along with the consequences of vegetarianism for colonial subjects.[73] Those who are receptive to health ideologies focused on the strong and inviolate body see Ayurveda very differently from the first group, who might see it as system of vegetarian diets, purity, and moral restraint. By portraying Ayurveda as rational and powerful, high protein diets and sexual tonics emerge as powerful symbols of the West that contemporary print versions have to appropriate if they are to make their case for healthy, American bodies.

SACRED COMMERCE AND PROSPERITY CONSCIOUSNESS

A third segment of American society, and perhaps the largest audience, targeted by Ayurveda in the print media are the educated but often somewhat conservative, middle classes who look for a middle way marked by success in both "traditional" and "modern" terms. This includes South Asian immigrants who epitomize the kind of synthesis suggested by Vivekananda—the "material" wealth of the West combined with the "spiritual" wealth of India—although this cultural path is not confined to immigrants. A large number of these articles are targeted at *American* audiences that are attracted by the adaptation of these spiritual means toward material goals. Many of these articles focus on dispelling yet another popular myth about Ayurveda: that it is irrational, overly traditional, and has nothing to do with material life. The strategy they use is one that authenticates traditional Ayurvedic knowledge through an ingenious blend of Eastern and Western thought that has a long legacy in ""harmonial" philosophies such as the early-twentieth-century New Thought movement.[74]

The main tactic in these print articles is Ayurveda's promotion for the modern business world. One of the first popular advocates of Ayurveda's *timeliness* for the modern business age was Deepak Chopra, as part of his early pitch to increase Ayurveda's popularity in America. One of his articles in *Better Nutrition* begins with the following diatribe: "Ayurveda. Just say the word and see what images come flashing through the mind. Fasting. Austerity. Discipline. Purity. Enlightenment. Forests. Detachment. Mantras. Observances. No wonder not many find the time! Given the values of the modern age, Ayurveda does not seem to fit. **Misconception**. Given the values of the modern age, Ayurveda is right on time."[75] Articles on Chopra in *Money* and *BusinessWeek* go on to suggest that regular use of Ayurveda is a good way to ease the stress of modern business lives. A 1997 article on Ayurveda in *BusinessWeek* shows an "executive lifestyle" profile in which a young manufacturing executive undergoes an Ayurvedic oil massage that is supposed to eliminate humoral "imbalances." This young executive, the picture of capitalist success, attests that Ayurveda and regular *Pancakarma* treatments not only help him avoid the stresses of modernity, keep him physically fit, and eliminate stress from his business life, but also aid his mental concentration in enhancing business and corporate goals. He is presented as a model for exactly the kind of material/spiritual synthesis suggested earlier by Vivekananda—an Ayurvedic ethic that simultaneously encourages capitalist spirits as well as ""healthy" bodies.[76]

This theme is occasionally taken a step further in magazines, such as *Forbes, Success,* and *Fortune,* explicitly aimed at young managers and investment bankers. Articles in these magazines discuss Ayurveda's uses toward attaining economic goals. Many of these pieces draw on an important historical legacy in American New Age thought called "prosperity consciousness"—essentially a set of spiritual techniques and strategies for attracting wealth—that connects the morality of the market with the capitalist uses of spirituality. An early article on Ayurveda in *Money,* for instance, claims that the discipline of Ayurvedic lifestyles would immediately transform "material lack into abundance." Another article in *Success* on Ayurvedic spas, aptly titled "Master your economic destiny" makes a link between regular therapeutic massage and corporate success.[77] The premise here is that the Ayurvedic philosophies and the Hindu ethics underlying health are far from incompatible with capitalist success, and are indeed responsible for it. Chopra's own various books fall within this genre and his popular dictum—that "health and happiness lead to success"—was taken to heart by some management schools and business companies. The enormous popularity of Chopra's blend of East and West, ancient wisdom, pop science and common sense, rests on its appeal to the large group of aging baby boomers who seek both the fountain of youth as well as a sound financial investment.[78]

Sociologist Glenn Rupert's essay "Employing the New Age" looks at the penetration of the American business community by the New Age in the form of New Age-inspired training seminars and entrepreneurial workshops.[79] Businesses have found such programs to be remarkably effective at improving the productivity and output of their employees. While certain health techniques are presented without reference to a particular worldview or value system, it has become common to indoctrinate workers into the New Age vision of the world. Conversely, practitioners who carry the message into the business world also indicate that the New Age movement itself has evolved into a "marketed social movement."[80] Indeed, Gordon Melton observes that the New Age movement "has welcomed a large number of entrepreneurs—alternative health practitioners (from chiropractors to masseurs), publishers, organizers of retreat centers, independent writers and teachers, health-food storeowners etc."[81]

Print articles on Ayurveda stress how these training seminars improve performance and efficiency. While business productivity in an increasingly competitive marketplace is the main goal here, many of these articles also tend to emphasize creativity in business settings. Do-it-yourself procedures for oil massages and simple herb remedies and recipes sit next to lessons on how to meditate, do yoga, and in one case, even "contact a spirit guide."[82] These are possibly the 1990s versions of the human potential groups and est seminars that were such an important feature of business training in the 1970s. In all of these images, the predominant moral lesson to be learned is this: because man is a deity equal to God he can do no wrong, and thus there is no sin and no reason for guilt in life. It is this philosophy that provides the context for the general health principles of "rewarding oneself with treats," "pampering oneself," and "being good to oneself." In this view, Ayurvedic spa treatments and *Pancakarma* retreats aimed at executives, busy professionals, and those in the heady, stressful world of business, are to be seen as important rewards for a job well done. Eastern-style health treatments, in other words, may be necessary detoxification packages for the all-important Western Protestant work ethic and capitalist spirit.

NATURAL WOMEN AND DOMESTIC CULTURE

The fourth group I consider comprises women, both American and South Asian, who are targeted by a number of publications such as *Good Housekeeping* and *Mademoiselle*, traditionally aimed at female readers. Many of the articles on Ayurveda build on well-understood trends such as the overwhelmingly middle-class and female clientele for alternative medicine in the United States or women's role as agents of change in the professionalization of Asian medical systems. However, what is most interesting in these articles are the cultural stereotypes that distinguish between "modern" American or non-Asian women and "traditional" South Asian women. While articles on Ayurveda appeal to American or non-Asian women as agents of progressive change and reform who might need some help in their professional lives, those that target South Asian women picture them as repositories of traditional knowledge responsible for keeping it alive in a modernizing world.

Articles in *Good Housekeeping* suggest that if the modern American woman of the 1990's chooses to use Ayurveda, the rewards are beauty, perfect skin, and compatibility with a demanding professional, vegetarian lifestyle. An appeal to beauty seems to be the dominant theme, and in some of these magazines, big business seems to have heard the message. With titles that proclaim "Beauty is only skin deep" they mine the Ayurvedic armamentarium for "secrets that are centuries old" and catch the eye with exotic remedies tailored for the season. Gramflour face packs, lemon-cumin eyewashes, and yogurt shampoos only scratch the surface in a list of beauty tips that are neither Ayurvedic nor even typically Indian, but are claimed as such.[83] In other alternative magazines, such as *East West* and *Natural Health* that rely on a more loyal readership, many of the articles call for the more disciplined virtues of a long-term, thoroughly *individualized* beauty regimen. In an article titled "What's Your Dosha?" a leading Ayurvedic "aesthetician" begins by claiming that one's Ayurvedic *dosa* (humor) is the building block for perfect skin. "Finding out your body type and *exactly* the right exercise regimen and beauty treatment is a must for professional women." She insists that the process cannot happen overnight, but once the beauty regimen is learned, "there can be no going back, the difference is miraculous, it is the secret wisdom of the ages."[84] Surprisingly, among all the articles on Ayurveda in the print media, these are the only ones to consistently take into account the notion of individualized body types and humoral typologies (*dosas*) that form such a central part of traditional Ayurvedic diagnostics and practice. Articles on Ayurvedic beauty care offer detailed do-it-yourself *dosa* charts as well as exercises that are tailored to different skin types.[85] It is particularly ironic that this "personalizing" of Ayurveda through body types and humoral classifications is only mentioned in the print media under self-help routines for skin care.

In some specialty magazines geared to niche audiences such as new mothers, or menopausal women, Ayurveda embodies a "natural" body ethic in which women are the supposed repositories of a superior, instinctual knowledge and philosophy of nature. In an article in *Mothering*, for instance, the author compares postpartum practices around the world, and gives Ayurveda high marks for "being in tune with harmonious Nature," for knowing that a "woman's body is not a machine but a "pot brimming gently with oil." The article continues by claiming that Ayurveda only echoes what we already know by instinct. "Natural births call for natural remedies. If we listen to our bodies, we get some answers. Ayurveda reaffirms what we know in the womb. It feels right because it *is* right, because it is natural."[86]

Similarly, at least some of the many articles on Ayurvedic cooking in the print media tread the same path. They are dominated by discussions of "healing cuisines" that, used intelligently, can always "heal, balance the *dosas* and integrate the body."[87] Articles on these "primordial, centered cuisines" make their way into publications that range from *Glamour* to *Health,* and they lay claim to multiple sources of legitimacy—traditional "female" goals such as nurturing and caring as well as cosmopolitan links with global food trends and fusion cuisine. In all of these images, the target audience appears to be the thirty or forty-something American single woman whose only stresses seem to be the juggling of professional schedules with beauty routines and healthy menus. Curiously, there seems to be no room in this picture for the problems of daily life, domesticity, children, or chronic illnesses.

On the other hand, visuals accompanying articles in publications for Indian immigrants, such as *Little India* and *Maitri* strike a different note. The advertisements in these limited-circulation magazines appear to target mature, married women seemingly responsible for their families' health and happiness. Recipes for traditional Ayurveda-inspired cooking abound, as do household remedies for common ailments. One article offers a pullout table of Ayurvedic first-aid remedies for various contagious diseases that can be picked up "either in the day-care or through contact with poison ivy."[88] Another more recent article focused on the "living tradition" of Ayurveda that is handed down "from mothers to daughters" and needs no more than a "well-stocked spice rack and Indian kitchen." Almost without exception, these articles suggest that the woman can play an important role as the repository of the Ayurvedic tradition within the family. All of them also suggest that using Ayurveda is a matter of cultural pride as well as an intelligent way of dealing with immigrant life in America.

This tactic in the American print media echoes larger historical processes that have already been shown to be part of the nationalist struggle in South Asia. In most popular reform movements in colonial and postcolonial contexts, it is now well understood that the woman's body is often narratively structured as the repository of national identity by their male counterparts, whether they are Indian nationalists or Dutch colonialists.[89] In South Asia, the attempt to popularize Ayurveda as part of the nationalist agenda included what Ashis Nandy has called, pace Foucault, the "feminization" of Ayurvedic medicine within the family.[90] With professionalizing Ayurveda, this accompanied a general understanding of the harmful and debilitating power of Western biomedicine, with a related attempt to strengthen "domestic medicine" as a revivalist tactic for household and village self-sufficiency in rural areas. This same ideological tactic appears to be important in how Ayurveda "takes" among diasporic South Asians. What is most interesting here is that these diasporic images of Ayurveda differ to some extent from nationalist representations. While early nationalist reform movements, as described by Partha Chatterjee, distinguished between Nature, seen as residing in women and indigenous tradition, and Culture, seen as residing in men and Western rationality, the South Asian diaspora consistently conflates the two. Women, especially immigrant women, appear to simultaneously embody both Nature and Culture, and must therefore straddle the worlds of Western modernity and Eastern tradition.

REJUVENATION TONICS AND LONGEVITY

A fifth group of media articles on Ayurveda revolves around the promotion of Ayurvedic health "tonics" for rejuvenation in the new collective health arena of commodified alternative medicine. These articles tend to target those populations who are traditionally considered "weak," such as the elderly and children, who are particularly vulnerable to the hot and powerful system of biomedicine and would therefore benefit from the "rejuvenating" qualities of Ayurvedic tonics.

The idea of rejuvenation, or *Rasayana*, holds a special place in the classical Ayurvedic armamentarium. *Rasayana* is one of the *Astanga*, the eight traditional limbs of classical Ayurveda, and it connotes the alchemy or the radical transformation of aging bodies into all but ageless beings. Rasayana medications and formulae, derived from Sanskrit texts such as the *Caraka Samhita* and *Susruta Samhita*, promise results of longevity and youthful existence. The adminstration of these drugs is often encompassed by other therapies, such as *Pancakarma,* and the texts describe the entire process as a literal reduction of the old body to its skeletal essentials in order that it can then be rebuilt.

Many classical texts inform us that given the potential violence of its transformative therapeutics, *Rasayana* is not always for the old, whose bodies are not only weak but, in Ayurvedic terms, "hot and dry" and in particular need of replenishment. Several commodified *Rasayana* tonics, however, are exceptions, most notably the product known as *Chyawanprash*—a bittersweet herbal concoction whose main ingredient is the vitamin-rich *amla* fruit, which is explicitly allowed for old people. While commodified *Chyawanprash* is big business in India, and is administered widely to the elderly, children, and the constitutionally weak, American print media versions of the product differ on one important count. They present commodified Ayurvedic *Rasayana* tonics such as Chyawanprash as *primarily* suitable for aging populations in need of energy boosts and increased immunity and describe them as "excellent energy givers for aging body systems" and as "the Ayurvedic secret to longevity and total health."[91] Many of these magazine articles also attribute to *Rasayana* tonics positive effects *beyond* "rejuvenation." One article in a magazine called *Midlife* targeted at baby boomers presents Ayurvedic *Rasayana* products as having prophylactic properties for disease in older bodies—the "strong anticancer and antioxidant properties reverse toxicity in bodies most prone to these illnesses."[92] Still others present popular Ayurvedic botanicals, such as a*shwagandha, Sida cordifoilia* and *Coleus forskohli*, as "alchemical energy-givers" and as "critical for increasing resistance and energy."[93] "Energy" in fact seems to be the single most important appeal to the elderly Ayurvedic user. In this view, the inevitable process of aging and degeneration is somehow "reversed" or "kept at bay" with the incredible energy-boosting qualities of Ayurvedic *Rasayana*.[94] A recent article on Ayurvedic *Rasayana* tonics even mythologizes this image of "stolen time" and "discovery": "If Prometheus stole fire from the gods, Ayurveda was the one that seized the energy."[95]

Another set of articles on *Rasayana*'s anti-aging properties target the oldest baby boomers, who may have reached the age where they are concerned about the memory loss and cognitive degeneration that naturally accompany aging. Many Ayurvedic *Rasayana* products, herbs, and rejuvenators, such as *ashwagandha, bacopa monnieri (brahmi), gingko biloba, Siberian ginseng*, are actively promoted as "brain tonics" or "cognitive enhancers" that are thought to improve brain function, "clear the fog," sharpen the mind, and actually promote longevity.[96] In the late 1990s, with the gradual incorporation of alternatives into the new integrative medicine, the print media was quick to announce these Ayurvedic *Rasayana* products among the new "smart drugs," "smart nutrients" or "nootropics" (Greek for "mind-turning"). Many articles interpret them in modern medical terms as "adaptogens" or substances that help correct imbalances in the body's immune system, restoring its natural ability to respond to stress, and promoting overall vitality. Interestingly, while these drugs typically have to be obtained from overseas by mail-order because they are not approved by the Food and Drug Adminstration for the purpose of "cognitive enhancement," the print media articles tend to deemphasize their exotic Indian or classical origins. Instead, Ayurvedic *Rasayana* medications emerge as the source of several *natural* "brain" nutrients that serve as cognitive aids for the middle-aged and the aging.[97]

In some popular accounts, these print media articles on Ayurvedic *Rasayana*'s "cognitive value" are responsible for popularizing these "smart supplements" and making them such a popular market item on the health food circuit. Gingko and ginseng, not part of the classical Ayurvedic armamentarium, have been appropriated as such in advertisements. A range of brain foods and health enhancing tonics—products with names such as GinkgoIQ, Thinker's Edge, MegaMind, and Brain Booster—claim to have Ayurvedic roots, or at least "non-Western" ones that are peculiarly ahistorical. The ingredients of a product called Remind, developed by a Seattle Ayurvedic nutritionist, includes among others a smattering of the top-rung "smart" ingredients: the herbs ginkgo biloba and Siberian ginseng as well as substances such as acetyl-L-carnitine and DMAE, thought to be important for "energy-generating mitochondria in cells" and for the fluidity and flexibility of brain cell membranes. Legitimizing Ayurvedic *Rasayana* products as biomedicines as well as natural medicines, and marketing them as cognitive aids for the soon-to-be elderly, appears to be a common ideological strategy in the commodification of many "Eastern pharmaceuticals" in late 1990s America.[98]

As described earlier, many *Rasayana* products are also being marketed to a young male market with more macho sounding names such as *Chyawanshakti* that suggest replenishment for loss of vigor and vitality. However, unlike the explicit Ayurvedic sexual tonics referred to earlier, *Chyawanshakti* and the other neo-*Chyawanprashes* on the market offer a more generalized power that often encompasses sexuality but is not reduced to it. Print media articles promoting and advertising these neo-Chyawanprashes and *Rasayana* products can be found in magazines such as *New Look, Men's Fitness,* and *Vitality,* which cater to middle-class audiences looking to build bodies as well as memory power and disease resistance. The language of the advertisements weaves together mental, sexual, and economic indices of strength, promotes *Rasayana* as particularly useful for events that require peak mental and physical alertness, or promises economic success in things such as competitive examinations and job interviews. The print media articles offer images of successful businessmen "on the go" in which Ayurvedic *Rasayana*-takers distinguish "those who have it all."[99] While the effectiveness of Ayurvedic *Rasayana* tonics cannot be presented here as a medical triumph, these articles emphasize *Rasayana* as a "solution" for those audiences who have to face the daily grind, competition, and the stresses of work, and who need optimal health if they are to succeed.

All in all, these five groups point to the several ways in which the print media represents Ayurveda and makes the East more appealing to Americans. The consumers of Ayurveda as ideology and practice constitute very different audiences, whose receptivity to Ayurveda as a valuable tool for countering stress and achieving health has been determined by specific contexts and backgrounds. In the context of these self-help media, Ayurveda appears as a set of ideas and practices geared toward the construction of *new* audiences as well as healthy, modern selves. The practice of Ayurveda seems to support the acquisition of a distinctively non-Western modernity by satisfying at least three goals at once: the modern goals of health and fitness geared toward economic success, the New Age goals of personal responsibility and transformation in a millennial age, and the traditional Hindu pursuit of *moksa* or spiritual salvation, which can be used to save souls in a troubled modern age. At the same time, these goals and ideological strategies all draw on a distinctive form of American Orientalism that has enjoyed almost unbroken popularity throughout the twentieth century. If Ayurvedic print representations reveal anything, it is that New Age healing may have emerged in the late twentieth century but that its ideological origins are neither new nor necessarily radical.

As sociologist Meredith McGuire has suggested, in its popular form alternative healing may represent a statement against the rationalization of body and emotions in contemporary society.[100] If so, the New Age Ayurvedic users among the ill have protested rationalization even as they have embraced scientific metaphors or notions of transformative individualism or ascetic health practices. Although there is no single trend that emerges in print presentations of Ayurveda, what is significant is not merely that it is transformed into a New Age variant, but rather that the New Age influence on popular audiences is both so pervasive and so varied. Much as James Lewis has described, the New Age movement is characterized by constantly changing subjects of interest and foci.[101] At any given time, Ayurveda print images might reflect the dominant incarnation adopted by the New Age, just as they might also incorporate minor elements of the New Age in order to appeal to different audiences. In the end, whether Ayurveda is portrayed as a New Age scientific metaphysics, or as the new alchemy, as eastern holism or as domestic medicine, it relies for its popular legitimacy on a powerful form of New Age Orientalism. As contemporary Ayurveda variously plays out in the politics of the contemporary multicultural medical arena, it becomes clear that this neo-Orientalism is simply the most recent inheritor of a long historical tendency to domesticate the East for popular consumption.

CAM CANCER THERAPIES IN TWENTIETH-CENTURY NORTH AMERICA

The Emergence and Growth of a Social Movement

David J. Hess

THERE IS LITTLE DOUBT that popular interest in complementary and alternative medicine (CAM) in North America, not to mention other world regions, has grown during the 1990s. The studies of physician David Eisenberg and colleagues were the most prominent in a survey literature that drew attention to the size of expenditures, the scope of therapeutic utilization, and the growth in patient interest during the 1990s.[1] CAM providers have also gained increasing access to insurance coverage and the protections of licensing.[2] The U.S. government has responded to patients' interest with dramatic increases in funding for research on CAM therapies as well as a comparatively open regulatory policy on food supplements under the Dietary Supplement Health and Education Act of 1994. Popular magazines and Web sites on CAM therapies have proliferated, and the new politics of evidence-based medical integration has in some situations displaced the older politics of quack-busting and suppression. In short, the many changes that can be charted for the 1990s in the United States as well as other countries shore up a claim that there has been a "CAM revolution."

However, the focus on the dramatic events of the 1990s may tend to overstate the depth of the transformation. For example, regarding the claim that interest in CAM from patients grew explosively during the 1990s, it would be interesting to document patient utilization and interest throughout the decades of the twentieth century. Although studies for early decades are hard to find, one survey of YWCA members during the 1930s is suggestive of a long-standing interest in CAM. The very sketchy results suggested that an equivalent number of members were seeing chiropractors and medical doctors, and even more were going to Christian Science practitioners and osteopaths.[3] Likewise, the essays in this volume show that interest in CAM in the United States has been sustained and substantial throughout the twentieth century.

One of the arenas in which the politics of healing have been most intense during the twentieth century is cancer treatment. There is no known cure for most types of cancer, and yet patients with many of the more common cancers can survive for years before dying. Those factors, together with the growth of cancer morbidity and mortality during the twentieth century, provide a fertile ground for the continued development of alternative cancer therapies. Today, cancer patients are potentially able to access a vast number of alternative or complementary therapies, clinicians, and advocacy organizations.

Before discussing the growth, diversification, and politics of the CAM cancer therapy movement in the United States, it is helpful to begin with some definitions and categories. First, the terms *complementary* and *alternative* are used here to refer to adjunctive interventions (complementary) or replacements (alternative) for conventional therapies such as chemotherapy, radiation, surgery, and standard immunotherapies (such as the interleukins). The same therapy may be complementary or alternative depending on how it is used or what the point of reference is. For example, a nutritional program following a lumpectomy is complementary or integrated with respect to the surgery, but it may be used in a way that is either alternative or complementary to a follow-up course of chemotherapy or radiation. Second, there are various classifications of CAM therapies. At the influential Chantilly, Virginia, conference of 1992, seven categories of CAM were articulated: mind-body interventions, bioelectromagnetics, alternative systems (such as Ayurveda), manual healing methods, pharmacological and biological treatments, herbal medicine, and diet and nutrition.[4] In my own research on CAM cancer therapies, I found most useful four general groupings of therapies: mind-body, immunological and pharmacological, dietary and nutritional, and herbal.[5] Manual healing methods are relatively unimportant in the CAM cancer field, and bioelectromagnetics have a minor, historical place that will be noted below.

The history of the therapies, research, clinicians, and political conflicts is still largely a product of advocates or critics, and the history is largely organized around single therapies and clinicians. The studies are rich and colorful, but with some exceptions there is a frustrating lack of documentation, comparative perspective, and social science analysis. This essay will attempt a broad sweep of the more visible and prominent CAM cancer therapies in the United States during the twentieth century; the goal is to develop some preliminary understanding of the pattern of social organization, politics, and diversification of the social movement that developed. Specifically, three types of organizational form are examined: (1) networks that developed around specific clinicians and therapies, which characterized most of the early and mid-twentieth century and continue to exist today; (2) the emergence of a broad-based social movement, especially emerging from the laetrile politics of the 1970s; and (3) the development of medical integration, especially during the 1990s. The analytical framework proposed here can help avoid two types of analytical error: the belief that CAM activity in the United States went through a period of quiescence during the mid-twentieth century, and the view that there was no significant transformation during the late twentieth century.

CLINICIAN-BASED NETWORKS

Among the early-twentieth-century alternative cancer therapy traditions, two of the most influential in the United States were inaugurated by John Beard and William Coley. Beard, a professor of embryology at Edinburgh University, developed the theory that aggressive, undifferentiated embryonic cells (trophoblasts) were placed under control by pancreatic enzymes, but cancer could emerge from remaining undifferentiated cells.[6] The theory led to a long series of enzymatic treatments of cancer. Although Beard did not have a significant contemporary following in the United States, his theory influenced subsequent generations of American clinicians and researchers, including the dietary programs of dentist

William Kelley and physician Nicholas Gonzalez, the bacterial program of physician Virginia Livingston, and the laetrile research of physician Ernst Krebs Sr. and scientist Ernst Krebs Jr.

In the 1890s the New York–based physician William Coley inaugurated another research and therapy tradition in the United States, when he used live Streptococcus bacteria in cancer patients to create a febrile skin reaction (Erysipelas) that, in some cases, led to long-term survival.[7] Coley's therapy has subsequently been reinterpreted in immunological terms, and he has been recuperated historically as a founder of cancer immunotherapy.[8] However, he was also interested in nutritional approaches to cancer as well as the controversial theory that cancer was an infectious disease caused by a pleomorphic (form-changing) microbe that would be described today under the rubric of cell-wall-deficient bacteria.[9] At the time stable categorizations of fungi, bacteria, and viruses were less well accepted than today, and some scientists and clinicians believed that microbes could undergo phases of development that stretched from "filterable" (viral-like) phases to full-blown fungi. At the height of the bacterial revolution in medicine, many mainstream clinicians believed that cancer was an infectious disease, but the theory fell out of favor by the 1920s. One reason for the decline in support for the infectious theory is that microbial cultures of tumor samples did not yield a stable specimen, and consequently many researchers came to interpret the cultures to be the result of secondary infection or contamination rather than a pleomorphic infectious carcinogen. Another reason is that by the 1920s hereditary and environmental interpretations of cancer etiology were beginning to congeal alongside the growing practice of radiation therapy; together they provided a theory-therapy package that was an alternative to biological treatments based on the infection theory.[10]

During the 1920s one of, if not the, first substantial North American networks of CAM cancer therapies emerged around the infection theory. The Canadian physician Thomas J. Glover and his partner Tom Deaken developed a serum and, with the support of a surgeon named Michael Scott, had a substantial network of clinicians using it, with some success, on cancer patients.[11] Given Coley's affiliation with Memorial Hospital (today Memorial Sloan-Kettering Cancer Center) in New York, his support of Glover and his interest in the serum were critical. Although Coley mobilized some critical support in the cancer field, including interest from Charles Mayo, he eventually parted ways with Glover due to the latter's secretive approach to his work and his almost paranoid concern with gaining fame and fortune from his serum. Coley's toxins, which evolved into a killed mixed bacterial vaccine, had a more lasting impact. During his lifetime the vaccine was used not only at Memorial Hospital but also at the Mayo Clinic and by clinicians in both in the United States and Europe. After his death the vaccine continued to be used at Memorial Hospital until the 1950s and is still used today in some locations.

Both Glover's serum and Coley's toxins did not die a "natural death" in the sense of losing a following due to negative clinical studies or to displacement by a clearly more efficacious therapy. Instead, both became early instances of what the sociology of science literature refers to as suppression.[12] In other words, elite and powerful medical networks worked actively to halt the development and use of the therapies.[13] The details are narrated elsewhere, but it is sufficient to say that by the 1920s and 1930s radium-based therapy and surgery were institutionalized to the point that immunologically based therapies posed professional and financial challenges to the dominant networks.[14] Coley had the position and potential influence to alter the direction of cancer research and treatment, but his death in 1936 foreclosed that possibility. Although his son continued to use the therapy at Memorial Hospital, during the 1950s Cornelius Rhoads, the director of the hospital and a leading chemotherapy advocate, ordered the cessation of the treatment. Due largely to the efforts of Coley's daughter, Helen Coley Nauts, the therapy continued to be used in some places, including China.

Another prominent but more controversial network that emerged during the 1930s was the group of supporters around Royal Raymond Rife, an inventor who had investigated foreign laboratories for the U.S. government during World War I and who subsequently developed a non-ionizing electronic frequency device and a high-powered microscope.[15] He claimed that the microscope allowed him to follow microbial pleomorphism and to identify tumor viruses, and likewise that his machine was able to kill the infectious agents without harming the patients. Rife's work attracted researchers at prominent institutions such as Northwestern University, the Mayo Clinic, McGill University, and the University of Southern California, particularly those who still advocated a microbial etiology of chronic diseases such as cancer and arthritis.[16] By the late 1930s Rife's medical colleague Milbank Johnson had opened three clinics in California, and Rife was manufacturing the electronic frequency instrument for more general distribution. After a period of suppression, Rife again began leasing out machines, and before the second wave of suppression in the 1960s Rife's company had leased out ninety machines across the country. The network was therefore quite large, but it was also so heavily suppressed that very little work in Rife's tradition survives today.

After World War II another generation of figures in the bacterial/vaccine tradition became prominent. Physician Virginia Livingston was at the center of a substantial network of researchers who published peer-reviewed literature on the topic of a pleomorphic cancer microbe, mostly from the 1950s to the 1980s.[17] Livingston and colleagues also developed an approach to cancer treatment that combined her autogenous vaccines with dietary interventions; the clinic that she founded remains open today in San Diego. Less prominent but still in the bacterial tradition was the work of Gaston Naessens, a French biologist who developed a high-powered dark-field microscope and studied what he believed were blood-borne microbial flora (a continental European variant of the research tradition of cancer and microbial etiologies). After experiencing problems with the French authorities during the 1960s because of his therapies, he moved to Quebec, where he developed an injectable formula that he claimed was efficacious in cancer treatment.[18]

The bacterial etiology/bacterial vaccine group of networks represents only one strand in the pre-laetrile networks of alternative cancer therapies. There was also a wide variety of pharmacological/biological therapies for cancer.[19] During the mid-twentieth century the most prominent was Krebiozen, a drug that was extracted from the serum of horses that had been injected with the bacterium *Actinomyces bovis*. The therapy had been introduced into the United States by a Yugoslavian physician and his brother, but it gained popularity only when a respected scientist, Andrew Ivy of the University of Illinois, supported it in 1951.[20] Ivy's battles to gain support for clinical trials of the drug and Food and Drug Administration approval for its use lasted into the 1960s, and he continued the struggle until his death in 1978, even though the advocacy left him isolated and discredited. At its peak the network of supporters included Illinois legislators and labor leaders, patients and clinicians, and members of the U.S. Congress. In 1961 a data set submitted to the National Cancer Institute included four thousand patients, a figure that gives some indication of the size of the network.[21] Yet Ivy did not set up an out-of-country clinic, as occurred for the Hoxsey therapy (discussed below), and unlike the laetrile movement, the extensive network of supporters did not crystallize into a social movement with organizations that were capable of surviving changes in leadership. As a result, Krebiozen is more or less a historical phenomenon, unlike many of the other therapies discussed in this section.

Another of the influential pharmacological/immunological group of therapies is the work of Emanuel Revici, a Romanian physician who in 1947 came to New York via Mexico.[22] Revici pioneered a nontoxic, lipid-based chemotherapy and has increasingly received historical recognition for his original research and thinking, especially as a pioneer in research on the therapeutic potential of selenium.[23] In the hospital that he ran from 1955 to 1978, Revici also provided an opportunity for Lawrence LeShan to develop his pioneering approach to the psychotherapy of cancer.[24] Revici, like the other advocates discussed here, suffered from various forms of suppression, including in his case a temporary loss of license shortly before his death in 1998 at the age of 102. He left behind a small network of supporters as well as widespread recognition in the CAM cancer therapy movement for his role as an innovative pioneer. However, because of the complexity of his therapy, its portability to other clinicians and clinical settings was limited, and I suspect that the long-term legacy of his work will be as a source of piecemeal insights for other research programs and therapeutic protocols rather than an influential system that is diffused intact.

In the dietary field, the most influential clinician was the German physician Max Gerson, who moved to New York after the Nazis came to power. He had developed a complex dietary therapy that was continually modified in light of new research and clinical experience. The therapy included juicing, a potassium-based diet, colonic irrigation (the famous coffee enemas used to open bile ducts to aid in liver detoxification), and other therapeutic interventions that continue to be influential today.[25] Although the New York Medical Society suspended his license in 1958 and he died in 1959, his ideas remained influential, and his daughter Charlotte Gerson helped revive the therapy. Today, variants of the Gerson therapy are offered both in the United States and in Tijuana.

Gerson's therapy also influenced the dietary program developed in the 1960s by the dentist William Donald Kelley, who claimed to have cured himself of pancreatic cancer through a special diet.[26] Kelley added to the Gerson program two central elements: a greater focus on dietary enzymes, which represents another strand of alternative cancer therapies that dates back to Beard's work and was more prominent in Europe at the time, and a belief in biological typing that lacks credibility in the form that he articulated it but in some ways predates the emergent field of nutragenomics. Kelley's dietary approach influenced several clinicians, including the midwestern chiropractor Jack Taylor and a group in Washington State known as Healthexcel.[27] While a medical student in the 1980s, Nicholas Gonzalez analyzed a sample of Kelley's cases and subsequently developed his own nutritional program, which today is being tested in a clinical trial for pancreatic cancer patients at Columbia University, for which oncologist Gonzalez is principal investigator.[28] Other dietary traditions came to vie with the ones listed here, but in my experience they have had less influence in the CAM cancer therapy field in North America.

Among the herbal formulas, the most prominent in North America were those of coal miner Harry Hoxsey and nurse Rene Caisse. Both formulas are now recognized to have pharmacologically active plant ingredients, but again clinical efficacy has not been documented in clinical trials. Hoxsey's great-grandfather developed a formula for cancer treatment after watching a horse with cancer eat selected plants in the fields and then attain a long-term remission or cure.[29] By the 1950s Hoxsey's clinic in Dallas, Texas, was the largest private cancer clinic in the United States, with branches in seventeen states.[30] The extensive network provided a solid base of support for his legal battles against the American Medical Association and Food and Drug Administration that were even more epic than those of Rife and Ivy. In fact, Ivy had investigated Hoxsey's therapy in 1949, with a negative report, but Hoxsey later flew to Ivy's aid when he encountered suppression during the Krebiozen controversy.[31] Mildred Nelson, a nurse who at first was very skeptical but became interested in the therapy after her mother underwent treatment at the clinic in 1947, moved the clinic to Tijuana in 1963, where it continued to operate even after her death in 1999.[32]

A second major herbal therapy for cancer was developed by Canadian nurse Rene Caisse in the 1920s, when a patient told her about an Ojibwa herbal tea formula. She treated hundreds of patients and eventually attracted the usual medical censure. Although a petition to allow her to continue to provide the formula for free gained fifty-five thousand signatures in 1938, the network around Caisse and the herbal therapy was smaller than some of the others discussed here in terms of number of clinical facilities, research projects, and patients treated.[33] She did attract the support of a major mainstream physician—Charles Brusch, the former physician for President Kennedy—who eventually helped convert the therapy to an over-the-counter herbal tea called Flor-Essence (see Clow's essay in this volume for more on Essiac).[34] Many other variants of Essiac are on the market, or patients can make it themselves from the four main ingredients.

There are many more CAM cancer therapies and attendant networks that existed during the early and middle decades of twentieth-century North America, but the ones discussed above represent the most influential in terms of the size of the network of supporters at the time. The lack of institutionalization meant that many of the therapies suffered a major setback after the primary architect and advocate died, unless there was an heir apparent, as in the case of Mildred Nelson for Harry Hoxsey. This "charismatic" pattern of social organization is still commonplace today among the many clinician-researchers with innovative therapies and a supporting network of colleagues and patients.

Two general patterns might also be noted from this early period. First, as has been noted, most of the advocates of alternative cancer therapies met with some form of suppression. The suppression generally came from leaders of the medical profession, such as Morris Fishbein of the American Medical Association, but the medical profession could mobilize government agencies, the media, and other institutions in its support. Elsewhere I have developed a typology of suppression mechanisms.[35] One group involves legal or formal sanctions (restraining orders, criminal charges, raids on clinics, FDA warnings, FDA denials or stonewalling of permit applications, hostile tax audits, and revocation of hospital privileges, licenses, or insurance), a second group involves more informal channels (media campaigns, dismissals from organizations, loss of funding, publication blockage), and a third group involves bias in research investigations (protocol modifications, exclusion of advocates from research teams, ignoring favorable data supplied by advocates, biased interpretations of equivocal data). In some cases, the suppression occurs in what some students of CAM history has called a "pincer movement," in which a series of mechanisms are mobilized at the same time.

Given the career and prestige risks associated with CAM cancer therapies, one might wonder why so many well-credentialed people have, over the years, become involved. To answer this question properly, one would need to undertake a detailed comparative biographical study, so at this point I can venture only a hypothesis. In my years of interviewing and observing the CAM cancer therapy movement, it appears that two motivating forces are paramount: the lure of historical glory to anyone who develops a significant breakthough in cancer treatment, and the personal satisfaction of being able to save lives and help terminal patients. Because most of the advocates claim to have some impressive cases of long-term remissions, they feel that any well-intended and open-minded researcher should explore the possibility of less toxic and potentially more efficacious alternatives. Most of the advocates have a relatively naive sociological model of science and medicine, and when they discover that science and medicine are highly political, their dismay can turn either to withdrawal or to confrontation. The flip side of this question is the many physicians who suspect that CAM therapies do work for cancer but remain quiet for fear of personal reprisal.

THE EMERGENCE OF A CAM SOCIAL MOVEMENT

If there is a formative event that marked the transition from relatively precarious networks of clinicians, patients, and researchers to a more lasting mass social movement, it is arguably the controversy that erupted around a single laetrile doctor in California. Originally following the model described in the previous section—that is, a network of patients, clinicians, and researchers around a single therapeutic agent or program—advocacy for laetrile had by the end of the 1970s become a social movement. One crucial event was the arrest and subsequent court trials in 1972, and then again in 1976, of physician John Richardson for his use of laetrile.[36] Because Richardson happened to be an articulate member of the John Birch Society, the medical profession arguably made a strategic mistake in selecting him as a target for suppression. According to Michael Culbert, a journalist who covered the Richardson trial and later became a leader in the alternative wing of the CAM cancer therapy movement, about half of the original members of the Committee for Freedom of Choice in Cancer Therapy (today the Committee for Freedom of Choice in Medicine) were Birchers.[37] The linkage was the basis for the popular image of the laetrilists as extreme right-wingers; however, the history is much more complicated, in ways similar to what Gregory Field has shown for the perception of anti-fluoridationists during the 1950s and 1960s as merely right-wingers.[38] By 1977 the Committee for Freedom of Choice in Cancer Therapy claimed five hundred chapters and over thirty thousand members.[39]

Another wing of the laetrile movement developed in 1975 in a research setting around an organization that became known as Second Opinion.[40] Consisting mainly of employees and former employees of the Memorial Sloan-Kettering Cancer Center, this group began discussing a cover-up of animal experiments that had provided evidence in support of laetrile. In November 1977 the group released a forty-eight-page report that led to the famous dismissal of Ralph Moss, who had worked in the public affairs office. In 1980 Moss published the first edition of his exposé of the suppression of CAM cancer therapies that was later republished as the influential book *The Cancer Industry*. Moss became one of the leaders of the CAM cancer therapy movement, particularly those who wanted to have more funding and fairness for research, and today he writes both a column on CAM cancer therapies in the *Townsend Letter for Doctors and Patients* and the Moss Reports, which are individually tailored guides for cancer patients who wish to explore alternatives.

As the laetrile movement grew, its politics and membership became more diversified. Culbert noted that the Richardson trial in Berkeley drew out not only right-wing sympathizers but also "McGovern-for-president left-wing hippies."[41] The left-right polarities were noted in sociological work by James Petersen and Gerald Markle, although a member of the CAM cancer therapy movement who read the essay told me that he felt that the emphasis on right-left political differences, particularly the association of Second Opinion with left-wing politics, was an exaggeration.[42] Indeed, the friendships that spanned the political spectrum even led to jokes among colleagues in the movement about favoring "right-handed" or "left-handed" laetrile, a reference both to the political leanings of the advocates and to the optimal chemical structure of the molecule.

The laetrile movement had other organizational bases that came together in the formation of a social movement. The National Health Federation had a longer history of involvement in the politics of healing in the United States. Founded in 1955 by Fred Hart, the president of a company that had been prosecuted for selling unconventional medical devices, and by Royal Lee, a dentist whose company sold vitamin supplements and whose foundation published nutrition information,[43] the organization's first representative in Washington, D.C., was one of Harry Hoxsey's lawyers.[44] In the late 1970s the National Health Federation became active in some prominent court cases in defense of laetrile.[45] The organization was also a strong opponent of fluoridation, therefore providing one point of contact between the CAM cancer therapy movement and the anti-fluoridation movement that I have seen repeatedly flagged in conferences during the 1990s (see Reilly's essay in this volume).

One of the more significant developments toward institutionalization during this period was the founding of what is today called the Cancer Control Society. The society began around the work of Cecile Hoffman, a laetrile patient who convinced Mexican physician Ernesto Contreras to offer her the drug on a compassionate basis.[46] Suffering from late-stage, metastatic disease, she underwent a remission in 1964 after treatment with laetrile. As often happens, she began offering information to other late-stage patients, and in 1965 she founded the organization Cancer Victims and Friends (today Cancer Victors and Friends), which by the late 1970s had fifty chapters and eight thousand members.[47] Under the leadership of Norman Fritz, an engineer and friend of Hoffman, the organization became financially healthy, and a polarization on the board developed.[48] As a result he, Lorraine Rosenthal, and Betty Morales left to found the Cancer Control Society. Among the organization's activities today is an annual convention in Los Angeles, which I would characterize as the more alternative, populist wing of the social movement. Prominent among the speakers are representatives of some of the larger Tijuana clinics.

The hospitals and clinics in Tijuana provided another important institutional basis for the laetrile movement. In the mid-1970s a wealthy Canadian, Andrew McNaughton, who had long been a leading laetrile advocate, established manufacturing and clinical facilities in Tijuana.[49] Laetrile is still offered at some of the major hospitals in Tijuana, such as the Contreras family's Oasis of Hope Hospital and the American Biologics Integrative Medical Center, for which Michael Culbert became director of information. Today those two hospitals offer a wide spectrum of therapies that are usually combined in complex packages and tailored to each individual. More generally, Tijuana provided a clinical home not only for laetrile, but for the continuation and reestablishment of other therapies that were suppressed in the United States, such as the Gerson therapy (which Norman Fritz played a role in reestablishing along with Gerson's daughter), the Hoxsey therapy (which Hoxsey's nurse Mildred Nelson led until her death), and the therapy of biologist Harold Manner (which included laetrile, enzymes, and vitamins). Over time the leaders of several of the larger clinics and hospitals tested many alternative, nontoxic therapies, although not in the form of clinical trials, and they drew on their clinical experience to sort through which ones were most efficacious under which circumstances. Thus the clinical setting in Tijuana, and to some extent in other non-U.S. sites (especially Germany), provided another impetus to the diversification of the social movement. The international dimension of the social movement is crucial to understanding the survival of the alternative wing of the movement and several of the therapies that were effectively closed down in the United States.

In the 1970s and early 1980s a number of other organizations were founded or became publicly much more visible in ways that contributed to the growing diversification of the social movement and to its dense network of cross-therapeutic relationships. In the early 1970s followers of Michio Kushi founded the *East-West Journal* and the East-West Foundation,[50] and in 1975 the foundation co-sponsored the first New England symposium on macrobiotics and natural foods.[51] In 1981 the movement's leader published *The Macrobiotic Approach to Cancer*; that publication and a book by a doctor who claimed to have recovered from cancer through a macrobiotic diet signaled the movement's growing influence in the CAM cancer therapy field.[52] Although in my experience the macrobiotic diet has been less influential than Gerson-derived diets, particularly in the large cluster of Tijuana clinics, a very modified version of the diet has had some influence at the more complementary end of the spectrum, as in the work of oncologist Keith Block, a leader in the integrative therapy movement of the 1990s (whose worked is discussed below); John Boik, a specialist in Oriental medicine who has written a significant textbook on the mechanisms of nutritional interventions in cancer;[53] and Jeffrey Bland, a biochemist who has educated thousands of doctors in his "functional medicine" seminars, in which he has described the macrobiotic diet as a good place to start.[54]

Other organizations and networks during the 1970s and early 1980s contributed to the diversification of the movement. In the Pacific Northwest the major naturopathic schools and the growing holistic health movement contributed some leaders to the CAM cancer therapy movement, and the *Townsend Letter for Doctors and Patients* carries many articles on CAM cancer therapies. In 1983 Patrick McGrady Jr. established his CanHelp service after his father, himself a major cancer journalist, succumbed to cancer. In Washington, D.C., cancer patient Robert DeBragga founded Project Cure in 1979; the organization laid some of the groundwork for the changing currents in Washington, D.C., and published an influential critique of bias in cancer therapy evaluation by journalist and researcher Robert Houston.[55] In Philadelphia in 1977 linguist Susan Silverstein founded the Center for Advancement in Cancer Education after her husband died of cancer. In Virginia U.S. government physicist Arlin Brown held six conferences in the 1970s and 1980s on alternative cancer therapies. Brown had founded his organization, the Arlin J. Brown Information Center, in 1963. He had become interested in herbal approaches to cancer when stationed in Panama, but he found that the National Cancer Institute was uninterested in his calls for research.[56]

In addition to the development of organizational diversity, during the 1970s a wider range of CAM cancer therapies were pioneered or developed. The pattern of a core researcher/clinician with a network of supporters discussed for earlier in the century continued, but the new therapies and advocates were being developed in an environment with greater organizational diversity and a potential to draw mass support from the diversifying laetrile movement. Only a few examples of the more prominent of the recent networks will be mentioned here. Physician Joseph Gold was developing work that started in the 1960s on hydrazine sulfate; the drug appeared to block gluconeogenesis, a metabolic process in the liver that was associated with the extreme weight loss of late-stage cancer known as cachexia. [57] In the early 1970s scientist Linus Pauling and physician Ewan Cameron started testing their vitamin C therapy,[58] oncologist O. Carl Simonton and psychologist Stephanie Simonton were developing their visualization therapy for cancer,[59] and physician Judah Folkman published a paper on the antiangiogenesis implications of cartilage.[60] Later in the decade physician Stanislaw Burzynski began testing his antineoplaston therapy in humans, and scientist Lawrence Burton became involved in controversies over the testing of his immuno-augmentative therapy.[61]

By the beginning of the 1980s the terrain had shifted tremendously. The laetrile movement had merged or spilled over into a more general alternative cancer therapy movement, in turn part of the broader holistic health movement. The wide range of alternative health organizations was increasingly having an effect on national policy in both the regulatory and research arenas. For example, in 1976 the National Health Federation's lobbying efforts led to the passage of the Proxmire Amendment to the Food, Drug, and Cosmetics Act.[62] The amendment limited the Food and Drug Administration's ability to regulate supplements and predated the Dietary Health Supplements and Education Act of 1994.[63] The National Health Federation had also supported work that led to a court decision in 1977 to allow the importation of laetrile for terminally ill patients; the appeals process lasted nearly a decade.[64] In the research arena, the National Cancer Institute developed a protocol to evaluate Burton's immuno-augmentative therapy in 1975, but he rejected it because it violated the ethics of equipoise; that is, it did not offer treatment to the control group.[65] After this event and continued stonewalling from the Food and Drug Administration for his investigational new drug approval, Burton decided to move his work on immuno-augmentative therapy to the Bahamas. Given the epic controversies that Linus Pauling was to have after the results of the first clinical trial for vitamin C trial were published in 1979[66] and the controversies over the clinical trial for laetrile that were published in 1982,[67] Burton's decision not to proceed with an NCI-run clinical trial may have been prescient. Although the clinical trials of the late 1970s and early 1990s represented the first moves of the research establishment toward an evidence-based approach to CAM therapy evaluation and away from the quack-busting mode, unfortunately the trials excluded the advocates from participation in the study design and implementation. As a result, the negative results or failures to agree on protocols only increased the gap between the research establishment and the CAM cancer therapy advocates, and led to charges that suppression was ongoing, only now through the mechanism of biased protocol modifications.

The gap intensified after the raids on the Burton clinic in the Bahamas and the Burzynski clinic in Houston, which occurred in July 1985, a second galvanizing date in the CAM cancer therapy movement.[68] Due largely to grassroots lobbying by patients and advocates, in 1986 U.S. Representative Guy Molinari and eventually about forty other members of Congress requested that the Office of Technology Assessment (OTA) study Burton's treatment. The office was unable to come to an agreement with Burton over a protocol, and criticism of the OTA from the CAM movement eventually became heated.[69] The final study, which was published in 1990, is still considered to be deeply flawed. Scholar and journalist Robert Houston found two hundred errors in the study; half were corrected.[70]

According to Ralph Moss, the public affairs officer of the Memorial Sloan-Kettering Cancer Center who went on to become one of the leading figures in the CAM cancer therapy movement, in the year following the OTA report several members of Congress became convinced that the National Cancer Institute was unwilling to carry out the report's recommendations to investigate CAM cancer therapies.[71] The frustration led to a bill introduced by Senator Tom Harkin, based on conversations with Representative Berkley Bedell, to establish an Office of Alternative Medicine within the National Institutes of Health.[72] The first year's appropriation was $2.2 million—a homeopathic dose (to use the phrase of journalist Peter Barry Chowka)[73]—but a decade later the budget had grown to about $100 million, no longer an infinitesimal financial dose but still less than 1 percent of the full budget of the National Institutes of Health. Furthermore, the office had been transformed into the National Center for Complementary and Alternative Medicine, a more than nominal change that signaled authority over funding decisions. Perhaps more than the funding, the symbolic importance of the growth of a precarious toehold within the NIH into a center represented to many the "coming of age of CAM" or the "CAM revolution." This leads to the third phase or type of politics of healing in the CAM cancer therapy field.

THE POLITICS OF INTEGRATION

As mentioned at the outset of this essay, on a number of grounds—patient utilization patterns, insurance, regulatory changes, research funding shifts, and so on—significant changes did occur with respect to the politics of complementary and alternative medicine during the 1990s. Advocacy for CAM cancer therapies not only influenced the shifts but also benefited from the more general advocacy coming from other quarters of the CAM or holistic health movement. By the end of the twentieth century NCCAM was funding studies of CAM cancer therapies, including a clinical trial of the Gonzalez dietary and enzyme protocol. The trial itself was a significant event, because (1) unlike the previous trials of laetrile, vitamin C, and hydrazine sulfate, the key advocate had control over the protocol, so controversy over experimental design could be limited; (2) the trial took place at a prestigious university rather than a cancer or medical center that had lost credibility as a site for fair testing due to previous clinical trial controversies; and (3) if successful, the Gonzalez protocol could replace chemotherapy as the standard of care for pancreatic cancer patients. However, even though the politics of cancer had driven the OTA study and to some degree the founding of the OAM, by the late 1990s CAM cancer research had to compete with the funding needs of many other CAM therapeutic traditions and diseases. Furthermore, there were signs that the funding portfolios themselves were being oriented toward the more complementary uses of CAM cancer therapies and to the idea of "integrative oncology practice."

The older politics of suppression, which characterized most of the history of alternative cancer therapies in the United States, had given way partially to a new politics of integration based on the model of evidence-based research (with the catch of low funding to support the needed research).[74] Suppression continued as a strategy of social control, as was evident in the continued attempts to close down Burzynski's therapy[75] in the 1990s and the closure of several Tijuana clinics in 2001.[76] However, as has occurred with other successful social movements, increasingly the politics of CAM cancer therapies involved integration with the mainstream.

In addition to the name change of the Office of Alternative Medicine to the National Center for Complementary and Alternative Medicine, another bellwether of the shift was a revised operational statement of the American Cancer Society in 1999.[77] The organization had long been reviled in the alternative cancer therapy movement for its list of "unproven" therapies; having a therapy added to the list has in several cases coincided with the pincer movement of suppression that involved media campaigns, closures of clinics, loss of license, and so on. In the new statement *alternative* is defined as unproven, and *complementary* is defined as supportive or adjunctive. The role of CAM therapies for cancer is repositioned as primarily palliative care, which is targeted to receive funding for evaluation. Although the change represents a tremendous shift from the older quack-busting policy and the unproven-methods list, there should be little doubt that if this statement accurately represents the cancer establishment's new stance, it is intended to divide the CAM cancer therapy field into acceptable adjunctive therapies and unacceptable alternative therapies. In this context the closure of several Mexican clinics in 2001 may be less a return to an older policy than a new articulation of an unchanged policy that continues to limit head-on alternatives to chemotherapy and radiation therapy. The Gonzalez trial, which could lead to a replacement of chemotherapy as a standard of care for pancreatic cancer patients, therefore takes on a special political significance.

Organizationally, the new politics of CAM cancer therapies are evident in the annual conferences that began in 1998 under the leadership of psychiatrist James Gordon of the Center for Mind-Body Medicine in Washington, D.C. The registration fee structure, availability of continuing education credits, and generally high scientific quality of the research reflect the orientation toward the health care professions, in contrast with the populist, patient-to-patient advocacy orientation of the Cancer Control Society's annual meeting. The Washington, D.C.–based conference also has higher participation from federal research agencies (including the armed forces, NCI, and NCCAM), from nutritional and mind-body researchers, from oncologists who were increasingly adding nutritional and mind-body protocols to their practices, and from major cancer hospitals that were adding off-site CAM facilities. Although the alternative strand was represented at these conferences, the more complementary perspective was foregrounded. Gordon has been a crucial reformer inside the system; he chaired the White House Commission on Complementary and Alternative Medicine Policy, and he is more open to bona fide alternative therapies than the American Cancer Society. I would therefore classify him as a mediating voice that retains an open door to the alternative side of the complementary/alternative spectrum within an emergent policy field that is oriented toward complementary rather than alternative therapies.

Increasingly, oncology practices and some oncology hospitals within the United States are moving toward integrative care. One leading institution is Cancer Treatment Centers of America, which was founded in 1988 and now includes multiple centers and affiliated oncologists across the country.[78] Another leading force is Keith Block, a Chicago-based oncologist who in 2002 founded the journal *Integrative Cancer Therapies*.[79] Block has brought conventional therapies such as chemotherapy and surgery together with complementary approaches that include dietary modification, nutritional and herbal supplements, massage therapy, mind-body therapy, acupuncture, and other alternative modalities.[80] The new models of integrative care emphasize treating the patient humanistically as a whole person, strengthening the body through nutritional and other programs, and reducing toxicities and side effects of conventional therapies while attempting to retain some of their benefits. The models are probably a harbinger of what will become the standard of care of twenty-first-century cancer therapy, although there is still a huge gap between the sophistication of, for example, Block's practice and the very limited adjunctive offerings at the major conventional cancer hospitals.

CONCLUSIONS

Cancer patients who have the financial and physical resources to travel now have more options available to them than at the beginning of the century. They may receive the best of conventional care at a major oncology center with some nutritional and mind-body support at an adjunctive facility; they may be lucky enough to find one of the pioneering integrative clinicians who understand the details of nutritional therapeutics in the context of compassionate care; or they may travel to Mexico, the Bahamas, or Germany for access to bona fide alternative therapies that can replace chemotherapy, radiation therapy, and even in some cases surgery, although at a risk of uncertainty regarding efficacy and in some cases safety. The last option represents optimal "medical freedom," as the phrase in the movement goes, because the out-of-country clinics have (at least until very recently) been able to offer therapies that are not available in the United States. Yet those therapies are often (though not always) the least investigated, and it takes a great deal of knowledge to be able to separate out the more credible out-of-country clinics and therapies from the less credible ones.

In general social movements that grow and diversify tend to develop reformist and radical wings as well as shades of difference in between. The development of the CAM cancer therapy movement in the twentieth century is no exception to the general pattern. The different wings have their own strengths and weaknesses, and together they contribute to a diversification in the politics of healing, from the medical freedom issue to the more complex politics of medical integration and research funding priorities.

The historical developments also lead to a normative question that lies behind this essay and, I hope, this volume: the issue not only of what the politics of healing have been and are in North America during the twentieth century, but also of what they should be during the twenty-first century. Certainly the issue of "medical freedom," of access to alternative treatments, is a crucial public good that holds out the potential to help many patients. However, choice is almost meaningless in the absence of meaningful research to guide the choices, and in the absence of regulatory changes that would allow patients and clinicians a full spectrum of choices that historically has been available only outside the United States and Canada. It seems clear, to me at least, that a broader public interest will be served by providing more research funding for the bona fide alternative traditions discussed here and by legalizing the rights of patients to choose them—and clinicians and other health care providers to offer them—if they see fit. Thus, the twenty-first century promises to be a time of ongoing negotiations and confrontations over the rights of access to complementary and especially more alternative therapies, and over the release of funding for their proper evaluation. The lessons of history suggest that the so-called CAM revolution of the 1990s is only a beginning.

BEYOND THE CULTURE WARS
The Politics of Alternative Health

Matthew Schneirov and Jonathan David Geczik

IN THIS ARTICLE WE EXPLORE the political potential of alternative health, focusing on two alternative health networks we have studied, one New Age (or what some call "holistic health")[1] and the other a conservative Christian cancer support group and a group that provide resources on agricultural practices and dietary habits. Among the New Age groups we studied, Art Sutton is an activist who embodies this sensibility. He no longer believes in marriage, traditional religion, or conventional ways of making a living. He believes that the purpose of life is to break through boundaries and open oneself to a wide range of experiences. Following his divorce, he has traveled widely in a spiritual search for an enlarged self-definition. In contrast, Lenny Gamulka, head of the Committee for Freedom of Choice in Cancer Therapy (CFC), describes himself as a "conservative born-again Christian." He has been married to the same woman his whole adult life and organizes his life in accordance with biblical principles. He opposes abortion and believes that New Age forms of spirituality are expressions of dark forces, almost satanic in character.

Despite these differences, Art and Lenny are engaged in some sense in a common project around health and illness. They share a commitment to "taking responsibility for one's health," in contrast to reliance upon medical expertise. They also share a suspicion of allopathic medicine and its institutional roots in the pharmaceutical industry. Finally, they share a project that aims to create a space in everyday life in which people can exchange information, support one another, and bring their message to a larger audience.

Such an improbable connection between two individuals rooted in different conceptions of life and its purpose suggests larger questions that we will take up in this article. How do we account for the ability of alternative health to bring together people from different traditions? How does participation in an alternative health community politicize participants by forging a new language that bridges the divide between left and right? What are the larger political implications of the reemergence of alternative health as a social movement? We argue in this chapter that alternative health is a new social movement providing a cultural laboratory where new ideas and identities emerge. These identities and an oppositional stance toward political and medical authority bridge the ideological divide between right and left.

HISTORICAL CONTEXT

We have studied two alternative health subcultures or networks in the Pittsburgh area over the past ten years. The first consists of health care practitioners, activists, and patients who have a New Age sensibility, centered around various Eastern spiritual and healing disciplines, and who by their own self-descriptions root themselves in 1960s social movements, from the ecology and alternative food movement to the antiwar movement, feminism, and the counterculture. Within this network can be found the local food co-op and various alternative health organizations that practice macrobiotics, energy medicine, homeopathy, massage therapy, colon therapy, naturopathy, therapeutic touch, crystal healing, and herbal medicine, among others. We can also find an organization (Holistic Living Quest) that tries to provide meeting points where various practitioners and activists can share ideas and information.

Various movements such as organic farming, natural foods, and therapies inspired by Eastern and Western metaphysical traditions have circulated throughout our history, but they reemerged with a renewed vitality in the context of the growing resistence to all forms of authority during the 1960s. While all of these movements had a utopian sense that they were participating in a world-transforming project, alternatives to allopathic medicine were at best marginal to the social energies of this period. The counterculture aimed to unbind the self in order to escape the restrictions of conventional middle-class morality. The focus in large part was on ecstatic experience and on eroticizing more and more aspects of personal life. The New Age movement emerged out of the defeat of the utopian impulses of the sixties. The effort was to keep alive small embers within narrowly cultivated contexts such as the alternative foods movement (which started, or at least gained national attention, in Berkeley), intentional communities, and various Eastern and Native American spiritual traditions. All this provided seeds for the eventual emergence of an alternative health care movement. Alternative health continued what remained of the utopian project of the sixties because it confronted the costs of "progress" in the form of chronic disease or, to put it another way, the way the body registers the costs of modernity.[2]

The Committee for Freedom of Choice in Cancer Treatment (CFC) reaches back into a significantly different history. The CFC is part of a network of alternative health groups that includes the Natural Foods Group and a local affiliate of a national organization, the National Health Federation. Most participants characterize themselves as "conservative Christians," are older, come from working-class backgrounds, and tend to live in more rural areas compared to New Age participants. Of the seventy-four people surveyed at a recent CFC meeting, the average age was fifty-nine, only 20 percent were college graduates, and most characterized themselves as Christians who go to church at least once a week. More than a third are retired or are full-time housewives. Of those who are employed outside the home, the vast majority are clerical or blue-collar workers. The average household income of CFC members (as of 1998) is $24,800, which is below the national average and substantially lower than the consumers of alternative medicine in David Eisenberg's now famous study.[3]

The CFC is a support group for cancer patients and their families but reaches out also to patients who suffer from a range of chronic illnesses. Since its inception, the CFC has held monthly meetings attended by 120–400 people. Meetings begin with an opening prayer and feature a speaker, often brought in from outside the city, who explains some alternative approach to treating chronic disease. Patient testimonials are also quite common. In one instance, a cancer survivor who has written a book on her experience recounted to more than four hundred people her ordeal and eventual cure through alternative treatments. Typically one hour is devoted to questions from the audience. It is common for participants at the meeting to exchange phone numbers and to make themselves available to others in order to spread information about their own experiences and share their knowledge. Often whole families will attend, and it is common to see two or three generations of a family sitting and taking notes or tape-recording the lecture. In the 1970s the CFC was part of a national coalition of groups organized to support a physician in California who was a proponent of laetrile as a cure for cancer and who was prosecuted for his activities. Most of these groups are no longer active, but the CFC has survived.

The Natural Living Group (NLG) has more of an emphasis on organic farming and disseminating alternative nutritional advice. Speakers at the monthly meetings give talks such as "The Fats in Our Lives: Then and Now," "Hypoglycemia, Diabetes, and Emotional Disorders," "Pollution Most Likely Culprit for Latest List of Ills," and "Dealing with Candidiasis and Allergies," among many other topics. The speakers are typically advocates of nutritional approaches for maintaining health or for addressing particular health problems. Members of the NLG are also invited to attend a yearly organic food festival where they can sample and buy organic food, see "natural living displays," and view demonstrations of health products and programs. The NFG was part of the health foods movement, which emerged in the 1930s as an alternative approach to the discoveries of nutritional science. In the view of the NLG, food has been "devitalized" or depleted of its minerals and essential nutrients by modern agricultural practices and by the application of chemicals—fertilizers, pesticides, and preservatives.[4]

Participants in the NLG and CFC believe that the road to health requires strict obedience to biblically based dietary regimes that must be faithfully followed. In this way they continue the tradition of nineteenth-century botanical medicine and dietary regimes of Thomson, Graham, and Kellogg, among others who promoted an ascetic approach to health that prohibited alcohol, processed foods, and meat, grounding these prohibitions in religious doctrine.[5] Graham's regime, for example, was promoted as a natural alternative to the moral and material excesses of "civilized society." Here, "natural" meant a corset that one put on in order to discipline the body into health. This clearly diverges from the New Age sensibility, which has an aesthetic orientation of releasing the self and its energies.[6]

The dietary regimes followed by NLG and CFC members are varied, but by and large they are understood as in accordance with biblical principles. A newsletter published by one frequent speaker at CFC meetings and a prominent Christian health activist, *God's Plan for Good Health*, demonstrates the role of biblical principles for CFC members. The front page of the newsletter reports on a new "deadly virus" spread by rodents, with cases throughout the South and Northwest. The short article concludes with a citation from Corinthians: "Know ye not that ye are the temple of God and that the spirit of God dwelleth in you? If any man defile the temple of God, him shall God destroy: For the temple of God is holy, which temple ye are." The clear implication is that disease is a result of straying from God's law. While one rarely hears speakers at CFC and NLG meetings blaming patients for their own illness, a common refrain is that God made us perfect and only "people can screw it up." But the more positive side of the message is that obedience to dietary principles consistent with the Bible can cure most any disease. This, along with faith in God, can restore the damage humans have done to our bodies and to nature.

In the same newsletter, the authors condemn the FDA for threatening to "take three to five hundred vitamins and minerals off the market." This effort to restrict the public's access to vitamin and mineral supplements "couldn't come at a worse time in history."

> We are being bombarded with mutant viruses caused by a long time use of antibiotics (drugs) that are actually killing some people within 24 hours. Our immune systems are in a weakened condition and only those [who] start building up their immune systems are going to survive the upcoming plagues. The only recourse we will have if they do take away our supplements is to get back to growing and eating God's food without the pesticides and artificial fertilizers. We will need to eat organic meat and make juice from organic vegetables for added supplementation.

Speakers at NLG and CFC meetings make the same point repeatedly: that we have damaged nature and our own bodies through the use of drugs and the growing of food that has been depleted of minerals and contaminated by pesticides. A return to a more natural condition in accordance with biblical dietary principles is the only way to restore an original condition of perfection. While the details of the dietary regimes recommended by various speakers come from a wide range of alternative health modalities, from naturopathy to oxidation approaches to various cleansing regimes that focus on the colon, in most cases it is asserted that these regimes are in accordance with biblical principles.

In another newsletter the same authors get more specific. Here, they assert a biblical warrant for their rejection of white sugar, Proverbs 24:14: "My son, eat thou honey, because it is good." Honey, it is argued, is naturally occurring, while refined sugar is depleted of nutrients and harmful to the body. This passage concludes with Hosea 4:6: "My people are destroyed for lack of knowledge." The idea here, that adherence to biblical principles obligates us to take control of our health, is in clear contrast to the tradition of faith healing. God will not cure us unless we "walk toward the temple," or take responsibility for our health.

In the New Age or holistic health network, religion has to do with ever new experiential states, whereas in the Christian network religion has more to do with conformity to rules. This is what Max Weber called "inner worldly" asceticism, which he argued was predominant in Western societies, in contrast to the emphasis on transcendent experiences or "outer worldly asceticism" in the East.[7] Despite their divergent histories, however, both traditions shared an adversarial relationship to state power, because, given the dominance of allopathic medicine, they have both been objects of repression. In this way both traditions have been forced into a common space by virtue of what opposed them rather than what they shared. The common repression of state power has, in turn, provided the basis for emerging interconnections between the traditions.

THE TRANSFORMATION OF IDENTITIES

We interviewed sixty practitioners, patients, and activists from both the New Age and Christian networks. We also observed and participated in a wide range of meetings, lectures, study groups, and health fairs. Our approach is to conceptualize alternative health not as an expression of health consumer preferences but as a social movement with socially transformative potential. The social movement literature within sociology has evolved from an emphasis on movements as strategic actors within the polity to a broader focus on social movements as cultural laboratories in which people explore new ways of looking at the world and defining themselves. In this sense everyday interactions become as relevant to the study of social movements as organized efforts within the polity. In fact, in new social movement theory these two levels are crucially linked, with an emphasis on culture as the "pacemaker of change."[8]

Yet alternative health is largely unstudied as a social movement. The reason for this may well be that health and illness are thought of as private matters and are therefore are captured by disciplines that are more likely to explore the institutional domain of health care, such as medical sociology.[9] Because alternative health is not as visible as other movements, engaging in disruptive activities such as marches, demonstrations, and sit-ins, its grassroots base and political potential are not always appreciated.

A good way to highlight the movement character of alternative health is to adopt Claus Offe's discussion of three levels of power in modern societies that can also be understood as the sources of social transformation.[10] At the most visible, in the sense of being the most studied and open to media scrutiny, is the level of political elites, where concrete decisions are made, resisted, and negotiated. This is the level of the polity, or what political scientists call authoritative decision making. The second or intermediate level refers to the space where interest groups and other collectivities form coalitions and contest with one another over the distribution of resources and over competing discourses. The third level is interwoven in the texture of everyday interactions. Here, struggles directly relate not to decision making or interest groups but to questions of who people are and what they want to become. This is often expressed in the demand for autonomy or for a space protected from the polity. On this level the quest for self-definition is not a purely private or personal project but involves people entering into new interactions, forming new institutions, and experimenting with new modes of communications. In new social movement theory this third level is emphasized as the precondition for fundamental change in the other levels.

To what extent are the two networks that we are studying involved in a common cultural project at the level of everyday life? On one level our mention of Lenny and Art seems to show that they are not. Our study of these groups also suggests obvious differences in cultural style, religious beliefs, level of education, class background, and political allegiances. Participants in the CFC invoke God repeatedly, during an opening prayer and in discussing the path to recovery, which typically involves religious faith as an essential companion during every step toward recovery. On the other hand, New Age participants typically rebelled against the religion of their parents and had a more diffuse sense of spirituality. In addition, while both networks are well aware of the existence of the other, there is considerable suspicion and even a desire to build fences between them. One nurse we have interviewed told us she was afraid to go to a CFC meeting because they might think of her as demonic. The leader of the CFC does welcome New Age people to his meetings but not "if they bring their crystals." One fundamentalist Christian health activist who writes his own newsletter explicitly prohibits New Age enthusiasts from coming to a health resort clinic that he runs.

From our point of view, though, what is significant is what they have come to share despite their different worldviews. All of the people we interviewed in both networks shared a set of practices: following a health regime; attending meetings, cooking classes, seminars and workshops, and health fairs; reading alternative health literature; and seeing an alternative health care practitioner. These practices generate a common language that binds them together. They both share a discourse that is anti-bureaucratic and that partially critiques the commodification of everyday life. Health care, they argue, should not be limited to a narrow set of rules that constrain the personal freedom of alternative health care providers and patients in experimenting with different health care regimes. For example, both groups oppose government regulations of alternative health products and treatments and believe that patients have the right to pursue and even self-administer unconventional treatments that have not been approved by the FDA. In addition, both groups emphasize self-care in which the patient works on herself through regimes that are in large part self-designed and self-administered. The common refrain of "taking responsibility for one's health" can also be understood as part of this anti-bureaucratic ethos. A number of patients we interviewed stressed the differences between the active role of alternative health patients, who educate themselves about their illness and treatment regime and who see themselves as partners with their practitioners, and the medical patient who passively absorbs expertise.

The qualified critique of commodification is often expressed as a concern about the pressure to consume, stresses connected to overwork, and the emptiness of lives that revolve around the pursuit of material things—all of which have health consequences. This critique of commodification also involves an institutional critique. Both sides believe that modern medicine is driven by the financial interests of pharmaceutical companies, resulting a drug-based culture that is not unlike the quick fix inherent in the consumption of commodities. Latent within both themes—anti-bureaucratization and the critique of commodification—is a distrust of the promises of "progress." While a critique of progress comes from a variety of quarters, ranging from radical economists who question the correlation between economic growth and general social well-being to environmentalists who talk about the impossibility of generalizing Western forms of life to the entire planet without jeopardizing the ecosystem, in alternative health this critique is literally embodied in the experience of disease and by virtue of this has a certain tenacity.[11] Progress, in this view, is directly in collision with the well-being and happiness of the person. The populism that unites both networks in a shared critique of consumerism and bureaucracy (especially the regulatory state) is reminiscent of Christopher Lasch's discussion of the "petit-bourgeois tradition" in American history. This tradition, among other things, is rooted in the "producerist" ideology of artisanal and working-class radicalism as well as the populist movement's defense of family farming and rural traditions.[12] For Lasch, this tradition of social protest is important because it challenges the "ideology of progress."

Most of our informants entered into the world of alternative health as a result of a life crisis, usually an illness accompanied by unsatisfactory treatment by conventional medicine. At first they began to see an alternative health care practitioner and then to use alternative health products. At this stage their allegiance is divided; they are willing to go in several directions at the same time. But what tips the balance for the activists and practitioners we interviewed is the pull that is exerted on their consciousness by their relationships with their practitioners and others in the community. These relationships pull them into deeper involvement. The ever deepening immersion in an alternative health network provides the experience of nonbureaucratic and noncommodified relationships, which solidifies their commitments. In addition, for those who are ill, the daily practice of staying on a demanding health regime serves to distance them from the practices of their prior life. These regimes therefore serve to remind people of the threats to personal health coming from "eating on the run," eating fast food, working too much, and having poor nutrition.

Our interviews with members of a macrobiotic study group, part of the New Age network, illustrate some of these processes of identity formation. Two participants had recurrent problems of drug addiction and eating disorders. They experimented with various recovery groups but they found these groups to be too "negative," with too much of an emphasis on the person's "powerlessness." Instead, through macrobiotics, they were encouraged by an approach that satisfied their desire to actively work on becoming healthy. Once they became active in this study group and in other alternative health activities, their commitment was reinforced by the personal relationships they formed with their practitioners, the pleasure of shopping at the co-op where they felt a sense of community, and by the associations with like-minded patients. One member of the study group formed a barter relationship with her practitioner, while most of the others are involved in their own program of wellness education, where they met others with similar interests. All of the participants we interviewed found themselves drawn to the slower-paced life, with its close attention to seasonal changes in nature and sense of solidarity and community they found in this study group and the larger alternative health community. A number told us that the source of their interest in feminism and ecology came from their alternative health activities. Here is an example of one devotee of macrobiotics who describes the importance of the larger alternative health community, which for her revolves around Whole Health Resources, whose director started the macrobiotic study group.

> When you go to Whole Health Resources there are people that you may have conversations with, there's a small library and I will ask if this is a good book, and have some conversations about some of that. So there's a network that revolves around Whole Health Resources. And through my yoga class, there's a woman there that practices macrobiotics and the yoga teacher herself, and every once in a while I'll ask her an odd question. And then the co-op. I know where to go. I know who has good books. I know who can give me advice, if I have a question. I had a question last week about whether I should brew barley in a coffeepot to make barley tea, so I asked someone in my yoga class because I couldn't find it in any of my books. The biggest support that I have found probably has been just my whole lifestyle change, just making the time to make it important. So I'm happy to be part of that, that network of people and organizations.

What is happening here can be conceptualized in light of Putnam's concepts of bridging and bonding social capital. "Social capital" refers to the benefits that accrue to individuals and communities as a result of social connections and networks. When social capital is of the bonding sort, strong in-group loyalty and boundaries are created, whereas bridging social capital creates linkages between groups. What we are referring to thus far is the creation of bonding social capital between alternative health activists and patients, but the other kind is present as well.[13]

We discovered that alternative health provided a space where activists came into contact with other progressive communities. This was the case with people in the Christian as well as New Age networks. Shopping at the local co-op, relationships with practitioners, health fairs, and classes unavoidably result in alternative health activists coming into contact with people who have had experiences in peace movements, those involved in the gay and lesbian rights movement, ecology activists, and feminists, among others. One practitioner of applied kinesiology we interviewed was also active in gay and lesbian rights groups and was especially interested in treating people with AIDS.[14] A nurse-midwife we interviewed was also involved in the peace movement. The multiple political allegiances of many practitioners means that their patients will be exposed, in many cases, to oppositional movements other than alternative health.

Quite a few of the patients we interviewed said that their association with an alternative health care practitioner led to an interest in other social movements. One college student, suffering from candidiasis, established a barter relationship with her naturopathic practitioner and became active in the alternative health community. This led to a change in her own career plans as she rejected her parents' strong urging to major in business. She also became an activist in the ecology movement. One leader of the NLG, who describes herself as a conservative Christian, has become interested in ecology and "sustainable agriculture" through her involvement in an organic food co-op, which, in turn, led to associations with groups outside her community such as the Western Pennsylvania Solar Energy Society, the Green Party, and the candidacy of Ralph Nader, who, she says, is "on the right track." This is interesting because it shows that alternative health provides a nondogmatic space that seems to pull members of the Christian network toward points of view, people, and experiences that undermine their biblically grounded certainties. For instance, the same Christian health activist who excluded New Age people from his retreat spoke at the local co-op in Pittsburgh, where aging hippies and long-haired counterculture types freely asked questions and seemed enthusiastic about his lecture on oxygen therapies. The local food co-op and its café is one gathering place for many activists as well as for people who are just interested in their health (it has a large alternative health section). As one food co-op worker told us, "Most of the alternative-thinking people are into alternative food. The main connection between progressive communities is food."

Patients and activists come into contact with a wide range of healing traditions as well as progressive communities as they seek a path to health. Many of the conservative Christian activists we interviewed combined in eclectic ways elements of an evangelical Christian discourse with references to meditation, energy fields, and acupuncture. As stated earlier, the NLG and CFC are in the ascetic tradition in which health must be grounded in biblical law, emphasizing certain dietary practices and restrictions. Nevertheless, these activists often come into contact with others outside their own network as well as a variety of healing traditions that do not easily fit within the biblical tradition. In practice, they learn to combine ascetic and aesthetic perspectives, much as their New Age associates also combine a belief in connecting to sources of energy beyond the self with ascetic regimes that require self-discipline. The result is an opening up of a space where Christian activists become exposed to non-Western healing traditions and progressive political perspectives.

For most of the activists we interviewed, involvement in alternative health introduces them to various non-Western healing traditions, from macrobiotics and acupuncture to meditation and tai chi, that in many cases become part of the fabric of their lives. For these people, the selective appropriation of diverse healing traditions provides them with a resource for critical reflection about the world around them and in many cases a resource for change. For one member of a macrobiotic study group we interviewed, macrobiotic cooking was a way for her to slow down and become more aware of nature and seasonal change. This was an important part of her recovery from various addictions and more broadly from a life in which she had lost herself in trying to live up to the demands of others. A patient who began her "accidental journey" into alternative medicine with a family tragedy eventually changed her career path and outlook on life through her relationship with a homeopathic physician and yoga instructor. She has cut back on her hours at work in order to appreciate what is valuable in her life and is a critic of the "male-dominated medical profession" and the way advertising tells us how to live.

Alternative health, in short, is a social movement that is embedded in the texture of everyday life. It involves a set of practices that are ongoing and tenacious in character, it throws people into new relations with one another, and it crystallizes new forms of life. It precipitates new identities and, finally, opens participants to other oppositional cultures that are also rooted in everyday life.

THE POLITICS OF ALTERNATIVE HEALTH

How does alternative health as a cultural laboratory connect with the polity and the traditional divisions between left and right that inform the debate within it? As mentioned earlier, from a conventional point of view the politics of the New Age and Christian networks could not be more different. In terms of issues such as abortion, the death penalty, gun control, gender equality, gay rights, and welfare, members of both groups have diametrically opposed points of view. But if we adopt the broader view of politics suggested by Offe's discussion of levels of power, a different picture emerges.

At the level of everyday life, the practices of members of these two networks reveal an emerging set of values and ideas that link them together in surprising ways. For both networks there is a shared commitment to the autonomy of their health practices from bureaucratic intervention and, in a more qualified way, commodification. The belief that everyone is responsible for his or her health is rooted in what can be called "the care of the self."[15] This phrase, which seems commonplace on one level, has rich political implications. The care of the self involves, for patients and activists, a schedule of self-administered routines or "disciplines" that have the potential to reorganize the totality of a person's life. Shopping for organic food, drinking only distilled water, mixing food in proper combinations, learning how to prepare and use herbal remedies, utilizing cleansing regimes that are quite elaborate and require extensive periods of free time, and reading health books and newsletters in order to refine the schedule and menu of treatments make up the fabric of this practice of self-care. As mentioned earlier, these practices serve to create a boundary between the patient or activist and the outside world. In a more positive sense, these practices embody an embryonic politics. Shopping for organic food suggests a critique of the commercially prepared system of food production, involving preservatives, pesticides, and antibiotics. Mixing herbal remedies suggests a return to "nature's pharmacy" rather than the products of the drug industry. Food preparation and proper food combining requires elaborate effort in shopping and food preparation. All of these activities suggest a slowing down of time. If, as Teresa Brennan suggests, the essential feature of modern capitalist societies is the speeding up of all levels of social life in order to increase the velocity at which goods and services circulate, then these practices involve a bodily informed resistence to this acceleration of time.[16] This experientially based critique of time is embedded in everyday life and only on occasion reaches the level of consciously articulated discourse. For example, one meeting of Wellness 2000 concluded with a discussion of how modern life creates too much stress because of the overabundance of useless information and because people have to run around to do too many things in too little time. But this discussion was more the exception than the rule.

This slowing down of time is bound up with a trust in the "natural" that provides a normative justification for these practices and a source of guidance for their direction. For example, herbal remedies and organic food are thought to be superior to drugs and processed food because they are closer to the rhythms of nature. The celebration of the natural also has a political implication in addition to its connection to the slowing down of time; it provides a resource for resistence to commodification.[17] Natural remedies, in the sense of products that have not been processed and transformed by human agency (or at least have undergone only a minimal level of processing), cannot be made into private property. Garlic cannot be sold by a pharmaceutical company unless it is chemically transformed and subjected to their proprietary control. Natural remedies, therefore, provide an experience of access to things that are inherently common. Of course, "nature" is often deployed as a marketing strategy in order to sell various products. But the common use of the word *nature* in advertising is, for the most part, a commercialized expression of the more fundamental changes we are describing here. The slowing down of time and the celebration of the natural suggest the rudiments of a value shift on the level of everyday life. To put in another way, from what experiences would a critique of progress and its costs be derived? What would give that critique staying power or tenacity? We have suggested at least the beginning of an answer to these questions.

The anti-bureaucratic impulse and alternative health's partial critique of commodification can be taken up in different ways or assume different social forms. The central tendency in the New Age network is for the anti-bureaucratic impulse to be expressed through the conquest of new social, political, and cultural territories and the creation of new ways of living (such as intentional communities) and new associations. Communal living, which many in the holistic health have experimented with, as well as experiments in personal relationships and organizational forms (such as alternative health HMOs), are examples of such efforts to create new ways of living and new associations. In other new social movements, "prefigurative politics," or creating the forms of life that embody elements of a desired future, is a central task.[18] For the CFC and NLG, on the other hand, the anti-bureaucratic impulse is in large part expressed through a commitment to entrepreneurship and the market, a more conservative expression of the opposition to bureaucratic intervention. But this valorization of the market is always embedded in some conception of an organic community and the values within which market relations operate. No member of the CFC or NLG would say that the purpose of life is buying and selling. Instead, buying and selling are a vehicle of the expression and perpetuation of a way of life that is religiously grounded.

Alternative health's critique of commodification, which takes the form of practices of mutuality and sharing, is contradicted by tendencies going in a different direction. Both networks are emeshed to a significant degree in small commodity production and entrepreneurship. Natural products are promoted and sold, health activists frequently promote their own products and services, and even alternative health dot-coms have sprung up. While in the New Age network entrepreneurship is practiced but not publicly proclaimed as a goal (the food co-op that looks and functions like a supermarket also claims to be a communal enterprise based upon noncommercial values), in the CFC entrepreneurship is more enthusiastically celebrated. Much of what typically occurs in both networks is the exchange of money for products and services. Moreover, in the CFC new products are continuously displayed and promoted as solutions to a wide range of illnesses. In fact, alternative health is, in part, a cottage industry for the emergence of a host of new companies.

From this point of view, opposition to the "medical industrial complex" expresses a conflict between a monopoly and an emerging entrepreneurial sector, a feature of capitalism from its very beginning. But when all is said and done, alternative health is not distinctive because it is entrepreneurial. What is more fundamental is the way it serves to reorient our notions of time and the natural world through its ongoing body-based practices. Today, with the triumph of the market and the way it dominates all discourse within the public sphere, it is not surprising that alternative health would share elements of this dominant discourse and its related practices. But what is more fundamental for the purposes of social change is the way alternative health's practices reorient our notions of time and the natural world. In this way, it "brushes history against the grain."[19]

The implications of this value shift in everyday life depend on the way these values and ideas are transformed and mediated at the second level of power, where discourses circulate and organizations operate. Here advocates of alternative health pressure policy makers in different directions. Conservatively oriented groups such as the CFC and NLG advocate deregulation of the health care market and oppose any model of universal health insurance because they fear the restriction of their autonomy with respect to health care. It is quite common to hear, following the opening prayer, a speech informing the audience of efforts to restrict access to vitamins and to herbal and other natural remedies as well as efforts to restrict alternative health care practitioners from operating. The audience is encouraged to sign petitions and call their congressional representatives to prevent this from happening. This suspicion of the state's regulatory power has been a defining characteristic of alternative health ever since the biomedical model became hegemonic through state enforcement. Many speakers, during the period of intense discussion of health care reform that followed President Clinton's initiative in the early nineties, came out against national health insurance because they believed that the government in principle should not be providing or regulating health care services. More progressively oriented groups, such as the New Age network we studied, are more open to regulation and universal health care provided it allows for choice of health care providers. The discourse that resists regulation (the conservative discourse) is coupled with a defense of a traditional way of life rooted in biblical values. For the New Age network, diversity and self-invention are embraced as cultural ideals. The point here is not to protect an existing way of life rooted in tradition but to invent new spaces of autonomy and community.

However, these divisions, if reframed, can be bridged at higher levels of power. The value shift at the level of everyday life creates the condition, which both networks share, for a critique of progress and an appreciation of its costs. One expression of how this value shift works its way into higher levels of power is an openness to and potential support for positions such as sustainable economic development. A number of economists, such as Herman Daly, have tried to develop models of sustainable development that would involve a radical transformation of the economic system in relation to the environment. This includes new measures of economic development, distinct from measures of GDP, that incorporate the depletion of natural capital, as well as a conception of development that moves beyond the notion of quantitative growth.[20] Discussions of sustainable development, however it is conceived, would have no impact if they remained within the boundaries of technical analysis. The analysis of sustainable development by experts must be adopted by social movements for it to have a socially transformative effect. We are suggesting that the experiences that are rooted in self-care, the slowing down of time, and the valorization of nature within alternative health provide a basis for an ongoing receptivity to these ideas about sustainable development that come from experts located in a variety of settings. The notion of sustainable development has a complex lineage. Elements of the "new left" during the 1960s as well as religious liberals and, more recently, some communitarians have developed a systematic critique of industrial civilization that focuses around the fixation of industrial societies on "economic man" and on quantitative growth as the only measure of progress. These ideas, floating around for some time in intellectual circles, have been taken up by the ecology movement as well as by segments of the alternative health care movement.[21]

The traditional left-right divide does not capture adequately what is going on here. The debate between the left and the right is about how to equitably distribute the fruits of progress, but neither questions the desirability of progress itself. We suggest that at the level of everyday life both alternative health care networks share certain practices that move them beyond this consensus. Despite the real differences between a biblically grounded defense of autonomy and tradition and one that embraces the modern values of self-creation and invention, the deeper affinities between these networks should not be ignored.

CONCLUSION

Robert Burger, a chiropractor whose practice includes a wide range of alternative therapies, is also one of the organizing directors of the CFC. He has a daily radio program where he answers questions about health and illness from people in the greater Pittsburgh area. In response to one question Burger articulated a general analysis of problems in American society and, surprisingly, on the dangers of too much corporate power over our lives. In this respect he mentioned favorably the Green Party and the presidential candidacy of Ralph Nader. This may be surprising to some, because conservatives, religious or otherwise, tend to focus exclusively on the dangers of state power and see the economy only as a sea of entrepreneurs and consumers involved in spontaneous networks of market transactions.

From another point of view, Burger's remark is not so surprising. As we have pointed out, alternative health leads people into a nondogmatic space where they are exposed to a variety of cultural and political influences such as other social movements and healing traditions. As a result, it is difficult for them to focus only on state power as the threat to their autonomy. It is not government, after all, that puts pesticides into food or pollutes the atmosphere or makes drugs the magic bullet for all health problems. To be sure, government may support and reinforce some of these activities, but it is not the source of them.

The growing receptivity to Green politics among religious conservatives in the alternative health movement shows that alternative health can be conceived at its core not as a resistance to modernity but as a significant permutation of it. While drawing upon premodern health traditions, alternative health engages with modernity through its reflective appropriation of diverse health traditions, as well as its linkage with other political movements. This breaks down the bonding social capital that can lead toward dogmatism in groups that are not so permeable to other traditions and movements. What is tenacious about this openness and makes it more than just a matter of belief and ideas is "the body in pain," which gives rise to a set of practices that reorient a person's life, her relations to others, and—wider still—the community as a whole.[22] The radical impulse in alternative health toward social reconstruction therefore is rooted paradoxically in the private experience of the body and its afflictions. The body registers the costs of progress and becomes the enduring source of efforts at social reconstruction.

CONCLUSIONS

CONTEMPORARY ANTI-VACCINATION MOVEMENTS IN HISTORICAL PERSPECTIVE

Robert D. Johnston

AT THE END OF THE MILLENNIUM, *The Simpsons*—as always—tapped the pulse of the American nation like no other cultural production. In December 2000 Homer finally discovered the joys of virtual reality, quickly becoming an investigative reporter on the Internet. Our intrepid breadwinner proceeded to uncover a vast conspiracy behind the flu vaccine. This finding put Homer in grave danger. The conspirators, using *The Prisoner* as their inspiration, took Homer to an island where they placed him under complete isolation, thereby preventing him from spreading The Truth. Yet his kidnappers ultimately did confess. Why, after all, are influenza shots given right before Christmas? Because . . . they contain a serum that heightens the impulse to shop.[1]

Nor should I fail to mention that Agent Dana Scully of *The X-Files* discovered one day, during the course of her duties, the likelihood that some government agency has for decades been tagging all Americans with a special alphanumeric code during their immunizations.[2]

A jaundiced view of vaccination became a staple of popular culture during the 1990s. Yet real-life concerns about this miracle medical procedure also became, during the same period, intensely political. And to the immunization establishment, anti-vaccination sentiment was—rather is—no laughing matter. For in the last decade, even in just the last half decade, skepticism about vaccinations, and in particular their compulsory nature, has become epidemic in North America.[3]

Indeed, as I write during the middle of 2003, President Bush, secretary of Health and Human Services Tommy Thompson, and members of the federal medical establishment in Washington, D.C., are as stymied as they have ever been in matters relating to vaccination. Fearing a bioterrorist attack, Thompson promised in late December 2002 to vaccinate half a million health care workers against smallpox within thirty days. A month after the program began, however, less than 1 percent of the targeted subjects had volunteered for the risky immunization, and the figure had not even reached ten percent by July 2003. Before the war with Iraq a former Massachusetts health commissioner commented that the president's project was "as close to stalled as you can get"; after the war, national security officials feared that the program was "all but dead." Moreover, powerful voices within the public health elite, as well as among rank-and-file health workers, have effectively—and with few if any consequences—encouraged opposition to official government vaccination policy.[4]

We should, though, ask: how historic is this massive resistance? Is it truly a phenomenon we have never seen before? On one hand, nothing like it occurred during the midcentury golden decades of vaccines, when immunization became a "sacrament" that received only rare public questioning. On the other hand, opposition to compulsory vaccination runs quite deep in the currents of this continent's history. We might be surprised by these present-day vaccination reactions. But, looking to the past, we really shouldn't be.[5]

The Politics of Healing begins with an essay on anti-vaccination-related issues, and for good reason. Immunization was the focus of intense controversy throughout the nineteenth and early twentieth centuries, galvanizing many concerns about medicine held by unorthodox healers and ordinary people alike. This means that the effective shutting down of current smallpox vaccination efforts has plenty of direct parallels in North American history. The primary purpose of this essay is to make these parallels meaningful by putting current anti-vaccination efforts into historical perspective. First I will briefly outline the scope and scale of earlier anti-vaccination crusades; then I will provide a sketch of the movement that has developed over the last two decades. I seek to highlight both similarities and differences between past and present in terms of medical rhetoric, attitudes toward science, and political ideology. One fundamental difference is immediately apparent: the remarkable legitimacy of latter-day vaccine skeptics in the eyes of the media, parts of the political elite, and even to some extent the medical establishment. When so-called anti-vaccinationists (and their naming is a crucial part of the story) receive such a high level of respect, intellectual engagement, and at times celebration in the common public culture, this alone justifies our recognition that we live in a historic era in the realm of the politics of healing.

THE LONG HISTORY OF NORTH AMERICAN ANTI-VACCINATION MOVEMENTS

Just as writers for the *New York Times* and anchors on ABC News have come to admit vaccination skeptics into the acceptable civic landscape, so too have historians finally begun to take anti-vaccinationists seriously. This has not always been the case. As recently as 1991, one historian labeled those who resisted vaccination "the deluded, the misguided, the ignorant, the irrationally fearful." Yet at least a few scholars now understand that the genuine power of previous crusades against compulsory vaccination demands, if not sympathy, at least a modicum of respect.[6]

What have we learned from these historians? First, that the roots of resistance reach far down in American soil, playing a role in our very origin stories. The symbolic precursor to today's struggles is a conflict in colonial Boston in 1721–22, when shopkeepers and artisans used threats of violence against Puritan cleric Cotton Mather. Mather sinned, according to the plebeian portion of the populace, by attempting to introduce into the continent inoculation against smallpox. The result was, in the words of Perry Miller, a "grim struggle" over political and cultural authority throughout New England. In the next century, within the medical ferment of nineteenth-century America, opposition to vaccination itself was even fiercer. Upset about the procedure was rife among free blacks; Frederick Douglass was himself an anti-vaccinationist. Native Americans, Mexican Americans, and a variety of immigrant communities were also at the forefront of resistance. This fit the worldwide pattern, where struggles against vaccination among lowly "subaltern" peoples—whether in the Philippines, India, or Ghana—were an integral part of the fight against European imperialism.[7]

Yet displeasure with smallpox vaccination (the only immunization widely available until the early twentieth century) was just as intense within the North American mainstream. Communities from Niagara Falls, New York, to Muncie, Indiana, convulsed with conflict. The western states were the least susceptible to the vaccinators' appeals. Arizona voters actually outlawed compulsory vaccination in a 1918 popular referendum. Two years earlier, Oregon voters had come within 374 votes of doing the same, with voters in the state's cultural and political center, Portland, favoring the measure by a 55 to 45 percent margin. The legislatures in California and Washington repealed compulsory vaccination laws in 1911 and in 1919, respectively. As a result, renowned public health official Charles Chapin despaired in 1913 of the United States' status as "the least vaccinated of any civilized country." If anything, though, that honor would have gone to Canada ahead of the United States. In early-twentieth-century Toronto, to take just one example, two mayors denounced compulsory vaccination, the school board removed vaccination regulations, and the city council refused to allow city health officials to carry out Ontario's law requiring vaccination of all citizens.[8]

Uniting all these laypeople, whether Polish immigrants in Milwaukee or small-business owners in Portland, was a hostility toward the *compulsory* nature of vaccination. As social scientist Paul Greenough has commented, "The modern state is in a position to demand that its citizens surrender their immune systems as a public duty." Anti-vaccinationists, however, refused to accept this increasingly powerful public health idea, often declining to sanction their governments' compelling of any health measure for the supposed common good.[9]

Such a sentiment frequently differed little from a primal libertarianism—an extreme individualism that demands that the state always and ever keep its coercive hands off the bodies of the citizenry. Yet frequently the anti-vaccinationists developed a considerably more complex, and indeed more fundamentally democratic, philosophy. In matters of state, for example, anti-vaccinationists such as Portland's Lora C. Little insisted that the people as a whole were wise enough to vote on scientific policy. Most emphatically, they held that *parents* had the wisdom to take full charge of the medical affairs of their children. Anti-vaccinationists thus repudiated the cult of the expert blossoming into full flower during the Progressive era. Often they allied themselves as well with advocates of direct democracy, a powerful movement that during the first two decades of the century brought the initiative, referendum, and other electoral reforms to (primarily) the West. In 1913, for instance, Little led a successful campaign to overturn, by popular referendum, Oregon's new eugenic sterilization law, which would have put to the knife "habitual criminals, moral degenerates and sexual perverts."[10]

Many citizen-activists were, in addition, fully anti-*vaccinationists*, meaning that they objected not just to state coercion, but to vaccines themselves. Anti-vaccinationists pointed—correctly—to the significant risks of the smallpox vaccine, which if contaminated at times transmitted syphilis and other virulent infections; even when free of bacteria it could cause fatal cases of encephalitis. Also, those who received the vaccination could spread a related infection to close contacts. Protests were only infrequently religious, at least in the public realm, with some objecting to tampering with God's handiwork in the form of the human body. Much more common were concerns about the poisoning of the blood and the introduction of impurities into an otherwise healthy body. Such thinking frequently flowed from a comprehensive philosophy of natural healing. Lora Little, along with many others, believed that individuals could best heal themselves through close attention to diet, exercise, and right thinking and living. In turn, governments should focus on sanitation. Anti-vaccine activists complained as well about corrupt connections between the state, vaccine manufacturers, and the medical profession. Many of these themes would carry through straight into the twenty-first century.[11]

All in all, the anti-vaccinationist crusades of the nineteenth and early twentieth centuries were a crucial part of an overall movement for full "medical freedom," against the tyranny of "state medicine." What happened to that movement after the 1920s, with the collapse of Lora Little's Chicago-based American Medical Liberty League, remains mostly a mystery—and a subject very much worthy of study. On the surface, the lack of much overt protest against vaccination fits the dominant model in the history of medicine, which posits a midcentury golden age for orthodox medicine. Still, there are traces that cry out for further examination.

We must first appreciate that, outside of this volume, little—really, almost no—research has been done on mid-twentieth-century movements against orthodox medicine. What we will find when we start exploring this unknown world could be quite surprising. For example, the only sustained work on the subject, Eric Juhnke's *Quacks and Crusaders*, reveals the surprising strength of figures such as goat-gland doctor John Brinkley and alternative cancer entrepreneur Harry Hoxsey. In 1932 Brinkley received 240,000 votes when he ran for governor of Kansas. Anti-vaccinationism was an integral part of this world of attempted sexual revitalization and anti-Semitism. Activist Norman Baker decried the "horrors of vaccination" of both children and livestock; Hoxsey in turn warned of the dictatorial power—greater than that of Hitler or Stalin—of the American Medical Association, which sought to vaccinate all children as part of its "medical straitjacket." The rabidly anti-communist organization American Rally, which staunchly supported Hoxsey, denounced with equal fervor the United Nations and "totalitarian health powers" that sought to inject an untested polio vaccine "in their mad scramble to launch a new money-making empire." Anti-fluoridationists also carried forth many anti-vaccination ideas during alternative medicine's supposed years in the wilderness, as Gretchen Ann Reilly's essay in this volume reveals.[12]

By no means were the little-known theorists of midcentury anti-vaccination efforts all right-wing extremists. In 1935, Annie Riley Hale penned what turned out to be the most powerful anti-vaccine treatise written between the Wall Street crash and the age of Reagan. Besides presenting a case against immunizations based on a well-developed theory of natural healing, Hale, in *The Medical Voodoo*, decried "medical experimentation" on "the inmates of jails and orphanages" and castigated the "militarization of medicine" that resulted from increased cooperation between public health authorities and the armed forces. Hale also pointed out that the "rich and powerful" could fend off "medical overlordism" in the form of compulsory vaccination, quarantining, and inspection, but that "the helpless classes" of children, workers, and soldiers could not so easily defend themselves. Arguing for a full "democracy in the healing art" that would allow a genuine choice of different kinds of healers, Hale defended "common-sense reasoning which any lay intelligence can grasp" against the supposed authority of would-be "experts."[13]

That said, by the 1950s extreme and conspiratorial anti-communist agitators were apparently at the forefront of anti-vaccination activities. One flyer asked of those behind vaccine "terror": "The Master Minds, who are they? REDS, seeking our destruction?" Another broadside named the "Unholy Three" as fluoridation, "mental hygiene," and polio serum. As for the latter, the "vaccine drive is the entering wedge for nation-wide socialized medicine, by the U.S. Public Health Service (heavily infiltrated by Russian-born doctors, according to Congressman Clare Hoffman). In enemy hands it can destroy a whole generation." The Keep America Committee concluded its screed: "FIGHT COMMUNISTIC WORLD GOVERNMENT by destroying THE UNHOLY THREE!!!" Still, even moderates—including polio vaccine pioneer Albert Sabin—could, and did, question the safety of specific vaccines, especially after the so-called Cutter incident, in which a batch of the new Salk polio vaccine containing live virus caused over 200 cases of polio, with eleven deaths.[14]

Recognizing that a strong, and still largely undiscovered, anti-vaccination underground survived in the years from 1930 to 1980 helps us make much more sense of the 1945 statement of leading public health authority Wilson Smillie. Smillie complained that year about how vaccination was still "gradually losing ground. Its enforcement meets with constant opposition from the general public." Indeed, by the 1930s, four states (Arizona, North Dakota, Minnesota, and Utah) had laws explicitly prohibiting compulsory vaccination, and just nine states and the District of Columbia had compulsory vaccination legislation. The rest of the country effectively rejected coercion—at least most of the time—by leaving the matter to local authorities, who generally acted only during epidemics. Overall, public acceptance for vaccinations became much more solid over the course of the twentieth century. Just as clearly, though, such a strongly rooted tradition of dissent on the vaccine issue by no means simply disappeared.[15]

THE CURRENT ERA: THE ORIGINS OF DISSATISFIED PARENTS TOGETHER

If it is currently difficult to establish an effective chronology of anti-vaccination activity during the middle of the twentieth century, it is much easier to date the beginnings of the current movement.[16] In April 1982, WRC-TV in Washington, D.C. aired a documentary produced by Lea Thompson titled *DPT: Vaccine Roulette.* Repeated on the *Today Show* and later the recipient of local Emmy awards, *Vaccine Roulette* focused on the apparently deadly or life-threatening reactions of children who received the combination diphtheria-pertussis-tetanus (DPT) vaccination. Within a week of the documentary, a group of parents in the Washington area founded Dissatisfied Parents Together (DPT). These citizens, most of whom had children "damaged" by the pertussis component of the DPT vaccine, immediately began to contact federal and state legislators in order to seek official recognition of vaccine dangers, to obtain better information from physicians, and to support the development of a safer vaccine.[17]

Characterizing themselves as an all-volunteer "grassroots movement," DPT activists moved into the political arena with stunning speed and considerable success. By May 1982 Paula Hawkins, a Republican senator from Florida, chaired subcommittee hearings where those who testified included DPT co-founder Kathi Williams. At the first public meeting of DPT later that month, influential Democratic congressman Tony Coehlo greeted its members with open arms. From the very beginning, DPT fashioned itself as a group critical of, but willing to cooperate with, the medical mainstream. DPT met right away with representatives of the American Public Health Association, the Food and Drug Administration, and the Centers for Disease Control. The group also initiated talks with the American Academy of Pediatrics (AAP) to discuss the creation of a federal program to compensate families with children who suffered adverse reactions to the pertussis vaccine. "In a remarkable show of agreement," DPT and the AAP then both testified before the Senate Labor and Human Resources Committee in June 1982, reaching consensus on the need for federal legislation that would not restrict the right of families to sue vaccine manufacturers. AAP spokesman Martin H. Smith even went so far as to praise, in front of Congress, his group's "extensive and productive discussions with members of . . . DPT . . . . We have been impressed by the skill and knowledge of the parents, and frankly we have learned a great deal from them."[18]

Although at first DPT worked within the medical establishment, it also without delay displayed a populist orientation toward science. "You don't need a Ph.D. or an M.D. to understand the medical and scientific literature," the organization proclaimed. Rather, parents should go to the local hospital or university medical library to investigate what doctors and public health officials would not tell them—or perhaps didn't even know. DPT frequently supplied to its members accounts of mainstream medical studies, generally ending such reports not with its own lessons but rather with the moral that parents should draw their own conclusions. "We must educate ourselves about vaccines, start asking questions and demanding answers" the group's first vice president and co-founder, Barbara Loe Fisher, declared in an inaugural editorial. And those associated with the organization made it clear that their views would be potentially unpredictable. Assuring her audience that "we don't want to see the return of the kind of pertussis disease that ravaged American households in the early part of the twentieth century," Fisher refused to be categorized as anti-medicine. "No matter what some may want the public to believe, concerns about the vaccine and the disease are not mutually exclusive." Rather, a "40-year conspiracy of silence" suppressing the known risks of the pertussis vaccine must come to an end, as citizens "reassert our rights as parents to protect the mental and physical health of our children" and mothers in particular stand up to "intimidat[ion] by physicians."[19]

In the four years after its founding, DPT concentrated its political efforts on the creation of a federal vaccine injury compensation system. While eventually successful, the organization found the ways of Washington to be deceptive and ever-changing. The alliance with the American Academy of Pediatrics would fray and then break, while the patronage of conservative senator Orrin Hatch and liberal congressman Henry Waxman would prove fickle but ultimately productive. DPT had a fair amount of political skill at its disposal; president Jeff Schwartz was a lawyer and lobbyist who had worked for the Environmental Protection Agency, as well as for a congressional committee where he drafted amendments to the Clean Air and Safe Drinking Water acts. Yet when up against the power of organized medicine within the government, as well as the clout of pharmaceutical companies, DPT—which had only recently gained its first part-time employee (Kathi Williams) and donated storefront space (from Kathi Williams' parents' small business) and which still in the spring of 1984 raised a considerable amount of money at a yard sale—had to accept a painful compromise.[20]

What DPT wanted was simple. Activists sought a no-fault, nonadversarial system in which parents with vaccine-injured children could go to the government and receive compensation. Opponents such as the AMA and vaccine manufacturers, on the other hand, hoped to get an "exclusive remedy" that would not only strictly limit damage awards from the government but also legally prevent parents from suing for vaccine injuries. They disagreed with DPT in the first place about the relative risks of the pertussis vaccine, but even more they argued that a DPT-style compensation system would drive the cost of vaccine production so high that manufacturers would have to withdraw from the market, causing a severe shortage of vaccines.[21]

Nevertheless, DPT gained powerful establishment allies. Despite consistent opposition from the Reagan administration, conservatives Paula Hawkins and Orrin Hatch remained sponsors of DPT-inspired legislation, joined by Democrats John Stennis, Ted Kennedy, Jay Rockefeller, and Al Gore. The American College of Physicians and the American Nurses Association joined with the March of Dimes and the Epilepsy Foundation of America to endorse the bill. Yet DPT had to endure many "long and often frustrating struggles" along the way before seeing Ronald Reagan sign into law the National Childhood Vaccine Injury Act of 1986. A multitude of congressional hearings over the course of more than four years, along with a last-minute vigil in front of the White House, proved necessary. As the triumphant but somewhat chastened story in the *DPT News* put it, "Like David against Goliath, DPT represented essentially powerless vaccine injured victims pitted against three of the most powerful and wealthy segments of our society: the pharmaceutical industry, organized medicine, and the federal government."[22]

First along the road to the passage of the 1986 act came the collapse, amid rounds of mutual recrimination, of the "fragile coalition" with the American Academy of Pediatrics. Then Henry Waxman temporarily abandoned DPT after Lederle, one of the primary man-ufacturers of pertussis vaccine, in 1986 increased the price of its vaccine a staggering 10,000 percent over its cost just four years earlier. Waxman, though, still brought DPT into negotiations over the bill's future. DPT fought hard, and ultimately successfully, to make sure that the compensation system covered children of all ages. While Waxman was willing to back away from a provision that would have removed children older than four years from the program, he extracted a price from DPT: its agreement to support an amendment that would cover only future unreimbursed medical expenses for children injured prior to the bill's enactment. This was a bitter pill for many activists, who would end up seeing their own vaccine-injured children denied "money for pain and suffering, loss of future earned income, or past medical expenses."[23]

The drama was not yet over, however. Although the bill passed unanimously in the Democratic-controlled House, once it reached the Senate its fate was in the hands of key Reagan allies Strom Thurmond and Orrin Hatch. Thurmond, working in cooperation with Attorney General Ed Meese, remained implacable in his opposition. But Hatch was trying hard not to alienate either side. First, he reached a "great compromise" with Wax-man that saw the inclusion of the bill in an omnibus health act that, among its provisions, gave pharmaceutical companies authority to export to certain countries drugs that had not yet been approved by the FDA. Second, Hatch used his political skills to convince the Reagan administration not to veto the bill. He did so through intense private lobbying of Meese, as well as in conjunction with the very public agitation of DPT and its allies. During a press conference Hatch, who had reportedly wept (in private) at the fate of the bill, held aloft a vaccine-injured child, Stacy Scholl, who in turn hugged the Utah senator. Perhaps Hatch realized the power of the social movement that DPT had mobilized; apparently no other measure received so much public comment during the 99th Congress as the vaccine injury bill.[24]

Although Dissatisfied Parents Together had been caught up in the middle of a serious game of political hardball that it could not control, the organization effectively used its popularity, along with its organizing skills, to score a major political victory. Indeed, the passage of the 1986 National Childhood Vaccine Injury Act was the first time that a movement critical of the vaccine establishment had ever helped enact federal legislation, and for that reason alone the bill's passage was historic. A not insignificant reason for DPT's visibility was the publication, in the middle of the fight for the compensation system, of *DPT: A Shot in the Dark*. Co-authored by Barbara Loe Fisher and prominent homeopath and historian of alternative medicine Harris Coulter, and published by a major New York publishing house, the book alternated between an accessible account of the scientific knowledge about the hazards of the pertussis vaccine and wrenching portraits of children either killed or brain-damaged by the vaccine.[25]

Coulter and Fisher put front and center the many dangers that they insisted were associated with the pertussis vaccine. Besides the common localized pain and swelling at the site of the shot, reactions ranged from high fever to intense screaming, from brain damage to death. Coulter and Fisher argued that medical authorities had known about these hazards for four decades but had engaged in a "conspiracy of silence" to deny the risk. Indeed, the whole vaccine system was broken, from stem to stern. Vaccines went on the market without proper scientific testing, public health officials who were supposed to be monitoring vaccine safety were caught up in conflicts of interest because of their connection to drug companies, and doctors (who themselves received confusing and conflicting information from vaccine manufacturers and regulators) refused to listen to parents who expressed concerns about their children's possible susceptibility to vaccine injuries. Furthermore, a safe pertussis vaccine was available, and already in use in Japan, but the American medical establishment refused to even consider developing a safer vaccine.[26]

Coulter and Fisher also made a case against government medical compulsion, being sure to point out, in the context of renewed Cold War tensions, that western European countries did not compel vaccination but totalitarian Eastern European states did. They foretold a "revolution" in which they envisioned ordinary citizens so well educated in healing matters that medical decision making would become "truly a shared responsibility between parents and doctors." Parents would then realize that "medicine cannot and should not be legislated." Still, contesting state mandates was a relatively minor part of Coulter and Fisher's mission. Rather, replete with heart-rending stories of babies dying hours after their immunizations, *DPT: A Shot in the Dark* was above all a remarkably effective work in the best muckraking tradition. And the book had a real effect: seasoned vaccine policymaker Sam Katz argued that it "to a real degree threatened the entire immunization program of this country."[27]

VACCINE SKEPTICISM HITS THE BIG TIME IN THE MEDIA AND IN THE CULTURAL ESTABLISHMENT

In the more than two decades since the organization's founding, Barbara Loe Fisher has remained the chief public spokesperson and driving force of DPT and its successor, the National Vaccine Information Center. Along with her primary partner, Kathi Williams, Fisher has fashioned an image that is equal parts dedicated parent, determined activist, and dogged seeker after the truth. In a battle increasingly fought out in the realm of public opinion, Barbara Loe Fisher is the movement's media icon, appearing everywhere from *People* to the *New York Times Magazine*.[28]

Raised in a military family, Fisher earned her B.A. in English from the University of Maryland. She then worked as a writer and editor, and in public relations, at New York Life

Insurance Company, a New Jersey hospital, Lockheed, and the city of Alexandria, Virginia. Recognizing her prominence among activists, the secretary of Health and Human Services appointed her to serve from 1988 to 1991 on the National Vaccine Advisory Committee, where she chaired the subcommittee on adverse vaccine events. Fisher has also been a member of the National Academy of Sciences' Institute of Medicine's Vaccine Safety Forum, and from 1999 to 2003 she was the voting consumer representative on the FDA's Vaccines and Related Biological Products Advisory Committee. Most importantly, Fisher's oldest son, Christian, has had, ever since his fourth DPT shot at the age of two and a half, multiple learning disabilities and attention deficit disorder.[29]

Fisher and her many allies spent much of the decade after the passage of the National Vaccine Injury Compensation Act defending and consolidating their victory. Because of their persistence, the leaders of the National Vaccine Information Center were perfectly poised to take advantage of a relatively sudden burst of media interest that came at century's end. DPT and the NVIC had always been media-savvy, and from its earliest years, the organization had been featured prominently on programs such as *Nightline*, *20–20*, and the *CBS Evening News with Dan Rather*. Nothing in previous years, however, matched the efflorescence of attention that the vaccine issue, and the NVIC in particular, received from 1999 on.[30]

Never before had so-called anti-vaccinationists received such sustained, respectful attention from the mainstream media. Indeed, even NVIC, which tends to present itself as constantly embattled, announced gleefully that "this year, the last of this century, has . . . been a turning point in public recognition." On television alone, NVIC or its associates were prominently featured in January on *20/20*, in February on the *ABC Evening News*, in August on the Fox News channel, again that month on the *ABC Evening News*, and in October on CNN, MSNBC, and *Nightline*. All of the shows went out of their way to be fair to the NVIC crusade, presenting the concerns of anti-vaccine activists accurately and often allowing Fisher, dissident physicians, or parents themselves to make their case at length in their own words. Only two of the programs were clearly slanted—mildly—against the NVIC position: Fox News put up pro-vaccine "Fox Facts" behind Fisher as she spoke, while *Nightline* reporter John Donvan accused activists of placing anecdote above science and the clear rational thinking of experts.[31]

The other newscasts simply varied in their level of sympathy toward the cause. While *20–20* did not mention NVIC on its segment about hepatitis B, it devoted a great majority of the program's airtime to parents and their vaccine-injured children, including at least one family closely associated with NVIC, Michael and Lorna Belkin. One of NVIC's dissident scientists, Bonnie Dunbar, coolly presented her scientific case, while representatives from the CDC and Merck had a minute amount of time to advance their side of the story. And at that, the Merck spokesman came off as advocating secrecy when he admitted to fear that the controversy was being aired at all, because the result might be the decline of public confidence in and use of vaccines. *20–20* allowed an ordinary parent to gently make the opposing case, for the virtue of providing full information for all citizens to make their own decisions. The concluding words of Barbara Walters then provided the kind of legitimacy that previous vaccine activists could only have dreamed of. Observing that parents had an extremely difficult choice to make because of all the conflicting information, Walters noted that while the World Health Organization still recommended the hepatitis B vaccine, France had just lifted its requirement because of the potential risks. In turn, MSNBC's feature nearly dripped with sarcasm as reporter Linda Vester attempted to file an adverse-reaction report under a supposedly user-friendly system. Her difficulties, and her visible frustration, spoke volumes about which side the American public was supposed to be on in the coming vaccine battles.[32]

The attention and respect that the NVIC cause received was by no means due simply to its skillful tugging of hearts as middlebrow viewers wept at the fate of beautiful young children killed and disabled in the flower of their youth. The chattering classes also began to pick up the virus of skepticism toward vaccines. Nothing demonstrates this better than the sympathetic attention granted to two highly controversial books, *Darkness in El Dorado* (2000) and *The River* (1999). Although these two works did not directly connect to current debates over childhood immunizations, their reception still had much to say about a cultural atmosphere that no longer granted automatic honor to these lifesaving interventions.[33]

Both of these books propounded extremely bold theses that, not too many years before, would in all likelihood have been dismissed without delay by the cultural establishment. Indeed, both volumes veered toward the conspiratorial. Patrick Tierney's *Darkness in El Dorado* was the more sensational, arguing—in the words of the subtitle—"how scientists and journalists devastated the Amazon." Tierney contended that scholars, above all the famous anthropologist Napoleon Chagnon, had wreaked havoc on their Yanomami subjects through a whole host of unethical behaviors ranging from illegal trading in weaponry to sexual abuse.

The charge that received the most attention in *Darkness in El Dorado* had to do with the misuse of vaccines. Tierney maintained that University of Michigan geneticist James Neel, along with Chagnon, acted with potentially genocidal malice aforethought in contributing to—perhaps even causing—a 1968 measles epidemic among the Yanomami. Neel brought with him to the Amazon "one of the most primitive measles vaccines," Edmonston B, even though contemporary medical authorities believed that this vaccine strain was too crude and dangerous to be used, especially among indigenous populations, without an additional shot of gamma globulin—and even at that it was still quite hazardous. So why did Neel select Edmonston B, especially when he could have used a less reactive measles vaccine, and when he did not have permission from the Venezuelan government for any kind of vaccination project in the first place? Because, according to Tierney, Neel was an unabashed advocate of eugenics who wished to perform a grand experiment on the Yanomami, testing genetic adaptation by coming as close as possible to seeing how a virgin population's immunity would function when confronted with a wild measles epidemic. By vaccinating a large population—often without the necessary gamma globulin, and at times by only selectively vaccinating within a village—Neel and his associates set off a kind of disease devastation never before seen among these "fierce people." In the end, Tierney suggests that the Edmonston B vaccine might have not just caused its recipients dangerous reactions, but even helped spread measles itself to others. This is a tentative conclusion, he admits, and at the same time Tierney recognizes that James Neel also "genuinely wanted to help the Yanomami and sincerely thought he was doing so." All the same, Tierney indicts Neel and his fellow scientists for reckless use of a "dinosaur vaccine" and for placing scientific experimentation far ahead of the welfare of indigenous peoples.[34]

For our purposes, what exactly happened among the Yanomami is of less concern than the fascinating debate engendered by *Darkness in El Dorado*. Much of the main action occurred even before the book broke into print. *The New Yorker* carried an excerpt containing even stronger charges, and Leslie Sponsel of the University of Hawaii and Terence Turner of Cornell University—longtime Chagnon foes who had seen the book in galleys—alerted the American Anthropological Association (AAA) to the depth of the upcoming scandal. Sponsel and Turner contended that Neel and Chagnon's behavior was so horrific that "[i]n its scale, ramifications, and sheer criminality and corruption it is unparalleled in the history of anthropology." Josef Mengele served as an appropriate comparison. As charges and countercharges flew fast, with "raw fury," across the Internet, the AAA agreed to launch a full-scale investigation.[35]

During the fray that followed, many commentators made compelling points against Tierney's vaccine-related charges. The American Anthropological Association found one of Tierney's main claims completely "without foundation," although some members of the investigating commission found it impossible to refute the idea that Neel's research objectives—set in significant part by the Atomic Energy Commission—at times trumped his humanitarian goals during the vaccine episode. The overall evaluation of the AAA, in fact, was that *Darkness* "served anthropology well."[36]

Despite the energetic and frequent criticism of Tierney's book—indeed, even more because of the hostility it engendered—the favorable response *Darkness in El Dorado* received is nothing short of remarkable. Tierney's tome was a finalist for the National Book Award, and it earned accolades as one of the best books of the year from the *New York Times*, the *Los Angeles Times*, and the *Boston Globe*. John Horgan argued in the Sunday *New York Times Book Review* that "Tierney's exhaustively reported book . . . makes a powerful case" against Chagnon and Neel. Horgan did note the controversy over the vaccination accusations, but rather than condemning Tierney, Horgan merely stated that he "should have worked harder to prove this horrific charge." The final moral of the story, according to Horgan: the book's "faults are outweighed by its mass of vivid, damning detail. My guess is that it will become a classic in anthropological literature."[37]

So, while it had not become completely fashionable in the heart of the cultural establishment to believe the very worst possible accusations against vaccines and the vaccine complex, the reaction to *Darkness in El Dorado* vividly demonstrated the intellectual respectability of skepticism toward vaccines. The reception of Edward Hooper's *The River: A Journey to the Source of HIV and AIDS* provided an even more powerful exhibition of the new cultural politics surrounding vaccination.[38]

Hooper's 1000-page tome was epic in consequence as well as scale. If his argument was anywhere near correct, then much of modern medicine, and certainly much of the modern vaccine complex, was on trial for one of the worst crimes possible against humanity. For Hooper, a former BBC radio correspondent, claimed to have discovered, through years of dogged research, that vaccines had caused AIDS. Or, to qualify this statement significantly: that a particular strain of oral polio vaccine (CHAT) had contained chimpanzee simian immunodeficiency virus. This SIV transformed into HIV when, between 1957 and 1960, it crossed the species barrier during the administration of the vaccine to a million subjects of Belgian-ruled African territories. While Hooper made it clear that the contamination of the polio vaccine was inadvertent, he was emphatic that those involved in the African vaccine experiments, particularly distinguished researcher Hilary Koprowski, had since been involved in a cover-up.[39]

Such is the stuff of popular conspiracy theories, and indeed Hooper's hypothesis built on an underground dissident scientific culture that flourished on talk radio, the Internet, and *Rolling Stone* magazine. Indeed, it should come as no surprise that since 1992 Barbara

Loe Fisher's NVIC has been reporting on similar hypotheses about the origins of AIDS. Previously, the intellectual and media establishment had by and large dismissed these ideas as crackpot. Yet Hooper, while far from winning over scientific elites, received remarkable acceptance as someone purveying ideas worthy of consideration and further exploration. Even some of those most opposed to his ideas went out of their way to praise him. One of Hooper's chief antagonists, Robin Weiss, wrote in *Science* that *"The River* is a towering achievement." Another leading AIDS researcher remarked in *Nature* that "*The River* is, in many ways, superb. It is scholarly, thoroughly researched, well (if densely) written and deserves, indeed demands, to be taken seriously." And Charles Gilks, head of tropical medicine at the Liverpool School of Tropical Medicine, praised *The River* as a work of "immense scholarship, providing what will surely be the definitive chronicle of the opening of the AIDS era."[40]

Hooper and his ideas also received extraordinarily sympathetic attention in mainstream cultural organs. The on-line magazine *Salon* extensively excerpted the book. Lawrence Altman, the chief medical reporter for the *New York Times*, called the book "remarkable" and granted Hooper considerable legitimacy by arguing that he "builds a sufficiently detailed case to require serious examination of his theory." The *New York Review of Books* gave *The River* a largely favorable review, categorizing it as "among the best surveys to appear on the epidemiology of AIDS." And Roy Porter, the dean of Anglo-American historians of medicine, provided a powerful endorsement in the *London Review of Books*. Porter credited Hooper with "meticulous tracking" and "impressively precise correlations," noting that the theory linking the oral polio vaccine and AIDS now "has all the requisites of a legitimate hypothesis." *The River* even brought conspiracy theories out of the closet, as Porter, the quite cosmopolitan academic, observed that "a cover-up is not implausible."[41]

Surely, the battle for cultural legitimacy of vaccine skepticism is far from over. Curt and easy dismissals of those who argue against the vaccine status quo still come readily from the pens and tongues of many members of the media elite. Jane Brody of the *New York Times*, for example, has attributed vaccine skepticism to "ill-informed hysteria." In a similar manner, Randy Cohen, the *Times*' influential "Ethicist," counseled someone working in an anti-vaccinationist chiropractors' office to practice "counterleafleting" to bring to the masses the easily distinguished truth about vaccines. Better yet, Cohen invited his anonymous correspondent to move to a different job by asking: "Are you prepared to keep silent when they begin treating patients by bloodletting? Maybe it's time to look for work at another clinic, preferably one conveniently located in the 21st century." And Leon Jaroff unleashed a barrage in *Time*, calling concerns about vaccines "laughable" and "preposterous," pushed by "quacks or fanatics" who "demonstrate both medical illiteracy and an appalling ignorance of history." Even such authoritative pronouncements, however, increasingly seem to be taking on a wistful tone, implicitly recognizing that the masses are no longer falling into line behind the standard pro-vaccine messages.[42]

THE CONSOLIDATION OF THE NATIONAL VACCINE INFORMATION CENTER

Perhaps it is pure coincidence that the level of vaccine skepticism among intellectuals has spread like a contagion at just the same time that grassroots activists have been most successful in pressing their claims in the realms of politics and public culture. It is much more likely, however, that there are concrete reasons for such a convergence between high and middlebrow cultures. Just as many scholars and critics have over the last couple of decades become more dubious of the imperial claims of science, so have the opponents of compulsory vaccination become considerably more pro-scientific in their attitudes. Hostility to vaccinations themselves has hardly disappeared, especially (but not exclusively) in the fringes of the movement. Yet in a historic transformation, the mainstream of so-called anti-vaccinationism has moved far away from such antagonism, toward an emphasis on what it views as the best traditions of modern medicine: better vaccines, better science, and informed consent.

Of course, what the NVIC and other organizations mean by these common values is often radically different from the interpretations given to them by the vaccine establishment. Often, but not always. With significant changes on both sides of the vaccine debate, we are entering another historic era in which we may be witnessing the birth of a new possibility, that of genuine dialogue—and therefore of a truly democratic science.

We can only see how close we might be coming to such democratic dialogue by coming to grips with the evolution of vaccine activism since 1986. One of the primary triumphs of Dissatisfied Parents Together was passage in that year of the federal vaccine compensation system, and one of NVIC's on-going and most difficult tasks has been the system's defense. Pharmaceutical companies and the governmental vaccine establishment have, in the eyes of activists, frequently tried to undercut the system by denying it adequate funding, making the system more adversarial, failing to publicize its provisions, and refusing to enforce the law's mandates for reporting and monitoring adverse vaccine reactions. Not only has DPT become the compensation system's chief legislative defender, the organization has also become the primary conduit for parents with vaccine-injured children seeking to navigate its increasingly labyrinthine structure. DPT has gone so far as to file lawsuits against two different secretaries of Health and Human Services for failing to issue the brochures describing vaccine risks and benefits that the 1986 law requires be given to parents each time a child is vaccinated, and also for arbitrarily restricting the system's eligibility rules. "We were betrayed," sighed Barbara Loe Fisher in 1999.[43]

So embattled was NVIC, primarily over issues relating to the compensation system, that Barbara Loe Fisher and Kathi Williams had by 1993 decided to shut down the organization. The NVIC had only $2000 to its name, and the hostility of the vaccine establishment was so toxic that the activists felt as if their mission was doomed to failure. But as Fisher recounts the story, her spirits were revived when she received an enthusiastic reception among a group of chiropractors, who donated $8000 to the cause. "That was probably the biggest turning point in our history," Fisher notes, "because we understood our fight was part of a larger fight for freedom of choice in health care that was being waged by a brave and outspoken segment of the professional health care community." Indeed the NVIC, although never making alternative medicine its focus, has increasingly become open to advocates and practitioners of chiropractic, homeopathy, and other forms of integrative healing. A special issue of the organization's *The Vaccine Reaction* solely devoted to chiropractic, for example, begins with the statement: "the vaccine safety and informed consent movement is coinciding with a broader revolution occurring in American health care today, which is causing a paradigm shift away from sole reliance on the allopathic medical model for preventing disease and maintaining health."[44]

Soon after that 1993 nadir, the NVIC picked up considerable steam. By 1995, the organization had sufficient funds to pay Fisher as the second full-time member of the office staff. A year after that, the NVIC finally won the battle it had been fighting since its inception when the FDA at last licensed for infants a pertussis vaccine that promised to be less reactive than the traditional "whole cell" vaccine. This acellular vaccine had been in use for many years in Japan, but government regulators held up its usage in the United States until they felt that a complete research regime had demonstrated its effectiveness and relative safety.[45]

During the long-standing battle over the pertussis vaccine, the NVIC displayed one of its most interesting characteristics: its ability to recruit a loyal corps of dissident scientists willing to speak out against the vaccine establishment. Generally these scientists had respectable scholarly credentials, but their views had either partially or radically departed from the scientific mainstream. Arguably the most prominent is John H. Menkes, professor emeritus at UCLA's School of Medicine and former director of pediatric neurology at Cedars-Sinai Medical Center. A Jewish refugee from Nazi-controlled Vienna, Menkes went on to become one of the pioneers in the field of pediatric neurology, authoring a standard textbook in the field. Yet although he was distinguished enough to have had a disease named after him, by the end of the 1980s Menkes had become a genuine vaccine rebel. He insisted, against many voices within the vaccination complex, that there was a concrete link between the pertussis vaccine and serious brain injuries, and also that there was an urgent and compelling necessity for more research. Menkes even went out of his way to testify on behalf of parents in cases of "shaken baby" syndrome. Where prosecutors blamed overly aggressive parents for neurological damage, Menkes blamed vaccines. The result of Menkes' dissidence was NVIC's bestowal of a Courage in Science Award on him at its 2000 International Public Conference for being "one of the first pediatricians to dissent from the widely held a priori assumption in infectious disease medicine that all neurological adverse events following DPT vaccination are only coincidentally and not causally related to the . . . vaccination."[46]

Respectable, even distinguished, medical researchers such as Menkes gave the vaccine safety movement a crucial legitimacy as the grounds of battle rapidly moved from, primarily, pertussis to a rapidly expanding number of vaccines. Over the past decade, the number of required vaccines has significantly increased, and many more immunizations are in the pipeline. The response of NVIC has been to question the need for each vaccine, to make sure that risks as well as benefits are properly researched and acknowledged, and to insure that the victims of vaccine injury have a forum for publicity and redress.

Activists indict every vaccine, for a variety of reasons. Oral polio vaccine, for example, has been the source of all recent cases of polio in this country. The NVIC proudly took credit when this live polio vaccine was recently phased out in favor of a killed version. (Along with the change to the acellular pertussis vaccine this was, according to one writer, "a move that backhandedly acknowledged the activists' claims"; NVIC also crowed when the CDC suspended the use of the rotavirus vaccine because of evidence that it caused bowel obstruction.) The vaccination for hepatitis B can supposedly cause a variety of neurological and immunological disorders, and it is given to newborn babies despite the disease's transmission primarily through sexual contact and dirty needles. Those who take the vaccine for Lyme disease might be at risk for severe arthritis. Even the vaccine for chicken pox can, by providing non-permanent immunity, drive a disease that is almost always harmless in childhood into the adult population, where it has much more serious consequences. Moreover, the sheer number of vaccines, many of them given to infants all at one time, is itself allegedly a problem, with no good scientific studies showing the level of risk either of immediate injury or of longer-term effects on the immune system. Finally, the most common additive used in vaccines, at least until 2000, was thimerosal, a mercury-based preservative. Even the American Academy of Pediatrics and the FDA for a time admitted to the possibility that thimerosal could be the source of childhood neurological impairment and recommended its removal from vaccines, although there was no requirement that vaccines containing the additive be taken off the market immediately.[47]

No vaccine, however, has stirred as much recent passion as has MMR. A triple shot meant to immunize against mumps, measles, and rubella, critics have insisted that it, perhaps in conjunction with a general overdose of vaccines, is responsible for the current epidemic of autism. There is, after all, complete consensus about the deeply troubling rise of autism: the number of autistic children has increased ten-fold since the 1980s. Where the consensus falls apart is in trying to explain the increase. Expanded definitions and better diagnoses account for only part of the swelling autistic population. Federal officials and the medical elite have vigorously denied a connection between vaccinations and autism, and they have several scientific studies to back up their claims. Parents, in turn, insist that they have literally been able to witness the connection, as bright and healthy children have fallen grievously ill immediately after their MMR shots. In addition, activists claim that the scientific record is not nearly so clear-cut, with establishment science incomplete and likely corrupt, and dissident science (particularly as practiced by the controversial medical researcher Andrew Wakefield, another winner of NVIC's Courage in Science Award) pointing inconclusively but insistently toward a significant relationship between MMR and autism. The controversy has become so heated that conservative Indiana congressman Dan Burton, the chair of the House Government Reform Committee, started holding a series of hearings in 1999 to investigate autism and other vaccination issues. Burton has brought all viewpoints to his meeting room, but he himself blames the MMR vaccine for his grandson's autism, and he is clearly on the side of vaccine-injured children. Indeed, Burton has worked so closely with the NVIC that in 2000 he was the featured keynote speaker at the organization's Second International Public Conference on Vaccination.[48]

A theme that runs through all the criticisms of specific vaccines is an insistence that individual experience, even if highly emotional, has just as compelling a claim on public attention as the cool, rational claims of science. Injured children—often labeled as "damaged"—make up a huge part of the iconography of the movement. Almost all occasions, whether they are fundraising dinners or testimony before august scientific advisory boards, include vivid and wrenching testimony about dead and injured children. Activists justify this focus on the individual child in part because they believe mainstream scientists to be fraudulent and unwilling to confront the genuine hazards of vaccination. The establishment will only be forced to face up to vaccine risks if parents continue to speak out forcefully on behalf of their beloved children.

Yet this is not the whole story. Even if science, in a full and fair fashion, did conclusively determine that vaccine risks were low, vaccine activists would still insist that the life of each individual child is sacred, not to be sacrificed on the utilitarian altar of herd immunity. If NVIC has one favored slogan, it is the phrase that has appeared on the masthead of the organization's newsletter from the very first issue: "When it happens to your child, the risks are 100%." This focus on the individual child has concrete political and ethical dimensions. While serving on various governmental immunization policy boards, Barbara Loe

Fisher has insisted that scientists pay heed not just to academic researchers, but to parents describing their grief and loss. Fisher once reported how gratified she was that an Institute of Medicine panel "listened carefully to the case histories of deaths and injuries following childhood vaccinations which many parents presented to them." NVIC activists have come to expect as almost a fundamental right the ability to have authorities take their stories and viewpoints seriously. They complained bitterly, for example, when the formulation of policy for chicken pox occurred without "meaningful public debate" or "vote of the people." And beyond issues of the *way* that public policy is formulated, Barbara Loe Fisher has articulated the parental perspective in a compelling philosophical fashion, arguing for "man's human right to be free from the tyranny of any government policy that employs the utilitarian rationale, judged to be immoral at Nuremberg 50 years ago, which justifies the sacrifice of individual human lives without their informed consent for what the majority has determined to be 'the greater good.'"[49]

NVIC's validation of parental and citizen experience and civic involvement has led to a dramatic rise of activism among the parents most responsible for taking care of children, especially disabled children: mothers. While the dissident scientists who increasingly are NVIC's public face are largely—but by no means exclusively—male, those dedicating themselves to the cause of vaccine safety have been overwhelmingly female. Most of these women do not, however, embrace a traditional maternal role. Consider the composition of NVIC's board. Men have served as officers and board members, as have stay at-home moms, but the great majority of those elected to the board—while visible and proud mothers—also have backgrounds in business or the professions. For example, Barbara Loe Fisher's co-leader in the organization, Kathi Williams, is a partner in her family's glass company, having also been a cosmetologist and a teacher's aide.[50]

Or consider the slate of NVIC board members elected in 1987. Gerrie Cohen, the president, was an accountant and financial manager as well as the single mother of a severely brain-damaged teenager. Vice President Maryl Levine was president of a Washington, D.C. management consulting firm, previously having worked in the Office of Management and Budget and as the assistant director of a public policy institute at Duke University. Jo George, the treasurer, was a registered physical therapist who also did corporate accounting and computer work. Secretary Jacqui Middaugh had put in 14 years as a management analyst at the State Department after working for the Federal Reserve and the state of Missouri. An interior designer, a nurse, and an attorney joined them on the board. The 1993 NVIC board had roughly the same composition. First Vice President Janet Ciotoli organized for a nurses' union, while secretary Judy Braiman had a quarter century experience as a well-recognized consumer advocate.[51]

DAWN RICHARDSON

Although this essay has focused on the one full-fledged national vaccine safety organization, it would be a mistake to discount activism at the state and local levels (not to mention on the Internet). The most prominent of state activists is also a mother with professional experience. Dawn Richardson began to play a prominent role in vaccine safety circles during the late 1990s when she and a small circle of associates stymied the Texas Department of Health's attempts to include all children in a computerized registry that would track their immunization records. Fearing an unconstitutional intrusion on civil liberties through governmental access to citizens' medical records, Richardson took her fight to the legislature. She was able to claim victory when the health department was forced to make the registry an "opt-in" system, where the state had to ask permission to include citizens, rather than an "opt-out" system, where citizens had to request not to be included. From that time on, Richardson has thrown herself nearly full-time into vaccine safety advocacy, counseling parents who are unsure about what to do about the children's vaccinations, helping many to formulate religious exemptions; lobbying legislators, who have come to know her well; and operating an active Internet site that politically mobilizes Texans and that brings together "Parents Requesting Open Vaccine Education" throughout the nation. (PROVE is the name of her organization.)[52]

Dawn Richardson had some pre-existing cultural commitments that predisposed her to becoming involved with the movement. Yet as she tells the story, her transformation into an activist had more to do with thoughtful parenting than ideology. (Indeed, having vaccine-injured children, or fearing for the safety of one's children, is the clearest common denominator of vaccine safety activism.) When Richardson was pregnant with her first daughter, Alexa, she started reading about the birth process. The fact that "women were taken out of control of childbirth" bothered her. Toward the end of her pregnancy, Richardson had decided to refuse the vitamin K shot and the hepatitis B vaccination that her newborn would be routinely given while still in the hospital. Nurse after nurse tried to talk her out of such crazy ideas, one even raising the level of guilt by saying that Richardson would be personally responsible for helping to halt the global eradication of hepatitis B. When, in contrast, Richardson called the Texas Department of Health to check on the possible ramifications of withholding such treatment, she had the chance to talk to a sympathetic bureaucrat who told Richardson that if she was interested in such issues, she should get in touch with Karin Schumacher, a local woman already involved in the vaccine safety movement.[53]

Richardson hooked up with Schumacher, and in the weeks before the birth they worked together to investigate children's death records to see if they might confirm a relationship between vaccinations and Sudden Infant Death Syndrome. Richardson saw more than enough to concern her. She proceeded to question her mother, and with the help of her baby book she proceeded to reconstruct life-threatening reactions that she had had as a child to the measles and smallpox vaccinations. The rest of her family had a similar history of allergies and reactions to shots. So, it turned out, had her husband Scott, who suffered from a variety of autoimmune problems. When they reviewed his medical records, they noticed what seemed like a significant relationship between his vaccinations and his medical woes. "We both come from a scientific background. We're both electrical engineers," Richardson notes, and the empirical evidence seemed clear: their children would be predisposed to having serious reactions to vaccines. Soon they decided not to vaccinate their children at all—although Richardson notes that if she believed her children might be predisposed to specific diseases themselves, she would seriously consider vaccination. Predictably, they had difficulties finding a sympathetic pediatrician. One of the twelve they interviewed called Richardson a "child abuser" for failing to vaccinate. No wonder that one of Richardson's main forms of activism is hooking up—often in a kind of underground fashion—sympathetic pediatricians with vaccine-skeptical parents.

Richardson moved quickly up a largely self-created ladder from lone concerned parent to energetic political activist. When she discusses her trajectory as an activist, she mentions the six loads of laundry piling up on her floor as well as the burdens of running an organization on a shoestring budget that flies under the government's radar by refusing to claim tax exempt status because that would restrict its ability to lobby, if necessary, in a partisan fashion. Each time she thinks of giving up her vaccine safety work, however, she receives a call from a panicked, or desperate, or simply inquisitive parent, and she realizes the very concrete help that she can render to a family. Yet Richardson is quite savvy on an organizational level as well, particularly in her use of the Internet (which she characterizes as "the great equalizer"). In 2000, she estimated her email list went out to 2,000 people and was reprinted for several thousand more on other vaccine email lists. Exhaustive lobbying also pays off. Richardson believes that Texas legislators have found it extremely refreshing to encounter parents without any apparent agenda other than the protection of their children. The way that the vaccine machine works is through "Power, Position, and Profits," according to Richardson, whereas her organization has no material self-interest.

Despite her disavowal of politics-as-usual, Dawn Richardson is hardly shy of ideology. Gradually, she has evolved into a self-identified conservative, although one who is flexible and open to alliances with other groups. Up through college, she was a Democrat and a liberal, although not, she says, a particularly reflective one. And her brother was a big supporter of Ralph Nader during the 2000 election. Once Richardson entered the rough and tumble world of politics, however, she gravitated toward conservatism because it promised a fuller respect for parents' thoughtfulness and rights. When Richardson went to the state house to talk about the dangers, indeed lunacy, of hepatitis B mandates for infants who would not, at worst, be sexually active for another dozen years, the conservative legislators understood this "common sense." More generally, a "one size fits all" vaccination policy goes against the grain of the best of conservatism's respect for individual rights, whereas such uniformity fits right into liberals' glee in changing the world. Richardson carefully chooses how not to alienate supporters, being willing to cooperate openly with the ACLU, for example, in defense of the privacy of medical records but being much more cautious about connections with anti-abortion activists concerned about fetal cells used in vaccines and during vaccine research. Above all, those on the right offer a respect Richardson finds lacking on the left side of the political spectrum: "instead of assuming I'm too dumb to decide, and that the government needs to help me decide," conservatives trust parents to make up their own minds.

Richardson's political philosophy has interesting practical consequences when it comes to matters of race and class. For example, she has not had much luck working with Hispanic legislators, whom she considers to be too tied into the liberal establishment. Yet, on the ground, Richardson notes a considerably higher level of sympathy among ordinary Hispanics, especially given the strong family values enshrined in Catholic culture. Like vaccine activists, Hispanics seem to instinctively fear meddling in such matters as, for instance, whether children should sleep in bed with their parents—an important tenet of most natural parenting advocates. Moreover, Richardson decisively rejects the culture of entitlement that she believes both poor people and their political representatives have bought into. The health of children in poor communities is a mess, Richardson argues, at least in part because parents have given over their responsibilities to the government, figuring that Medicaid doctors would cure their asthma and diabetes. Instead, the only ones who really benefit are the pharmaceutical companies that produce the drugs that are be administered to the poor children in the absence of a systematic attempt to solve underlying cultural and economic problems. For example, Richardson notes that public health officials in Texas, when confronted with an epidemic of water-borne hepatitis A in a poor border area that lacked public water treatment, mandated vaccines but did not even take the elementary step of bringing in bottled water.

Richardson admits to being torn on these difficult issues. On one hand, she declares that "I really am wanting a safety net for abused and neglected kids; I feel for them." On the other hand, she makes it clear that the safety net cannot come at the expense of other ordinary parents, the ones who are working hard to take good care of their kids. "I don't want us to be dolphins swept up into a net" as the state targets abusive parents. Richardson notes that this distaste for state involvement is in line with the kind of economic and political values that are at the core of her activist community, where, on the whole, college-educated moms stay at home while the dads own their own businesses. "It's a kind of entrepreneurial free spirit," Richardson notes, where "they've had to rely on themselves to be successful instead of relying on the ideologies of others." She guesses that the median family income of the parents who support her cause is between $40,000 and $50,000. Richardson comments: "I'd describe it as a middle-class movement, definitely."

And it is a middle-class movement that is remaking the political landscape in dramatic fashion. Richardson has had to do constant battle on a wide variety of fronts. She remains especially vigilant about the immunization registry, along with the privacy of medical records generally. She and her allies scored an astounding victory in June, 2003, when the Texas legislature voted to loosen the compulsory nature of vaccinations. At a time when some top officials in the federal government were making it seem as if contesting mandatory vaccinations was unpatriotic, Richardson's group, PROVE, worked successfully to allow for parents to claim a conscientious exemption against vaccinations. Previously, only religious and medical exemptions were possible. This is just one small sign that when Richardson calls her movement a "revolution in the making," such phrasing does not seem like too much of an overstatement.[54]

FROM ANTI-VACCINATIONISM TO VACCINE SAFETY ADVOCACY

Dawn Richardson is a proud member of the Greek Orthodox church, and she volunteered for George W. Bush in 2000. Indeed, many of the most visible vaccination activists are proudly Christian and conservative. Evangelical homeschooling families provide many of the shock troops for letter writing campaigns on the vaccine issue. As noted in the book's introduction, Phyllis Schlafly has become a fierce enemy of the vaccine establishment. And Dan Burton has been that establishment's most powerful stinging nettle. The deeply conservative Indiana congressman has been joined by many of his fellow Republicans in sponsoring hearings and championing anthrax-vaccine-injured Gulf War veterans in their search for justice. All in all, it might seem that anti-vaccinationism has become part and parcel of the libertarian conservative agenda during a right-wing age.[55]

Yet below the surface, vaccine activism clearly transcends the left-right divide, as does the politics of alternative medicine as a whole. For example, the NVIC works actively to welcome both left- and right-wing activists into its spacious tent; when I attended NVIC's Second International Public Conference on Vaccination during September 2000, I was struck by how the meeting might have been the only place in America where those opposed to Ralph Nader could speak civilly to supporters of the Green Party insurgent. Such ability to work together does not flow merely, it seems, from a blind putting aside of principled differences as activists single-mindedly concentrate on one narrow issue. Rather, vaccine safety activists have cultivated a comprehensive philosophy that allows for equal opportunity criticism of Democrats and Republicans, those on the left and those on the right.

This has became quite clear in the last two years as vaccine safety activists have turned bitterly on George W. Bush, becoming some of his chief critics as the president placed vaccination at the center of his homeland security program. Yet this tradition of political creativity and independence long predates September 11th. For example, it is not often that Phyllis Schlafly works with the Los Angeles Coalition against Racist Child Experimentation or the Afrikan Center of Well Being, yet that is exactly what Barbara Loe Fisher and NVIC did when minority children in L.A. and Houston were targeted with what appeared to be racially discriminatory vaccine mandates. The NVIC has also spoken out vigorously against the delay in removing all older vaccines from the market once a new and improved one has begun use, fearing that the out-of-date and less safe varieties will be dumped on free clinics where the clients are predominantly poor and people of color. Nor would it be likely for Orrin Hatch or Dan Burton to join a coalition organized by the AIDS Coalition to Unleash Power (ACT UP). Yet once again, this is what Barbara Loe Fisher did, getting up in front of an avowedly queer audience at the Dissenters' Forum at the 11th International Conference on AIDS to call, during her talk on "Medical Tyranny and the AIDS-Vaccine Connection," for an end to the blaming of medical victims—whether they be vaccine-injured children, Gulf War soldiers, or gay men.[56]

It should be instructive that we can not easily label NVIC and associated activists as either Left or Right. The difficulty we have in categorizing them should help us keep in mind that some of the most interesting and creative political phenomena in American history moved "beyond left and right." But the issue of labeling this movement does not end with its ideologies. Indeed, the very name that we give to these activists goes a long way toward indicating how we consider their legitimacy in a culture that, at least rhetorically, seeks to honor both democracy and science.[57]

I have been self-consciously inconsistent in giving Barbara Fisher, Dawn Richardson, and their allies a uniform name. I have generally either said that they are "anti-vaccinationists" or "vaccine safety activists." From certain angles, this inconsistency might be justifiable. Consider the label "anti-vaccinationist." Historically, those who agitated on this issue were almost all proudly anti-vaccinationist, meaning that they detested vaccines themselves along with government compulsion. Today's activists clearly have a lineage in that tradition. Furthermore, there are many genuine anti-vaccinationists today, either calmly formulating the case against all vaccines as medically problematic, or offering up conspiracy theories about the conscious imposition of the disastrous vaccine complex. A lengthy anthroposophical treatise, for example, mentions the space travelers who came to earth thousands of years ago to take over human life with the help of "black brotherhoods." One of the methods they used was to vaccinate "the Christ out of the Human Body." Finally, there is no doubt that even in the mainstream of the movement, visceral suspicion toward vaccines is so great that it often quickly moves into a position of total hostile negation.[58]

That said, the NVIC and other members of the "anti-vaccination" mainstream have gone out of their way to repudiate that label. For good substantive reasons, we should take them at their word, noting their position on this issue as yet another historic quality of today's movement. From nearly its very beginning, Dissatisfied Parents Together went out of its way to make it clear that "We are not 'anti-vaccine.'" Emphatic statements of this sort soon became common in the NVIC literature. In 1992, NVIC director Ann Millan noted that the organization "is not against vaccines[;] we want safer vaccines on the American market and we want educated parents to have the right to choose which vaccines their child should have." NVIC rearticulated the party line in 1998, declaring: "we are not anti-vaccine nor do we oppose vaccination requirements. We are pro-information and support the human right of all citizens to informed consent to any medical procedure which carries the risk of injury or death, including vaccination."[59]

One of the interesting issues for mainstream vaccine safety activists is what to do with the full-blown anti-vaccinationists in their ranks, the people whom Dawn Richardson calls the "fringies." At NVIC's International Public Conference in 2000, I saw Barbara Loe Fisher skillfully position herself as a voice of reason, bridging the political divide between the portions of her rank-and-file who were considerably more radical and the mainstream media set to pounce on any sign of cultural deviance. For example, Fisher made no attempt to keep anti-vaccinationists from the microphones during the conference's open comment sessions, but she did make sure that they were tightly timed, and politely cut off if she deemed it necessary. In turn, there was more than a bit of grumbling at the tables from people concerned about the leaders of the movement selling out. Dawn Richardson provides an intriguing perspective on this subject. She herself is impatient with many outright anti-vaccinationists, noting that they are much more likely to be childless holistic health practitioners. Their ideological purity prevents them from making the kinds of compromises that get laws passed—and children saved. Still, unlike Barbara Loe Fisher, who sees the anti-vaccinationists as a significant threat to her carefully managed movement, Richardson celebrates the radical edge that they bring to the movement. Just as Malcolm X made it much easier for Martin Luther King, Jr. to get the attention of those in power, so too do the anti-vaccinationists compel the vaccine establishment to listen to the cooler heads that prevail at NVIC.[60]

Barbara Loe Fisher's management of her camp's extremists is by no means merely a matter of public relations. Rather, it flows from a deep ideological commitment that the mainstream movement has made to science. It is simply impossible to describe the advocates of vaccine safety as know-nothing anti-modernists who have chosen to reject the scientific worldview. Quite the contrary, for NVIC has embraced science with a vengeance. The organization simply believes that current vaccine science is hopelessly compromised by a whole host of conflicts of interest. Rather than throwing the baby out with the bathwater, NVIC demands *better*, more genuinely objective, science. The counts of the indictment run like this. First, "immunizations are big business," and what Fisher and Coulter called in *A Shot in the Dark* the "blinding effect of money" will always win out unless actively resisted. Second, the government can not protect the public from the predations of big corporations because of "the inherent conflict of interest in the federal government's role in developing new vaccines, promoting mandatory vaccination and monitoring vaccines for side effects." Third, the academic scientists who serve on advisory policymaking panels are no better than corporate and government officials, because almost all of them have direct financial ties to the vaccine industry, which pays them hundreds of thousands of dollars for their consultative services and funds much of their research. Even the most angelic scientist would find it difficult not to—at best—subtly twist his or her findings to downplay or deny vaccine risks. All in all, the NVIC critique, and defense, of science fits comfortably inside the long-standing

American anti-monopoly tradition, where the common people fight for the truth and justice against powerful and corrupt government-business connections.[61]

THE OUTSIDE EDGE OF THE MOVEMENT: ANTHRAX-NO

One set of vaccine skeptics, while connected to the larger movement, is distinct enough that it warrants separate consideration. Those who oppose the compulsory administration of the anthrax vaccination to military personnel have formed their own virtual community, with concerns different from, but not necessarily opposed to, those who focus on childhood immunizations. The anthrax agitators have likewise been remarkably successful in presenting their case to the media and to Congress. In fact, there was no sign more powerful that the anti-vaccination cause had reached deep into the very heart of the American mainstream than the example of patriotic soldiers willing to give their lives to die for their country but also willing to resist the medical dictates of what they increasingly view as a cruel and corrupt government.

The anthrax vaccine was originally licensed by the FDA in 1970 for protecting workers, such as ranchers, livestock veterinarians, and wool-mill laborers, who might come into contact with naturally occurring anthrax. Yet the extreme rarity of the disease meant that few civilians were ever inoculated. By 1997, the sole U.S. producer of the vaccine was the state-owned Michigan Biologics Products Institute. In March of that year, FDA inspectors warned the facility that the agency would revoke its manufacturing licenses for a variety of products, including the anthrax vaccine, if it did not correct multiple safety violations. A year later, the plant shut down for renovations and was slated to reopen under new ownership. The purchaser, BioPort Corporation of Michigan, counted among its board members Admiral William Crowe, former chairman of the Joint Chiefs of Staff.[62]

In May of 1998, Secretary of Defense William Cohen mandated a series of six shots to vaccinate all 2.4 million active and reserve military personnel against anthrax, at that time widely considered the frontrunner among potential biological weapons. The mass inoculation was to have been accomplished in three stages, with the first beginning in 1998, the second scheduled for January of 2000, and the final one for lower priority personnel in subsequent years. BioPort faced no competition for a $24 million Pentagon contract, but repeated delays and cost overruns in the plant renovation meant that the company could only supply the military with stockpiled vaccine manufactured in 1997 and 1998. An $18.7 million advance payment was agreed to in August of 1998 in order to speed up the reopening, but new lots continued to fail quality control tests.

Meanwhile, troop refusals and an April 1999 report from the General Accounting Office provided fuel for the increasing controversy over the shot series. The result was congressional hearings on the vaccine's safety and necessity during the fall of 1999, with two slightly different House bills being introduced to halt the anthrax immunization program, or at least make it voluntary. In December 1999, the Pentagon announced that the second phase of the vaccination program would have to be postponed almost a year because of the manufacturer's inability to supply the vaccine; only troops facing deployment to the highest risk zones—Korea and the Persian Gulf—would now complete a full series of shots. Gradually, as congressional hearings continued, the program was curtailed so that just researchers and soldiers on special missions received the shots. The mail scare during the fall of 2001 brought anthrax to greater public attention, but the military vaccination campaign only picked up with preparations for war in Iraq in 2003. Overall, approximately a million service members have received the vaccine since 1991, with nearly 600 soldiers refusing the shots. FDA package inserts acknowledge the deaths of five military personnel after receiving the shots.[63]

Opposition to the vaccination grew out of the fertile soil of the movement to recognize "Gulf War Syndrome," a cluster of symptoms such as fatigue, joint pain, and suppressed immune response that activists argue derive from some form of chemical or biological exposure suffered by troops during the 1990 Persian Gulf War. One hypothesis blames soldiers' symptoms not on Iraqi weapons but on the prophylactic drugs, including the anthrax vaccine, administered—often without consent—to both deployed and non-deployed troops. While the Pentagon has disputed the entire notion that Gulf War vets demonstrate higher illness rates than the general population, the persistent lobbying efforts of soldiers and their families have won a small measure of official response to their complaints.[64]

Anti-anthrax activists do not eschew traditional methods of organizing: holding rallies, addressing committee hearings, and contacting newspaper reporters. Yet where they come together is, most fundamentally, the Internet. And their chief site is Anthrax-no. Anthrax-no provides emotional comfort to those who associate their physical problems with the vaccine; it offers practical advice on how to avoid shots while staying in the military; and it gives support to those who refuse the vaccination, even if this means that their discharges will be other than honorable.[65]

In order better to understand the reasons why those who are most conditioned to obey orders are disobeying them, or at least attempting to subvert them, it is important to examine the interior world of Anthrax-no and its members. Few if any markers highlight race, but posters to the list do provide some clues to their class positions. Of those who state their military ranks, virtually all are enlisted folk or NCOs, although one of the most prominent activists, Sonnie Bates, was a major. Moreover, the military posters seem to assume an audience of non-officers, for example by frequently making hostile references to military brass. While a few activists are nurses, MDs, or lawyers, a more typical poster is an airline pilot who brings in an extra income through the Air National Guard or the ex-soldier who now works as a prison guard. Money is never far from participants' minds: when discussing individual decisions to refuse the vaccine and leave the service, they consider bills, moving expenses, health insurance, and pensions. In short, most of those who gave any indication of their occupations or financial status are making it (they are, after all, wired), but not by a big margin.[66]

Education levels as an overt topic come up considerably less often, but a few indicators stand out. First of all, the many postings contain serious errors in spelling, grammar, and punctuation. Heavy-handed irony, repetition, and clichés predominate. Participants sometimes seem very self-conscious about their writing ability, apologizing for expressing themselves inelegantly or reassuring one another about writing letters. A representative participant explained that her husband "holds a position with the Guard that pays a lot more money than he used to make . . . great money for a guy with an 11th grade education and a G.E.D." Technical training, on the other hand, is evidently a common experience among Anthrax-no-niks, and many are justifiably proud of their ability to navigate the Internet. They also show a marked orientation toward self-education, favorably comparing their own intelligence to that of physicians, lawyers, and the Pentagon elite.[67]

Class concerns do not surface often in their communiqués; rather than attacking the status of their enemies in the Department of Defense or the scientific establishment, they are more likely to talk about the usurpation of power. Occasionally someone will indict "the aristocrats who rule this country." The author of this remark elaborated: "they look on us as pawns (lower class=disposable) and don't care how many of us are disabled or die from the vaccine as long as there is a sizable force left who can protect them and their wealth." Another time this same poster questioned in class terms whether the top Washington military officials pictured in the media receiving their anthrax shots were actually getting injected with the same substance as their subordinates. "I will never believe," he declared, that "they will risk taking the exact same shots that they test on us. I'm sure they will rationalize this by saying they are 'mission essential,' but it is really just an aristocratic social class thing—poor folks are expendable." In neither instance, however, did other correspondents rise to the bait.[68]

In spite of their relative inattention to socioeconomic class, Anthrax-no members—like NVIC activists—constantly exhort one another to "follow the money," especially in reference to Bioport. In their more generous interpretations of their opponents' motivations, the list members routinely cite money as the main factor—the harsher options being simply tyranny or pure evil.

One of the most attention-grabbing features of Anthrax-no—a list primarily concerned with military personnel—is the preponderance of women in the ranks of the posters. Some of them are soldiers themselves, or reservists, but more are wives or mothers of service members. What becomes clear from these women's postings is that while their menfolk are the ones imperiled, the women themselves are more likely to research the vaccine and to become activists against it. Several serve as the e-mail link for husbands stationed on ships at sea, relaying information in both directions; one of these stamps her outgoing mail with the tag "Well behaved women rarely make history!" The wives encourage one another to stand by their men, while aggressively taking on that most masculine of institutions, the United States military.[69]

Even the postings that encourage the most traditional of gender relationships within marriage, however, assume—indeed celebrate—the presence of brave young women in the military. Male and female posters heap praise on female activists without any reference to sex. Moreover, the unappointed leader of the movement is a female doctor, Meryl Nass. While the women express relatively few gender-specific concerns, they do voice fears of the vaccine's potential effect on their own reproductive health, as well as on the health of babies of inoculated fathers.[70]

The arena of Anthrax-no members is much less disciplined than the world of NVIC. As befits an open Internet chat group, the variety of political ideas, as well as the level of sheer eccentricity, is often considerably greater. Yet on one issue the professional-class NVIC mothers and the rough-and-tumble enlisted men's wives of Anthrax-no easily agree. That is: the new homeland security regime of George W. Bush and John Ashcroft is one of the most dangerous threats to civil liberties in our nation's history.

THE RETURN OF THE REPRESSED: SMALLPOX VACCINATION TAKES CENTER STAGE IN AN AGE OF HOMELAND SECURITY

Vaccine safety activists are equal opportunity critics when it comes to matters of medical liberty. As soon as the Clintons unveiled proposals for health care reform, for example, the NVIC started attacking their plan for a universal health care identifier number and medical tracking system as an unconstitutional threat to the freedom of American citizens. Throughout the Clinton presidency NVIC worked with groups, ranging from Phyllis Schlafly's Eagle Forum to the ACLU, fighting to preserve the privacy of medical records.[71]

Yet NVIC did not worry about mortal dangers to the republic until the aftermath of September 11th. That is when George W. Bush decided to push for sweeping powers in all realms of American life—and, not incidentally, in matters relating to vaccination. The resulting clash saw Barbara Loe Fisher and Dawn Richardson mobilizing their troops so effectively that they nearly brought the president's entire homeland security program to a halt.

History turned full circle when, at the beginning of a new century, smallpox returned to center stage in the battle over vaccination. As Americans struggled to come to grips with terrorism, President Bush and his advisors immediately moved to medicalize the conflict. Despite the successful worldwide eradication of smallpox—one of the great triumphs of global public health—officials in the United States government feared that rogue states such as Iraq or North Korea might have obtained stockpiles of the virus that they could use for bioterrorism. Federal health officials in turn moved to accumulate as much smallpox vaccine as possible. Health and Human Services secretary Tommy Thompson then announced his plans to vaccinate those who would first respond to any possible attack. The result, as mentioned at the beginning of this essay, was a nearly total defeat for the administration as nurses, physicians, and their unions acted on concerns about the dangers of this relatively crude vaccine and successfully resisted the new government dictates.[72]

Bush and public officials then moved in a different direction. Portions of their showcase Homeland Security Bill granted federal officials the right to force vaccinations for smallpox on citizens in case of a declared emergency. Also, manufacturers received a complete exemption from liability for any injuries caused by their smallpox vaccines. Those hurt could sue only the federal government, and because of pre-existing federal law, their chances of success in the courts would be close to zero. Vaccine safety activists immediately started mobilizing to strip section 304 from the bill, contending that a medical emergency declared by the secretary of HHS would unnecessarily override all state laws providing for religious, medical, or conscientious objection to vaccinations. As Barbara Loe Fisher put it, the bill raised the possibility of "Vaccinating America at Gunpoint."[73]

Theirs was a relatively lonely crusade, however, until an obscure amendment was slipped into the bill just before it came up for a vote in the House in November 2002. The mystery rider promised to grant manufacturers of vaccine additives, especially the mercury-based preservative thimerosal, complete protection from liability, even though the almost exclusive use of that preservative had been in childhood immunizations with no visible connections to the terrorist threat. "In a Washington whodunit worthy of Agatha Christie," no one would take credit for the amendment. A mad scramble to uncover the sponsor ensued, but not until weeks after the bill's passage did outgoing House majority leader Dick Armey proudly own up to having inserted the clause. Armey asserted that national security demanded the protection of pharmaceutical companies from frivolous lawsuits that might well drive them out of the vaccine business.[74]

The main beneficiary of this amendment would prove to be Eli Lilly, one of the largest pharmaceutical companies and a corporation with extremely close ties to the Bush administration. What appeared to be a transparent give-away to Eli Lilly inspired outrage from many mainstream politicians. Democrats, in particular, reacted with great anger. Senators Joseph Lieberman, Tom Daschle, and Robert Byrd proposed an amendment to delete the thimerosal provision from the bill. (Their amendment, though, left in place the government's emergency smallpox powers.) Lieberman and his colleagues held good cards. The president was desperate to get the homeland security bill signed before Congress adjourned for the session. If the Lieberman amendment passed, the bill as a whole would have had to go back to a House-Senate conference committee, likely killing off any prospects for passage until the next session and thus placing a crucial stumbling block in Bush's plans to fight terror. Bean counters realized that the vote would be quite close, with the outcome dependent on which way senators Lincoln Chafee, Susan Collins, and Olympia Snowe decided to cast their ballots—and these liberal Republicans were "incensed" about the rider protecting vaccine manufacturers. In the end, though, president Bush put enormous political pressure on the three solons, who agreed to vote against the Lieberman amendment if the congressional leadership promised to change the bill to their liking upon the opening of the new session. The Lieberman amendment went on to fail narrowly, 52–47, and the overall homeland security bill then passed by an overwhelming margin.[75]

Still, for a brief moment it looked as if vaccine safety concerns would be holding up the entire war on terrorism. That was due primarily to the political skill and power of NVIC, PROVE, and the entire brigade of vaccine safety activists. Closely monitoring the homeland security bill from the beginning, they launched their most intensive lobbying effort since the 1986 crusade to convince Ronald Reagan to sign the federal compensation law. Forming an "informal coalition" with groups like the ACLU, Barbara Loe Fisher decried not only the continued gutting of the vaccine compensation system and the draconian medical powers that the bill gave federal officials, but also a whole host of other civil liberties and privacy violations. Under the bill, for example, the government would have much easier access to citizens' email, bank account information, and medical records. Vaccine safety advocates also condemned the bill's severe weakening of the Freedom of Information Act. More generally, critics feared that the measure would unconstitutionally change the balance of power between the executive and legislative branches, giving even greater authority to the imperial presidency.[76]

NVIC and its allies ultimately lost this latest round in the battle for vaccine safety and freedom. Yet they seemed to recognize that their narrow loss meant, perhaps even more than sheer defeat, the coming of age of their collective power in what was, according to Dawn Richardson, "an incredible grassroots fight." Not that vaccine safety activists moderated their rhetoric as they got nearer to power; instead, the closer vaccine safety activists came to having influence over the most important issues in national politics, the more they came to sound like left-wing critics of a corporate-government police state. Moreover, these battles show no signs of letting up. As I write in the middle of 2003, conflicts over the federal vaccination compensation system reach toward their second decade, with Senate majority leader Bill Frist increasingly taking on the visage of the prince of vaccine darkness. And while it was only because of a peculiar conjunction of partisan political forces that vaccine safety activists were able to play such an important role in the debate over the homeland security bill, the headlines about smallpox, anthrax, and vaccines generally show few signs of abating. No longer can anyone claim that vaccines are a sideshow that a lunatic fringe grasps onto to distract the polity from more substantive issues. They are, in fact, at the heart of our democracy as well as at the foundation of our immune system, and vaccine safety activists have begun to settle—albeit a bit uncomfortably—into the center of national political culture.[77]

CONCLUSION: THE POSSIBILITIES OF DIALOGUE AND
A DEMOCRATIC MEDICINE

The vaccine establishment clearly has a painful, but potentially quite fruitful, decision to make about how to respond to vaccine safety activists—and, for that matter, to anti-vaccinationists—as they continue to grow stronger. Even the brief historical sketch provided in this article shows that, if the past has any hold at all, challenges to mass vaccination policies will maintain their power, perhaps regardless of how the government and medical officials react. Indeed, we do not even need to look to the past: prominent anthropologist Emily Martin has found in the present age a common "reluctance to vaccinate across age, gender, ethnic, and class lines."[78]

Those involved with immunization policy can certainly write off activists as demagogic cranks and concerned parents as ignorant members of the herd. Members of the vaccination establishment have done this plenty of times before, and plenty continue to do so. A personal anecdote from 2002: when I was asked to present some of my research on early-twentieth-century resistance to vaccination to the CDC's Vaccine Risk Communication workgroup, I was surprised to hear the level of respect that the so-called opponents of vaccination were receiving from officials from the FDA, CDC, and other public health agencies. Then, suddenly, one member on the conference call boomed in, saying (with apologies for her language) that "this is all *bullshit*" and that Barbara Loe Fisher and the NVIC were mortal enemies of the entire vaccination complex. Fisher and her associates were indeed, and most emphatically, full-blown *anti-vaccinationists*, and to call them "vaccine safety advocates" granted them a legitimacy that directly endangered the health of young children.

The resulting conversation was heated but inconclusive. Frankly, though, I was delighted to know that this kind of discussion was occurring within the very heart of the vaccine policy-making complex. It is a sign of the kind of deliberation that keeps bureaucracies flexible and creative. And it points toward an understanding that all citizens, and not just the so-called experts, can—in fact, should—engage in such democratic dialogue with a democratic government in a democratic country.

As I suspected, the discussion I heard was clearly the continuation of many previous conversations. For, it turns out, bubbling up from within the vaccine establishment in the new millennium is the most remarkable set of proposals for public participation in vaccine policy making in American history. Roger Bernier, the Associate Director for Science at the National Immunization Program, has received support from the Johnson Foundation to bring together government officials, pharmaceutical industry executives, and members of the public to discuss how to improve and increase the quality and quantity of democratic dialogue on the vaccine issue. Some of this "public," such as members of the League of Women Voters, is self-consciously neutral, but other segments are forthrightly critical of the current administration of vaccines. And that is, in fact, why they have been invited into the process. Bernier and his fellow officials explicitly wish to figure out how to get the most powerful vaccine safety activists—among them Barbara Loe Fisher and the NVIC, Dawn Richardson and PROVE, and Rick Rollens (the most prominent autism-vaccine activist)—involved as "stakeholders" in the very heart of the vaccine policy making process. Never before have the farmers invited into the chicken coop, and with such open arms, the anti-vaccinationist wolves.[79]

The Wingspread Public Engagement Planning Group, or Wingspread for short, has so far propounded a staunchly democratic vision. Those involved are emphatic that bringing the public into a "Vaccine Policy Analysis Collaborative" (VPAC) is not just a way to transmit information from experts to the masses at a time of heightened skepticism toward vaccines in particular and government in general. Rather, public participation is "right" in and of itself, and it also provides policy makers the opportunity to "make better decisions" by seeking "citizens' ideas and the wisdom of the group." And the concrete issues proposed for a VPAC to tackle lie at the heart of the vaccine safety agenda: should pediatricians refuse care to children who are not fully immunized? should all states have philosophical exemptions to vaccinations? should the federal compensation program loosen its requirements for proving a vaccine injury?

A healthy majority of the identified stakeholders have stayed active in the Wingspread process as discussions have evolved. Yet even though the explicit goal of the group is to find some way to reach a new and more robust *pro*-immunization consensus, it is, ironically, some pro-vaccine and industry representatives who have either jumped ship or expressed their concern that the search for public participation has taken the wrong path, becoming too "critic friendly." These advocates of mass immunization fear that what looks like real dialogue is actually pre-determined to reach an outcome that focuses an inordinate amount on safety and risk issues in order to "appease vaccine critics." Still, Bernier and his fellow high-level vaccination officials continue on with their attempt to shift "the paradigm to see the public as a resource[,] not a drag." Ultimately, whatever form the Wingspread process takes if it ever becomes institutionalized, they hope to see it extended "to other programs where citizens distrust government and feel disenfranchised." In particular, Bernier and his colleagues hope it proves "useful for the conduct of science in democratic societies where the science is complex, citizen support and consent is needed, and scientists and citizens must interact."[80]

The Wingspread process, while still in its infancy, helps to confirm that what vaccine safety activists have accomplished over the last quarter century is, in some ways, nothing short of astounding. They have suffered many setbacks, and quite legitimately they often emphasize their frequent defeats. Still, the anti-vaccinationists of a century ago could have only dreamed of appearing before Congress as honored witnesses, having mainstream journalists knocking down their door to make sure that their side of the story was well and fully told, and being actively sought out for consultation by those at the peak of the national vaccine policy making process. This is, in my mind, all for the good. No group of citizens is perfect, and of course today's vaccine safety advocates are not. Yet they have consistently brought intelligent, informed, and urgently important ideas to the public square. It is even safe to say that, without them, vaccines would be more dangerous, and that they have thus done something directly beneficial for those implementing mass immunization. Furthermore, it should now also be safe to say that vaccine safety advocates have greatly enriched the intellectual and political worlds of public health, creating the possibilities of a truly democratic medicine.

Americans have been justly proud of our tradition of conquering disease. We should be just as proud of our vigorous tradition of medical dissent.

FROM CULTISM TO CAM

Alternative Medicine in the Twentieth Century

James C. Whorton

IN THE AUTUMN OF 1994, a *New Yorker* cartoonist imagined a clinical scene in which a patient who is literally radiant with health, basking within a veritable halo of wellness, is nevertheless being sternly admonished by his physician because he has achieved his health the wrong way: "You've been fooling around with alternative medicines, haven't you?" the doctor scolds.[1]

New Yorker cartoons constitute the most sensitive of barometers to shifting currents in America's cultural atmosphere. And in truth, whatever one chooses to call it—alternative medicine, fringe medicine, unconventional medicine, holistic medicine—a lot of people were fooling around with unorthodox forms of therapy by the end of the twentieth century. In a now legendary survey published in 1993, Harvard's David Eisenberg and colleagues reported that one in three Americans had used one or more forms of alternative medicine in 1990, and they expressed surprise at the "enormous presence" of healing alternatives in American society. When Eisenberg and colleagues repeated the survey in 1997, they found that "alternative medicine use and expenditures have increased dramatically" since the first study. Now 40 percent of the population employed such procedures.[2]

That alternative methods were so widespread in the presumably enlightened 1990s was a startling revelation to the medical profession. It shouldn't have been, for as this volume has shown, Americans had been fooling around with alternative medicine for a long time. That such activity is mere foolishness has been the opinion, of course, of conventional, or "allopathic," physicians. From the start, allopaths have scorned alternative systems of treatment as a hodgepodge of inert (when not dangerous) therapies foisted upon gullible hypochondriacs by scientifically uncritical quacks. Alternative practitioners, Spalding Gray has joked on behalf of M.D.'s, believe that "*everything* gives you cancer," but there's no need to worry, because they also believe that "everything else heals you of it."[3]

Yet scarcely three years after that New Yorker cartoon, in December 1997, the *Journal of the American Medical Association (JAMA)* announced that unconventional medicine had been ranked among the top three subjects for American Medical Association (AMA) journals to address in the next year, and that the topic would be the focus of a special issue of the *JAMA*. That issue appeared in November 1998. It included reports on clinical trials of seven different alternative therapies (including chiropractic, acupuncture, yoga, and herbs); four of the seven trials found positive benefits from the tested treatment.[4] Now, it would seem, allopaths were going to start fooling around with alternative medicine themselves.

To be more accurate, conventional medicine was by 1998 showing a greater receptivity to *complementary* medicine. *Alternative*, which became the standard designation for unconventional systems of therapy in the 1970s, steadily yielded ground during the 1990s to *complementary*, a term that suggested use in conjunction with, rather than in place of, orthodox treatments. This transformation of outlook was demonstrated with particular clarity by the 1998 renaming of the Office of Alternative Medicine (OAM), opened at the National Institutes of Health (NIH) in 1992, to the National Center for Complementary and Alternative Medicine (NCCAM). Even before then, however, a new acronym had been born—CAM, for "complementary and alternative medicine"—to express the growing acceptance that nonorthodox therapies might be used either in combination with or as substitutes for allopathic methods, depending on a patient's needs. CAM was a culmination, the climax of a century in which furious conflict between mainstream and marginal medicine had gradually subsided and been replaced by entente, sometimes cordial, more often wary, but in any event a state of affairs impossible to have foreseen at the beginning of the 1900s.

Conflict was concentrated on differences in practice and philosophy, of course, but politics was inextricably bound up with both sets of questions. Indeed, the history of alternative medicine in the twentieth century is, almost by definition, the story of outsiders fighting the establishment, and, awkward though it sounds, there is considerable merit in another of the names that has been suggested for unconventional practice: "counterhegemonic medicine."[5] The challenging of orthodox medical hegemony is in fact a theme of all the chapters in this volume. Some have examined distinct schools of practice (homeopathy, Native American healing); more have focused on single-issue protest movements (anti-vaccination, anti-fluoridation). This chapter will deal with alternative medicine in the form of organized systems of therapy and theory that were initially intended to displace the established system of practice but which have evolved into would-be complements to allopathic care. The chapter's themes apply to all the century's unorthodox systems, but I will illustrate those themes primarily with three schools of practice that have not yet received much attention in this book: osteopathy, chiropractic, and naturopathy, therapeutic programs that in the early 1900s set themselves apart as systems of "drugless healing."

At the turn of the twentieth century, alternative systems of medicine were commonly referred to—by allopaths, at any rate—as "irregular medicine." Irregular practice had begun a full century earlier, with Thomsonianism, a program of botanical practice developed by New Hampshire farmer Samuel Thomson that started to attract attention in the first decade of the nineteenth century and grew to considerable strength by the 1830s. Thomsonianism faded after the death of its founder in 1843, but a number of other systems stood ready to take its place: homeopathy, hydropathy, magnetic healing, eclecticism, and physio-medicalism, to name just the most popular. Those all survived, though some just barely, into the twentieth century, where they were joined by a second generation of unorthodox systems. Osteopathy, formulated by Andrew Taylor Still in the 1870s, was a method of musculoskeletal manipulation that claimed to relieve impediments to the free flow of blood. Chiropractic, the creation of D. D. Palmer in the 1890s, likewise employed skeletal manipulation, in this instance to correct subluxations, or minor dislocations, of the vertebrae and thereby restore the nervous system to full functioning. Naturopathy, organized by Benedict Lust in the late 1890s and early 1900s, utilized various agents from the natural world to stimulate the patient's natural recuperative powers. Each of these systems employed its own distinctive therapies, and each had its own distinctive theoretical rationales. At the level of philosophy, however, there was unanimity, a shared doctrine that had as its basic tenets trust in the body's innate reparative mechanisms to accomplish healing, a holistic interpretation of illness as a confluence of psychological and physical factors, and reliance on clinical experience instead of theory as the path to therapeutic discovery. Those principles were all prominent in the medical legacy of Hippocrates, the ancient Greek "father" of orthodox medicine, so one might think of the various irregular systems as Hippocratic heresies.[6]

That they were heresies brooked no doubt, although the term preferred by medical orthodoxy through most of the twentieth century was *cults*. A typical characterization of irregular medicine as cultism was presented in a 1932 book published by the Committee on the Costs of Medical Care. "The founder of each sect launched his theory as an explanation of all disease," the author of *The Healing Cults* began, "and taught a procedure . . . of treatment which he claimed to be a cure for all disease." Narrow- and simple-minded believers in the all-encompassing truth of their healing revelation, adherents of medical cultism "cling to their particular beliefs with a fervor more characteristic of an evangelistic than a scientific group." Winning converts among the uneducated and uncritical through enthusiastic hellfire-and-brimstone preaching, they exalted themselves as the saviors of the disease-ridden world from the treacherous snares of the allopathic Satan. It was this uncompromising hatred of scientific medicine, "this close-mindedness, this devotion to" their peculiar "dogmas," that "justifies the title, 'cult' or 'sect,' for all these groups."[7]

There was more than a little truth in that depiction. A certain cult of personality had formed around the charismatic founders of osteopathy, naturopathy, and chiropractic, particularly the last, which was dominated by D. D. Palmer and B. J. Palmer, father and son, "The Discoverer" and "The Developer." Practitioners of all the systems had made sweeping theoretical generalizations ("Discoverer" Palmer maintained that 95 percent of all disease was caused by subluxated vertebrae) and extravagant claims of healing potency. Naturopathic leader Lust averred with a straight face that half the seriously ill patients treated by allopaths died, while those who sought out naturopathic help were lost at the rate of only 5 percent (and most of those only because of the damage that had already been done by M.D.'s). Chiropractors prided themselves on routinely curing infantile paralysis, a disease that had allopaths stymied. Nor did they experience any special difficulty treating influenza during the great pandemic of 1918–19, which killed more than half a million Americans. "The mortality rate under routine medical treatment" during the outbreak, a chiropractic publication observed, "was exceedingly high." Chiropractic, however, rang up numbers of cures that "were truly startling in their revelations." Of more than twenty thousand flu patients treated with adjustments, the death rate was a miniscule 0.14 percent, meaning "that Chiropractic is from ten to thirty times as effective in the treatment of influenza as any other method that has been employed." Not so, countered naturopaths, who were capable of a 0.00 percent mortality rate. "Not one of my influenza patrons had the fever over three days," one naturopath reported; "not one had to remain away from work more than a week, not one had any bad after-effects or any complications. And of course, there were no deaths."[8]

Allopaths had still other reasons for thinking of alternative practitioners as deluded cultists, not the least of which was the sorry state of their educational institutions. To be sure, the famous Flexner Report of 1910 had revealed that few orthodox institutions had any reason to be proud; "utterly wretched" and "a hopeless affair" were typical Flexner evaluations of most of the conventional schools. But he had been even less sparing of irregulars' feelings, scornfully rejecting homeopaths, osteopaths, chiropractors, naturopaths, and other "drugless healers" as at best members of "medical sects" and at worst as "unconscionable quacks" who were properly dealt with by "the public prosecutor and the grand jury." The strongest flattery he could come up with for their educational institutions was "utterly hopeless" and "fatally defective."[9]

The result of Flexner's bombshell was that nearly half the country's allopathic schools closed over the next few years, and the survivors upgraded their standards drastically. Irregular colleges, on the other hand, continued merrily along their utterly hopeless way. An M.D. who made "A Visit to a Chiropractic School" in 1922, for example, reported that most of the students he met there "had not bridged the stage between the grammar school" and their supposed medical course. A physician discoursing on "where chiropractors are made" dismissed the schools as devoted "entirely to financial and not at all to scientific standards" and the students as "intellectual refuse" whose "mental equipment" was in a state of "extreme wretchedness." A New York practitioner who in the early 1920s actually enrolled in the Palmer School of Chiropractic to get a look at "Chiropractic From the Inside" found that the only educational requirement enforced was to "insist that you must be able to write. If not, it would lead to all kinds of trouble to cash your check." Finally, a Texas doctor went undercover in the guise of a widow who wrote a chiropractic school in Oklahoma City lamenting that "she" had had only three years of schooling yet wondered "if I can be kirpatic dr. if you can make a kirpatic dr. for how much money I got about 2 thousand dolers." "You have the intelligence . . . and sufficient education to understand the English language," the head of the school promptly replied, and "you would have no difficulty in getting a knowledge of this subject so that you could go out and practice and be efficient. You can enter at any time and in eighteen months, upon making your grades, can be graduated." B. J. Palmer himself confirmed chiropractic's dubious educational standards by admitting in courtroom testimony that while anatomy was the basis of chiropractic science, his students' dissection experience was limited to an occasional sheep anatomized in a barn behind the school and the odd cadaver examined at Ed Horrigan's funeral parlor; dissection may have been irrelevant, however, since Palmer also professed to adhere to a system of anatomy that differed from the allopathic standard, *Gray's Anatomy*, "very materially."[10]

Naturopathic schools fared no better in allopathic appraisals, being shrugged off as "small affairs of a fly-by-night character" operated "by men untrained in and antagonistic to medical science" who taught "fantastic forms of assault . . . devised by the paranoic brains of a hundred cultist prophets." Only too typical was the graduate of a Seattle school who put down responses such as the following on his drugless healing licensing examination.

Q.   What foods are rich in iron, sulphur, proteids?

A.   Beets, lecttes, spenat, carets is very rich in iron. Eggs is rich in sulphur meats is rich in proteids also brad and of corce meny other foods.

Q. Why are some of the heartiest eaters thin?

A. One reason may be that they eats to much more than they can digest and they don't eat the wright combination also eat too fast.

The dietitian's physiology and orthography were worrisome enough, but even more disturbing was the fact that his exam had been passed by the state drugless board with a score of 90 percent.[11]

Lest these commentaries be read as unjustified expressions of allopathic bias, it must be pointed out that the leaders of the different systems of alternative medical practice often said the same things. Lust, for example, bemoaned the miserable standards of education and practice of many naturopaths throughout his long career as the profession's paterfamilias: in the very first volume of *The Naturopath,* in 1902, he complained of the many "pseudo-naturopaths" and "abortioners of naturopathy"; more than four decades later, less than a week before his death, he dictated an address to be read at the American Naturopathic Association convention in which he lamented the number of "woeful misfits" and "outright fakers and cheats masking as Naturopaths." Through the years in between, he was joined by many other naturopaths indignant over "the hundreds of so-called drugless healers who are a disgrace to our calling," all the "money changers [who] clutter up our ranks and despoil our temples," and the fact that "there are as many quack methods prevalent in the Nature Cure as there are in the drug business."[12]

Some early-century alternative healers were equally ready to speak against their discipline's theories as simplistic and its therapies as something less than the panaceas they were touted to be. More than one osteopath renounced the founder's original formulation as "a creed," that is, a cult, that inhibited the profession's advance toward "a complete system or science," and at least one referred to it as "fanaticism." Many chiropractors likewise came to acknowledge by the 1910s that "many conditions ... are beyond the reach of spinal technic" and some elements of Palmer's theory "beyond the scope of truth or reason."[13]

But however much intramural dissension occurred in any system (and within chiropractic there existed a great deal indeed), the bulk of irregulars' wrath was directed toward allopathic medicine. From their perspective, it was orthodoxy that was cultism; it was the allopaths who clung blindly to a simplistic creed (treat all patients the same, with drugs and the knife) and who refused to even consider the wisdom of other ways. This allopathic "science" was further discredited by basing itself on cruelty (animal experimentation) and coercion (compulsory vaccination). The whole pathetic jumble of orthodox medicine was summed up lyrically by a naturopath:

Sing a song of doctors, A satchel full of dope,
Four-and-twenty patients, A hundred miles of hope.
When the satchel opens, the doctors start to guess;
The patients are about to get some nauseating mess.
Dosem's in the parlor, Analyzing frogs;
Cuttem's in the kitchen, Vivisecting dogs;
Prickem's found another Serum for disease.
But there's no disagreement When they figure up their fees.[14]

Offensive as all those components of allopathic medicine were, what truly enraged irregular practitioners was allopathic *politics*, the determination of the majority profession to impose its depraved standards on the public through legislation. Allopaths would have described their standards differently, of course, but they freely admitted that they were becoming more politically active, working "to stimulate, to restrain, or otherwise to control the law-making power" at every level of government in order to preserve and elevate the health of the public (the position of the medical profession throughout the twentieth century was that it "has an obligation to expose cultist practices" that arises "not out of animosity toward the cultists, but from dedication to the welfare of the public"). Leadership in these efforts came from the American Medical Association, in existence since 1847, but not particularly involved politically until the beginning of the twentieth century. One of the AMA's most ambitious projects in the years prior to World War I was the establishment of a national health bureau to implement and coordinate an array of public health programs (including vaccination and medical inspection of schoolchildren) nationwide. AMA lobbying resulted finally in Oklahoma's Senator Robert Owen introducing in 1910 a bill to create a cabinet-level department. That first bill did not get past committee, nor did two subsequent attempts by Owen (in 1911 and 1913) succeed in becoming law. The mere threat of enactment, however, was enough to rally all unorthodox practitioners—homeopaths, eclectics, osteopaths, chiropractors, naturopaths, Christian Scientists, even patent medicine manufacturers—to join arms in resistance to what they saw as an onslaught of allopathic tyranny. Uniting under the banner of the National League for Medical Freedom, they worked tirelessly to stir up the public to fight back against the schemes of M.D.'s to assume complete control of all matters medical and hygienic ("To defeat paternal, unnecessary, extravagant, un-American medical legislation is the purpose of the National League for Medical Freedom").[15]

"Senator Owen of Oklahoma is the tool by which this monster evil [the AMA] hopes to become master of the medical field in the United States," an affronted naturopath charged. "No kingdom or monarchy throughout the world has ever had such a cursed monster to exercise iron sway over the people. It is the infamy of the infamous. It is the horror of this world—the 'Black Hand' of medical robbery and murder." It was, according to this same critic, the desperate ploy of "medical peanut politicians," "intellectual degenerates and moral perverts," "vampires and vandals," a "primping grafting affected conglomeration of masculine inanity," "effeminate dudes . . . fops and idiots," and "medical turntits [of] hyena heartlessness." If all that seems a bit hyperbolic, then hyperbole was the norm. Consider the words of a speaker at "the monster mass-meeting for medical freedom" held at Carnegie Hall in 1911: "no bolder or more audacious demands for monopolistic privileges were ever put forward" than by these seekers after "pelf and power," these "political doctors" so deranged by "selfishness, greed and arrogance" as to think they can set up "a sanhedrin of medicine, from which there is to be no appeal" and then "cast into utter darkness" anyone "who will not bow down and worship the god of allopathy."[16]

There was no question among irregulars but that "pelf and power," the one of course serving the other, were the true motivations behind organized medicine's desire for a national department of health. It seemed equally clear that the allopathic plan to get the government to "supply fat jobs for all this army of incompetent political doctors" stemmed as well from fear of competition from more skilled irregular healers. The proposed federal health department was most threatening, therefore, because it portended a prohibition of unorthodox practice enacted from the national level. A chiropractor foretold what would happen:

> The devilish doctors now laugh and grin and chuckle in their ghoulish glee:
> "Oh, we are the only, only ones, now, who can touch the sick for a fee.
> We can charge as we wish, and do what we like with poison and knife and saw,
> And should we by chance kill a patient or two, it's in the name of the law;
> The Chiropractors, altho [*sic*] they have brains, we have to acknowledge that fact,
> If they practice, will be heavily fined by our Medical Practice Act."[17]

The "Medical Practice Act" was code for a number of legislative acts at the state level that outlawed the practice of medicine without a license. Such laws had a long and turbulent history, dating to the early 1800s, when allopaths had won licensing legislation in virtually every state restricting the practice of medicine to graduates of medical schools or those who could pass an examination on allopathic theory and practice. Those laws came under attack in the 1830s, the heyday of Jacksonian democracy, as undemocratic restrictions on the patient's right to choose his or her form of healing and on the healer's right to choose a career. By 1850, all but two states had responded to the campaign for medical democracy by repealing their licensing statutes; the arena of healing was open for all schools to compete freely.[18]

With the advent of the germ theory in the 1870s, however, and particularly the explosive growth of surgery following the introduction of asepsis, state legislatures became once more agreeable to allopaths' argument that would-be practitioners of the healing arts should be forced to demonstrate their competence before being allowed to practice. During the 1880s and 1890s states revived their licensing requirements. The resurrection of licensing did not, however, drive irregulars from the field, for by the last quarter of the century two unorthodox groups—homeopaths and eclectics—were too well established, attracting too many patients, to be outlawed. The regular profession's victory in reviving licensing restrictions, in short, was a bit of a Pyrrhic one, obtainable only by accepting that homeopaths and eclectics be granted their own licensure acts too.[19]

The extension of licensing to those old-school irregulars did not, of course, carry over to new systems still struggling to get themselves established. As osteopathy, chiropractic, naturopathy, and other newcomers appeared, their practitioners found themselves in the same position as homeopaths and Thomsonians had been in during the 1830s: guilty of practicing medicine without a license. Actually, their position was worse, as the licensing laws of the early nineteenth century had not been vigorously enforced, and punishment had usually been nothing more than denial of the right to sue for uncollected fees. Late-nineteenth-century laws were applied more seriously, however, and the penalties for violation were more severe: fines and time in jail.

The new circumstances provoked an angry political reaction, both from individual members of the various healing schools and from national organizations formed expressly to fight for "medical freedom": such were the aforementioned National League for Medical Freedom, as well as the American Medical Liberty League and the Constitutional Liberty League of America. The case made for medical freedom was based primarily on the need to protect constitutional liberties, including first of all the liberty of citizens to choose the treatments they thought best for their own bodies. Americans were guaranteed the right to elect representatives in government according to their political beliefs, and the right to choose a religious faith according to their spiritual beliefs. Why, then, it was often asked, should they not have the right to choose physicians according to their medical beliefs? The allopathic profession did not have "any more moral right to impose its peculiar therapeutic methods upon an unwilling individual than a Baptist majority in any state would have to require universal immersion."[20]

The second constitutional liberty being challenged was that of the freedom of every person to follow a calling. "I don't know that I cared much about these osteopaths," Mark Twain testified to the New York legislature in favor of a bill to license osteopathic practitioners, "until I heard you were going to drive them out of the State; but since I heard this I haven't been able to sleep." No one who treasured freedom should be able to sleep, irregular practitioners argued, as long as there was a profession that behaved as if it were the "National Established Church of Medicine" empowered "to weed out dissent" through "harsh and vindictive measures." There was considerable popular sympathy at the beginning of the twentieth century for the charge that "medical orthodoxy has always been as intolerant and bigoted as religious orthodoxy, and about as ready to torture and destroy."[21]

"Destroy" seems a bit strong, though it was reported that among naturopaths one "committed suicide . . . in despair, several died with broken hearts in the struggle and many happy homes were ruined" by the enforcement of allopathic licensing laws. Of "torture," however, there can be no doubt: "What the drugless doctors suffered in those days only those who were pinched can tell." Hundreds, if not thousands, of irregular practitioners were fined and/or jailed for unlicensed practice, and, a naturopathic journal opined, even "Jesus Christ would be arrested for practicing medicine without a license were He to come to New York State to-day and begin healing the sick and making the blind see." The founder of naturopathy himself was hauled into court as early as 1899, after a man to whom he had administered a bath reported him to the authorities. Fortunately, the judge who heard the case was taking the cure himself at a New Jersey establishment on weekends and dismissed the charges. Lust didn't always come out on top the numerous other times he was arrested, however, and once his fine was as stiff as $500. D. D. Palmer also spent time "in Bastile [*sic*]," but even though it cost him twenty-three days and $39.50 in fines and court costs, the experience had been worth it, he declared, because newspaper publicity given his incarceration had "stimulated the growth of our business," and consequently "thousands will be benefitted."[22]

Palmer's story would be repeated time and again over the next several decades ("some chiropractors are such confirmed jailbirds that incarceration is no novelty for them whatever"), though it seems that, more often than not, juries were sympathetic toward alternative practitioners in their self-appointed role as champions of health liberty. In the 1920s novelette *Health and Love à la Chiropractic*, the exoneration of Dr. Justor for practicing medicine without a license is hailed as "another victory for humanity, another step toward medical freedom," and the scene played out in real life with regularity. To cite the most striking example, a Texas chiropractor was taken before a jury sixty-six times—and acquitted all but once. Occasionally, there were even rulings from the bench in support of medical freedom, an Illinois judge, for instance, pardoning an osteopath on the grounds that "the people seemed to want to try this new humbug."[23]

One could not be certain of supportive judges and juries, however, so for the long term the key to survival for alternative medicine in the early twentieth century was to obtain permanent freedom from legislators. It was in irregular practitioners' struggle to win licensing provisions of their own, bitterly contested by the orthodox profession in state after state, that so much of the animosity and distrust between the two camps was generated. Allopaths' animus was only intensified, of course, when irregulars won legislative contests. Osteopaths' first victory was in Vermont, in 1896; naturopaths obtained their first licensing statute in California, in 1909; chiropractors were the last to succeed, being first recognized by Kansas, in 1913. Other states steadily fell into line for all three systems, though it was not until well into the second half of the century that osteopathy and chiropractic achieved legal protection in every state; naturopathy, licensed by a majority of states by the 1940s, is presently recognized in only eleven, but additions to the list will likely be made soon.[24]

Already by the 1920s, however, enough state legislatures had capitulated to alternative practitioners' appeals for medical democracy as to force the orthodox profession to adopt a new strategy, a campaign for so-called basic science laws. While opposition to the licensing of any practitioners other than M.D.'s could indeed appear monopolistic and tyrannical, allopaths recognized, there was a good amount of disinterested reason to be seen in the argument that any person presuming to treat the diseased human body should have at least some knowledge of the basic biological sciences. The argument was especially compelling in the wake of the Flexner Report, which had profoundly impressed the public with the ideal of a new medicine grounded in the modern biological sciences of bacteriology, biochemistry, physiology, pathology, and the like (what in the early years of the century the medical profession self-consciously referred to as "scientific medicine"). Consequently, mainstream practitioners in many states began lobbying for new laws that would require applicants for a license in any school of practice to pass an examination in anatomy, physiology, pathology, and other areas of science fundamental to understanding health and disease before taking the licensing test in their special system of therapy. To M.D.'s, it was as straightforward a matter as could be. Our "cards are placed upon the table face-up," Oregon's physicians announced, "and the fight is clear-cut as being between scientific and unscientific medicine."[25]

Alternative practitioners fought back, not surprisingly, but it was not so easy to paint basic science legislation as an assault on individual freedom as it had been to put restrictions against nonallopathic therapies in that light. Irregular doctors were not, after all, being barred from practice altogether, but simply were being asked to demonstrate more clearly that they knew what they were doing. "With the education necessary to pass such a board," it was pointed out, "the sincere therapeutic enthusiast, be he osteopath, chiropractor, electrotherapist, faith-healer, or herb-doctor, will probably not do much harm to the individual, or be a source of danger to the public health." The first basic science act was signed into law in 1925, in Wisconsin; within four years, six states and the District of Columbia had followed suit, and ultimately twenty-three states would adopt such laws.[26]

At first the laws produced the effect desired by allopaths. In Washington State, for example, in the two years preceding the 1927 statute there had actually been more chiropractors licensed than M.D.'s (47 allopaths, 48 chiropractors, 44 sanipractors [naturopaths], and 38 osteopaths). In the two years following the act, the numbers were 80 doctors of medicine, 6 osteopaths, 1 chiropractor, and no drugless healers (it should be noted that it was the rule in all states to preclude bias by blinding examiners to the school of practice of individual test takers). In Nebraska, 122 osteopathic licenses had been granted during the eight-year period immediately before the basic science law, but only 21 were issued for the eight years after; for chiropractors, the numbers were 290 before and zero after. For all states with boards in the late 1920s and early '30s, the rates of success on the basic science exam were 90 percent for allopaths, 63 percent for osteopaths, and 27 percent for chiropractors.[27]

As time passed, however, the allopathic profession became disgruntled with basic science laws for several reasons, not the least being the problems they posed for allopathic licensing reciprocity between states in which the examinations tested on different subjects. The laws backfired in another way, though, by forcing alternative healers to sink or swim. They chose to swim, and that meant they had to elevate the level of instruction they provided their students in medical science. Although it was a slow process, osteopaths, chiropractors, and naturopaths did steadily improve their pass rates, and basic science exams became a less effective sieve for separating "cultists" from scientists. Beginning in 1967, one state after another repealed its basic science law, until the last three disappeared in 1979.[28]

The most rapid progress in educational improvement was achieved by osteopathy, which in the early twentieth century steadily expanded its range of therapies to include first surgery, then drugs. By the time educational reform was undertaken in a serious way, in the mid-1930s, osteopathy was well along on the path to becoming a duplicate of allopathic medicine with osteopathic manipulation techniques attached. The reform effort was risky, it should be borne in mind, because unlike allopathic schools, osteopathic institutions received no public funding; they were financed almost entirely (more than 90 percent) by tuition fees, and by raising entrance requirements to the M.D. standard of two or more years of college, they would sharply decrease the size of their applicant pool. But with the basic science exam movement gathering momentum, they had little choice. Between 1936 and 1940 all six osteopathic schools adopted a two-years-of-college prerequisite. Concomitantly, facilities were expanded, the curriculum lengthened to four years, and more highly qualified instructors in the basic sciences hired. The schools managed to stay afloat financially by intensified fund-raising within the profession and aggressive recruiting of college students, and the evident commitment to improvement paid off in the decade following World War II with the first allocations of funds for osteopathic schools and hospitals from the federal government. Osteopaths' success rate on basic science exams shot up between 1942 and 1953, from 52 percent to 80 percent (the allopathic rate was 87 percent in the early 1950s), so forcefully demonstrating the profession's educational advancement as to attract the attention of the American Medical Association.[29]

In 1954, the AMA proposed to conduct inspections of osteopathic colleges comparable to the evaluation visits used for accrediting allopathic schools. One osteopathic institution declined the proposal as condescending, but the rest agreed to the survey, which was carried out early in 1955. The inspection committee, which included three medical school deans, determined that while osteopathic schools were still inferior to allopathic ones in several ways, they nevertheless were providing a "sound medical education." Students' records had been examined, and it had been found "that all had completed the education requirements for admission to medical school"; even more of a surprise was that "the records indicate that a considerable number could have obtained admission to medical school." Further, the committee observed, since osteopathic manipulative therapy now played only a subordinate, and declining, role in theoretical and clinical instruction, "the teaching in these colleges does not fall into the 'cultist' category."[30]

Chiropractic underwent a similar evolution, efforts to upgrade education beginning in the 1910s but making little headway until the 1930s and the appearance of the profession's own Flexner, one John Nugent. Nugent had particular reason to shoulder the task of educational reform—in the early 1920s he had been expelled from the Palmer School of Chiropractic for "disrespect and insult to the President." In 1935, the National Chiropractic Association appointed Nugent director of education and charged him with overhauling the profession's training system. For the next quarter century he pressed for entrance requirements of at least a high school education and standardization of programs at four years of instruction, with more and better educated faculty and expanded clinical facilities. Nugent pushed for smaller schools to close or merge, and for all institutions to be made nonprofit. The nonprofit part did not sit well with many schools' administrators (Nugent became "the most hated name in chiropractic," one observer commented), but over time he got his way. By 1960 most schools of chiropractic had adopted the Nugent standards, and the quality of training would continue to rise through the rest of the century.[31]

Naturopaths were initially less successful at raising professional standards, but by 1940 leaders of the American Naturopathic Association had resolved to rid their profession of "driftwood from wrecks of poor schools," and to that end had organized a National Board of Naturopathic Examiners to work for standard requirements of a high school diploma for entrance and a full four years of coursework for graduation. As with chiropractic, however, the higher standards program encountered resistance from the affected schools; "indeed," one leader of the reform effort lamented as late as 1951, "their direct opposition is surprisingly considerable." That opposition reflected an internal disarray following the death of leader Benedict Lust that was for a time, at least, the undoing of naturopathy (at one point in the 1950s there were six separate national organizations for naturopathy). The situation did not begin to be reversed until the 1970s, and not until 1980, with the founding of the American Association of Naturopathic Physicians, would some measure of cohesion be brought to the field and educational standards be significantly raised. Bastyr University, established in 1978 as John Bastyr College of Naturopathic Medicine, has been the pacesetter in the modernization of naturopathic education.[32]

In the meantime, the rising tide of osteopathic medicine was lifting all alternative medical boats. As has been seen, by the 1950s osteopathic medical schools had so successfully achieved the Flexnerian standard of education as to be recognized as more or less the equals of allopathic institutions. A more concrete and dramatic demonstration of having transcended cultist status came about in 1961, when the state medical and osteopathic associations in California agreed to a merger in which the osteopathic medical school in Los Angeles was converted into an allopathic school, and more than two thousand osteopathic physicians, hoping for enhanced social and economic status, had their D.O. degrees transformed into M.D.'s. The medical society's rationale for the measure was that the two professions were now essentially identical, and merging would eliminate confusion and inefficiency; others suspected allopathy of promoting its own economic interests by gobbling up the competition. Whatever the balance of motives, for a period it did indeed seem that, in California at least, osteopathic medicine might be fully absorbed by the majority profession. That failed to occur, but the fact that the California osteopathic school had overnight and with little change been turned into an accredited M.D.-granting institution impressed both state and federal legislators and officials as evidence that there was no longer any basis for thinking of osteopathy as an inferior form of medical practice. One of the most important demonstrations of newfound respect was the opening of state-supported schools of osteopathy, beginning with Michigan State University College of Osteopathic Medicine in 1969; during the 1970s several more state-funded schools were established. At the national level, the U.S. Civil Service Commission announced in 1963 a new policy of considering D.O. and M.D. degrees as equal, referring specifically to the California merger as justification for the decision.[33]

Three years later, Secretary of Defense Robert McNamara brought an end to one of osteopaths' longest-standing grievances, their exclusion from medical practice in the armed forces. This in fact had been a century-long sore spot for all the alternative systems: in World War I, Lust accused the federal government of "treason" for "keeping drugless physicians out of the country's service." Osteopaths had protested most loudly, though, and after being shut out of two world wars and the Korean conflict, they finally won acknowledgment of their acceptability for military practice just as the American involvement in Vietnam began to escalate. A more telling sign of acceptance had come the year before, in 1965, when osteopathic medical services were specified for reimbursement under the newly established Medicare system.[34]

Chiropractic and naturopathy also appealed for inclusion in Medicare but were denied at first on identical grounds: the secretary of Health, Education and Welfare determined for each that their "theory and practice are not based upon the body of basic knowledge related to health, disease, and health care that has been widely accepted by the scientific community." That determination was applauded most loudly by the American Medical Association, which only shortly before, in 1963, had established a Committee on Quackery whose chief assignment was "to contain and eliminate chiropractic" (naturopathy, on the wane at the time, seemed to be on the verge of eliminating itself). Three years later, the AMA's House of Delegates reaffirmed that position by decreeing that "chiropractic is an unscientific cult whose practitioners lack the necessary training and background to diagnose and treat human disease." Subsequently, the association's members were regularly reminded that "all voluntarily associated activities with cultists are unethical."[35]

Chiropractors refused to surrender. Their first counterattack was launched against the Medicare system; then they went after organized medicine itself. On the Medicare front, chiropractors used the tactic that had worked so well early in the century in keeping unlicensed practitioners out of jail, that of mobilizing satisfied patients to demand justice. "Manufactured mail campaigns" (the phrase is the AMA's) deluged federal legislators with an estimated twelve million letters and telegrams. "Congressional aides were reportedly astonished over the sacks of prochiropractic mail, which never seemed to diminish"—and which demanded "health freedom," the right of the public to choose the type of care they received. "The fallacy of such an argument appears obvious," critics of chiropractic retorted; "should we license and give Medicare dollars to alchemists, witches, herbalists, health food therapists, faith healers, etc., on the assumption that the consumer will be wise enough to choose the proper kind of care?" If chiropractors did somehow manage to win coverage, another suggested, they should be dealt with in the same manner as other unquestioned threats to public health: since "chiropractic constitutes a hazard to the public at least as great as smoking cigarettes," practitioners should be required to prominently display in their office a sign stating "Warning: The Department of Health, Education and Welfare Has Determined That the Chiropractic Method (Unscientific Cultism) Is Dangerous to Your Health." Chiropractic nevertheless was granted admission into the Medicare system in 1974, and over the course of the next decade chiropractic services came to be covered by virtually every major health insurance carrier and to be included in all states' workmen's compensation plans; even the Internal Revenue Service began to allow taxpayers to deduct the costs of chiropractic care as a medical expense.[36]

Two years after overcoming allopathic opposition to inclusion under Medicare, chiropractic turned the tables on the AMA, filing suit against the association (along with the American Hospital Association, the American College of Surgeons, and nine other medical organizations, including the American Osteopathic Association) for violation of the Sherman Antitrust Act. The intent of the AMA's Code of Ethics, particularly its renewed consultation clause, it was alleged, was primarily economic, an effort to restrain competition. The court battle was a protracted one, dragging on until 1987, but in the end, the U.S. District Court for the Northern District of Illinois decided against organized medicine in the case of *Wilk v. AMA* (C. A. Wilk was one of five Illinois chiropractors who initiated the action). Although the court allowed that the AMA had fought chiropractic out of "a genuine concern for scientific methods in patient care," it found that the belief that adjustments were unscientific was insufficient to justify "a nationwide conspiracy to eliminate a licensed profession." Further, the court ruled that the association had failed to prove that its repudiation of chiropractic as unscientific was "objectively reasonable." An injunction was issued permanently forbidding the AMA "from restricting, regulating or impeding" any of its members or any hospitals or other medical institutions from associating professionally with chiropractors. The final slap was the requirement that the association publish the injunction order in its journal, and send copies—"first class mail, postage prepaid"—to all its members. The AMA appealed the decision but was refused by the United States Supreme Court in 1990.[37]

Even before the unfavorable judgment was handed down, however, the AMA had retreated from its exclusionary stand on chiropractic. In 1979, the association adopted a new policy that acknowledged that some chiropractic treatments might indeed be of benefit despite the unscientific theory behind them, and allowed that not all chiropractors "should be equated with cultists. It is better to call attention to the limitations of chiropractic in the treatment of particular ailments than to label chiropractic an 'unscientific cult.'" The following year, all restrictions on consultation were lifted, members now being left "free to choose whom to serve, with whom they associate, and the environment in which to provide medical services." To be sure, the association backed off not so much because of a change of heart on the merits of chiropractic care as out of a desire to avoid costly lawsuits and unfavorable publicity. The effect was nonetheless the same, a new level of legitimacy for practitioners of chiropractic.[38]

Chiropractors were not alone. By the 1980s, alternative healers generally were enjoying a degree of popular acceptance unequaled since the mid-1800s, benefitting on one hand from public frustration with mainstream medicine and on the other from the fallout from what Norman Cousins called, in 1979, "the holistic health explosion." The decade of the 1970s bore witness to an extraordinary outpouring of frustration and exhausted patience with conventional medicine. A wave of books such as Illich's *Medical Nemesis*, McKeown's *The Role of Medicine*, Carlson's *The End of Medicine*, and Millman's *The Unkindest Cut*, not to mention numerous articles in lay periodicals, repeatedly took the profession to task for a catalogue of sins of both commission and omission.[39]

Prior to that time, allopathic medicine and the American public had enjoyed an extended honeymoon that dated back to Flexner and the era of "scientific medicine" and had strongly intensified with the introduction of sulfa drugs in the 1930s and antibiotics in the 1940s. So enamored was society with the "wonder drugs" that by the 1950s it could be fairly stated that "most patients are as completely under the supposedly scientific yoke of modern medicine as any primitive savage is under the superstitious serfdom of the tribal witch doctor." Yet by then it was already becoming evident that wonder drugs were not in-variably wonderful, that they could produce side effects of quite serious proportions. That was unsettling enough, but a good bit more disturbing was the realization that many physicians were dispensing the potentially hazardous substances indiscriminately, pre-scribing penicillin as if it were synonymous with panacea. "Antibiotic abandon" was the way an American authority on adverse drug effects described his colleagues' behavior dur-ing the 1950s, while the British journal *Lancet* spoofed the profession's heedless enthusi-asm by announcing "yet another wonder drug," the compound "3 blindmycin."[40]

The dangers of untoward reactions to drugs would be imprinted upon public awareness even more forcefully by the thalidomide tragedy of the 1960s, after which it became com-monplace to attack allopathic medicine as dangerous. Illich's first sentence in *Medical Nemesis*, for example, accused "the medical establishment" of having become "a major threat to health"; shortly after, he referred to doctor-induced illness as an "epidemic." Alternative practitioners of course exploited the new drug anxiety, chiropractors of the 1970s, for example, distributing pamphlets with titles such as *Drug-Caused Diseases* and *Drugs—Dangerous Whether Pushed or Prescribed.*[41]

Medicine's critics were bothered not simply by the physical threat posed by new drugs, however, but equally by what antibiotic abandon appeared to say about the physician-patient relationship. Blindmycin could be thought of as the successor to the bleeding and purging favored by nineteenth-century allopaths: it seemed antibiotics were routinely ad-ministered for any and all physical complaints, without attention to a patient's individual-ity. As early as the 1950s complaints were already accumulating that physicians were giving less time to physical examinations and patient histories because the treatment was likely to be the same whatever the diagnosis: this "new generation" of practitioners, an infectious-diseases expert objected, was "substituting antibiotics for thinking."[42]

Until the 1970s, however, such misgivings were effectively drowned out by all the huzzahs for scientific medicine. Only then did there at last erupt a full-scale revolt against not just routine prescribing of drugs and physician indifference toward patients, but above all against the mind-set of biological reductionism that fostered such attitudes. As with any revolt, there was an archvillain to be overthrown. In this instance it was the renowned French philosopher René Descartes, ingloriously exhumed from the seventeenth century for having drawn a rigid distinction between mind and body that, it was charged, had turned medicine onto a path of denying any influence of the psyche upon the material body. As Carlson, for example, asserted in *The End of Medicine*, allopaths had, thanks to Descartes, "divided the body and mind and chosen the body as [their] focus," and from there "it was only a small step to equate the working of the human organism with the pre-cision of machine function."[43] Machines did not have minds, nor did they have emotions or spiritual qualities. The fundamental meaning of 1970s holism was medicine that repu-diated Cartesian dualism to embrace an understanding of human beings as organisms whose mental, emotional, and spiritual powers were fully integrated with, and affected the functioning of, their bodies.

That core meaning was conveyed by the use of the word *wholism,* as commonly em-ployed as *holism* in the early 1970s. The alternative spelling soon all but disappeared, how-ever, as the reaction widened to include so many other objections to the allopathic orientation beyond neglect of the whole patient. Taken singly, most of these objections were not new; many had been voiced since the 1950s at least. But under the heading of holism they were now combined into a single unified brief against the medical establishment.

First, it was argued, physicians trained as biomedical scientists were unable or unwilling to communicate with patients in terms the lay person could understand, and tended to be aloof and superior (the complaint was an old one, a Chicago woman of the 1920s, for example, relating that a physician she had recently seen "was as pompous as a New Zealand devil dancer"). The situation worsened as the century wore on, for the infectious diseases that had previously constituted the most common type of health threat came to be replaced in large measure by chronic ailments such as heart disease, cancer, and diabetes. Infection was an acute problem that usually could be quickly cured with the right antibiotic. Not only were chronic complaints difficult or impossible to cure, but by their protracted and disabling nature they imposed a severe emotional toll on sufferers. Physicians educated according to the model of "scientific medicine," trained for prompt and decisive physical interventions, were ill-equipped to provide the sensitive management of personal miseries needed by victims of chronic conditions. One of the memories that haunted an allopathic physician dying of cancer was all the time he had had to spend "upbraiding the medical profession for its callous conduct at the bedside."[44]

Sensitive personal handling of the sick was further handicapped, it was often charged, by the fragmentation of care resulting from medical specialization, a trend that had accelerated dramatically from the 1930s on. In 1930, more than 80 percent of allopathic physicians were general practitioners; by 1960, that percentage had fallen to 45, and the downward trajectory in numbers of generalists was so steep as to augur extinction of the species. Specialist care, by its nature, was episodic, restrained from providing the ongoing personal attention inherent to general practice. The fact that decreasing personal attention was being paralleled by increasing costs and that physicians' income was climbing while organized medicine was steadfastly opposing proposals for national health insurance further alienated the public from mainstream medicine. The growing expense of medicine figured into public dissatisfaction in still another way, as the 1970s witnessed more and more objections that all that money was not buying all that much health. America, it was pointed out repeatedly, possessed the most technically advanced medical system in the world, yet by measures such as life expectancy and infant mortality the nation finished well down on the list of industrialized countries. Even what improvements in health had occurred, critics now argued, were due much more to limitation of family size, improved nutrition, and environmental hygiene than to wonder drugs and miracle surgeries. "When contrasted with all the other factors that demonstrably affect health," Carlson wrote, "medicine plays a minor role, despite being cast for lead"; the contribution of medical care to improved health, in fact, was one of an "insignificance [that] cannot be overemphasized."[45]

Broader social forces pushed the process of alienation forward as well. The "secular humanism" counterculture of the 1960s, with its rebellion against authority, distrust of science and technology, concern for individual rights, and promotion of consumerism, necessarily aroused hostility toward establishment medicine. At the same time, counterculture rhetoric extolling the virtues of the simple, natural life and toleration of diverse lifestyles and cultures (particularly of the oppressed) burnished the appeal of the medical counterculture.[46]

All these concerns and values went into the molding of a remarkably broad medical philosophy. Details varied somewhat from one advocate to the next, but one can nevertheless identify certain principles central to essentially all versions of holism. Relating to and treating the whole patient was the cornerstone, of course, but just as fundamental was recognition of the healing power of nature. The holistic physician "uses therapeutic approaches that mobilize the individual's innate capacity for self-healing," one of holism's

pioneers explained; "practitioners view themselves as midwives to the body's own resources." Similarly, the 1978 *Holistic Health Handbook* was actually dedicated "to the search
for the universal healer within us all," while one of the best-selling books in the nonfiction
category in the 1970s was Norman Cousins' *Anatomy of an Illness*, in which the editor of
the *Saturday Review* told the inspirational story of how he overcame a degenerative illness
diagnosed as incurable through the stimulating effects of laughter on his "life-force" (it
might be noted that Cousins had been anticipated by a naturopath in the 1910s who had
written a book titled *The Laugh Cure*; in the 1920s another drugless healer put forward
"phobiotherapy," or the "fear-cure").⁴⁷   Cousins' wife was dosing him homeopathically +
he didn't know it

Engaging the healer within implied a deeper involvement of the patient in diagnosis,
treatment, and recovery than was usually encouraged or allowed by allopathic physicians.
In his widely read *The Role of Medicine*, McKeown submitted that one of the chief reasons
conventional medicine should be thought of as "sinister" was that "it usurps the right of the
individual to face, deal with, and bear his own health problems." Biomedicine was inclined
to dictate to the patient and impose treatment upon him or her rather than invite a collaboration. Already in the 1920s, a patient had protested that "medicine treats you merely as
an objective—a clod of a thing to be worked upon," whereas irregular doctors "make you a
factor in your own healing." True healing could not occur, holists maintained, until the
patient was enlisted as an ally and made to feel responsible for bringing him- or herself
back to health by acting on the healer's guidance and encouragement. "The principal contribution" of his physician, Cousins asserted, "was that he encouraged me to believe I was
a respected partner with him in the total undertaking." Emphasis on prevention, and the
interpretation of health as "high level wellness" instead of the mere absence of disease,
were still other aspects of the multifaceted philosophy of medical holism.⁴⁸

By 1980, *holistic* had become one of American culture's hottest buzzwords, an obligatory descriptor of anything new and good and nonallopathic that was thrown around in
conversation and print, one observer quipped, "as enthusiastically as a frisbee in the
springtime." Novel as it seemed, however, it was only an updated statement of principles
that had formed the core of the alternative medical heresy for two centuries. What was new
was the interest in holism being shown by the orthodox school of practice. The 1970s provided fertile soil not just for the resurgence of alternative systems, but also for a revolt
within allopathic medicine against the reductionist "biomedical model" of disease and
treatment that had ruled the profession throughout the century. Thanks primarily to insights developed within the fields of family medicine and psychosomatic medicine, critics
of biomedicine succeeded in establishing a "biopsychosocial model" of illness that blended
mental, emotional, and social factors with the patient's organic pathology.⁴⁹

The biopsychosocial movement came to a head in 1979 with the founding of the American
Holistic Medical Association (AHMA), an organization of mainstream practitioners who
announced themselves to be "dedicated to the concept of medicine of the whole person
which emphasizes integration of body, mind, and spirit with the environment." Espousal
of such an orientation was no longer news in allopathic circles, of course, but organizing a
professional society primarily to advance that viewpoint was. Even more striking, however,
was the AHMA's acceptance that "this process of integration may demand combination of
both orthodox and non-damaging unorthodox approaches." That hint that the door might
be opened to alternative therapies to collaborate in the holistic care of patients was soon
made explicit. As early as the third issue of the association's *Journal of Holistic Medicine*, the

editor listed ten "interrelated fields of knowledge" that were acceptable as subject matter for articles; these included predictable items (nutrition, exercise, psychotherapy) but also two surprises, acupuncture (which had only occasionally been discussed seriously in mainstream journals before) and homeopathy (hitherto mentioned by allopaths only for purposes of derision). Further, the editor immediately added that the journal would give "special emphasis" to any of the "less well-known and non-traditional methods of diagnosis and treatment which are safe and effective."[50]

Receptivity to alternative approaches was a characteristic as well of the holistic health centers that allopathic physicians established in significant number from the mid-1970s on. In part an outgrowth of the free clinics opened in Haight-Ashbury and elsewhere to serve the disaffected youth of the 1960s, holistic health centers publicly professed to a medical philosophy essentially identical to that of alternative medical systems: addressing the psychological and spiritual needs of patients, catering to the unique needs of each individual, giving preference to therapies that encourage self-healing, promoting wellness through patient education, and the like, including the employment of alternative methods where useful.[51]

M.D.'s advocating holistic medicine met with skepticism from colleagues, of course, and much of it was justified. As the definition of *holistic* expanded, after all, it came to be thought of as a synonym for *nonallopathic*. The result was that the holistic explosion was not just a burst of interest in the tenets of holism, but an explosion of megaton proportions in the number of therapies set before the public with the label of "holistic medicine" affixed. Reflexology and Rolfing, suggestology and shiatsu, megavitamin therapy and dream work, Native American medicine and Tibetan medicine: all manner of practitioners devoted to freeing one's inner healer rushed to link arms under the holistic umbrella, and many—the empathologists, for example ("Empathology facilitates your Personal Truth . . . finds and clears the underlying causes of your life and health issues")—possessed dubious skills. There was good reason for one of allopathic medicine's most prominent spokesmen to complain that while there was "a valuable message in the holistic movement," the principle of treating the whole patient was "distorted by the palpable quackery and silliness of much that calls itself holistic."[52]

Among the laity, however, enthusiasm for holistic remedies grew unabated; sales of homeopathic remedies, for instance, increased a full 1,000 percent during the decade of the 1980s. That burgeoning public support, coupled with mounting evidence that certain alternative methods were truly effective and the hope that low-tech alternative therapies might be a way to rein in runaway medical costs, culminated at last in the most remarkable political endorsement of alternative medicine in the century. In 1991, the United States Senate committee responsible for funding the National Institutes of Health, convinced that "the conventional medical community" had not "fully explored the potential that exists in unconventional medical practices," instructed the NIH to appoint a panel to develop a research program to evaluate the efficacy of "the most promising" alternative therapies. This panel, christened the Office of Alternative Medicine, convened in June of the following year, greeted by some as "the Berlin wall [of medicine] coming down," denounced by others as akin to an "Office of Astrology."[53]

Though provided with a budget of only $2 million ("a homeopathic level of funding," the director of the office joked), the OAM was soon inundated with more than four hundred applications for research support. Initially, only two proposals were funded (1994), one from the University of Minnesota Medical School, the other from Bastyr University, the leading naturopathic school. The following year, OAM grants were awarded to eight more institutions, all allopathic medical schools, including such prestigious representatives of orthodox medicine as Harvard, Columbia, and Stanford. Critics could protest that the government was "buying snake oil with tax dollars," wasting money studying "superstition masquerading as science," but funding for OAM grew rapidly nonetheless, increasing sevenfold by 1996 (for 2001, the appropriation was $110 million, some fifty-five times the original budget for the office). Meanwhile, tax support for alternative medicine was appearing at the local level as well. In February 1995, the council for Washington State's King County (which encompasses Seattle, long a hotbed of alternative medicine) unanimously approved the establishment of a clinic to provide naturopathy, acupuncture, and other alternative treatments in conjunction with orthodox therapy. The King County Natural Medicine Clinic opened in 1996, the first publicly funded alternative medical institution in the country; the contract for organizing and managing the clinic was awarded to Bastyr University.[54]

A major consideration in King County's adoption of alternative medicine was the hope that expenditures for medical care would be lowered. "We want insurance companies to see how effective natural medicine is," stated the council chair, who had a Ph.D. in chemistry; "we want to give patients more effective options and in doing that, reduce the overall cost of health care." Soon the state was cooperating with the county, enacting a law that took effect January 1, 1996, requiring every health insurance plan in Washington to cover claims for services provided by all licensed practitioners, including chiropractors, naturopaths, acupuncturists, and massage therapists. This was the first such law in the United States, but already health maintenance organizations (HMOs) throughout the country were including some alternative procedures (most frequently chiropractic) among their services; by 1999, nearly two-thirds of the nation's HMOs offered coverage of at least one alternative method.[55]

Examples of growing acceptance of alternative medicine, and of increasing collaboration between mainstream and heretofore fringe practitioners, could be multiplied several times over. Certainly one of the most remarkable is the establishment, in 1996, of the Program in Integrative Medicine within the Department of Medicine at the University of Arizona, a major allopathic medical school. Designed to provide two-year fellowships for allopathically trained physicians who have completed residencies in family medicine or internal medicine, the program "seeks to combine the best ideas and practices of conventional and alternative medicine into cost-effective treatments. . . . It neither rejects conventional medicine nor embraces alternative practices uncritically." In short, the two-century-old battle between allopaths and irregulars seems to be ending, and concluding not in a truce but in an alliance. Suddenly "we find ourselves," the editor of *The Integrator* has recently written, "in an era beyond the polarization of alternative medicine and conventional medicine," with "an opportunity to become a seamless part of an integrated system that might rightfully be called, simply, *health care.*"[56]

Numerous practical obstacles to integration remain, but there is a spirit of cooperation about overcoming them that could scarcely have been imagined before the last quarter of the twentieth century. One wishes that a certain naturopath from the early 1900s could have somehow survived to the present to witness the new environment. In 1918, trying to picture what the best of all medical worlds would be like, he proposed that it would include exchanges between the American Medical Association and the American Naturopathic

Association in which each might "appoint a representative or committee whose sole duty will be to ascertain the points of greater wisdom and excellence *in the other association.* The A.M.A. could say to the A.N.A.—'We are doubtless making serious mistakes, which your superior knowledge would enable us to correct. Please inform and reform us.' Then the A.N.A. would reply to the A.M.A.—'Not so, brothers. We, verily, are the bunglers—will you not graciously condescend to show *us* the better way?' Each would thus become a regular Alphonse of courtesy to the other's Gaston of humility." At that point, he came to his senses, realizing how absurd a vision he had conjured up. "I have to stop here," he sighed; "such a spectacle takes my breath entirely away, and I must needs recover from the shock."[57]

CONTRIBUTORS

Michael Ackerman is a graduate student in the Department of History at the University of Virginia. He is currently working on a Ph.D. dissertation on the contested and fluid reception given to the newer knowledge of nutrition in the United States between the 1910s and the 1970s.

Amy Sue Bix is an associate professor in the History Department at Iowa State University and assistant director of ISU's Center for Historical Studies of Technology and Science. Her book *Inventing Ourselves out of Jobs?: America's Debate over Technological Unemployment, 1929–1981* was published by Johns Hopkins University Press in 2000. She has also published on the history of breast cancer and AIDS research, on the history of eugenics, on the history of home economics, and on post–World War II physics and engineering, among other subjects. She is currently finishing a book entitled *Engineering Education for American Women: An Intellectual, Institutional, and Social History.*

Barbara Clow is a social historian of medicine, specializing in twentieth-century North America. She has published on various aspects of the history of medicine, including the history of cancer, doctor-patient relations, alternative medicine, and illness metaphors. Her book *Negotiating Disease: Power and Cancer Care, 1900–1950* was published in 2001 by McGill-Queen's University Press, and she is currently working on a history of thalidomide in North America. Dr. Clow is director of the Atlantic Centre of Excellence for Women's Health, Dalhousie University, Halifax, Canada.

Nadav Davidovitch, M.D., M.P.H., is a lecturer in the Department of Health Systems Management, Ben Gurion University. He has recently submitted his Ph.D. dissertation to the Cohn Institute for the History and Philosophy of Science, Tel Aviv University. His thesis, on the relationship between homeopathy and scientific medicine, is titled "Framing Scientific Medicine: American Homeopaths Quest for Professional Identity, 1870–1930." His current research is on the social history of resistance to vaccination and on health and immigration in Israel.

Wade Davies is an assistant professor of Native American studies at the University of Montana in Missoula. He earned a B.A. from Indiana University and then studied American Indian history at Arizona State University, where he earned a Ph.D. After completing his book *Healing Ways: Navajo Health Care in the Twentieth Century* (2001), Davies spent three years teaching at San Juan College in Farmington, New Mexico, near the Navajo Nation.

Otniel E. Dror, M.D., Ph.D., is lecturer and head of the Section for the History of Medicine at the Hebrew University of Jerusalem, Israel. He received his M.D. from Ben-Gurion University (1989) and his Ph.D. in history from Princeton University (1998). His contribution to this collection is part of a new project on the cultural history of modern excitement and death. His book *The Science of Passion: Modernity, Excitement, and the Study of Emotions, 1880–1950* is forthcoming with Stanford University Press. Recent publications have appeared in *Isis* (1999), *Configurations* (1999), *Social Research* (2001), and *Science in Context* (2001).

Georgina Feldberg is an associate professor of social science at York University, Toronto, where she teaches in health and society, women's studies, and history. Her book *Disease and Class: Tuberculosis and the Shaping of Modern North American Society* (1995) received the Hannah Medal from the Royal Society of Canada. Her recent work explores the history of women and health in late-twentieth-century North America. She is co-author of *Women, Health and Nation* (2003). From 1992 to 2001 she was director of the York University Centre for Health Studies and academic director of the National Network on Environments and Women's Health.

Jonathan David Geczik was a professor of political science at the Community College of Allegheny County. Along with Matthew Schneirov he is the author of *A Diagnosis for Our Times: Alternative Health—From Lifeworld to Politics* (2003).

David J. Hess is professor of Science and Technology Studies at Rensselaer Polytechnic Institute. He has published a dozen books and numerous articles that make contributions to social studies of medicine, the environment, science, and technology. Among his projects is research on the movement for less toxic and more efficacious cancer therapies in the United States, which resulted in books such as *Women Confront Cancer* (with Margaret Wooddell, New York University Press), *Can Bacteria Course Cancer?* and *Evaluating Alternative Cancer Therapies.* He is currently working on issues of health, sustainability, and social movements, for which some publications are available at his Web site, http://home.earthlink.net/~davidhesshomepage. Hess is the recipient of the Diana Forsythe Prize for his work in the anthropology of science, technology, and medicine, and his recent work has been supported by the National Science Foundation and Fulbright Commission.

Velana Huntington is an adjunct assistant professor in the Department of Anthropology at the University of Iowa. Her research has focused on notions of embodiment, health, and healing within Orisha, a Yoruba-derived religion, as it is encountered in the midwestern United States. Her current research interests include health and healing, feminist medical anthropology, embodiment, and the narratives of homeless children and families.

Robert D. Johnston is associate professor and director of the Teaching of History Program in the History Department at the University of Illinois at Chicago. His book *The Radical Middle Class: Populist Democracy and the Question of Capitalism in Progressive Era Portland, Oregon* (2003), which contains a section on anti-vaccination movements, won the 2002 President's Book Award of the Social Science History Association. He has taught at Buena Vista College in Storm Lake, Iowa, and in the history department at Yale University, where he was also an associate fellow in the History of Medicine Program at Yale Medical School. During 2001–2002, he was a visiting lecturer in the American Studies program at the Hebrew University in Jerusalem. Johnston delivered a paper at the National Vaccine Information Center's Second International Public Conference on Vaccination in 2000, and he is a member of the Centers for Disease Control's Vaccine Risk Communication workgroup. He is also co-editor of *The Middling Sorts: Explorations in the History of the American Middle Class* (Routledge, 2001, with Burton J. Bledstein) and *The Countryside in the Age of the Modern State: Political Histories of Rural America* (2001, with Catherine McNicol Stock).

Anne Taylor Kirschmann is an independent scholar and lecturer in American history at the University of Massachusetts, Dartmouth. Her research interests include nineteenth-century health reform and twentieth-century alternative medicine, as well as women in the health professions. She is the author of *A Vital Force: Women in American Homeopathy* (2003).

Michelle M. Nickerson is a visiting professor of history in the William P. Clements Jr. Department of History at Southern Methodist University. She is completing her Ph.D. in the American Studies Program at Yale University. Nickerson has delivered conference papers and published essays relating to her dissertation, "Domestic Threats: Women, Gender and Conservatism in Cold War Los Angeles."

Sita Reddy is an independent scholar and sociologist whose research lies at the intersections of alternative medicine, sociology of science, and museum studies. She received a Ph.D. in sociology from the University of Pennsylvania for her thesis on the reinvention and professionalization of New Age Ayurveda in contemporary America. Most recently, she was a postdoctoral fellow at the Penn Center for Bioethics as part of an interdisciplinary project on the history, ethics, and politics of genetically modified foods. Her current work ranges from the history of cultural defense in criminal courts to the politics of display and representation in contemporary museums.

Gretchen Ann Reilly is a professor of history at Temple Junior College, Temple, Texas. She received her Ph.D. from George Washington University in 2001. She is currently working on a detailed history of the fluoridation controversy.

Naomi Rogers is an assistant professor in the Section of the History of Medicine and the Women's and Gender Studies Program at Yale University. She is the author of *Dirt and Disease: Polio before FDR* (1992) and *An Alternative Path: The Making and Remaking of Hahnemann Medical College and Hospital of Philadelphia* (1998). She is currently working on a book on Sister Kenny, with the working title of *Healer from the Outback: Sister Elizabeth Kenny and American Medicine, 1940–1952.*

Matthew Schneirov is an associate professor of sociology at Duquesne University in Pittsburgh. He is the author of *The Dream of a New Social Order: Popular Magazines in America: 1893–1914.* Along with Jonathan David Geczik, he is also the author of *A Diagnosis for Our Times: Alternative Health—From Lifeworld to Politics* (2003). His current work explores health concerns in turn-of-the-century American popular culture.

James C. Whorton received a BS in chemistry from Duke University in 1964 and a Ph.D. in history of science from the University of Wisconsin in 1969. He has taught medical history at the University of Washington School of Medicine since 1970, and is the author of four books and numerous articles on various aspects of the history of medicine. His most recent publication is *Nature Cures: The History of Alternative Medicine in America* (2002).

NOTES

Introduction

My thanks to Nadav Davidovitch, David Hess, Michelle Nickerson, and Naomi Rogers for their helpful comments.

1. Paul Starr, *The Social Transformation of American Medicine: The Rise of a Sovereign Profession and the Making of a Vast Industry* (New York: Basic Books, 1984), 127.

2. Just one sign that scholars are starting to recognize alternative medicine's contested chronology is Rennie B. Schoepflin's excellent *Christian Science on Trial: Religious Healing in America* (Baltimore: Johns Hopkins University Press, 2003). Schoepflin seeks to "challenge the sunny assumptions made by many historians regarding the confidence of the medical profession about who would control the future of American health care" during the early twentieth century. He argues that rather than a "death struggle," "a relationship of complexity or convergence had evolved between spiritual healing and medical practice." Overall, Schoepflin observes, "American physicians lacked a strong position of cultural authority over health care until after the 1920s" (2–3). An earlier statement of this perspective came from James Cassedy, who highlighted "[t]he flourishing of medical diversity between 1865 and 1940." Noting "the remarkable . . . failure of the regular medical establishment, despite its new strength, to prevent the emergence of new sects," Cassedy argues that these "came to play far more than token roles in fostering a continuing skepticisim of, if not actual resistance to, orthodox medical authority." See James H. Cassedy, *Medicine in America: A Short History* (Baltimore: Johns Hopkins University Press, 1991), 96, 99. On the other hand, Hans Baer, while emphasizing pluralism in the overall history of American medicine, still adopts Starr's chronology, as well as his assumptions about the "dominance" of orthodox medicine. See Hans A. Baer, *Biomedicine and Alternative Healing Systems in America: Issues of Class, Race, Ethnicity, and Gender* (Madison: University of Wisconsin Press, 2001), esp. 31–49.

3. Although the other primary works in the history of American alternative medicine have not completely neglected politics, neither have they explored the political realm as much as they might have. See Norman Gevitz, ed., *Other Healers: Unorthodox Medicine in America* (Baltimore: Johns Hopkins University Press, 1988) and James C. Whorton, *Nature Cures: The History of Alternative Medicine in America* (New York: Oxford University Press, 2002).

4. David M. Eisenberg et al., "Unconventional Medicine in the United States: Prevalence, Costs, and Patterns of Use," *New England Journal of Medicine* 328 (1993): 246–52; David M. Eisenberg et al., "Trends in Alternative Medicine Use in the United States, 1990–1997," *Journal of the American Medical Association* 280 (1998): 1569–75. For Harvard Medical School faculty member Eisenberg's effective canonization in the popular media as *the* authority on alternative medicine, see the special report "The Science of Alternative Medicine" in *Newsweek*, December 2, 2002, 45–75.

5. Louis S. Reed, *The Healing Cults: A Study of Sectarian Medical Practice: Its Extent, Causes, and Control* (Chicago: University of Chicago Press, 1932), 1.

6. Reed, *Healing Cults*, 3, 61, 106, 117; Annie Riley Hale, *"These Cults": An Analysis of the Foibles of Dr. Morris Fishbein's "Medical Follies"* (New York: National Health Foundation, 1926), 16, 14, 15, 19; E. C. Levy, "Reciprocity Between the Health Officials and the Medical Profession," *American Journal of Public Health* 13 (December 1923): 994; Edwards J. G. Beardsley, "Why the Public Consult the Pseudo Medical Cults," *Journal of the Medical Society of New Jersey* 21 (September 1924): 277; Irvin Arthur, "The Medical Profession and the People," *Journal of the Indiana State Medical Association* 16 (November 1923): 369. The results of the Chicago study appeared originally in the *Illinois Medical Journal* and received prominent public play in "What People Think of Their Doctors," *Literary Digest* September 22, 1923, 25–26.

Also worth noting is how concerned establishment officials were that "it seemed frequently to be the case that the more enlightened, in other knowledge than medical science, and apparently more progressive citizens of the various communities were the citizens who were consulting the representatives of the cults"; see Beardsley, "Why the Public," 276. Finally although lacking quantitative evidence, the screeds of chief AMA publicist Morris Fishbein against "medical follies" can be read not just as partial declarations of victory against quackery, but also as exasperation at the continued popularity of healing cults. See, for just one example, Fishbein's cataloguing of all the legislative attempts to legalize alternative medicine in

1931 alone in Morris Fishbein, *Fads and Quackery in Healing: An Analysis of the Foibles of the Healing Cults, with Essays on Various Other Peculiar Notions in the Health Field* (New York: Blue Ribbon Books, 1932), 200–2. In turn, Annie Riley Hale's response to Fishbein, *"These Cults,"* is an explicit and not necessarily fanciful celebration of "the medical world's scared realization of its waning supremacy over the minds of the masses" as well as "an emphatic protest against State Medicine" (viii, 13).

7. A critical perspective on Harkin's role in shaping the OAM comes in James Harvey Young, "The Development of the Office of Alternative Medicine in the National Institutes of Health, 1991–1996," *Bulletin of the History of Medicine* 72 (1998): 279–98.

8. Tom Harkin, "The Third Approach," *Alternative Therapies in Health and Medicine* 1, 1 (1995): 71; Orrin G. Hatch, "Alternative Medicine: Who Decides?" *Alternative Therapies in Health and Medicine* 1, 5 (1995): 96; Alex Stone, "Overtreated," *The New Republic*, February 10, 2003; "Orrin Hatch: Presidential Candidate, Chiropratic Advocate," http://www.chiroweb.com/archives/17/23/09.html; Stephanie Mencimer, "Scorin' with Orrin," *Washington Monthly*, September 2001; Paul Kurtz, "White House Commission on Complementary and Alternative Medicine Is Biased," *Skeptical Inquirer*, May/June 2001; Leon Jaroff, "Wasting Big Bucks on Alternative Medicine," *Time*, May 15, 2002; Jaroff, "Save Us from Alternative Medicine," *Time*, January 7, 2003. For a powerful account of Harkin's farm politics, see Mary Summers, "From the Heartland to Seattle: The Family Farm Movement of the 1980s and the Legacy of Agrarian State Building," in Catherine McNicol Stock and Robert D. Johnston, eds., *The Countryside in the Age of the Modern State: Political Histories of Rural America* (Ithaca: Cornell University Press, 2001), 304–5.

9. Michael S. Goldstein, *Alternative Health Care: Medicine, Miracle, or Mirage?* (Philadelphia: Temple University Press, 1999), 10–11 (see also for the same point at greater length 146–59 and 173–74); David A. Horowitz, *Beyond Left and Right: Insurgency and the Establishment* (Urbana: University of Illinois Press, 1997).

10. Phyllis Schlafly, *A Choice Not an Echo* (Alton, Ill.: Pere Marquette Press, 1964). For an early account of Schlafly's non-medical political activities, see Carol Felsenthal, *The Sweetheart of the Silent Majority: The Biography of Phyllis Schlafly* (Garden City, N.Y.: Doubleday, 1981).

11. See especially Schlafly, "Can Courts Order Kids to Take Drugs?" September 13, 2000, and "Is Ritalin Raising Kids to Be Drug Addicts?" June 21, 2000, both available on Schlafly's Ritalin Web page, http://www.eagleforum.org/topics/ritalin/ritalin.html; "Follow the Money on Vaccines," September 5, 2001; "Conflicts of Interest About Vaccines," February 2001; "Government Experiments on Humans?" February 2000; "Congressional Hearing Exposes Conflict of Interest," June 28, 2000; "No, We Can't Trust the Government," September 1999; all available at http://www.eagleforum.org/topics/vaccine/vaccine.html. For Roger Schlafly's Web page, go to http://www.mindspring.com/~schlafly/vac/.

12. For a short biography, see the Beyt Tikkun Syngagogue Web site, http://www.beyttikkun.org/bios.htm. For Lerner's perspective on the Clinton episode, see Michael Lerner, *The Politics of Meaning: Restoring Hope and Possibility in an Age of Cynicism* (Reading, Mass.: Addison-Wesley, 1997), 309–21.

13. Lerner, *Politics of Meaning*, 4–6, 16.

14. Lerner, *Politics of Meaning*, 273–74, 277, 279.

15. Many of the essays in this volume make substantial contributions to the study of feminism and/or populism. See in particular the articles by Bix, Feldberg, Rogers, Nickerson, Schneirov and Geczik, and Johnston. For an excellent recent exploration of populism and alternative medicine, see Eric S. Juhnke, *Quacks and Crusaders: The Fabulous Careers of John Brinkley, Norman Baker, and Harry Hoxsey* (Lawrence: University Press of Kansas, 2002). Juhnke too notes the "left/right" political connections of alternative medicine, although his focus is more on the right side of the spectrum (see especially 150–52). I also trace the populist foundation of alternative medicine in Robert D. Johnston, *The Radical Middle Class: Populist Democracy and the Question of Capitalism in Progressive Era Portland, Oregon* (Princeton: Princeton University Press, 2003), 177–220.

Negotiating Dissent

This research was partially funded by the Resident Research Fellowship of the Francis Clark Wood Institute for the History of Medicine of the College of Physicians of Philadelphia. An earlier version of this article was presented at the annual conference of the American Historical Association, San Francisco, 2002. I am grateful to the various librarians and archivists whose help was crucial for this work, especially Barbara Williams from the Archives and Special Collections of Allegheny University of the Health Sciences and Jack Eckert from the Rare Books and Special Collections Department, Countway Library of Medicine. Special thanks to Allan Brandt for his continuous support during my two-year stay in the History of Science Department at Harvard University, to the members of the History of Medicine Working Group there, and to Naomi Rogers for her encouragement and help. Finally, I would like to thank Robert Johnston for his patient and dedicated editorial work and for his vision and relentless efforts in putting this important volume together.

1. See, for example, "Ten Great Public Health Achievements—United States, 1900–1999," *Morbidity and Mortality Weekly Report* 48 (1999): 241–43.

2. For just few examples, see Judith Walzer Leavitt, *The Healthiest City: Milwaukee and the Politics of Health Reform* (Princeton: Princeton University Press, 1982), 76–121; Joan Retsinas, "Smallpox Vaccination: A Leap of Faith," *Rhode Island History* 38 (1979): 113–24; Nadja Durbach, "'They Might as Well Brand Us': Working-Class Resistance to Compulsory Vaccination in Victorian England," *Social History of Medicine* 13 (2000): 45–62.

3. Beyond the issue of smallpox vaccination in a time of potential bioterrorism, there are many current controversies surrounding vaccination in normal times, such as a possible tie between vaccination and autoimmune diseases and vaccination as a possible trigger of autism. See Robert D. Johnston's essay in this volume, "Contemporary Anti-vaccination Movements in Historical Perspective."

4. Edward Jenner, *An Inquiry into the Causes and Effects of the Variolae Vaccine, a Disease Discovered in some Western Counties of England, particularly Gloucestershire, and known by the Name of the Cow-Pox* (London, 1798). On the controversial character of Jenner and of the vaccine's discovery, see P. E. Razzel, *Edward Jenner's Cowpox Vaccine: The History of a Medical Myth*, 2nd ed. (Firle: Caliban, 1980) and Cyril William Dixon, *Smallpox* (London: Churchill, 1962).

5. In regard to the irrationality of opponents to vaccination, see Martin Kaufman, "The American Anti-Vaccinationists and Their Arguments," *Bulletin of the History of Medicine* 41 (1967): 471; Ann Beck, "Issues in the Anti-Vaccination Movement in England," *Medical History* 4 (1960): 317; and John Duffy, *The Sanitarians: A History of American Public Health* (Urbana: University of Illinois Press, 1990), 200.

6. See, for example, Robert D. Johnston, *The Radical Middle Class: Populist Democracy and the Question of Capitalism in Progressive Era, Portland, Oregon* (Princeton: Princeton University Press, 2003), 177–220, and Durbach, "'Might as Well Brand Us.'"

7. The most cited example is Kaufman's treatment of American anti-vaccinationists in the nineteenth century. See Kaufman, "American Anti-Vaccinationists." See also Judith Walzer Leavitt, "Politics and Public Health: Smallpox in Milwaukee, 1894–1895," *Bulletin of the History of Medicine* 50 (1976): 553–68 and n. 3.

8. See, for example, John Harley Warner, "Orthodoxy and Otherness: Homeopathy and Regular Medicine in nineteenth-Century America," in Robert Jütte, Guenter B. Risse, and John Woodward, eds., *Culture, Knowledge and Healing: Historical Perspectives of Homeopathic Medicine in Europe and North America* (Sheffield: European Association for the History of Medicine and Health Publications, 1998), 5–29.

9. International Hahnemannian Association Meeting of 1892, "Discussion on Vaccination," *Homoeopathic Physician* 12 (1892): 468–88.

10. C. A. Eaton, "Vaccins," *New England Medical Gazette* 52 (1917): 64–71.

11. See, for example, Kaufman, "American Anti-Vaccinationists"; Dorothy Porter and Roy Porter, "The Politics of Prevention: Anti-Vaccinationism and Public Health in Nineteenth Century England," *Medical History* 32 (1988): 231–52. An excellent criticism of past anti-vaccination historiography can be found in Johnston, *Radical Middle Class*, 179–185.

12. See Eberhard Wolff, "Sectarian Identity and the Aim of Integration: Attitudes of American Homeopaths Towards Smallpox Vaccination in the Late Nineteenth Century," in Robert Jütte, Guenter B. Risse, and John Woodward, eds., *Culture, Knowledge and Healing: Historical Perspectives of Homeopathic Medicine in Europe and North America* (Sheffield: European Association for the History of Medicine and Health Publications, 1998), 217–50.

13. Cited in Thomas Lindsley Bradford, *The Life and Letters of Samuel Hahnemann* (Philadelphia: Boericke and Tafel, 1895), 185–86. Sulphur was intended to counteract the possibility of transmitting "psoratic" or chronic influences from the source child.

14. Ibid.

15. See Constantine Hering, *The Homeopathic Domestic Physician* (Philadelphia: Boericke and Tafel, 1897), 387–92. See also Wolff, "Sectarian Identity," 221–22.

16. This question of how internal disputes within homeopathic circles on the vaccination question will be discussed further in the paper. Citation from D. H. Beckwith, "Vaccination," *Transactions of the American Institute of Homeopathy* 35 (1882): 342–62, discussion 363–77, 370, in Wolff, "Sectarian Identity," 233.

17. For one example, see Stuart Close, "The Truth and Error of Vaccination," *Homeopathic Physician* 12 (1892): 468–69.

18. D. P. Maddux, "The Significance of Bacteriological Discoveries to the Homœopathic Method of Treatment," *Hahnemannian Monthly* 28 (1892): 81–90.

19. S. Liliental, "Hahnemann, Hering and Swan: Pasteur and Koch," *Hahnemannian Monthly* 27 (1891): 91.

20. See, for example, Close, "The Truth and Error of Vaccination," 475–76.

21. J. Laurie, *An Epitome of the Homœopathic Domestic Medicine*, 41st ed. (London: Homoeopathic Publishing, 1914), 497–98.

22. See J. Compton Burnett, *Vaccinosis and Its Cure by Thuja, with Remarks on Homoeoprophylaxis*, 2nd ed. (1897; reprinted, New Delhi: B. Jain Publishers, 1999), 11. See also A. C. Cowperthwaite, *A Text-Book of Materia Medica and Therapeutics*, 11th ed. (Philadelphia Boericket Tafel, 1916): "Vaccination is more apt to cause bad results in sycotic constitutions, so we find Thuja a remedy for the bad effects of vaccination; especially when the pustules are very large, and the patient has diarrhea."

23. For a current discussion of Thuja, see Marianne Harling and Brian Kaplan, eds., *Studies of Homoeopathic Remedies* (Beaconsfield, Bucks, England: Beaconsfield Publishers, 1987), 512–17. On homeopathic domestic manuals and vaccination side effects, see also Wolff, "Sectarian Identity," 227–30.

24. See James Tyler Kent, *Lectures on Homoeopathic Materia Medica* (1904; reprinted with introduction by Jugal Kishore, New Delhi: B. Jain Publishers, 1992), 997.

25. See "Symposium on Smallpox," Homeopathic Medical Society of the County of Philadelphia, October 10th, 1901, Historical Library, College of Physicians of Philadelphia.

26. Such interactions could also sometimes take place in various state government vaccination inquiries. Usually a committee was composed of both pro- and anti-vaccination forces, as well as "neutral" participants. For example, see Pennsylvania State Vaccination Commission, *Report and Dissenting Reports* (Philadelphia: Allen, Lane and Scott, 1913).

27. On the history of smallpox vaccination, see Derrick Baxby, *Jenner's Smallpox Vaccine: The Riddle of Vaccinia Virus and Its Origin* (London: Heinemann, 1981); F. Fenner, D. A. Henderson, I. Arita, Z. Jezek, and I. D. Ladnyi, *Smallpox and Its Eradication* (Geneva: World Health Organization, 1988).

28. Even more time would elapse before the discovery of the virus that caused smallpox. For an analysis of the "inappropriate timing" of smallpox vaccine in relation to the germ theory, see Derrick Baxby, "Smallpox Vaccine: Ahead of its Time," *Interdisciplinary Science Reviews* 26 (2001): 125–38.

29. See Anne Hardy, *The Epidemic Streets: Infectious Disease and the Rise of Preventive Medicine, 1856–1900* (Oxford: Clarendon Press, 1993), 110–15. Anti-vaccination publications at the time were quick to pick up on these consequences of smallpox vaccination. For several examples published in the discussed period, see George William Winterburn, *The Value of Vaccination: A Non-Partisan Review of its History and Results* (Philadelphia: F. E. Boericke, Hahnemann Publishing House, 1886); J. M. Peebles, *Vaccination a Curse and a Menace to Personal Liberty* (Battle Creek, Mich.: Temple of Health Publishing, 1900); and Charles M. Higgins, *The Crime Against the School Child: Compulsory Vaccination, Illegal and Criminal and Non-enforceable upon the People* (Brooklyn, N.Y.: P. J. Collison, 1915).

30. On the rise of the laboratory, see Andrew Cunningham and Perry Williams, eds., *The Laboratory Revolution in Medicine* (Cambridge: Cambridge University Press, 1992) and W. F. Bynum, *Science and Practice of Medicine in the Nineteenth Century* (Cambridge: Cambridge University Press, 1994), 92–117.

31. Bert Hansen, "America's First Medical Breakthrough: How Popular Excitement About a French Rabies Cure in 1885 Raised New Expectations for Medical Progress," *American Historical Review* 103 (1998): 374.

32. John P. Sutherland, "Serum-Therapy, and the Animal Extracts," *New England Medical Gazette* 36 (1901): 339–50, citation from 342.

33. It is also important to make a clear distinction between opposition to vaccination on principle as a treatment strategy and opposition to coercion in administering vaccinations. In practice, in many cases the two are linked, but this does not have to be the case.

34. See also Nadja Durbach, " 'The Vaccination Vampire': Blood, Boundaries, and the Victorian Body," paper presented at the annual conference of the American Historical Association, 2002.

35. Ibid. As Nadja Durbach has emphasized, the "blood motif" appeared frequently in the rhetoric of anti-vaccinationists.

36. On Almroth Wright and his vaccine research, see Wai Chen, "Laboratory as Business: Sir Almroth Wright's Vaccine Programme and the Construction of Penicillin," in Andrew Cunningham and Perry Williams, eds., *The Laboratory Revolution in Medicine* (Cambridge: Cambridge University Press, 1992).

37. See, for example, "Serum Therapy in Its Relation to Homoeopathy" (editorial), *Journal of the American Institute of Homœopathy* 1 (1909): 392–93; George Royal, "The Relation of Toxins, Vaccines and Serums to Homœopathy," *Journal of the American Institute of Homoeopathy* 4 (1912): 1063–7.

38. On homeopathy and the opsonic theory, see also Harris L. Coulter, *Divided Legacy: A History of the Schism in Medical Thought*, vol. 4: *Twentieth Century Medicine: The Bacteriological Era* (Berkeley: North Atlantic Books, 1994), 390–416.

39. See, "Serum Therapy in Its Relation to Homœopathy," 392.

40. Ibid.

41. W. H. Watters, "A Pathologist's View of Homoeopathy," *New England Medical Gazette* 43 (1909): 415.

42. See Eaton, "Vaccins," 68–69.

43. See Josephine M. Danforth, "Opsonic Work with Children," *Journal of the American Institute of Homeopathy* 1 (1909): 526–39; W. H. Hanchett, "The Opsonins—Thermo-Therapy—Homoeopathy," *Journal of the American Institute of Homeopathy* 1 (1909): 560–65.

44. *Boston University School of Medicine Annual Announcement*, 1915, 19.

45. Bureau of Materia Medica, "Discussion," *Journal of the American Institute of Homœopathy* 4 (1912): 1068.

46. For an excellent treatment of this homeopathic dilemma, see Naomi Rogers, "American Homeopathy Confronts Scientific Medicine," in Robert Jütte, Guenter B. Risse, and John Woodward, eds., *Culture, Knowledge and Healing: Historical Perspectives of Homeopathic Medicine in Europe and North America* (Sheffield: European Association for the History of Medicine and Health Publications, 1998), 31–50.

47. "Homœopathy versus Serum and Vaccin treatment," *New England Medical Gazette* 52 (1917): 508.

48. For example, Hahnemann Medical College was one among other medical institutions in Philadelphia that endorsed the "resolutions confirming their belief in the efficacy of vaccination and urging that the integrity of the present vaccination statutes be not interfered with." See *Vaccination: A Message from the Medical Society of the State of Pennsylvania* (Harrisburg, Penn.: The Medical Society, 1908).

49. C. C. Teal, "Vaccination," *Journal of the American Osteopathic Association* 12 (1913): 304.

50. For the relation between homeopathy and social reform, see Rogers, "American Homeopathy" and Anne Taylor Kirschmann, "A Vital Force: Women Physicians and Patients in American Homeopathy, 1850–1930," Ph.D. dissertation, University of Rochester, 1999, esp. 118–167.

51. Rogers, "American Homeopathy," 38.

52. Close, "The Truth and Error of Vaccination," 469.

53. See William Jefferson Guernsey, "Some Letters Regarding Vaccination," *Homœopathic Recorder* 16 (1901): 544–53.

54. Ibid., 544

55. Ibid., 552–53

56. On *Life* and other publications involved in the debate, see also Susan Lederer, *Subjected to Science: Human Experimentation in America before the Second World War* (Baltimore: Johns Hopkins University Press, 1995), 41–42.

57. See, for example, "Medicine and the Serum Craze," *Journal of Zoöphily* 22 (1913): 72.

58. Edward Pollock Anshutz (1846–1918), the editor of the *Homoeopathic Envoy*, is a good example of a lay supporter of homeopathy promoting the cause of anti-vaccinationists. Anshutz was also a devoted Swedenborgian and the editor of the *New Church Life*, and in 1885 he joined the known homeopathic publishers, Boericke and Tafel, as literary editor. Several Swedenborgians were also anti-vaccinationists, and the relationship between homeopathy and Swedenborgianism is well established. See also Nadav Davidovitch, " 'To Save Science from Materialism:' Homeopathy, Swedenborgianism and American 'Shadow Culture,' " paper presented at the annual conference of the society for the Social History of Medicine, July 2000.

59. See, for example, B. O. Flower, *Progressive Men, Women, and Movements of the Past Twenty-five Years* (Boston: The New Arena, 1914), 298–316. Flower dedicates a whole chapter in his book to the issue of medical freedom. Flower was an active figure in various anti-medical establishment groups and the president of the National League for Medical Freedom, a short-lived movement established in 1910 that was active against the establishment of a national health bureau. The aim and purpose of the league was "the maintenance of the rights of the American people against the unnecessary, unjust, oppressive, paternal and un-American laws, ostensibly related to the subjects of health" (cited from *Prospectus of the National League for Medical Freedom*, Pamphlet 4440, Historical Library, College of Physicians of Philadelphia, 3). As the editor of the reform journal *Arena*, Flower attacked "organized" medicine as well as other evil economic and political monopolies.

60. On Lora Little and her involvement in resistance to vaccination, see Johnston, *Radical Middle Class*, 192–213.

61. "Diary of a Doctor," *Life* 40 (1902): 467. See also "Commercialism in Medicine" (editorial), *Journal of Zoöphily* 18 (1909): 95.

62. C. S. Carr, "Smallpox and Vaccination," *Medical Talk* 3 (1902): 209–10

63. Prospectus of the National League for Medical Freedom, 4–5.

64. Ibid., 12.

65. B. O. Flower, "The Battle for Medical Freedom," *Twentieth Century* 4 (1911): 656–657.

66. B. O. Flower, "Letter to the Editor of The Century," *Century Monthly Magazine* 85 (1913): 512–513.

67. "The Fight for Medical Freedom" (editorial), *Twentieth Century* 2 (1910): 367–68.

68. See David Arnold, *Colonizing the Body: State Medicine and Epidemic Disease in Nineteenth-Century India* (Berkeley: Univeristy of California Press, 1993) and Durbach, "Working-Class Resistance."

69. J. M. Peebles, *Vaccination a Curse and a Menace to Personal Liberty: With Statistics Showing Its Dangers and Criminality* (Los Angeles: Peebles Pub. Co., 1913), 55.

70. Dutch Doctor Barnes, "How to Produce a Scar Resembling Vaccination," *Medical Talk* 5 (1904): 308.

71. "False Vaccination Scars: A Vile Crime Encouraged" (editorial), *American Medicine* 7 (1904) and "Vaccination a Condition of Entrance to Almshouses, Hospitals, Etc." (editorial), *American Medicine* 7 (1904). See also "Mock Vaccine Scars," *Medical Talk* 5 (1904): 631.

72. William Jefferson Guernsey, "Some Letters Regarding Vaccination," *Homoeopathic Recorder* 16 (1901): 544–53, citation from 547.

73. "Against the League of Medical Freedom" (editorial), *Homoeopathic Recorder* 27 (1912): 92–93.

74. *Buck v. Bell*, 274 U.S. 200 (1927).

75. On eugenics in the legal arena, especially in the U.S. Supreme Court, see Paul A. Lombardo, "Medicine, Eugenics and the Supreme Court: From Coercive Sterilization to Reproductive Freedom," *Journal of Contemporary Health Law and Policy* 13 (1996): 1–25.

76. *Buck v. Bell*, 274 U.S. 200 (1927): 12–13. Holmes based his "public health rationale" on *Jacobson v. Massachusetts*, an important precedent in U.S. public health law decided in the wake of a smallpox epidemic in Boston, where the court upheld a Massachusetts statute that compelled citizens to receive smallpox immunizations or be fined if they refused. *Jacobson v. Massachusetts*, 197 U.S. 11 (1905). See also Michael R. Albert , Kristen G. Ostheimer, and Joel G. Breman, "The Last Smallpox Epidemic in Boston and the Vaccination Controversy, 1901–1903," *New England Journal of Medicine* 344 (2001): 375–79.

77. On homeopaths in the American political arena, see Naomi Rogers, "The Public Face of Homoeopathy: Politics, the Public and Alternative Medicine in the United States, 1900–1940," in Martin Dinges, ed., *Patients in the History of Homeopathy* (Sheffield: European Association for the History of Medicine and Health Publications, 2002), 351–72.

78. For an interesting contemporary call for an open discussion, see Anthony S. Fauci, "Smallpox Vaccination Policy: The Need for Dialogue," *New England Journal of Medicine* 346 (2002): 1319–20.

Making Friends for "Pure" Homeopathy

I would like to thank Julian Winston and the National Center for Homeopathy for allowing me use of the NCH archives in researching this topic. I am also grateful to the following people for generously granting me interviews, including Joseph Lillard, Richard Moskowtiz, Lisa Harvey, Allen Neiswander, Lia Bello, George Guess, Lauren Fox, Karl Robinson, David Wember, Nicholas Nossaman, Stephen Messer, and the late Henry Williams and Maeisimund Panos. A special thanks goes to Robert Johnston for his insightful and constructive criticism of earlier drafts. Portions of this chapter have been published previously in *A Vital Force: Women in American Homeopathy* (New Brunswick, N.J.: Rutgers University Press, 2003) and are used here with permission.

1. See Paul Starr, *The Social Transformation of American Medicine: The Rise of a Sovereign Profession and the Making of a Vast Industry* (New York: Basic Books, 1982), 79–144.

2. As Naomi Rogers shows, homeopathy maintained an important political presence as well as social acceptance during the first four decades of the twentieth century. See Rogers, "The Public Face of Homoeopathy: Politics, the Public and Alternative Medicine in the United States, 1900–40," in Martin Dinges, ed., *Patients in the History of Homoeopathy* (Sheffield: European Association for the History of Medicine and Health Publications, 2002), 351–71.

3. Charles E. Rosenberg, "Holism in Twentieth-Century Medicine," in Christopher Lawrence and George Weisz, eds., *Greater than the Parts: Holism in Biomedicine 1920–1950* (New York: Oxford University Press, 1998), 341.

4. See George Weisz, "A Moment of Synthesis: Medical Holism in France between the Wars," in Christopher Lawrence and George Weisz, eds., *Greater than the Parts: Holism in Biomedicine, 1920–1950* (New York: Oxford University Press, 1998), 68–111.

5. Rosenberg, "Holism," 342.

6. Samuel Hahnemann, *Organon of Medicine*, 6th ed., translated by William Boericke (1810; reprinted, New Delhi: B. Jain Publishers, 1992), 94–96. German physician and scholar Samuel Christian Hahnemann (1755–1843) developed homeopathy in the late 1700s, providing a medical system that competed with the harsh and often harmful therapeutics of "regular" physicians. See Martin Kaufman, *Homeopathy in America: The Rise and Fall of a Medical Heresy* (Baltimore: Johns Hopkins University Press, 1971) and Harris L. Coulter, *Divided Legacy: The Conflict Between Homoeopathy and the American Medical Association*, 2nd ed. (Berkeley: North Atlantic Books, 1982).

7. Hahnemann, *Organon*, 304–5.

8. Homeopaths, however, continued to maintain separate medical societies, hospitals, and medical journals at this time. See Naomi Rogers, *An Alternative Path: The Making and Remaking of Hahnemann Medical College and Hospital of Philadelphia* (New Brunswick, N.J.: Rutgers University Press, 1998). The 1941 *Directory of Homeopathic Physicians in the United States* lists approximately 6,600 homeopaths.

9. Viewing themselves the torchbearers of "true" homeopathy, Hahnemannians organized the International Hahnemannian Association in 1881 to prevent the "mongrelization" of their profession.

10. "What the Laymen Are Doing," *The Layman Speaks* (hereafter TLS) IX, 4 (1956): 134.

11. See Anne Taylor Kirschmann, *A Vital Force: Women in American Homeopathy* (New Brunswick, N.J.: Rutgers University Press, 2003). For explanations of the declining numbers of medical women in the first half of the twentieth century, see Regina Markell Morantz-Sanchez, *Sympathy and Science: Women Physicians in American Medicine* (New York: Oxford University Press, 1985), 232–65, and Mary Roth Walsh, *Doctors Wanted, No Women Need Apply: Sexual Barriers in the Medical Profession, 1835–1975* (New Haven: Yale University Pess, 1977).

12. Julia Minerva Green, M.D. 1871–1963 Scrapbook, Box 2, National Center for Homeopathy Archives (NCHA).

13. Mary Ware Dennett, AFH/IHA Meeting Report (June 26, 1925), 169, AFH Box 6, NCHA.

14. J. W. Waffensmith, M.D., "Economic Determinism in Homeopathy," *Journal of American Institute of Homeopathy* 37, 5 (1944) reprinted in *TLS* III, 3 (1949): 50.

15. G. Kent Smith, M.D., "Universality of Homoeopathy," *Pacific Coast Homoeopathic Bulletin* XVI, 2 (1958): n.p.

16. Robert H. Wiebe was one of the earliest to articulate this view. See *The Segmented Society: An Introduction to the Meaning of America* (New York: Oxford University Press, 1975).

17. *TLS* III, 1 (1949): 4.

18. Maisimond Panos, M.D., interview by author, Tipp City, Ohio, March 9–10, 1996.

19. "Medical Freedom," *TLS* I, 7 (1948): 12–13.

20. "Medical Freedom.," 12–13.

21. Rogers, *An Alternative Path*, 212.

22. "Medical Freedom," 12–13.

23. E. Underhill Jr., *Proceedings of the IHA 1931 and The Homeopathic Recorder* (hereafter *THR*) XLVII, 4 (1932): 258–59.

24. See Martin Kaufman, "The American Anti-Vaccinationists and Their Arguments," *Bulletin of the History of Medicine* 41 (1967): 463–78.

25. Alfred Pulford, M.D., "The Modern Medical Prevention Racket," *THR* LII, 5 (1937): 120, 127.

26. Pulford, "The Modern Medical Prevention Racket," 122.

27. *TLS* VIII, 8 (1955): 253. See also Naomi Rogers, *Dirt and Disease: Polio before FDR* (New Brunswick: Rutgers University Press, 1992), 165–90.

28. Eugene Underhill Jr., "Editorial," *THR* LVI, 5 (1941): n.p.

29. Eugene Underhill Jr., "Editorial," *THR* LVIII, 9 (1943): 467–68.

30. *TLS* III, 12 (1950): 332–36.

31. *TLS* I, 7 (1948): 7.

32. As Gretchen Reilly's essay in this volume explains, although anti-fluoridation campaigns were necessarily local, a very effective national network linked local activists with the broader movement.

33. "E Subcommittee on Constitutional Rights," *TLS* VIII, 10 (1955): 361.

34. Adah F. Sievert, "The Chicago Homoeopathic Layman's League," *TLS* VII, 2 (1955): 56.

35. "What the Laymen are Doing," *TLS* IX, 4 (1956): 135.

36. Mrs. Gladys Caldwell to Mr. Green, La Crescenta, Calif., July 5, 1969, NCHA.

37. Arthur Green to Mrs. Gladys Caldwell, July 24, 1969, NCHA.

38. Arthur Green to the Rt. Rev. Francis J. Lally, November 14, 1959, NCHA.

39. Kaufman, *Homeopathy in America*, 178.

40. Howard M. Engle, M.D., *THR*, LIX, 5 (1943): 232. For mainstream opposition to national health insurance proposals, see Starr, *Transformation*, 280, and Daniel M. Fox, *Health Policies, Health Politics: The British and American Experience, 1911–1965* (Princeton: Princeton University Press, 1986).

41. Eugene Underhill Jr. "The Post-War Medical World" (editorial), *THR* LIX, 3 (1943): 141.

42. *TLS* II, 6 (1949): 11.

43. See, for example, C. P. Bryant, "Shall Politics Control Medicine?" *THR* LIV, 5 (1939): 10–11.

44. *TLS* II, 6 (1949), 11.

45. Eugene Underhill Jr., "The Post-War Medical World," (editorial), *THR* LIX, 3 (1943): 142.

46. Mrs. A. L. Maynard, response to questionnaire, November 1970, "Comments: *TLS*" folder, NCHA. For an examination of the American consumer's enthusiasm for vitamins, see Rima D. Apple, *Vitamania: Vitamins in American Culture* (New Brunswick, N.J.: Rutgers University Press, 1996).

47. Dora M. Wilson to the AFH, St. Paul, Minnesota, March 20, 1958, NCHA.

48. Pierre Bouillette to the AFH, New York City, November 26, 1962, NCHA.

49. "Report to the Federation of Laymen's Leagues from the Delegate, April 11, 1970," "Federation of Laymen's Leagues 1970" folder, NCHA. In 1961 there were seven active leagues and six in the process of organizing. The increase in numbers of leagues, however, did not necessarily indicate growing interest in homeopathy. Rather, it was a response to the loss of homeopathic physicians and patients' desire to learn how to prescribe remedies for themselves and their family members.

50. Clara Strodel to Margery Lavelle, February 2, 1963, "Chicago Laymen's League" folder, NCHA.

51. "Report to the Federation of Laymen's Leagues from the Delegate, April 11, 1970," NCHA.

52. Useful histories on the health food movement include James C. Whorton, *Crusaders for Fitness: The History of American Health Reformers* (Princeton: Princeton University Press, 1982); Warren James Belasco, *Appetite for Change: How the Counterculture Took the Food Industry, 1966–1988* (New York: Pantheon Books, 1989); and Kristina Beyerman Alstar, *The Holistic Health Movement* (Tuscaloosa: University of Alabama Press, 1989).

53. Helen Pohlmer to Kay Vargo, February 13, 1971, "New York Laymen's League" folder, AFH Box 51, NCHA.

54. Elizabeth Wright Hubbard, "President's Page," *TLS* XIII, 8 (1960), 263–64, reprinted from the *Journal of the American Institute of Homeopathy/THR* LIV, 5–6 (1960). Wright was a trustee of the AFH for several years beginning in the late 1920s and an ardent Hahnemannian homeopath.

55. Hubbard, "President's Page," 263–64.

56. Harris L. Coulter, "Homoeopathy and Today's Youth," *TLS* XXIV, 7 (1971).

57. For an overview of the various social movements of the 1960s, see Todd Gitlin, *The Sixties: Years of Hope, Days of Rage* (New York: Bantam Books, 1993 [1987]) and Stewart Burns, *The Social Movements of the 1960s: Searching for Democracy* (Boston: Twayne Publications, 1990).

58. Joseph Lillard, interview by author, Washington, D.C., June 22, 2000. Lillard later became the first lay president of the NCH and is the founder and current head of Washington Homeopathic Products in Bethesda, Maryland.

59. See John Harley Warner, *The Therapeutic Perspective: Medical Practice, Knowledge, and Identity in America, 1820–1885* (Cambridge, Mass.: Harvard University Press, 1986) and "The Fall and Rise of Professional Mystery: Epistemology, Authority and the Emergence of Laboratory Medicine in Nineteenth-Century America," in Andrew Cunningham and Perry Williams, eds., *The Laboratory Revolution in Medicine* (Cambridge: Cambridge University Press, 1992). For a regional perspective, see Steven M. Stowe, "Seeing Themselves at Work: Physicians and the Case Narrative in the Mid-Nineteenth Century American South," *American Historical Review* 101, 1 (1996): 41–79.

60. Richard Moskowitz, M.D., "Why I Became a Homeopath," unpublished paper adapted from an article in the *Journal of the American Institute of Homeopathy* 89, 74 (1996): 6.

61. Moskowitz "Why I Became a Homeopath," 15. Also see Susan, Sontag, *Illness as Metaphor and AIDS and Its Metaphors* (New York: Anchor Books, 1988).

62. Moskowitz, "Why I Became a Homeopath," 15–16.

63. Ibid., 18.

64. Ibid., 28.

65. See also Lesley Doyal, "Women, Health, and the Sexual Division of Labor: A Case Study of the Women's Health Movement in Britain," in Elizabeth Fee and Nancy Krieger, eds., *Women's Health, Politics, and Power: Essays on Sex/Gender, Medicine, and Public Health* (Amityville, N.Y.: Baywood Publishing Company, 1994), 61–76.

66. According to many former members, women constituted a large majority of study group members during this period.

67. Lisa Harvey, M.D., telephone interview by author, August 17, 2000. Harvey received a B.S. from West Virginia University in 1975 and her M.D. from Wake Forest University in 1979. She currently practices medicine in western Massachusetts, focusing on family health care and homeopathy.

68. Lia Bello, R.N., telephone interview by author, November 17, 2000. Bello is currently a family nurse practitioner certified in classical homeopathy with a practice in Questa, New Mexico.

69. Lia Bello, interview.

70. Richard Moskowitz, "Dear Members and Friends of the National Center," *Homoeopathy Today*, April 1981, 1.

71. Dr. Wyrth Post Baker, chairman of the AFH board of trustees, in a letter to the homeopathic community, February 18, 1981, cited in Julian Winston, *The Faces of Homoeopathy: An Illustrated History of the First 200 Years* (Tawa, New Zealand: Great Auk Publishing, 1999), 524.

72. For specific details of "The Great Unpleasantness," see Winston, *The Faces of Homeopathy*, 522–27, and Moskowitz, "Dear Members," 1–2.

73. Richard Moskowitz, M.D., and George Guess, M.D., interviews by author, Washington, D.C., June 23, 2000. According to admirers, Vithoulkas was a charismatic teacher and master prescriber who possessed an "unparalleled understanding of homeopathy." His European seminars on homeopathy drew large numbers of students. See Winston, *Faces*, 357–362.

74. Moskowitz, "Dear Members," 1.

75. In March 1988, the NCH listed 2,750 members, and in 1997, it counted more than 7,000 members. By the year 2000, approximately 200 study groups were affiliated with the NCH.

76. See, for example, T. J. Jackson Lears, *No Place of Grace: Antimodernism and the Transformation of American Culture, 1880–1920* (Chicago: University of Chicago Press, 1981) and Christopher Lasch, *The True and Only Heaven: Progress and Its Critics* (New York: W. W. Norton and Company, 1991).

77. For a discussion of scholars' neglect of twentieth-century conservatism, see Alan Brinkley, "The Problem of American Conservatism," *American Historical Review* 99, 2 (1994).

78. Robert D. Johnston's recent reexamination of the middle class in the twentieth century provides a new context for understanding midcentury homeopaths. See Johnston, *The Radical Middle Class: Populist Democracy and the Question of Capitalism in Progressive Era Portland* (Princeton: Princeton University Press, 2003).

79. David A. Horowitz, *Beyond Left and Right: Insurgency and the Establishment* (Urbana and Chicago: University of Illinois Press, 1997), 311–12.

80. Naomi Rogers, "American Homeopathy Confronts Scientific Medicine," in Robert Jütte, Guenter B. Risse, and John Woodward, eds., *Culture, Knowledge, and Healing: Historical Perspectives of Homeopathic Medicine in Europe and North America* (Sheffield: European Association for the History of Medicine and Health Publications, 1998), 50.

Revisiting the "Golden Age" of Regular Medicine

Portions of this article are based on material from my book, *Negotiating Disease: Power and Cancer Care, 1900–1950* (Montreal and Kingston: McGill-Queen's University Press, 2001).

1. Tyrell Dueck's story is drawn from a selection of news articles: Leslie Perreaux, "Teen Refused Cancer Treatment under Influence of Father, Court Hears," *Canadian Press Newswire* (March 17, 1999); "Boy's Cancer Fight Sparks Legal Controversy," *Canadian Press Newswire* (March 18, 1999); Jonathon Gatehouse, "Teen's Chemo Postponed while Family Appeals Court Order," *National Post* 1 (March 20, 1999), A1, A2; Martin O'Hanlon, "Cancer Case Poses Ethical, Legal Dilemma," *Canadian Press Newswire* (March 21, 1999); David Roberts, "Boy's Cancer Spreads: MDs Give Up," *Globe and Mail* (March 22, 1999), A1, A10; Mark Nichols, "Faith or Medicine? A Judge Orders Chemotherapy after a Boy Says No," *Maclean's* 112 (March 29, 1999), 78; Marnie Ko, "Out with His Parents, Off with His Leg: A Saskatchewan Judge Takes Control of a Teenager's Cancer Treatment," *Alberta Report* 26 (March 29, 1999), 27–28; Marnie Ko, "Doubting the Diagnosis: The Duecks Weren't the First to Challenge a Saskatoon Cancer Clinic's Decisions," *Alberta Report* 26 (April 5, 1999); Eric Beresford, "Medical Choices Raise Issues of Human Dignity," *Anglican Journal* 125 (1999); Marnie Ko, "Maybe a Miracle, Maybe a Mistake: Either Way, Tyrell Dueck's Cancer Diagnosis Raises Questions About Saskatchewan Health Care," *British Columbia Report* 10 (May 3, 1999), 50; Marnie Ko, "You Can't Buy That Publicity: Saskatchewan's Tyrell Dueck Becomes the Poster Child for Alternative Medicine," *British Columbia Report* 10 (May 31, 1999), 49; Mary Rogan, "Acts of Faith: When Tyrell Dueck Said No to Chemotherapy and Amputation, He Started a Process That Tested Everyone's Faith; in Medicine, in the Legal System, in a Family's Love, in God," *Saturday Night* 114 (1999), 42–52; Deana Driver, "The Tyrell Dueck Dilemma," *Medical Post* 35 (November 23, 1999), 17, 20.

2. Miriam Shuchman, "Two Boys, Same Disease—Different Treatments," *Toronto Globe and Mail*, July 13, 1999, C7.

3. Rogan, "Acts of Faith," 44.

4. "Boy's Cancer Fight."

5. Ko, "Out with His Parents," 28.

6. Paul Starr, *The Social Transformation of American Medicine* (New York: Basic Books, 1982), 13–21.

7. Rogan, "Acts of Faith," 46.

8. Perreaux, "Teen Refused Treatment"; Driver, "Tyrell Dueck Dilemma," 17; Rogan, "Acts of Faith," 45.

9. Nichols, "Faith or Medicine," 78.

10. Ko, "Doubting the Diagnosis," 41. See also Beresford, "Medical Choices"; Art Willock, quoted in Ko, "Maybe a Miracle," 50; Robert Heckman and Kari Simpson, quoted in Ko, "Out with His Parents," 28; Rogan, "Acts of Faith," 42.

11. Ko, "Doubting the Diagnosis," 41.

12. Barbara Clow, "Swapping Grief: The Role of the Laity in Alternative Medical Encounters," *Journal of the History of Medicine and Allied Sciences* 52 (1997): 175–201.

13. Beresford, "Medical Choices."

14. John C. Burnham, "American Medicine's Golden Age: What Happened to It?" *Science* 215 (March 19, 1982): 1474–9. See also Edward Shorter, *Bedside Manners: The Troubled History of Doctors and Patients* (New York: Viking, 1985), 128, 231.

15. Burnham, "Golden Age," 1474–9; Starr, *Social Transformation*, 388–89; Shorter, *Bedside Manners*, 24, 228–30; David Rothman, *Strangers at the Bedside: A History of How Law and Bioethics Transformed Medical Decision Making* (New York: Basic Books, 1991), 127–47.

16. Rene Caisse's first name was pronouced "Wren," "Rain," or sometimes "Rainy."

17. *Unconventional Cancer Treatments* (Washington, D.C.: Government Printing Office, 1990), 169–70.

18. J.W.S. McCullough, "1910–1920: A Review of Ten Years' Progress," *Thirty-Ninth Annual Report of the Provincial Board of Health for 1920*, 21–23. See also Mary Powell, "Public Health Litigation in Ontario,

1884–1920," in Charles Roland, ed., *Health, Disease and Medicine: Essays in Canadian History* (Toronto: Hannah Institute for the History of Medicine, 1984), 412–35.

19. Glenn Sawyer, *The First 100 Years: A History of the Ontario Medical Association* (Toronto: Ontario Medical Association, 1980), 26–75; J. Castell Hopkins, *The Canadian Annual Review of Public Affairs*, 1919, 509, 668–69, and 1923, 580.

20. McCullough, "A Review of Ten Years' Progress," 33; Sir Charles G. D. Roberts and Arthur Leonard Tunnell, eds., *The Canadian Who's Who* (1938–39), 3: 378–79; "Address of the Honourable Harold J. Kirby, K.C., Minister of Health," *Ontario Medical Association Bulletin* 5 (May 1938), 93–94.

21. Elizabeth MacNab, *A Legal History of Health Professions in Ontario* (Toronto: Queen's Printer, 1970), 10–17.

22. R. J. Gidney and W. P. Millar, "The Origins of Organized Medicine in Ontario, 1850–1869," in Charles Roland, ed., *Health, Disease and Medicine* (Toronto: Hannah Institute for the History of Medicine, 1984), 84–86. See also MacNab, *Legal History*, 14–17; J. T. H. Connor, " 'A Sort of Felo-De-Sé: Eclecticism, Related Medical Sects and Their Decline in Victorian Ontario," *Bulletin of the History of Medicine* 65 (1991): 503–27; J. T. H. Connor, "Minority Medicine in Ontario: A Study of Medical Pluralism and Its Decline," Ph.D. dissertation, University of Waterloo, 1989.

23. Sawyer, *Ontario Medical Association*, 28; MacNab, *Legal History*, 38.

24. MacNab, *Legal History*, 47.

25. Randall White, Ontario, *1610–1985; A Political and Economic History* (Toronto: Dundern Press, 1985) 214–19; James Naylor, *A New Democracy: Challenging the Social Order in Industrial Ontario, 1914–1925* (Toronto: University of Toronto Press, 1991); Charles M. Johnson, *E. C. Drury: Agrarian Idealist* (Toronto: University of Toronto Press, 1986).

26. MacNab, *Legal History*, 48.

27. J. E. Bates, "Report of the Division of Pathology," *Seventh Annual Report of the Department of Health, 1931* (Toronto: King's Printer, 1931).

28. Madge Thurlow Macklin, "The Problem of the Increase in Cancer," *Canadian Medical Association Journal* 36 (February 1937): 192.

29. Charles Hayter, "Medicalizing Malignancy: The Origins of Ontario's Cancer Program, 1929–34," *Canadian Bulletin of Medical History/Bulletin canadien d'histoire de la médicine* 14 (1997): 198–201; "Medical Societies: The Western Ontario Academy of Medicine," *Canadian Medical Association Journal* 24 (April 1931): 573; "Government Control of Radium," "The Ontario Government and Cancer," and "Study of Cancer," Ontario Medical Association, Executive and Board of Directors Minutes (hereafter OMA Minutes), November 1929 to June 1932, Ontario Medical Association Archives, 96, 102, 113; "News Items: Ontario," *Canadian Medical Association Journal* 24 (June 1931), 890; "The Cancer Commission," *Canada Lancet and Practitioner* 77 (July 1931): 4–6; *Report of the Royal Commission on the Use of Radium and X-Rays in the Treatment of the Sick*, February 29, 1928, Royal Commissions of the Province of Ontario, RG 18–95, Box 1, Archives of Ontario, 1; Herbert A. Bruce, "Cancer Centres Abroad," *Canadian Journal of Medicine and Surgery* 71 (February 1932): 31; Robert Bothwell, *Eldorado: Canada's National Uranium Company* (Toronto: University of Toronto Press, 1984); "Radium and the Cancer Commission," *Canadian Journal of Medicine and Surgery* 72 (October 1932): 77.

30. J. M. Robb, quoted in "Medical Societies: The Western Ontario Academy of Medicine," *Canadian Medical Association Journal* 24 (April 1931): 573–47.

31. "Report of the Cancer Committee," April 18, 1932, and "Royal Commission on Cancer," June 1932, OMA Minutes, November 1929 to June 1932, 166, 196.

32. Hayter, "Medicalizing Malignancy," 203, 209. See also "The Cancer Commission," *Canada Lancet and Practitioner* 77 (July 1931): 4–6; "Radium and the Cancer Commission," *Canadian Journal of Medicine and Surgery* 72 (October 1932): 77; "Ontario's Royal Commission on Cancer," *Canadian Journal of Medicine and Surgery* 70 (July 1931): 5–7; George Henry, Premier, to W. H. Fyfe, Principal, Queen's University, June 11, 1931, and Memorandum, 1931, RG 3, Series 8, Box 136, File 03-08-0-059, Archives of Ontario; "Re Royal Commission on Cancer," May 1931, and "Royal Commission on Cancer," November 1931, OMA Minutes, November 1929 to June 1932, 140, 143; "Report of the Cancer Committee," April 18, 1932, "Royal Commission on Cancer," June 1932, and "Report of the Committee on Public Health," June 1932, OMA Minutes, November 1929 to June 1932, 166, 196, 214; "Report of the Advisory Committee on Cancer," November 23, 1932, OMA Minutes, November 1932 to May 1934, 5–6; *Report of the Royal Commission on*

the Use of Radium and X-Rays in the Treatment of the Sick, February 29, 1932, Royal Commissions of the Province of Ontario, RG 18–95, Box 1, Archives of Ontario.

33. Charles Hastings, "Cancer Is Not Incurable," *Health Bulletin* 18 (May 1927); "The Cancer Situation" and "Re Cancer Institutions," April 7, 1933, OMA Minutes, November 1929 to May 1934, 31, 48; A. G. Nicholls, "A Cancer Campaign for Canada," *Canadian Medical Association Journal* 32 (March 1935), 305; "Resolution Passed by Wellesley Hospital Clinical Society," February 23, 1937, OMA Minutes, August 1936 to June 1937, 94; "Cancer 'Cures,' " August 21, 1937, OMA Minutes, June 1937 to August 1937, 159. "Non-Medically Operated Cancer Institutions," May 30, 1933, OMA Executive and Board of Directors' Minutes, November 1932 to May 1934, 51.

34. James Faulkner, Minister of Health, quoted in Minutes, Advisory Cancer Committee, November 23, 1934, File 11.7, Archives of Ontario, 3–4, 12–14; Minutes, Advisory Cancer Committee Minutes, February 8, 1935, RG 10, Series 106, File 11.9, Archives of Ontario, 21–22; Faulkner to Mitchell Hepburn, Premier, May 4, 1935, RG 3, Series 9, Box 184, File 139.2, Archives of Ontario.

35. Faulkner to Hepburn, May 4, 1935, RG 3, Series 9, Box 184, File 139.2, Correspondence: Department of Health, Archives of Ontario.

36. Roberts and Tunnell, eds., *The Canadian Who's Who*, 3: 378–79; "Address of the Honourable Harold J. Kirby, K.C., Minister of Health," *Ontario Medical Association Bulletin* (hereafter *OMA Bulletin*) 5 (May 1938): 93–94; "Should Investigate This Claim of Cancer Cure," *Port Arthur Evening News-Chronicle*, December 11, 1937.

37. For more details on Caisse, see Clow, *Negotiating Disease* and Gary Glum, *Calling of an Angel* (Los Angeles: Silent Walker Publishing, 1988).

38. Glum, *Angel*, 18–19. According to available documents, Caisse did not articulate her theories on cancer causation and the pharmacological action of Essiac until well into the 1930s, when her work was under investigation by the Cancer Commission. R. C. Wallace and T. H. Callahan, "Proceedings of a Sub Committee Appointed by the Commission to Enquire into and Report upon Cancer Remedies—Evidence (Re Rene Caisse)," February 3–4, 1939, College of Physicians and Surgeons of Ontario, 6–7.

39. Glum, *Angel*, 18–21.

40. Ibid., 19–21; Sheila Snow Fraser and Carroll Allen, "Could Essiac Halt Cancer?" *Homemaker's Magazine*, June/July/August 1977, 14–16; B. T. McGhie, Deputy Minister of Health, Memo to File, July 25, 1935, RG 10, Series 106, File 14.1, Archives of Ontario.

41. Glum, *Angel*, 20–21; Fraser and Allen, "Essiac," 14.

42. Rene Caisse to Mitchell Hepburn, September 3, 1937, RG 10, Series 106, File 13.11, Archives of Ontario.

43. J.S. to Department of Health, March 12, 1938, RG 10, Series 106, File 13.11, Archives of Ontario; M.H. to Mitchell Hepburn, Premier, October 25, 1937, RG 3, Series 9, Box 207, Archives of Ontario. See also W.S. to Hepburn, August 5, 1937, RG 10, Series 106, File 13.11, Archives of Ontario; "Will Report on Cancer: Bracebridge Nurse's Treatment Still Not Recognized by Doctors," *Toronto Globe and Mail*, March 16, 1937; "Living Evidence of Benefits of Nurse Caisse's Cancer Treatment Deserves Consideration," *Toronto Telegram*, April 2, 1937.

44. "The Cancer Commission," *OMA Bulletin* 7 (January 1940): 7–9.

45. "Planning to Curb 'Quack' Treatment," *Toronto Daily Star*, March 2, 1937; "Visits Sir Frederick Banting about Cancer Treatment," *Toronto Telegram*, March 16, 1937; "Bill to Control Cancer Quackery," February 23, 1937, and "Cancer," OMA Minutes, August 1936 to June 1937, 94, 125; T. C. Routley, Secretary, OMA, to K. G. Gray, Solicitor, Department of Health, February 26, 1937, and Routley to Mitchell Hepburn, Premier, October 1, 1937, RG 3, Series 9, Box 271, Archives of Ontario.

46. Robert Noble, Registrar, College of Physicians and Surgeons, "Report of the Joint Advisory Committee," Minutes of the Medical Council, March 24, 1938, College of Physicians and Surgeons of Ontario. See also "Recent Medical Legislation in Ontario," *Canadian Medical Association Journal* 38 (June 1938): 612, and "News Items: Ontario," *Canadian Medical Association Journal* 39 (October 1938): 412.

47. "Orders-in-Council," Commission for the Investigation of Cancer Remedies, August 18, 1938, RG 10, Series 106, File 12.4, Archives of Ontario; "Cancer Commission Constituted," *Toronto Globe and Mail*, September 8, 1938; *Canadian Medical Directory and Physicians Handbook* (Montreal: R. Villecourt, 1927), 215, 232, 245, 252; Roberts and Tunnell, eds., *Canadian Who's Who*, 2:1107, 1165, 3:184, 266.

48. "Recent Medical Legislation in Ontario"; "News Items: Ontario"; J. G. Cunningham, Director of Industrial Hygiene, to B. T. McGhie, Deputy Minister of Health, January 14, 1937; K. G. Gray, Solicitor, to

B. T. McGhie, February 1, 1937, RG 10, Series 106, File 12.4, Archives of Ontario. See also "Bill 1937—An Act," March 5, 1937, RG 10, Series 106, File 12.4, clauses 4.(1), 6.(2), 9, and Cunningham to Harold Kirby, Minister of Health, October 17, 1938, RG 10, Series 106, File 15.6, Archives of Ontario; "An Act for the Investigation of Remedies for Cancer, Statutes of Ontario, 1938," *OMA Bulletin* 7 (January 1940): 7–9.

49. Cunningham to Kirby, October 17, 1938, RG 10, Series 106, File 15.6, Archives of Ontario.

50. The Department of Health kept many of the letters it received on behalf of Caisse. See RG 10, Series 106, File 13.11, Archives of Ontario. I am here quoting from Caisse to F.N., May 25, 1938. The College of Physicians and Surgeons of Ontario kept a scrapbook of news articles on Caisse that also captures the extent of popular support for her work in the summer of 1938.

51. "Nurse's Patients Ask Clinic Closing Ruling," *Toronto Daily Star*, June 27, 1938. Kirby quoted in "Patients Appeal for Reopening of Caisse Cancer Clinic," *Toronto Evening Telegram*, June 23, 1938.

52. "Miss Caisse Terms Probe 'Laughable,'" *Toronto Evening Telegram*, February 8, 1938.

53. Kirby responded to so many letters from irate patients and supports that eventually his office adopted a standard format for his response. See, for example, Kirby to W.R., June 2, 1938, RG 10, Series 106, File 13.11, Archives of Ontario. The press also reported popular outrage against the government. See "Nurse's Patients Ask Clinic Closing Ruling."

54. Kirby, quoted in "Patients Appeal for Reopening of Caisse Cancer Clinic."

55. Hepburn to Caisse, June 2, 1938, RG 10, Series 106, File 13.11, Archives of Ontario.

56. Mr. F.S. to Kirby, June 23, 1938, RG 10, Series 106, File 13.13, Archives of Ontario.

57. Both quotations attributed to Kirby can be found in "Nurse's Patients Ask Clinic Closing Ruling."

58. "Miss Caisse's Cancer Clinic Closed as New Law Takes Effect," *Bracebridge Gazette*, May 29, 1938.

59. Caisse quoted in "Miss Caisse to Re-Open Cancer Clinic," *The Huntsville Forester*, July 28, 1938. See also "Cancer Clinic Reopens Tomorrow," *Bracebridge Gazette*, August 4, 1938.

60. "Miss Caisse's Cancer Clinic Closed as New Law Takes Effect," *Bracebridge Gazette*, May 26, 1938.

61. J.G. Gillanders to Caisse, December 12, 1938, Wallace Papers, 1024a, Box 6, File 55, Queen's University Archives; Caisse, quoted in "Proceedings of a Sub-Committee of the Commission Appointed to Enquire into the Report upon Cancer Remedies," February 3–4, 1939, College of Physicians and Surgeons of Ontario, 119; Gillanders, quoted in Minutes of the Cancer Commission, October 26, 1938, and Caisse to Cancer Commission, October 27, 1938, Wallace Papers, 1024b, Box 1, File 1, Queen's University Archives; "Miss Caisse's Cancer Clinic Closed as New Law Takes Effect;" "Interim Report of Commission for the Investigation of Cancer Remedies," December 31, 1938, 6 (my emphasis).

62. E.S. to Hepburn, February 16, 1938, Wallace Papers, 1024b, Box 1, File 10, Case Book 5, Queen's University Archives; Gillanders to Kirby, February 27, 1940, RG 10, Series 106, File 13.13, Archives of Ontario.

63. R. C. Wallace and T. H. Callahan, "Report of Enquiry into the Caisse Cancer Clinic," 3–4 February 1939, 2, Wallace Papers, 1024b, Box 1, File 2, Queen's University Archives.

64. Wallace, quoted in "Proceedings of a Sub-Committee," 120, 122; Caisse to the Cancer Commission, December 3, 1940, Wallace Papers, 1024b, Box 1, File 3, Queen's University Archives; "Rene M. Caisse Close Cancer Clinic Here," *Muskoka Herald*, January 23, 1941. See also Caisse to F. Egener, Secretary, Commission for the Investigation of Cancer Remedies, March 13, 1941, Wallace Papers, 1024b, Box 1, File 3, Queen's University Archives.

65. A.J.W. to N. O. Hipel, MPP, May 9, 1943, Wallace Papers, 1024b, Box 1, File 4, Queen's University Archives; A.B.D. to Hett, July 10, 1944; W.H.E. to Hett, September 20, 1944, and E.M. to Whom It May Concern, September 20, 1944, RG 10, Series 138, Accession 1576/12, Archives of Ontario; Noble to C. J. Telfer, Secretary, Cancer Commission, April 21, 1949, Wallace Papers, 1024b, Box 1, File 5, Queen's University Archives.

66. Ed Zalesky, quoted in "Cancer Hope Reborn," *Vancouver Sun Saturday Review*, May 16, 1992.

67. Susan Pryke, "Essiac, Miracle Cancer Cure: Fact or Fiction?" *Bracebridge Herald-Gazette*, August 16, 1989.

68. Burnham, "Golden Age," 1479.

Science and the Shadow of Ideology in the American Health Foods Movement, 1930s-1960s

I would like to thank Joseph Kett, Karen Parshall, Gregory Field, and Robert Johnston for their helpful comments and support.

1. Joe D. Nichols, "What We Believe," in Natural Foods Associates, *Yesterday Today Tomorrow* (Atlanta, Tex.: NFA, [1959]); copy of pamphlet in American Medical Association, Department of Investigation Records, Box 577 (Correspondence), Folder 0577–06 (Nichols, Dr. Joe Daniel, 1954–61). Courtesy AMA Archives, Chicago.

2. "History of the American Academy of Applied Nutrition," *Catalog of the American Academy of Applied Nutrition*, 1951, 5.

3. Charles W. Crawford, FDA Commissioner, quoted in Arthur D. Morse, "Don't Fall for Food Fads," *Woman's Home Companion*, December 1951, 32.

4. Since members of the AAAN and NFA never felt a need to uniquely identify themselves or the ideas that they represented, I have coined the term "health foodist" to refer to all those who shared their views on food and health.

5. Robert McCarrison, "Faulty Food in Relation to Gastrointestinal Disorders," *Bulletin of the Pan American Union* 54 (April 1922): 328–43; E. V. McCollum and Nina Simmonds, *The Newer Knowledge of Nutrition: The Use of Foods for the Preservation of Vitality and Health*, 3rd ed. (New York: Macmillan Co., 1925), 528; Henry C. Sherman, *Food and Health* (New York: Macmillan Co., 1936), 156–60.

McCollum, a co-discoverer of vitamin A while employed by the University of Wisconsin in 1913 and the man who first assigned letters of the alphabet to the vitamins, pioneered the "biological method of analysis," a method of establishing human nutritional needs by feeding purified food substances to laboratory animals. He was also a leader in nutrition education, writing several textbooks and a column in *McCall's* magazine from the 1920s to the 1940s. After his retirement he wrote a number of works on nutrition history and an autobiography. See Elmer V. McCollum, *From Kansas Farm Boy to Scientist: The Autobiography of Elmer Verner McCollum* (Lawrence: University of Kansas Press, 1964) and Harry G. Day, "Elmer Verner McCollum," in National Academy of Sciences, *Biographical Memoirs*, vol. 45 (Washington, D.C.: National Academy of Sciences, 1974), 262–335.

6. Tom D. Spies, William B. Bean, and William F. Ashe, "Recent Advances in the Treatment of Pellagra and Associated Deficiencies," *Annals of Internal Medicine*, n.s., 12 (1938–39): 1830–44; Tom Douglas Spies, "The Vitamin B Deficiencies," *Transactions and Studies of the College of Physicians of Philadelphia*, 4th ser., 8 (1940–41): 12–26; Hazel K. Stiebeling and Esther F. Phipard, *Diets of Families of Employed Wage Earners and Clerical Workers in Cities*, USDA Circular No. 507 (Washington, D.C.: GPO, 1939). The most comprehensive statement on malnutrition is found in National Research Council (NRC), Food and Nutrition Board, Committee on Diagnosis and Pathology of Nutritional Deficiencies, *Inadequate Diets and Nutritional Deficiencies in the United States: Their Prevalence and Significance*, NRC Bulletin No. 109 (Washington, D.C.: NRC, 1943).

7. Thomas Parran Jr., "Nutrition and National Health," *Technology Review*, June 1940, 323; Lewis B. Hershey, "Selective Service and Its Relation to Nutrition," in Federal Security Agency, Office of the Director of Defense Health and Welfare Services, *Proceedings of the National Nutrition Conference for Defense* (Washington, D.C.: GPO, 1942), 63–67. For a discussion of the nutrition program, see Harvey Levenstein, *Paradox of Plenty: A Social History of Eating in Modern America* (New York: Oxford University Press, 1993), 64–79.

8. J. B. Orr, *Minerals in Pastures and Their Relation to Animal Nutrition* (London: H. K. Lewis and Co., 1929); E. C. Auchter, "The Interrelationship of Soils and Plant, Animal and Human Nutrition," *Science* 89 (May 12, 1939): 421–27; Kenneth C. Beeson, *The Mineral Composition of Crops with Particular Reference to the Soils in Which They Were Grown: A Review and Compilation*, USDA Miscellaneous Publication No. 369 (Washington, D.C.: USDA, 1941), 1–22.

9. N. Philip Norman, "Our National Nutritional Dilemma," *Transactions of the American Therapeutic Society*, 1942, 113–16; D. T. Quigley, *The National Malnutrition*, 3rd ed. (Milwaukee: Lee Foundation for Nutritional Research, 1959), 56–58.

10. Jane Holt, "News of Food," *New York Times*, October 31, 1942, 8; Jane Holt, "News of Food," *New York Times*, August 17, 1942, 18; "Food and Nutrition Board Adopts Resolution," *Food Industries* 15 (December 1943): 104–5; E. V. McCollum, "'How About Using Dry Milk?'" *McCall's*, March 1943, 50; "Promotion Urged for Health Foods," *New York Times*, August 27, 1941, 33.

11. Russell M. Wilder, "Nutritional Health of Adults," in United States Department of Agriculture, *Proceedings of the National Food and Nutrition Institute*, Agricultural Handbook No. 56 (Washington, D.C.: GPO, [1953]), 52–58; "Why Youths Are Getting Bigger: People Are Eating Better than Ever Before," *U. S.*

News and World Report, June 3, 1955, 64–66; W. J. Dann and William J. Darby, "The Appraisal of Nutritional Status (Nutriture) in Humans," *Physiological Reviews* 25 (1945): 332–34.

12. W. Coda Martin, *A Matter of Life: Blueprint for a Healthy Family* (New York: Devin-Adair Co., 1964), 5–6; James Rorty and N. Philip Norman, *Tomorrow's Food*, rev. ed. (New York: Devin-Adair Co., 1956), 244–45.

In a December 1961 speech on the poor physical condition of America's youth, President John F. Kennedy provided ammunition for the movement, when he announced that three out of every seven men drafted were being rejected as physically unfit. (Two out of seven were being rejected for mental disabilities.) Selective Service statistics also supported the notion that rejection rates were rising, albeit slightly; during World War II 29.7 percent of inductees failed their physical examination, and between 1948 and 1960 the figure had increased to 30.6 percent. John F. Kennedy, "Text of Kennedy Speech at Football Dinner Here," *New York Times*, December 6, 1961, 61; Lewis B. Hershey, *Outline of Historical Background of Selective Service and Chronology*, rev. ed. (Washington, D.C.: GPO, 1961), tables 4 and 8.

13. Martin, *Matter of Life*, 6–10; James Rorty and N. Philip Norman, *Tomorrow's Food: The Coming Revolution in Nutrition* (New York: Prentice-Hall, 1947), 53–56; Jonathan Forman, "What Has Been Learned about Soil-Health Relationships at These Conferences," in Jonathan Forman and O. E. Fink, eds., *Soil, Food and Health: "You Are What You Eat"* (Columbus, Ohio: Friends of the Land, 1948), 317–20.

14. Rorty and Norman, *Tomorrow's Food*, 1956 ed., 245–46; Royal Lee and Jerome S. Stolzoff, *The Special Nutritional Qualities of Natural Foods*, Report No. 4 (Milwaukee: Lee Foundation for Nutritional Research, 1942), 39–40, 51–57; W. Coda Martin, "A Report on the Health of the Nation," in *Natural Food and Farming Digest* (Atlanta, Tex.: Natural Food Associates, 1957), 14–24; Joe D. Nichols, "Scientific Suicide," *Natural Food and Farming*, April 1958, 6–7.

15. Lee and Stolzoff, *Special Nutritional Qualities*, 37–39; Martin, *A Matter of Life*, 77–82, 86–87; N. Philip Norman, "How to Eat Sensibly without Vitamin Charts," in Rorty and Norman, *Tomorrow's Food*, 1947 ed., 234–40; Quigley, *National Malnutrition*, 89–95, 97–99; Fred D. Miller, "Saving Your Face," *Esquire*, May 1941, 133; Rorty and Norman, *Tomorrow's Food*, 1947 ed., 69–81; Rorty and Norman, *Tomorrow's Food*, 1956 ed., 230–34.

16. Martin, *Matter of Life*, 79; Quigley, *National Malnutrition*, 95–97; Rorty and Norman, *Tomorrow's Food*, 1947 ed., 106–14; Jonathan Forman, "What About Vitamins?" *Medical Arts and Sciences* 5 (1951): 88.

17. Forman and Fink, "Friends of the Land and Its Annual Conferences on Conservation, Nutrition, and Health—an Historical Sketch," in Forman and Fink, *Soil, Food and Health*, 19–29; Russell Lord, *The Care of the Earth: A History of Husbandry* (New York: Mentor Books, 1963), 251–58; John Bainbridge, "Farmer Bromfield," *Life*, October 11, 1948, 111.

18. Forman, "What Has Been Learned," 71–73; Louis Bromfield, *Pleasant Valley* (New York: Harper and Brothers, 1945), 112–16; Louis Bromfield, *Malabar Farm* (New York: Harper and Brothers, 1948), 295–323; Fred D. Miller, *Open Door to Health: A Dentist Looks at Life and Nutrition* (New York: Devin-Adair Co., 1959), 52–64.

19. Albert Howard, *An Agricultural Testament* (New York: Oxford University Press, 1943); Rudolf Steiner, *Spiritual Foundations for the Renewal of Agriculture: A Course of Lectures Held at Koberwitz, Silesia, June 7 to June 16, 1924*, trans. Catherine E. Creeger and Malcolm Gardner (Kimberton, Penn.: Bio-Dynamic Farming and Gardening Association, 1993); Rorty and Norman, *Tomorrow's Food*, 1947 ed., 146–48; Bromfield, *Malabar Farm*, 274–94; Louis Bromfield, *Out of the Earth* (New York: Harper and Brothers, 1950), 51–79.

20. Kay K. Thomas, "Foreword," *Godfrey's Let's Live*, January 1951, 1; Nichols, "Scientific Suicide," 14; N. Philip Norman, "Fundamentals of Nutrition for Physicians and Dentists," *American Journal of Orthodontics and Oral Surgery* 33 (1947): 781; Jonathan Forman, "A Newer Concept of Disease—Curative vs. Creative Medicine," *Mississippi Valley Medical Journal* 77 (January 1955): 40–45.

The movement was essentially secular, in that it was founded by doctors and dentists inspired by the discoveries of science. Most health foodists, however, saw no conflict between religion and science, and for some of them the nutritional superiority of natural foods was proof of divine benevolence.

21. Martin, *Matter of Life*, 69–74, 76; Rorty and Norman, *Tomorrow's Food*, 1947 ed., 29–39; Quigley, *National Malnutrition*, 5–6; Norman, "Our National Nutritional Dilemma," 125; Miller, *Open Door to Health*, 124.

22. W. Coda Martin, "Evolution in Nutrition," *Journal of Applied Nutrition* 15 (1962): 183; Rorty and Norman, *Tomorrow's Food*, 1947 ed., 6, 154–73.

23. Ehrenfried E. Pfeiffer, "Commentary on Definitions," in *Natural Food and Farming Digest,* 137; Bromfield, *Out of the Earth,* 282–83, 289; Bromfield, *Malabar Farm,* 217; Jonathan Forman, "Current Thinking in the Field of Nutrition," *Ohio State Medical Journal* 38 (September 1942): 847; Forman, "What Has Been Learned," 48–49.

24. Rorty and Norman, *Tomorrow's Food,* 1956 ed., 225–30; William E. Smith, "Food Additive Legislation," in *Natural Food and Farming Digest,* 51–54; Lester A. Swan, "Are We Winning the War With Insects?" in *Natural Food and Farming Digest* (Atlanta, Tex.: Natural Food Associates, 1957), 55–62; Louis Bromfield, in U.S. Congress, House Select Committee to Investigate the Use of Chemicals in Food Products, *Chemicals in Food Products: Hearings Created Pursuant to H. Res. 74,* 82nd Congress, 1st Session (Washington: GPO, 1951), Part 1, 289–314. Organic farming advocate J. I. Rodale also testified against the use of pesticides (and chemical fertilizers) at these hearings. Ibid., 851–78.

Conservative publisher and NFA official Devin A. Garrity served as vice chairman of the Committee Against Mass Poisoning, which was formed to support a lawsuit filed by a group of Long Island homeowners in 1957 to halt the aerial spraying of DDT to eradicate the gypsy moth. This lawsuit was one of the key events that provoked Rachel Carson to write *Silent Spring.* Committee Against Mass Poisoning, "Bulletin," in *Natural Food and Farming Digest* (Atlanta, Tex.: Natural Food Associates, 1957), 92–94; Linda Lear, *Rachel Carson: Witness for Nature* (New York: Owl Books, Henry Holt and Co., 1997), 312–26.

25. Donald R. McNeil, "America's Longest War: The Fight over Fluoridation, 1950–," *Wilson Quarterly* 9 (summer 1985): 140–53; Gregory Field, "'Socialized Medicine Creeping through the Back Door:' Anti-Fluoridation and Postwar Conservatism in the United States," paper presented at the annual meeting of the German Association for American Studies, May 1999, 13–16; Rorty and Norman, *Tomorrow's Food,* 1956 ed., 234–43; Forman, "What Has Been Learned," 66; Granville F. Knight, "A Statement on Fluoridation," in *Natural Food and Farming Digest* (Atlanta, Tex.: Natural Food Associates, 1957), 143–44; Jonathan Forman, "A Statement on Fluoridation," in *Natural Food and Farming Digest,* 144–45; Miller, *Open Door to Health,* 103–15.

26. Miller, *Open Door to Health,* 119–27; Lee and Stolzoff, *Special Nutritional Qualities,* 49–50; N. Philip Norman and James Rorty, "Our 'Civilized' Food Habits," *Antioch Review* 4 (fall 1944): 434–48; Rorty and Norman, *Tomorrow's Food,* 1947 ed., 78–80, 93–96, 205–29.

27. Jonathan Forman, "Current Thinking in Nutrition," *Ohio State Medical Journal* 41 (1945): 811, 815, 818; Jonathan Forman, "The Curse of Industrialism," *Land,* autumn 1947, 391; Jonathan Forman, "The Summing Up," *Land,* autumn 1947, 400, 402; Jonathan Forman, "Creative versus Curative Medicine," in Lionel James Picton, *Nutrition and the Soil: Thoughts on Feeding* (New York: Devin-Adair Co., 1949), 23–25; Norman, "Fundamentals of Nutrition," 780–81, 785; Miller, *Open Door to Health,* 179.

28. Norman, "Fundamentals of Nutrition," 783, 785; Lee and Stolzoff, *Special Nutritional Qualities,* 39.

29. Quigley, *National Malnutrition,* 88–90; Lee and Stolzoff, *Special Nutritional Qualities,* 49–50; Martin, *A Matter of Life,* 74.

30. Joe D. Nichols, "A Concept of Totality," in *Natural Food and Farming Digest,* 8–9; Albert Howard, *An Agricultural Testament* (New York: Oxford University Press, 1943), 17–20, 219–20; Ehrenfried Pfeiffer, *Bio-dynamic Farming and Gardening: Soil Fertility Renewal and Preservation,* rev. ed. (New York: Anthroposophic Press, 1943), esp. iii–vii, 5–6, 16–41; Forman, "What Has Been Learned," 41–50.

31. For general discussions of the decentralist movement, see William E. Leverette Jr., and David E. Shi, "Herbert Agar and *Free America*: A Jeffersonian Alternative to the New Deal," *American Studies* 16 (1982): 189–206, and George M. Lubick, "Restoring the American Dream: The Agrarian-Decentralist Movement, 1930–1946," *South Atlantic Quarterly* 84 (1985): 63–80. For expressions of support for decentralism by health foodists, see Louis Bromfield, "To Clear the Dross," in Elmer T. Peterson, ed., *Cities Are Abnormal* (Norman: University of Oklahoma Press, 1946), 183–98; Jonathan Forman, "Biological Truths and Public Health," in Elmer T. Peterson, ed., 95–120; and Ehrenfried Pfeiffer, *The Earth's Face: Landscape and Its Relation to the Health of the Soil* (London: Faber and Faber, [1947]), 79–83, 116. For Borsodi's views on food and health, see Ralph Borsodi, *Flight from the City: An Experiment in Creative Living on the Land* (New York: Harper and Brothers, [1933]), 1–2, 20–24, and Ralph Borsodi, *This Ugly Civilization* (New York: Simon and Schuster, 1929), 84–90, 106–7, 301–2.

The writer, social critic, and organic farmer Wendell Berry currently espouses ideas very similar to those of the decentralists in the 1930s and 1940s. See Allan Carlson, *The New Agrarian Mind: The Movement Toward Decentralist Thought in Twentieth-Century America* (New Brunswick, N.J.: Transaction Publishers, 2000), 177–201. This book also discusses the decentralist views of Borsodi, Bromfield, and their contemporary Father Luigi Ligutti, a leader of the American Catholic Rural Life movement and an advocate of organic farming, pp. 55–98, 149–76. Also see Luigi G. Ligutti and John C. Rawe, *Rural Roads to Security: America's Third Struggle for Freedom* (Milwaukee: Bruce Publishing Co., 1940), 217–21.

32. For the official positions of the American Medical Association on the soil issue and the adequacy of the food supply, see Leonard A. Maynard, "Soils and Health," *Journal of the American Medical Association* 143 (1950): 807–12, and Leonard A. Maynard, "An Adequate Diet," *Journal of the American Medical Association* 170 (1959): 457–58.

33. Adelle Davis, *Let's Eat Right to Keep Fit* (New York: Harcourt, Brace and World, 1954), passim; Carlton Fredericks, *Living Should Be Fun* (New York: Institute of Nutrition Research, [1943]), 13.

34. Norman Jolliffe, "The Pathogenesis of Deficiency Disease," in Norman Jolliffe, ed., *Clinical Nutrition*, 2nd ed. ([New York]: Harper and Brothers, Hoeber Medical Books, 1966), 17–27; C. A. Elvehjem and Willard H. Krehl, "Imbalance and Dietary Interrelationships in Nutrition," in American Medical Association, Council on Foods and Nutrition, *Handbook of Nutrition*, 2nd ed. (New York: Blakiston Co., 1951), 383–408; NRC Committee on Food and Nutrition, "Recommended Allowances for the Various Dietary Essentials," *Journal of the American Dietetic Association* 17 (June-July 1941): 565–67.

35. Davis, *Let's Eat Right to Keep Fit*, 223; Fredericks, *Living Should Be Fun*, 25–26; Roger J. Williams, *Biochemical Individuality: The Basis for the Genetotrophic Concept* (New York: John Wiley and Sons, 1956), 135–65; Roger J. Williams, *Nutrition in a Nutshell* (Garden City, N.Y.: Doubleday, 1962); Adelle Davis, *Let's Get Well* (New York: New American Library, Signet Paperback, 1965), 346; Carlton Fredericks and Herbert Bailey, *Food Facts and Fallacies: The Intelligent Person's Guide to Nutrition and Health* (New York: Arc Books, 1965), 106.

Williams had discovered, isolated, and named the vitamin pantothenic acid in the 1930s. After the war, while investigating a possible link between nutrition and alcoholism, he formulated the theory that "some individuals, because of their genetic makeup, require more of certain nutrients than they are likely to get from ordinary food (especially the stored and processed food of an industrial civilization) and for this reason, they tend to become deficient, and unwell as a result." He speculated that hundreds of diseases of unknown etiology, including alcoholism and many major chronic illnesses, were caused by nutritional deficiencies and would someday be treated with vitamins and minerals. See Roger J. Williams, "The Genetotrophic Concept—Nutritional Deficiencies and Alcoholism," *Annals of the New York Academy of Sciences* 57 (May 10, 1954): 794–809; and Roger J. Williams, "The Expanding Horizon in Nutrition," *Texas Reports on Biology and Medicine* 19 (summer 1961): 245–58.

36. E. M. [*sic*] McCollum, "The Relation of Vitamins to Disease," *New York State Journal of Medicine* 26 (September 18, 1926): 280; Henry C. Sherman, "Food and Health," *De Lamar Lectures, 1928–9* (Baltimore: Williams and Wilkins Co., 1929), 14–16; NRC Committee on Food and Nutrition, "Report of Subcommittee on Standards for Dietary Requirements," [1941], 1, in Box 8, Subject File, Enriched Foodstuffs, Robert R. Williams Papers, Library of Congress, Washington, D.C.; Jonathan Forman, "The Trace Mineral Elements in Nutrition," *Ohio State Medical Journal* 38 (October 1942): 937.

37. Tom D. Spies, "Influence of Pregnancy, Lactation, Growth, and Aging on Nutritional Processes," *Journal of the American Medical Association* 153 (September 19, 1953): 185; "Food Facts and Fables," *Science News Letter*, July 20, 1957, 38. The writings and discussions of health food popularizers were filled with references to medical articles. For example, see Davis, *Let's Get Well*, and Fredericks and Bailey, *Food Facts and Fallacies*.

38. Institute of Medicine, Food and Nutrition Board, Standing Committee on the Scientific Evaluation of Dietary Reference Intakes, *Dietary Reference Intakes for Calcium, Phosphorus, Magnesium, Vitamin D, and Fluoride* (Washington: National Academy Press, 1997); Paul Walter, Dietrich Hornig, and Ulrich K. Moser, eds., *Functions of Vitamins beyond Recommended Dietary Allowances*, Bibliotheca Nutritio et Dieta, no. 55 (Basel: Karger, 2001); Joanne L. Slavin et al., "The Role of Whole Grains in Disease Prevention," *Journal of the American Dietetic Association* 101 (July 2001): 780–85. For a discussion of the role of knowledge gaps in scientific controversy, see S. Holly Stocking and Lisa W. Holstein, "Constructing and Reconstructing Scientific Ignorance," *Knowledge: Creation, Diffusion, Utilization* 15 (1993): 186–210.

39. Charles E. Rosenberg, "Pathologies of Progress: The Idea of Civilization as Risk," *Bulletin of the History of Medicine* 72 (winter 1998): 714–30. For the antimodernism of the popular conservation movement, see Stephen Fox, *The American Conservation Movement: John Muir and His Legacy* (Madison: University

of Wisconsin Press, 1981), 352–55. The history of the post-1966 health foods movement is told in Warren J. Belasco, *Appetite for Change: How the Counterculture Took on the Food Industry*, rev. ed. (Ithaca, N.Y.: Cornell University Press, 1993).

As the subtitle of his book indicates, Belasco focuses on the radical anti-business views of post-1966 health foodists. He does not seem to think that the pre-1966 and post-1966 movements had much in common, and he studiously avoids all mention of the well-known right-wing associations of the earlier movement. It is my contention, however, that aside from the latter's advocacy of vegetarianism, the views of pre-1966 and post-1966 health foodists were essentially the same.

"Voodoo Death"

This research was supported by the Israel Science Foundation (grant no. 0325229). I would like to thank Robert Johnston for his numerous helpful suggestions and comments.

1. Zora Neale Hurston, *Mules and Men* (Bloomington: Indiana University Press, 1935), 193. To include: Preface by Franz Boas, introduction by Robert E. Hemenway, this edition 1978.

2. Paul K. Feyerabend, *Against Method: Outline of an Anarchistic Theory of Knowledge* (London: Verso, 1975), 50.

3. Walter B. Cannon, " 'Voodoo' Death," *American Anthropologist* 33 (1942): 169–81.

4. Claude Lévi-Strauss, "The Sorcerer and His Magic," in *Structural Anthropology* (New York: Basic Books, 1963), 167–85, citation to 167. In her study on the military occupation of Haiti, Mary A. Renda argues that there are "several alternative spellings of Vodou (e.g., Vodoun, Vodun)." "Voodoo," she argues, "refer[s] to the exotic phantasm that sensational writers constructed through their discourses on Haiti." In this essay, I follow the usage of the correspondents themselves. See Mary A. Renda, *Taking Haiti: Military Occupation and the Culture of U.S. Imperialism 1915–1940* (Chapel Hill: University of North Carolina Press, 2001), 317 n. 28.

5. Zora Neale Hurston, *Mules and Men*, 195.

6. Cannon's correspondents included physicians and several anthropologists from around the globe. He contacted Dr. Rudolph Fuszek, of Monrovia, Liberia, West Africa; Dr. George W. Harley, of the Peabody Museum, Cambridge, Massachusetts; Prof. R. F. A. Hoernle, of the University of Witwatersrand, Johannesburg, South Africa; Dr. Leslie J. Tarlton, of Safariland Ltd., Nairobi, British East Africa; and numerous other physicians from Australia, Haiti, Hawaii, Fiji, and Havana. Even the surgeon general, R. U. Patterson, Washington, D.C., provided valuable information. For Cannon's correspondence regarding voodoo death, see box 67, Walter Bradford Cannon Papers (H MS c40), Rare Books and Special Collections, Harvard Medical Library in the Francis A. Countway Library of Medicine, Boston (hereafter WBC).

7. Cannon to Dr. Daniel de la Paz, Manila, Philippine Islands, June 30, 1934, folder 889, box 67, WBC.

8. Laurie Sharpe, Australian National Research Council, Sydney, to Mrs. Cannon, November 3, 1934, folder 901, box 67, WBC; and C. S. Butler, U. S. Naval Hospital, Brooklyn, New York, to Cannon, October 15, 1934, folder 898, box 67, WBC.

9. J. B. Cleland, professor of pathology, University of Adelaide, to Cannon, November 22, 1934, folder 901, box 67, WBC.

10. M. E. Higgins, U.S. Naval Hospital, Brooklyn, New York, to Cannon, October 23, 1934, folder 898, box 67, WBC.

11. H. L. Arnold, M.D., Honolulu, to Cannon, July 11, 1934, folder 899, box 67, WBC.

12. R. P. Parsons, lieutenant-commander (Medical Corps), U.S. Naval Hospital, San Diego, to Cannon, November 5, 1934, folder 898, box 67, WBC.

13. G. W. Harley to Cannon, April 29, 1935, folder 900, box 67, WBC.

14. Kent C. Melhorn, captain, Train Squadron Two, United States Fleet (Canal Zone), to Cannon, October 22, 1934, folder 898, box 67, WBC.

15. M. E. Higgins, US Naval Hospital, Brooklyn, New York, to Cannon, October 23, 1934, folder 898, box 67, WBC.

16. R. P. Parsons, lieutenant-commander (Medical Corps), U.S. Naval Hospital, San Diego, to Cannon, November 5, 1934, folder 898, box 67, WBC. This is probably a reference to Captain John Houston Craige, author of *Black Bagdad: The Arabian Nights Adventures of a Marine Captain in Haiti* (1933) and *Cannibal Cousins* (1934).

17. Cannon to Dr. Leslie J. Tarlton, c/o Safariland Ltd., Nairobi, British East Africa, February 14, 1935; and Leslie J. Tarlton to Cannon, March 26, 1935. Both are in folder 900, box 67, WBC.

18. Renda, *Taking Haiti*; Robert Hemenway, "Introduction," in Zora Neale Hurston, *Mules and Men* (Bloomington: Indiana University Press, 1978 [1935]).

19. Boas, preface to Hurston, *Mules and Men*, p. x.

20. S. de la Rue to Cannon, October 25, 1934, folder 898, box 67, WBC.

21. Ralph Linton to Cannon, October 16, 1941, folder 904, box 67, WBC.

22. For additional supporting letters, see, e.g., S. D. Porteus, professor of clinical psychology, University of Hawaii, to Cannon, January 5, 1935; and S. M. Lambert (?), Western Pacific Health Service, Rockefeller Foundation, Colony of Fijito, to Cannon, January 8, 1934. Both are located in folder 899, box 67, WBC.

23. The title is an adaptation of Ralph Ellison's *Invisible Man* (New York: Modern Library, 1952).

24. This particular correspondent, however, argued against his colleague, asserting that alleged spell deaths were explicable by real pathological lesions discovered during autopsies. See James R. Judd, the Medical Group, Honolulu, to Cannon, July 16, 1934, folder 899, box 67, WBC.

25. Michael Edward Bell, "Harry Middleton Hyatt's Quest for the Essence of Human Spirit," *Journal of the Folklore Institute* 16 (1979): 1–27.

26. On Puckett, see Patrick B. Mullen, "Belief and the American Folk," *Journal of American Folklore* 113 (2000): 119–43, especially 122–25.

27. Claude Jacobs, "Folk for Whom? Tourist Guidebooks, Local Color, and the Spiritual Churches of New Orleans," *Journal of American Folklore* 114 (2001): 309–30.

28. Rachel Stein, "Remembering the Sacred Tree: Black Women, Nature and Voodoo in Zora Neale Hurston's 'Tell My Horse' and 'Their Eyes Were Watching God,'" *Women's Studies* 25 (1996): 465–83. There has been some controversy concerning the assumed contributory role of voodoo ritual in the Haitian revolution. For the classic study, see Alfred Métraux, *Voodoo in Haiti* (London: A. Deutsch, 1959 [1950]). For a reappraisal, see David Geggus, "Haitian Voodoo in the Eighteenth Century: Language, Culture, Resistance," in *Jahrbuch fur Geschichte von Staat: Wirtschaft und Gesellschaft Lateinamerikas* 28 (1991): 21–51.

29. Cheryl A. Wall, "Mules and Men and Women: Zora Neale Hurston's Strategies of Narration and Visions of Female Empowerment," *Black American Literature Forum* 23 (1989): 661–80, citations to 672, 679 n. 13. Cynthia Schrager and Daphne Lamothe have developed similar arguments in their respective analyses of W. E. B. Du Bois' spiritualism and Hurston's *Their Eyes Were Watching God*. See Cynthia D. Schrager, "Both Sides of the Veil: Race, Science, and Mysticism in W. E. B. Du Bois," *American Quarterly* 48 (December 1996): 551–86; Daphne Lamothe, "Vodou Imagery, African-American Tradition and Cultural Transformation in Zora Neale Hurston's *Their Eyes Were Watching God*," *Callaloo* 22, 1 (1999): 157–75. The challenge that nonwhite syncretism posed for the Western moral and racial order was also visible and explicitly addressed by conservative clergymen and educators, who "feared that nonwhite syncretism was also behind utopian declarations about the radical equality of all human souls." See Russ Castronovo, "The Antislavery Unconscious: Mesmerism, vodun, and 'equality,' " *The Mississippi Quarterly* 53 (1999–2000): 41–56. See also Rocky Sexton, "Cajun and Creole Theaters: Magico-Religious Folk Healing in French Louisiana," *Western Folklore* 51 (1992): 237–48.

30. Yvonnne Chireau, "Conjure and Christianity in the Nineteenth Century: Religious Elements in African American Magic," *Religion and American Culture* 7 (1997): 225–47.

31. Seward Hiltner, executive secretary, Federal Council of the Churches of Christ in America, New York, to Cannon, November 7, 1941, folder 903, box 67, WBC.

32. Cannon to Seward Hiltner, November 8, 1941, folder 903, box 67, WBC: "Of course the emotional conditions which might result in death are undoubtedly extreme. The subtler influences which surely have a profound influence in bringing on illness or restoring health are not easily determinable. Perhaps sometime in the future physiologists will be able to learn how they may operate." On Christian healing, see, e.g., Jonathan M. Butler and Rennie B. Schoepflin, "Charismatic Women and Health: Mary Baker Eddy, Ellen G. White, and Aimee Semple McPherson," in Rima Apple, ed., *Women, Health, and Medicine in America: A Historical Handbook* (New Brunswick, N.J.: Rutgers University Press, 1990), 329–57; Eric Caplan, *Mind Games: American Culture and the Birth of Psychotherapy* (Berkeley and Los Angeles: University of California Press, 1998); and Robert Charles Powell, "Healing and Wholeness: Helen Flanders Dunbar (1902–59) and an Extra-Medical Origin of the American Psychosomatic Movement, 1906–36," Ph.D. dissertation, Duke University, 1974.

33. Leslie J. Tarlton to Cannon, March 26, 1935, folder 900, box 67, WBC.

34. Alison Winter, *Mesmerized: Powers of Mind in Victorian Britain* (Chicago: University of Chicago Press, 1998). These contestations over alternative systems of knowledge took on various forms and often involved or implicated the state and its particular interests. See, for example, Jan Goldstein, *Console and Classify: The French Psychiatric Profession in the Nineteenth Century* (Cambridge: Cambridge University Press, 1987).

35. Martin S. Pernick, "The Calculus of Suffering in 19th-Century Surgery," in Judith Walzer Leavitt and Ronald L. Numbers, eds., *Sickness and Health in American: Readings in the History of Medicine and Public Health* (Madison: University of Wisconsin Press, 1985), 98–112; and Naomi Rogers, *An Alternative Path: The Making and Remaking of Hahnemann Medical College and Hospital* (New Brunswick, N.J.: Rutgers University Press, 1998).

36. Steve C. Martin, "'The Only Truly Scientific Method in Healing': Chiropractic and American Science, 1895–1990," *Isis* 85 (1994): 207–27; Rogers, *An Alternative Path*; Caplan, *Mind Games*.

37. There were many kinds of psychosomatic approaches. The term *psychosomatic* may be misleading. Psychosomatic medicine included many clinicians who often disagreed on the relationships between psyche, soma, pathology, diagnosis, therapeutics, etc. Though it is true that psychosomatic medicine as a whole took a turn in the direction of psychoanalysis, particularly during the second third of the twentieth century, its pre–Second World War history was dominated by an important physiological approach. Several authors writing about psychosomatic medicine have traced its history to Freud. But this emphasis on psychoanalysis as representing psychosomatic medicine is an artifact of the psychosomatic movement in its late institutionalized form.

38. Dora Hepner Moitoret to the Department of Medicine and Psychiatry, New York Hospital, October 29, 1942, folder 6, box 1, Harold G. Wolff Papers, Archives, New York Weill Cornell Center of New York Presbyterian Hospital, New York (henceforth HGW).

39. Arthur Whitcomb to H. G. Wolff, May 2, 1963, folder 3, box 4, HGW.

40. "Conditioned Responses—Lecture to 1st year class Physiology—June 2, 1938," folder 21 ("Conditioned Response: Lectures Outlines, Notes, Mss. Etc., 1930s"), box 8, HGW; and Franz Alexander, "Psychological Aspects of Medicine," *Psychosomatic Medicine* 1 (1939): 7–18, citation to 7. See also Theodore M. Brown, "Emotions and Disease in Historical Perspective," in *Emotions and Disease* (Bethesda: National Library of Medicine, 1997); and Brown, "Alan Gregg and the Rockefeller Foundation's Support of Franz Alexander's Psychosomatic Research," *Bulletin of the History of Medicine* 61 (1987): 155–82.

41. Otniel E. Dror, "Counting the Affects: Discoursing in Numbers," *Social Research* 68 (summer 2001): 357–78. See also Elizabeth Lunbeck, *The Psychiatric Persuasion: Knowledge, Gender, and Power in Modern America* (Princeton: Princeton University Press, 1994) for the argument that emotions belonged to domestic knowledge, and for her analysis of the tensions that ensued when men (American psychiatrists) appropriated this knowledge in the process of constructing the new profession of psychiatrist.

42. Rogers, *An Alternative Path*, 9; Pernick, "The Calculus of Suffering." The heroic reliance on massive doses and extreme measures, regardless of pain, was by no means limited to orthodox physicians.

43. Naomi Rogers, "Women and Sectarian Medicine," in Rima Apple, *Women, Health, and Medicine in America: A Historical Handbook* (New Brunswick, N.J.: Rutgers University Press, 1990), 273–302, citation to 295.

44. Butler and Schoepflin, "Charismatic Women."

45. Judith R. Walkowitz, *City of Dreadful Delight: Narratives of Sexual Danger in Late-Victorian London* (Chicago: University of Chicago Press, 1992), chapter 6. For the citation, see 172. Epistemological marginality also had its advantages. As recent literature on several women scientists has highlighted, marginality could serve as an empowering device, enabling women to hold epistemological positions or to cultivate ways of knowing that were different from the male community of knowledge producers. See, for example, Evelyn Fox Keller, *A Feeling for the Organism: The Life and Work of Barbara McClintock* (San Francisco: W. H. Freeman and Company, 1983), and Alison Winter, "A Calculus of Suffering: Ada Lovelace and the Bodily Constraints on Women's Knowledge in Early Victorian England," in Christopher Lawrence and Steve Shapin, eds., *Science Incarnate: Historical Embodiments of Natural Knowledge* (Chicago: University of Chicago Press, 1998), 202–39.

46. William James, *The Varieties of Religious Experience: A Study in Human Nature* (New York: Modern Library, 1902). These are the Gifford Lectures on natural religion delivered at Edinburgh in 1901–02. See especially Lectures IV and V, 77–124.

47. Cynthia D. Schrager, "Pauline Hopkins and William James: The New Psychology and the Politics of Race," in John Cullen Gruesser, ed., *The Unruly Voice: Rediscovering Pauline Elizabeth Hopkins* (Urbana and Chicago: University of Illinois Press, 1996), 182–209. See also Schrager, "Both Sides of the Veil," and Susan Gillman, "Pauline Hopkins and the Occult: African-American Revisions of Nineteenth-Century Sciences," *American Literary History* 8 (spring 1996): 57–82. For a different reading of James, see Walkowitz, *City of Dreadful Delight.*

48. R. Laurence Moore, *In Search of White Crows: Spiritualism, Parapsychology, and American Culture* (New York: Oxford University Press, 1977), chapters 3–4. Before the Civil War the Spiritualists were supported by men and women who also supported Fourierism, temperance, anti-slavery, health reform, and women's rights. It was not a coincidence that Karl Popper, in his famous discourse on demarcation, *Conjectures and Refutation*, refers to the anti-vaccination movement as one example of a nonscience. See Karl R. Popper, "Science: Conjectures and Refutations," in *Conjectures and Refutations: The Growth of Scientific Knowledge* (New York: Basic Books, 1962), 33–65.

49. Cannon to Dr. Daniel de la Paz, Manila, Philippine Islands, June 30, 1934, folder 889, box 67, WBC.

50. Cannon, " 'Voodoo' Death," 179.

51. On the history of the decerebrate cat, see Otniel E. Dror, "Techniques of the Brain and the Paradox of Emotions, 1880–1930," *Science in Context* 14 (winter 2001): 643–660.

52. "Conditioned Responses—Lecture to 1st year class Physiology—June 2, 1938," folder 21 ("Conditioned Response: Lectures Outlines, Notes, Mss. etc., 1930s"), box 8, HGW.

53. Cannon to W. Lloyd Warner, Department of Anthropology, University of Chicago, September 30, 1941, folder 903, box 67, WBC.

54. From Freeman to Cannon, January 5, 1939, folder 1554, box 112, WBC. For Freeman's chapter, see Norman E. Freeman, "Shock," in William D. Stroud, ed., *The Diagnosis and Treatment of Cardiovascular Disease* (Philadelphia: F. A. Davis Company, 1941), 2: 1381–412. In this chapter, Freeman refers to "[c]linical cases of shock precipitated by fear" and enlists "a surgeon of such wide experience as J. M. T. Finney [who] has emphasized the importance of the emotional attitude of the patient prior to operation." He also describes a woman who deteriorated to a state of shock from fear and later recovered. Cannon had spoken with Finney in 1934 "regarding some ideas he has concerning the dangers of operating on a person who has great fear of death from operation. I told him that I am very much interested in this phenomenon, particularly in relation to the casting of a spell by the 'medicine man' in primitive tribes and the death that is said to result there from." Cannon to Philip Bard, Department of Physiology, Johns Hopkins University, June 6, 1934, folder 1525, box 110, WBC.

55. Barbara W. Lex, "Voodoo Death: New Thoughts on an Old Explanation," *American Anthropologist* 76 (1974): 818–23; H. D. Eastwell, "Voodoo Death and the Mechanisms for the Dispatch of the Dying in East Arnhem, Australia," *American Anthropologist* 84 (1982): 5–18; Janice Reid and Nancy Williams, "'Voodoo Death' in Arnhem Land: Whose Reality?" *American Anthropologist* 86 (1984): 121–33.

56. For the exchange, see *British Medical Journal* (1965): 591, 700, 876, 1004, 1124, and 1186.

57. Mary Douglas, *Purity and Danger: An Analysis of Concepts of Pollution and Taboo* (London and New York: Routledge, 1996 [1966]).

58. George L. Engel, "Sudden and Rapid Death during Psychological Stress: Folklore or Folk Wisdom?" *Annals of Internal Medicine* 74 (1971): 771–82. This is a review of numerous articles.

59. Chris Rojek, *Decentring Leisure: Rethinking Leisure Theory* (London: Sage, 1995), 87, and Peter Stallybrass and Allon White, *The Politics and Poetics of Transgression* (London: Methuen, 1986), 25.

Western Medicine and Navajo Healing

This selection is drawn from Wade Davies, *Healing Ways: Navajo Health Care in the Twentieth Century* (Albuquerque: University of New Mexico Press, 2001).

1. Linda Richards, "Resident Healer," *Arizona Republic*, April 10, 1997, HL1–HL2.

2. Donald Sandner, *Navaho Symbols of Healing* (New York: Harcourt Brace Jovanovich, 1979); Clyde Kluckhohn and Dorothea Leighton, *The Navaho*, rev. ed. (Garden City, N.Y.: Anchor Books/Doubleday, 1962); Leland Wyman, "Navajo Ceremonial System," in Alfonso Ortiz, ed., *Southwest*, vol. 10 of *Handbook of North American Indians*, gen. ed. William C. Sturtevant (Washington: Smithsonian Institution, 1983), 536–57.

3. Paul Starr, *The Social Transformation of American Medicine* (New York: Basic Books, 1982); Jennie Joe, "Navajo Singers and Western Medical Doctors," paper presented at the annual meeting of the American Historical Association, Chicago, Illinois, December 27–30, 1991, 3–4.

4. John Adair, Kurt Deuschle, and Clifford Barnett, *The People's Health: Medicine and Anthropology in a Navajo Community*, rev. and exp. ed. (Albuquerque: University of New Mexico Press, 1988), 27.

5. Robert Trennert, *White Man's Medicine: Government Doctors and the Navajo, 1863–1955* (Albuquerque: University of New Mexico Press, 1998).

6. Robert Trennert, "White Doctors among the Navajos, 1868–1928," paper presented at the annual meeting of the Western History Association, Tulsa, Oklahoma, October 1993.

7. Trennert, *White Man's Medicine*, 26–33.

8. Clarence Salsbury with Paul Hughes, *The Salsbury Story: A Medical Missionary's Lifetime of Public Service* (Tucson: University of Arizona Press, 1969), 123.

9. Alexander and Dorothea Leighton, "Therapeutic Values in Navajo Religion," *Arizona Highways* 43, 8 (1967): 2–13. Also see Alexander and Dorothea Leighton, *The Navaho Door: An Introduction to Navaho Life* (Cambridge, Mass.: Harvard University Press, 1944; New York: R and R, 1967).

10. Adair, *The People's Health*, 23, 32.

11. Statements of Maunelito Begay, Minutes of the Navajo Tribal Council, February 8–12, 1954, 132–33.

12. Adair, *The People's Health*, 11–12.

13. Jerome du Bois, *Navajo Times*, April 27, 1978, 19.

14. United States Department of Health and Human Services, United States Public Health Service, Indian Health Service, "Dedication, Chinle Comprehensive Health Care Facility," August 28, 1982, Chinle, Navajo Nation, Folder 189, Virginia Brown, Ida Bahl, and Lillian Watson Collection, MS269, Special Collections, Northern Arizona University, Flagstaff.

15. Raymond Estrada, discharge planner, Rehoboth McKinley Hospital, interview by author, Gallup, New Mexico, December 3, 1993; John King, director of development, Sage Memorial Hospital, interview by author, Ganado, Arizona, October 2, 1992; Will Stapleton and Patricia Heredia, "A History: Churches Contribute to Navajo Nation Health Care," *Navajo Times*, April 8, 1976, B-10, B-13.

16. H. J. Hagerman, J. C. Morgan, et al., Minutes of the Fifth Annual Session of the Navajo Tribal Council, July 7–8, 1927, pp. 3–8, 68–72, 76–83, Roll 1, *Navajo Tribal Council Minutes, Major Council Meetings of American Indian Tribes* (Frederick, Md.: University Publications of America, 1991), microfilm (hereinafter cited as NTCM); "Health—Establishment of Committee on," January 18, 1938, *Navajo Tribal-Council Resolutions, 1922–1951* (Window Rock, Ariz.: Navajo Tribe, 1952), 133; Statement of W. W. Peter, et al., Proceedings of the Meetings of the Navajo Tribal Council and the Executive Committee, January 17–20, 1938, p. 160, Roll 1, NTCM.

17. Statements by J. M. Stewart, Thomas Dodge, et al., July 9–11, 1943, 17, Roll 1, NTCM; Statements by Scott Preston, Thomas Dodge, et al., Proceedings of the Delegation of the Navajo Tribal Council in Washington, D.C., May 13–25, 1946, p. 13, Roll 2, NTCM; *Statements on Conditions among the Navajo Tribe: Hearings before the Committee on Indian Affairs, House of Representatives*, 79th Cong., 2nd sess. (Washington, D.C.: GPO, 1946).

18. Statements by J. M. Stewart, Thomas Dodge, et al., July 9–11, 1943, 17, Roll 1, NTCM; Statements by Scott Preston, Thomas Dodge, et al., Proceedings of the Delegation of the Navajo Tribal Council in Washington, D.C., May 13–25, 1946, p. 13, Roll 2, NTCM.

19. Virginia Hoffman and Broderick H. Johnson, "Annie Dodge Wauneka: Tsennjikini Clan—house beneath Cliff People," in Virginia Hoffman and Broderick H. Johnson, *Navajo Biographies* (Rough Rock, Ariz.: Diné Inc. and the Board of Education, Rough Rock Demonstration School, Navajo Curriculum Center, 1970), 292–307.

20. Steven Spencer, "They're Saving Lives in Navaho Land," *Saturday Evening Post* 227 (April 1955): 96.

21. Ibid.; Journal of the Navajo Tribal Council, May 13, 1954, p. 2, 12 February 1955, pp. 1–4, Box 82, Folder 36, Dennis Chavez Papers, Center for Southwest Research (hereinafter cited as CSR), University of New Mexico, Albuquerque; Statements by Kurt Deuschle, Annie Wauneka, et al., February 12, 1954, Roll 9, NTCM.

22. *Navajo Times*, September 3, 1981, 10, 12; Peggy Nakai, special projects coordinator for Navajo Division of Health, Department of Operations, interview by author, Window Rock, Arizona, March 5, 1993.

23. *Navajo Times*, April 19, 1996, A2, A5; February 19, 1998, A10; August 13, 1998, A2; January 21, 1999, Al.

24. Dr. Lori Arviso Alvord, interview by author, August 5, 1997, Gallup Indian Medical Center, Gallup, New Mexico.

25. "Navajo Mental Health," *The Rough Rock News*, November 18, 1970.

26. Impressions taken from the Navajo Transcripts, American Indian Oral History Collection, 1967–72, MSS 314 BC, CSR, microfilm (hereinafter cited as AIOHC), and Broderick H. Johnson, ed., *Stories of Traditional Navajo Life and Culture* (Tsaile, Ariz.: Navajo Community College Press, 1977).

27. Adair, *The People's Health*, 161–79; Deescheeny Nez Tracy, interview in Johnson, ed., *Stories of Traditional Navajo Life*, 165.

28. Tracy, interview in Johnson, ed., *Stories of Traditional Navajo Life*, 164.

29. John Dick, interview in Johnson, ed., *Stories of Traditional Navajo Life*, 200.

30. Hosteen Klah shared ceremonies with Franc Newcomb; see Franc Johnson Newcomb, *Hosteen Klah: Navajo Medicine Man and Sand Painter* (Norman: University of Oklahoma Press, 1964); Howard Gorman, interview by Daniel Tyler, Ganado, Arizona, October 25, 1968, Tape 533, Roll 3, Navajo Transcripts, AIOHC.

31. Peter Iverson, *The Navajo Nation* (Westport, Conn.: Greenwood Press, 1981; 3d pbk printing, Albuquerque," University of New Mexico Press, 1989), 114–123; "Navajo Mental Health."

32. Dr. Robert L. Bergman, interview in Brad Steiger, *Indian Medicine Power* (Atglen, Penn.: Whitford Press, 1984), 51; "Navajo Mental Health"; Robert A. Roessel Jr., *Navajo Education in Action: The Rough Rock Demonstration School* (Chinle, Ariz.: Navajo Curriculum Center, Rough Rock Demonstration School, 1977), 83–85; Robert Roessel, former director of the Rough Rock Demonstration School and president of Navajo Community College, interview by author, Round Rock, Arizona, July 29, 1997.

33. Ibid. "Navajo Mental Health."

34. Ibid. "Navajo Mental Health"; Bergman, interview, 47–51.

35. *Navajo Times*, November 10, 1977, A4, and April 27, 1978, 19; Charlotte J. Frisbie, "Temporal Change in Navajo Religion: 1868–1990," *Journal of the Southwest* 34, 4 (1992): 496–97.

36. Charlotte J. Frisbie, *Navajo Medicine Bundles or Jish: Acquisition, Transmission, and Disposition in the Past and Present* (Albuquerque: University of New Mexico Press, 1987), 284–95.

37. *Navajo Times*, October 19, 1995, B16; December 31, 1996, A7; March 20, 1997, Al, A3; April 2, 1998, Al.

38. *Arizona Republic*, November 4, 1991, Al.

Sister Kenny Goes to Washington

My thanks for their helpful comments and suggestions to Margaret Ernst, Gina Feldberg, Susan Lederer, Robert Johnston, and the audience of the New York Academy of Medicine, where I presented this work in its earliest incarnation.

1. Elizabeth Kenny, May 14, 1948, *Hearings before the Committee on Interstate and Foreign Commerce, House of Representatives, Eightieth Congress, Second Session, on H.R. 977* [cancer and polio research] . . . *H.R. 3257* [cancer research commission] . . . *H.R. 3464* [cure of cancer, heart disease, infantile paralysis, and other diseases] . . . *May 13, 14, and 19, 1948* (Washington, D.C.: GPO, 1948), 97, 114. Hereafter *Hearings*.

2. Elizabeth Kenny, Report to Board of Directors of the Sister Elizabeth Kenny Foundation, May 24, 1948, 143-E-10-3(b), Box 1, Board of Directors, Elizabeth Kenny Papers, Minnesota Historical Society (hereafter Kenny-MHS); Kenny, *Hearings*, May 14, 1948, 115.

3. See Tony Gould, *A Summer Plague: Polio and Its Survivors* (New Haven: Yale University Press, 1995), 44–46; Jane S. Smith, *Patenting the Sun: Polio and the Salk Vaccine* (New York: William Morrow, 1990), 52–63.

4. Marion T. Bennett, *Hearings*, May 14, 1948, 108. Marion Tinsley Bennett (1914–2000) was a Missouri Republican in the House 1943–49.

5. There is no full history of the National Foundation, but see Gould, *A Summer Plague*, 41–126, and Smith, *Patenting the Sun*, 64–87. On the significance of the National Foundation in funding medical research, see Daniel J. Kevles, "Foundations, Universities, and Trends in Support for Physical and Biological Sciences, 1900–1992," *Daedalus* 121 (1992): 195–235, especially 217–19.

6. John C. Burnham, "American Medicine's Golden Age: What's Happened to It?" in Judith Walzer Leavitt and Ronald L. Numbers, eds., *Sickness and Health in America: Readings in the History of Medicine and Public Health*, 3rd ed. (Madison: University of Wisconsin Press, 1997), 284–94; see also Allan M. Brandt and Martha Gardner, "The Golden Age of Medicine?" in Roger Cooter and John Pickstone, eds., *Medicine in the Twentieth Century* (London: Harwood, 2000), 21–37.

7. See Susan E. Lederer, *Subjected to Science: Human Experimentation in America before the Second World War* (Baltimore: Johns Hopkins University Press, 1995); Norman Gevitz, *The D.O.'s: Osteopathic Medicine in America* (Baltimore: Johns Hopkins University Press, 1982); Naomi Rogers, *An Alternative Path: The Making and Remaking of Hahnemann Medical College and Hospital of Philadelphia* (New Brunswick, N.J.: Rutgers University Press, 1998); and James Whorton, *Nature Cures: The History of Alternative Medicine in America* (New York: Oxford University Press, 2002). On the important point that the American public continued into the twentieth century to support critics of medical science, see Ronald L. Numbers, "The Fall and Rise of the American Medical Profession," in Judith Walzer Leavitt and Ronald L. Numbers, eds., *Sickness and Health in America: Readings in the History of Medicine and Public Health* (Madison: University of Wisconsin Press, 1985), 232–34.

8. See, for example, Morris Fishbein, *The Medical Follies: An Analysis of the Foibles of Some Healing Cults, Including Osteopathy, Homeopathy, Chiropractic, and the Electronic Reactions of Abrahms, with Essays of the Antivivisectionists, Health Legislation, Physical Culture, Birth Control, and Rejuvenation* (New York: Boni and Liveright, 1925).

9. See James Harvey Young, *The Medical Messiahs: A Social History of Health Quackery in Twentieth-Century America* (Princeton: Princeton University Press, 1967), 149–50, 371–74, 381; Alton Lee, *The Bizarre Careers of John R. Brinkley* (Lexington: University Press of Kentucky, 2002), 119–50. Brinkley used his growing wealth to support the American Fascist Party, and when he ran for a Kansas Senate seat he was endorsed by Wichita Fascist fundamentalist Reverend Gerald B. Winrod, whose journal, *The Defender*, castigated "Darwinism moralism," scientific orthodoxy, and later fluoridation; Leo P. Ribuffo, *The Old Christian Right: The Protestant Far Right from the Great Depression to the Cold War* (Philadelphia: Temple University Press, 1983), 90–91, 119–21.

10. A 1947 study of all sources of American medical research funding that year found 45 percent from industry, 28 percent from federal, state, and local governments, and 13 percent from foundations; Homer W. Smith, "Present Status of National Science Foundation Legislation," *Journal of the American Medical Association* 137 (1948): 19.

11. Harry M. Marks, "Cortisone, 1949: A Year in the Political Life of a Drug," *Bulletin of the History of Medicine* 66 (1992): 429–32, quote from 421; see also Stephen P. Strickland, *Politics, Science, and Dread Disease: A Short History of United States Medical Research Policy* (Cambridge: Harvard University Press, 1972), 20–21.

12. See Michael Kazin, *The Populist Persuasion: An American History* (Ithaca: Cornell University Press, 1995), 165–90; Elton Rayak, *Professional Power and American Medicine: The Economics of the American Medical Association* (Cleveland: World Publishing Company, 1967), 16, 98; James G. Burrow, *AMA: Voice of American Medicine* (Baltimore: Johns Hopkins University Press, 1963), 316.

13. Young, *Medical Messiahs*, 360–89; Eric S. Juhnke, *Quacks and Crusaders: The Fabulous Careers of John Brinkley, Norman Baker and Harry Hoxsey* (Lawrence: University Press of Kansas, 2002), 76–86, 140–42.

14. William Langer, May 7, 1945, *Congressional Record Appendix, 79th Congress* (Washington, D.C.: GPO, 1945), vol. 91, part 2, A2110; see also Charles M. Barber, "A Diamond in the Rough: William Langer Reexamined," *North Dakota History* 64 (1998): 2–18, and David A. Horowitz, *Beyond Left and Right: Insurgency and the Establishment* (Urbana: University of Illinois Press, 1997), 151–52. Republican lawyer William Langer (1886–1959) was governor of North Dakota 1932–34 and 1937–39, and was in the Senate 1941–59.

15. Quoted in Smith, "Present Status," 18.

16. See J. Merton England, *A Patron for Pure Science: The National Science Foundation's Formative Years, 1945–57* (Washington, D.C.: National Science Foundation, 1982), 85, and Daniel J. Kevles, *The Physicists: The History of a Scientific Community in Modern America* (New York: Knopf, 1977), 363.

17. Clarence A. Mills, "Distribution of American Research Funds," *Science* 107 (1948): 127–30; reprinted in *Hearing before the Committee on Interstate and Foreign Commerce, House of Representatives*

Eightieth Congress Second Session on H.R. 6007 and S. 2385 [on a national science foundation] June 1, 1948 (Washington, D.C.: GPO, 1948), 138–42.

18. The NSF bill of 1947, for example, had included special disease commissions to be directed by eleven-member boards made up of six "eminent scientists" and five representatives of the general public; see Donald C. Swain, "The Rise of a Research Empire: NIH, 1930–1960," *Science* 138 (1962): 1233–1237, and Toby A. Appel, *Shaping Biology: The National Science Foundation and American Biological Research, 1945–1975* (Baltimore: Johns Hopkins University Press, 2000), 34–35.

19. See Appel, *Shaping Biology*, 34–35; Kevles, *The Physicists*, 324–66.

20. England, *Patron for Pure Science*, 91. Compare the policies of foundations like the American Cancer Society and the American Heart Association, which welcomed federal funding of "cure-oriented research" through the National Institutes of Health; Marks, "Cortisone," 429, 438 n. 88. On twentieth-century medical research, see also Harry M. Marks, *The Progress of Experiment: Science and Therapeutic Reform in the United States, 1900–1990* (Cambridge: Cambridge University Press, 1997); Strickland, *Politics, Science, and Dread Disease*; Roger L. Geiger, *Research and Relevant Knowledge: American Research Universities since World War II* (New York: Oxford University Press, 1993); Victoria A. Harden, *Inventing the NIH: Federal Biomedical Research Policy, 1887–1937* (Baltimore: Johns Hopkins University Press, 1986); and James T. Patterson, *The Dread Disease: Cancer and Modern American Culture* (Cambridge: Harvard University Press, 1987).

21. Kevles, *The Physicists*, 356–64; Appel, *Shaping Biology*, 18–37.

22. Gerald Gross, *Washington Report on the Medical Sciences* 57 (July 5, 1948), Washington Report file, 143-E-10-5(b), Kenny-MHS.

23. See Naomi Rogers, "Polio, Power and Film-Making: RKO's 'Sister Kenny' and American Medicine in the 1940s," in Leslie J. Reagan, Nancy Tomes and Paula Treichler, eds., *Medicine's Moving Pictures: Education and Entertainment through Film and Television in the United States* (Berkeley: University of California Press, forthcoming).

24. For useful discussions of Kenny, see Gould, *A Summer Plague*, 85–110; Victor Cohn, *Sister Kenny: The Woman Who Challenged the Doctors* (Minneapolis: University of Minnesota Press, 1975); John R. Paul, *A History of Poliomyelitis* (New Haven: Yale University Press, 1971), 330–38; Daniel J. Wilson, "A Crippling Fear: Experiencing Polio in the Era of FDR," *Bulletin of the History of Medicine* 72 (1998): 464–495; John R. Wilson, *Through Kenny's Eyes: An Exploration of Sister Elizabeth Kenny's Views about Nursing* (Townsville: Royal College of Nursing Australia, 1995); Philippa Martyr, "'A Small Price to Pay for Peace: The Elizabeth Kenny Controversy Re-Examined," *Australian Historical Studies* 28 (1997): 47–65; Naomi Rogers, "The Debate Considered [Historians and Sister Kenny]," *Australian Historical Studies* 31 (2000): 163–66.

25. Elizabeth Kenny with Martha Ostenso, *And They Shall Walk: The Life Story of Sister Elizabeth Kenny* (New York: Dodd, Mead and Company, 1943), 17.

26. Ibid., 50, 94, 200.

27. Ibid., 207.

28. Ibid., 211–13; Morris Fishbein, *Morris Fishbein, M.D.: An Autobiography* (Garden City, N.Y.: Doubleday and Co., 1969), 229–34.

29. Marvin Kline used a photograph of himself standing with Kenny at the dedication of her new institute as part of his reelection campaign, and in a 1942 parade rode with Kenny in a convertible so they could wave to the crowd together. Hubert Humphrey, the city's next mayor, similarly recognized the importance of courting her goodwill. See "The Record in Print," from "Continue Progress with Marvin Kline" brochure, Mayoralty Files, Kline Campaign Literature, 1941–45, Hubert H. Humphrey Papers, MHS; and Hubert H. Humphrey to Marvin Kline, May 28, 1947, Hubert H. Humphrey, Mayoralty Files 1945–1948, 150-A-6-2(f), box 10, Kenny Institute 1947, Kenny-MHS.

30. Wallace H. Cole and Miland E. Knapp, "The Kenny Treatment of Infantile Paralysis: A Preliminary Report," *Journal of the American Medical Association* 116 (1941): 2577–2580; John Pohl, "Kenny Treatment of Anterior Poliomyelitis: Report of the First Cases Treatment in America," *Journal of the American Medical Association* 118 (1942): 1428–1433; editorial, "The Kenny Method of Treatment in the Acute Peripheral Manifestations of Infantile Paralysis," *Journal of the American Medical Association* 117 (1941): 2171–2172.

31. Basil O'Connor, "A Statement," in Elizabeth Kenny and John Pohl, *The Kenny Concept of Infantile Paralysis and How to Treat It* (Minneapolis: Bruce Publishing, 1943), 9–10; see also Don W. Gudakunst, *The Importance of Research* (New York: National Foundation for Infantile Paralysis, 1942); *The Story of the*

Kenny Method (New York: National Foundation for Infantile Paralysis, 1944). Kenny quoted from O'Connor's preface; Kenny, *Hearings*, May 14, 1948, 122.

32. "My Report on Conferences with the Medical Profession in Fourteen Foreign Countries—Elizabeth Kenny," reprinted in *Hearings*, May 14, 1948, 153; [film transcript] in Kenny, *Hearings*, May 19, 1948, 198.

33. See Smith, *Patenting the Sun*; Nina Gilden Seavey, Jane S. Smith, and Paul Wagner, *A Paralyzing Fear: The Triumph over Polio in America* (New York: TV Books, 1998).

34. See, for example, one pamphlet during a 1931 epidemic: Monmouth County Advisory Committee, *Bulletin on Poliomyelitis (Infantile Paralysis) Designed for Use of Medical Men and Other Public Health Professionals* [1931], C. A. E. Winslow Papers, #749, series 3, box 85, folder 1318, Manuscripts and Archives, Sterling Memorial Library, Yale University; and see examples in Edmund Sass with George Gottfried and Anthony Soren, *Polio's Legacy: An Oral History* (Lanham, Md.: University Press of America, 1996), 71–91, 127–56, and Seavey, Smith, and Wagner, *A Paralyzing Fear.*

35. Robert M. Yoder, "Healer from the Outback," *Saturday Evening Post*, 214 (January 17, 1942), 19.

36. See Glenn Gritzer and Arnold Arube, *The Making of Rehabilitation: A Political Economy of Medical Specialization, 1890–1980* (Berkeley: University of California Press, 1985); and Howard Rusk, *A World to Care For* (New York: Random House, 1972). On the shift in polio care from the 1920s and '30s to the 1940s and '50s, see Daniel J. Wilson, "Crippled Manhood: Infantile Paralysis and the Constructing of Masculinity," *Medical Humanities Review* 12 (1998): 9–28, and Amy L. Fairchild, "The Polio Narratives: Dialogues with FDR," *Bulletin of the History of Medicine* 75 (2001): 488–534.

37. For more on this point, see Wilson, *Through Kenny's Eyes*, 68–70.

38. See Elizabeth Kenny to Gordon K. Safarias [executive secretary, District Council no. 2, United Chemical Workers/CIO], December 26, 1946, United Chemical Workers 1945, 143-E-10-5(b), Kenny-MHS; Charles F. Samelson [Program Committee, Association of Internes and Medical Students, Chapter of University of Illinois College of Medicine] to Sister Kenny, October 20, 1942, University of Illinois College of Medicine, 1942, 143-E-10-5(b), Kenny-MHS.

39. This was the title of chapter 6 of Kenny's 1943 autobiography.

40. Kenny, "My Report," 151.

41. On Kenny's theories see Wilson, *Kenny's Eyes*, 40–45, and Kenny and Pohl, *The Kenny Concept.*

42. See Margaret L. Grimshaw, "Scientific Specialization and the Poliovirus Controversy in the Years before World War II," *Bulletin of the History of Medicine* 69 (1995): 44–65; Rogers, *Dirt and Disease*; Paul, *History of Poliomyelitis.*

43. "Medical News: Chicago: New Exhibit on Infantile Paralysis," *Journal of the American Medical Association* 137 (1948): 1068. The exhibit opened on June 17.

44. Fishbein, *Autobiography*, 229–34.

45. D. M. Horstmann, "Problems in Epidemiology of Poliomyelitis" [abstract], *Lancet* (1948) in *Journal of the American Medical Association* 137 (1948): 1491.

46. Paul, *History of Poliomyelitis*; Smith, *Patenting the Sun.*

47. Kenny, *Hearings*, May 14, 1948, 116.

48. George H. Gallup, *The Gallup Poll: Public Opinion 1935–1971* (New York: Random House 1972), 1:537, 663.

49. Lois Maddox Miller, "Sister Kenny vs. Infantile Paralysis," *Reader's Digest*, 39 (December 1941), 1–6; Robert D. Potter, "Sister Kenny's Treatment for Infantile Paralysis," *American Weekly*, August 17, 1941, 4–13; Yoder, "Healer from the Outback," 18–19, 68, 70; "Sister Kenny: Australian Nurse Demonstrates Her Treatment for Infantile Paralysis," *Life*, 13 (September 28, 1942), 73–75, 77; Miller, "Sister Kenny Wins Her Fight," *Reader's Digest*, 44 (October 1942), 27–30; Miller, "Sister Kenny vs. the Medical Old Guard," *Reader's Digest*, 45 (October 1944), 65–71.

50. Van Riper, *Hearings*, May 13, 1948, 83.

51. See Smith, *Patenting the Sun*, and Seavey, Smith, and Wagner, *A Paralyzing Fear.*

52. Helen Waterhouse, "Akron No Polio Nest, County Doctors Told," *Akron Beacon Journal*, June, 2 1948.

53. Gudakunst, *Importance of Research*, 41–42.

54. On organized medicine and the Republican Party, see Rogers, "The Public Face of Homeopathy: Politics, the Public and Alternative Medicine in the United States 1900–1940," in Martin Dinges, ed., *Patients in the History of Homeopathy* (Sheffield: European Association for the History of Medicine and Health Publications, 2002), 351–71.

55. On medical politics in the 1930s and 1940s, see Elizabeth Fee and Theodore Brown, eds., *Making Medical History: The Life and Times of Henry E. Sigerist* (Baltimore: Johns Hopkins University Press, 1997); Burrow, *AMA*; Daniel S. Hirschfield, *The Lost Reform: The Campaign for Compulsory Health Insurance in the United States from 1932 to 1943* (Cambridge, Mass.: Harvard University Press, 1970); Rickey Hendricks, *A Model for National Health Care: The History of Kaiser Permanente* (New Brunswick, N.J.: Rutgers University Press, 1993); Monte Poen, *Harry S. Truman versus the Medical Lobby: The Genesis of Medicare* (Columbia: University of Missouri Press, 1979); Frank D. Campion, *The AMA and U.S. Health Policy since 1940* (Chicago: Chicago Review Press, 1984); and Jonathan Engel, *Doctors and Reformers: Discussion and Debate over Health Policy 1925–1950* (Charleston: University of South Carolina Press, 2002).

56. See Strickland, *Politics, Science and Dread Disease*, 55, and Rayak, *Professional Power and American Medicine*, 98–90.

57. Van Riper, *Hearings*, May 13, 1948, 79; Savage, *Hearings*, May 13, 1948, 71.

58. Savage, *Hearings*, May 13, 1948, 71.

59. John O'Connor, *Hearings*, May 13, 1948, 41. New York Democrat John Joseph O'Connor (1885–1960) had been in the House 1923–1939.

60. O'Connor, *Hearings*, May 13, 1948, 49–50.

61. Savage, *Hearings*, May 13, 1948, 71.

62. On Fishbein and the National Foundation, see Fishbein, *Autobiography*, 342–49; see also Allen G. Debus, "A Tribute to Morris Fishbein," *Bulletin of the History of Medicine* 51 (1977): 153–54, and Campion, *AMA since 1940*, 118–30.

63. Robert Potter to Don W. Gudakunst, June 13, 1941, Public Relations, Kenny files, January 1940–, March of Dimes Archives, White Plains, New York (hereafter March of Dimes); Fishbein to Potter, July 15, 1941, Public Relations, Kenny files, January 1940–, March of Dimes; Robert D. Potter to Dr. Fishbein, July 16, 1941, Public Relations, Kenny files, January 1940–, March of Dimes; Potter, "Sister Kenny's Treatment for Infantile Paralysis."

64. Joe W. Savage to Morris A. Fishbein, February 25, 1948, Public Relations, AMA files, October 1947–, March of Dimes; Fishbein to Savage, February 28, 1948, Public Relations AMA files, October 1947–, March of Dimes; Editorial, "Medical Research," *Journal of the American Medical Association* 137 (1948): 465.

65. See Engel, *Doctors and Reformers*, 209, 295–96.

66. For Fishbein's version of events, see his *Autobiography*, 208–23. For one analysis of AMA policy and its "persistent, essential negativism" in the 1940s, see Strickland, *Politics, Science and Dread Disease*, 55–74.

67. Dr. Allan M. Butler [Progressive Citizens of America], *Hearings before a Subcommittee of the Committee on Labor and Public Welfare, United States Senate, Eightieth Congress, First Session, on S. 545* [NIH funding] *and S. 1320* [National Health Program] . . . *Part 2, June 25, 26, 27, July 2 and 3, 1947* (Washington, D.C.: GPO, 1947), July 3 1947, 1089; Joseph A. Clorety Jr., *Hearings . . . on S. 545* [NIH funding] *and S. 1320* [National Health Program], July 2, 1947, 1002. For more on the American Veterans Committee, see Kazin, *Populist Persuasion*, 178–79.

68. See Patricia Spain Ward, "*United States versus American Medical Association et al.*: The Medical Anti-Trust Case of 1938–1943," *American Studies* 30 (1989): 123–53; Hendricks, *Model for National Health Care*, 97–98; Carl F. Ameringer, "Organized Medicine on Trial: The Federal Trade Commission vs. the American Medical Association," *Journal of Policy History* 12 (2000): 445–72; Burnham, "American Medicine's Golden Age." The second investigation lasted until 1951.

69. William O'Neill Sherman [M.D., Pittsburgh] to Morris Fishbein, January 17, 1947, Public Relations/8/1938, March of Dimes.

70. Gross, *Washington Report on the Medical Sciences* 50 (May 17, 1948), Washington Report file, 143-E-10-5(b), Kenny-MHS.

71. Joseph P. O'Hara in Van Riper's testimony, *Hearings*, May 13, 1948, 81. Joseph Patrick O'Hara (1895–1975), a Minnesota Republican, was in the House 1941–59.

72. Wolverton, *Hearings*, May 14, 1948, 107; Edwin D. Neff, "Kenny Polio Fund Denial Is Denounced," *Times-Herald*, May 15, 1948; see Gross, *Washington Report on the Medical Sciences* 50 (May 17, 1948). Charles Anderson Wolverton (1880–1969), a New Jersey Republican lawyer, was in the House 1927–59, and was chair of the House Interstate Committee during the 80th and 81st Congresses.

73. Kenny, *Hearings*, May 19, 1948, 193.

74. Kenny, *Hearings*, May 14, 1948, 103, 112.

75. Kenny, *Hearings*, May 19, 1948, 202.

76. Kenny, *Hearings*, May 19, 1948, 204; Elizabeth Kenny to Hon. Charles A. Wolverton, May 26, 1948, reprinted in Kenny, *Hearings*, May 14, 1948, 154.

77. John Heselton, *Hearings*, May 14, 1948, 111. John Walter Heselton (1900–62) was a Massachusetts Republican in the House 1945–59.

78. Jungeblut, *Hearings*, May 13, 1948, 67.

79. Jungeblut, *Hearings*, May 13, 1948, 69.

80. Jungeblut, *Hearings*, May 13, 1948, 68.

81. See Lederer and Naomi Rogers, "Media," in Cooter and Pickstone, eds., *Medicine in the Twentieth Century*, 487–502.

82. Wolverton in Jungeblut testimony, *Hearings*, May 13, 1948, 68.

83. O'Hara in Van Riper testimony, *Hearings*, May 13, 1948, 83.

84. C. W. Jungeblut to Elizabeth Kenny, February 24, 1948, Jungeblut, Dr. Claus W., 1945–1950, 143-E-10-3(b), box 1, Kenny-MHS; Kenny to Jungeblut, February 16, 1948, Jungeblut, Dr. Claus W., 1945–1950, 143-E-10-3(b), box 1, Kenny-MHS.

85. Van Riper, *Hearings*, May 13, 1948, 81. He showed the Committee copies of National Foundation checks paying for patient care at the Kenny Institute during Minneapolis's 1946 epidemic to prove "we have not argued about the quality of her treatment"; Van Riper, *Hearings*, May 13, 1948, 82.

86. Van Riper, *Hearings*, May 13, 1948, 82.

87. Van Riper, *Hearings*, May 13, 1948, 81.

88. Paul, *History of Poliomyelitis*; Smith, *Patenting the Sun*.

89. Kenny quoted by Langer, *Congressional Record* (1945), A2109.

90. Elizabeth Kenny to Bruce Gill, July 19, 1943, Kenny file 1943, Kenny-MHS.

91. Stanley Henwood to Marvin Kline, May 21, 1948, letter submitted by Kenny, *Hearings*, May 14, 1948, 155.

92. Virgil H. Moon with David G. Wittels, "They're Trifling with Your Life," *Saturday Evening Post*, 221 (July 24, 1948),16–17. I would like to thank Sue Lederer for showing me this article.

93. See Lederer, *Subjected to Science*; Gevitz, *The D.O.'s*; Engel, *Doctors and Reformers*.

94. Sister Elizabeth Kenny, "God Is My Doctor," *American Weekly*, April 2, 1944, 18.

95. See postcards sent to a Berkeley woman by Chicago's National Anti-Vivisection Society, attacking the National Foundation for its lack of support of Kenny; Leona Pease to K. F. Meyer [Medical Center, University of California, San Francisco], February 28, 1944; Public Relations, Kenny files, January 1944–, March of Dimes.

96. Kenny, *Hearings*, May 19, 1948, 205.

97. Mrs Virgil Dicke [Goodhue, Minnesota] to Sister Kenny, July 2, 1948, General Correspondence, July-December 1948, Kenny-MHS.

98. Secretary to Mrs. Dicke, July 20, 1948, General Correspondence, July-December 1948, Kenny-MHS.

99. Wolverton, during testimony of Dr. Leonard A. Scheele, Surgeon General, *Hearings*, May 13, 1948, 22.

100. Wolverton, *Hearings*, May 14, 1948, 118.

101. The National Heart Institute allowed laymen to serve on its advisory councils as the result of lobbying by Mary Lasker, and she rejuvenated the American Cancer Society and made it an advocate for research; Strickland, *Politics, Science, and Dread Disease*, 53; Geiger, *Research and Relevant Knowledge*, 180–81.

102. The quote is from "An Open Letter," Herbert Avedon to Sister Kenny, *San Fernando Sun*, October 14, 1948.

103. Herbert Avedon to Sister Kenny, October 29, 1948, Elizabeth Kenny, General Correspondence, July-December 1948, Kenny-MHS; Harry R. Sheppard to Herbert Avedon, October 21, 1948, in *San Fernando Sun*, October 28, 1948; "Sister Kenny Answers Sun Open Letter," *San Fernando Sun*, October 28, 1948.

104. "The Polio Controversy" (editorial), *San Fernando Sun*, October 28, 1948.

105. "Group Launches Federal Polio Research Drive" [newspaper name missing], September 30, 1948, Public Relations, Kenny files, Clippings 1947–, March of Dimes.

106. Petition by Citizen's Polio Research League, Public Relations, Kenny Foundation Files, November 1948–, March of Dimes; transcript, "Telephone Conversation between Dr. Van Riper and Dr. Huenkens, Medical Director, Kenny Institute, Minneapolis—Dec. 8, 1948," Public Relations, Kenny files, November 1948–, March of Dimes. Unfortunately we know little about this group, although postwar southern California had a

strong tradition of right-wing activism; see Kurt Schuparra, *Triumph of the Right: The Rise of the California Conservative Movement 1945–1966* (Armonk, N.Y.: M. E. Sharpe, 1998).

107. See Paul, *History of Poliomyelitis*, 322.

108. Paul, *History of Poliomyelitis*, 320–23, quotes from 320, 321. Paul compared these conferences to their "formidable rivals" the WHO Expert Committee on Poliomyelitis, whose meetings (begun in 1952) "in the eyes of the world had a truly authoritative ring," 323.

109. "Illinois: Film on Poliomyelitis," *Journal of the American Medical Association* 137 (1948): 1325; "Medical Motion Pictures," *Journal of the American Medical Association* 138 (1948): 1115.

110. Roland Berg to Roy Naftzger [chairman, executive committee of the Los Angeles County Chapter], November 23, 1948, in Public Relations, Kenny Foundation files, November 1948—, March of Dimes.

111. Mildred Freeston to R. A. Burcaw, December 16, 1948, Memorandum on Citizens Polio Research League Conference, Jersey City, December 16, 1948, Public Relations, Kenny Foundation files, November 1948–, March of Dimes.

112. Kenny, Report to Board of Directors, May 24, 1948.

113. Thurman C. Crook to Sister Elizabeth Kenny, April 23, 1949, Elizabeth Kenny General Correspondence, "C", MHS. Thurman Charles Crook (1891–1981) was a House Democrat from Indiana 1949–51.

114. See Poen, *Truman and Medical Lobby*, 142–44; Campion, *Since 1940*, 113–25, 131–37.

115. Fishbein, *Autobiography*, 312; for his version see *Autobiography*, 298–313. See also Engel, *Doctors and Reformers* 293–94, and Campion, *AMA since 1940*, 113–25.

116. "Memorandum," KBA to Dorothy Ducas, October 16, 1950, Public Relations, Kenny Foundation files, April 1950–, March of Dimes.

117. Marvin Kline, "The Most Unforgettable Character I'd Ever Met," *Reader's Digest*, August 1959, 203–8.

118. Wolverton and Kenny *Hearings*, May 14, 1948, 101.

119. Gallup, *Gallup Poll*, 1:775. The poll was done on December 26, 1948.

120. Fishbein, *Autobiography*, 234.

121. Fishbein, *Autobiography*, 231–32.

The Lunatic Fringe Strikes Back

This essay is dedicated to Shafali Lal, who commented on several of its incarnations in her careful, generous, and encouraging way. With her recent death I have lost a precious source of wisdom, strength, leadership, joy, and friendship.
The author would like to thank Robert Johnston for calling her attention to the Alaska Mental Health Bill in the first place. She would also like to thank Benjamin Harris for pointing out that there was a great deal more to the controvsersy than the legislation itself. And lastly, the author wishes to extend her gratitude to her fellow students in the twentieth-century U.S. history research seminar at Yale, and to Benjamin Johnson, David Hecht, Holly Heinzer, Nancy Godleski, Marc Lindemann, Lis Pimentel, Sarah Peterson, Kim Reilly, John Witt, Heather Williams and Linda Janke, all of whom gave valuable comments on drafts of this essay.

1. On September 17, 2002, city council members and residents of Santa Cruz, California, held a "pot giveaway" at City Hall to protest the arrest of two medicinal marijuana growers by federal officials. "In Santa Cruz, an Official Handout of Medicinal Pot," *Los Angeles Times*, September 18, 2002, Part 2, p. 1.

2. "If You're a Good Conservative American Patriot . . . Let's Face It . . . You're Nuts," *The Southern Conservative* (April 1957), reprint, personal collection of Marie Koenig, Pasadena, California.

3. Clause-M. Naske, "Bob Bartlett and the Alaska Mental Health Act," *Pacific Northwest Quarterly* 71, 1 (1980): 37.

4. Mrs. Leigh F. Burkeland, "Now—Siberia U.S.A," *The Register*, January 24, 1956, reprinted by Keep America Committee. Radical Right Collection, Box 45, Hoover Institution.

5. U.S., Congress, Senate, Subcommittee on Territories and Insular Affairs, Committee on Interior and Insular Affairs, An Act to Provide for the Hospitalization and Care of the Mentally Ill of Alaska, and for Other Purposes: Hearings on H.R. 6376, S. 2518, S. 2973, 84th Cong., 2nd sess., 20, 21 February and 5 March 1956, 158.

6. Naske, "Bob Bartlett," 39.

7. A. Robert Smith, "'Siberia, U.S.A.,'" *The Reporter*, June 28, 1956, 27–29.

8. Priscilla Buckley, "'Siberia, U.S.A.': The Rocky Road of H.R. 6376," *National Review*, July 25, 1956, 9–10.

9. Alaska Mental Health Hearings, 121.

10. Stephen Whitfield, *The Culture of the Cold War* (Baltimore: Johns Hopkins University Press, 1991), 17.

11. Kurt Schuparra, *Triumph of the Right: The Rise of the California Conservative Movement, 1945–1966* (Armonk, N.Y.: M. E. Sharpe, 1998), 27.

12. Community Relations Committee (CRC), Notes on American Public Relations Forum—Meeting Friday Evening, May 2, 1952, p. 1. The CRC was a Los Angeles organization, affiliated with the Jewish Community Federation, that monitored anti-Semitic and right-wing activity in southern California. CRC spies recorded the minutes of several APRF meetings in 1952. The CRC's spy reports are housed in the Urban Archives, located at California State University at Northridge.

13. Marie Koenig, interview with author, April 5, 2001.

14. Ellen Herman, *The Romance of American Psychology: Political Culture in the Age of Experts* (Berkeley: University of California Press, 1995), 241–44.

15. Ibid., 119.

16. Ibid., 244–49.

17. Ibid., 127.

18. Ibid., 59.

19. T. W. Adorno et al. *The Authoritarian Personality* (New York: W. W. Norton, 1950), 765–66.

20. Isidore Ziferstein, "Race Prejudice and Mental Health," *Frontier*, August 1956, 2.

21. Ibid., 1.

22. Herman, *Romance*, 198.

23. International Congress on Mental Health, *Mental Health and World Citizenship, London 1948* (New York: National Association for Mental Health [1951]), 8, personal collection of Marie Koenig, Pasadena, California.

24. Ibid., 27.

25. Richard Hofstadter, *The Paranoid Style in American Politics* (New York: Knopf, 1965), 49–53.

26. Don Carlton, *Red Scare: Right-Wing Hysteria, Fifties Fascism and Their Legacy in Texas* (Austin: Texas Monthly Press, 1985), 111–34.

27. Alaska Mental Health Hearings, 139.

28. For a fuller examination of how middle-class homemakers cultivated expertise in local policy matters to make themselves better grassroots activists, see Sylvie Murray, *The Progressive Housewife: Community Activism in Suburban Queens, 1945–1964* (Philadelphia: University of Pennsylvania Press, 2003).

29. United Nations Educational, Scientific, and Cultural Organization, *Mental Hygiene in the Nursery School: Report of a Joint WHO-UNESCO Expert Meeting Held in Paris, 17–22 September 1951,* (Paris: UNESCO, [1953]), 22.

30. Charlene Kirchner, *California State Bulletin of Minute Women of the United States of America, Inc.* [ca. 1955], p. 3. The author confirmed this defintion was correctly quoted. See *Webster's New International Dictionary*, 2nd edition, s.v. "psychopathic."

31. The author confirmed that this interpretation of the article is correct. John R. Seeley, "Social Values, the Mental Health Movement, and Mental Health," *The Annals of the American Academy of Political and Social Science* 286 (1953): 20.

32. Kirchner, *Minute Women*, 5.

33. Ibid.

34. For more on the postwar culture of expertise, see Elaine Tyler May, *Homeward Bound* (New York: Basic Books, 1988), 26–28; Herman, *Romance*.

35. American Public Relations Forum, *Bulletin* 41 (1955): 2.

36. Kirchner, *Minute Women*, 5.

37. California Legislature, Assembly Bill No. 1158 (January 14, 1955); California Legislature, Assembly Bill No. 1159 (January 14, 1955); California Legislature, Assembly Bill No. 3300 (January, 21, 1955).

38. "Are You Mentally Ill?," *The Ledger* 31 (March 1955), reprint, Marie Koenig Collection.

39. Freedom Club, *Your Freedom May Be at Stake!* (Los Angeles [May 17, 1955]), Marie Koenig Collection.

40. American Public Relations Forum, *Bulletin* 41 (1955): 2.

41. Alfred Auerback, M.D., "The Anti-Mental Health Movement," *American Journal of Psychiatry* 120 (August 1963): 106.

42. Naske, "Bob Bartlett," 31.

43. 84th Congress, 2d Sess., 1956, H.R. 6376, Senate Report 2053.

44. Ibid., 9.

45. Ibid., 5.

46. Ibid.

47. Ibid., 25.

48. American Public Relations Forum, *Bulletin* 47 (1955): 1, 2.

49. Buckley, " 'Siberia, U.S.A.,' " 10.

50. Alaska Mental Health Hearings 285.

51. "A Report to the American People on the Alaska Mental Health Act," *American Flag Committee Newsletter* 41 (1956): 1.

52. The 1967 Anti-Defamation League study, *The Radical Right*, reported that the circulation figures of the *Dan Smoot Report* stood at 31,000. Benjamin R. Epstein and Arnold Foster, *The Radical Right: Reports on the John Birch Society and Its Allies* (New York: Random House, 1966), 11.

53. "Mental Health," *The Dan Smoot Report* 2, 11 (1956): 3.

54. For information on *Williams Intelligence Summary*, see "Alaska Mental Health Hearings," 163.

55. Robert Williams, "Here's a Section-by-Section Analysis of Alaska Mental Health Bill, HR 6376," *Williams Intelligence Summary*, March 1956, 3.

56. Smith, " 'Siberia, U.S.A.,' " 29.

57. Alaska Mental Health Hearings, 262, 269.

58. Ibid., 264.

59. Ibid., 268, 270.

60. Ibid., 124.

61. Ibid., 136.

62. Ibid., 164.

63. Judd Marmor, Viola W. Bernard, and Perry Ottenberg, "Psychodynamics of Group Opposition to Health Programs," *American Journal of Orthopsychiatry* 30, 331 (1960): 340.

64. Ibid., 169.

65. Ibid.

66. Ibid., 145.

67. Ibid., 254.

68. Smith, " 'Siberia, U.S.A.,' " 29.

69. Naske, "Bob Bartlett," 39.

70. Epstein and Foster, *The Radical Right*, 109.

71. Ibid., 27.

72. Richard Hofstadter, *The Paranoid Style*, 117.

73. Marmor, Bernard, and Ottenberg, "Psychodynamics of Group Opposition to Health Programs," 338.

74. Ibid., 339.

75. Ibid., 110.

76. Ibid., 100.

77. Ibid., 106, 107, 110.

78. Lisa McGirr, *Suburban Warriors: The Origins of the New American Right* (Princeton: Princeton University Press, 2001), 189–90; Schuparra, *Triumph of the Right*, 117, 121.

79. For another example of how conspiracy theories have proved useful and rational for the purposes of galvanizing political movements, see Jeffrey Ostler, "The Rhetoric of Conspiracy and the Formation of Kansas Populism," *Agricultural History* 69, 1 (1995).

"Not a So-Called Democracy"

1. George A. Swendiman, "The Argument against Fluoridating City Water," ca. 1951, Wisc. Mss. 13 PB, folder 25, Edward A. Hansen Collection, WHSM, Madison, Wisconsin.

2. Donald R. McNeil, "Time to Walk Boldly," *Journal of the American Dental Association* 63 (1961): 336.

3. Frank J. McClure, *Water Fluoridation: The Search and the Victory* (Bethesda, Md.: National Institute of Dental Research, 1970), 109–10.

4. Ibid., 246.

5. Donald R. McNeil, *The Fight for Fluoridation* (New York: Oxford University Press, 1957), 104–5.

6. Bernard Ladouceur and unknown, "Letter from Bernard Ladouceur/Editorial 'Fluoridation and Winston Smith,'" ca. 1956, SC 923, Ethel B. Dinning Collection, WHSM, Madison, Wisconsin.

7. William D. Herrstrom, "75 Reasons Why Community Water Supplies Should Not Be Fluoridated," ca. 1957, Joseph B. Lightburn Collection, West Virginia University Library, Morgantown, West Virginia.

8. "Six Ways to Mislead the Public," *Consumer Reports* 43 (1978): 480–82; Leo Spira, "Poison in Your Water," *American Mercury*, 85 (1957): 70. Examples of these arguments include George L. Waldbott, *A Struggle with Titans* (New York: Carlton Press, 1965), and Leo Spira, *The Drama of Fluorine: Arch Enemy of Mankind* (Milwaukee: Lee Foundation for Nutritional Research, 1953).

9. Waldbott, *A Struggle with Titans*, 1–67.

10. Examples of these stories include William R. Cox, *Hello, Test Animals . . . Chinchillas or You and Your Grandchildren?* (Milwaukee: Lee Foundation for Nutritional Research, 1953); Spira, *The Drama of Fluorine*; U. L. Monteleone and unknown, "Editor's Mail: Fluorides/The Allentown Story—Phase Two," ca. 1971, SC 923, Ethel B. Dinning Collection, WHSM, Madison, Wisconsin.

11. Robert L. Crain, Elihu Katz, and Donald B. Rosenthal, *The Politics of Community Conflict: The Fluoridation Decision* (New York: Bobbs-Merrill Co., Inc., 1969), 86; McNeil, *The Fight for Fluoridation*, 122.

12. Examples of these publications include Cox, *Hello, Test Animals*; Isabel Jansen, *Fluoridation: A Modern Procrustean Practice* (Antigo, Wisc.: Isabel Jansen/Tri-State Press, 1990); "Fluoridation Hysteria Is Government-Inspired," in *Citizens Medical Reference Bureau Inc. October-November 1951 Newsletter*, vol. XXII, no. 6, Wisc. Mss. 27 PB, folder "Anti-fl Material," Alex Wallace Collection, WHSM, Madison, Wisconsin. No author or editor is identified.

13. Frederick B. Exner, "Why Not to Fluoridate: An Address to the People of Madison, New Jersey on November 1, 1956," bx. 2, "Fluoridation (newsletters) ADA-reviews," Donald R. McNeil Collection (M63-231), WHSM, Madison, Wisconsin, 2.

14. Exner, "Why Not to Fluoridate," 12.

15. Mary Bernhardt and Bob Sprague, "The Poisonmongers," in S. Barrett and S. Rovin, eds., *The Tooth Robbers: A Pro-fluoridation Handbook* (Philadelphia: G. F. Stickley, 1980), 216.

16. Exner, "Why Not to Fluoridate," 4.

17. Michael W. Easley, "The New Anti-fluoridationists: Who Are They and How Do They Operate?" *American Journal of Public Health* 45, 3 (1985): 139.

18. American Dental Association Bureau of Public Information, "Comments on the Opponents of Fluoridation," *Journal of the American Dental Association* 65 (1962): 696, 698; Don Matchan, "Fred J. Hart—Farmer, Scholar, Gentleman," *National Health Federation Bulletin* 6 (1960): 6; Lee Foundation for Nutritional Research, "Price List," 1954, Wisc. Mss. 13 PB, folder 43, Mrs. Merlin Meythaler Collection, WHSM, Madison, Wisconsin.

19. Crain, Katz, and Rosenthal, *Politics*, 86; McNeil, *The Fight for Fluoridation*, 162.

20. Easley, "The New Anti-fluoridationists," 135; H. Williams Butler, "Legal Aspects of Fluoridating Community Water Supplies," *Journal of the American Dental Association* 65 (1962): 654; R. Roemer, "Water Fluoridation: Public Health Responsibility and the Democratic Process," *American Journal of Public Health* 55 (1965): 1340. For examples of court cases, see Butler, "Legal Aspects."

21. Elena G. Koziar, letter to the editor, *New York Times*, April 12, 1974, 88; Frederick B. Exner, "Government by Laws, Not by Men," *National Fluoridation News* 14, 5 (1968): 1; Hans Moolenburgh, "Fluoride—The Freedom Fight," *National Fluoridation News* 32, 3 (1987–88): 1.

22. Royal Lee, "Foreword," in W. R. Cox, ed., *Hello, Test Animals . . . Chinchillas or You and Your Grandchildren?* (Milwaukee: Lee Foundation for Nutritional Research, 1953), 6.

23. "Letters to Editor: Flouridation [*sic*]," October 31, 1968, SC 923, Ethel B. Dinning Collection, WHSM, Madison, Wisconsin. This reprint consists of a number of letters to the editor from a variety of people. Where these letters were originally published is not noted, but from the content, at least some of them were probably written in 1968.

24. Examples of this argument include "Bottled Water Outlook Rosy," *National Fluoridation News* 15, 5, (1969): 2; "Waking up to a Nightmare," *National Fluoridation News* 14, 6 (1968): 4; Frederick B. Exner, "Why Fluoridating Water Supplies is Dangerous," in F. B. Exner and G. L. Waldbott, *The American Fluoridation*

Experiment, ed. J. Rorty (New York: Devin-Adair Company, 1957), 48; "Antihostility Water?" *National Fluo-ridation News* 15, 3 (1969): 2.

25. Rollin M. Severance, "Copy of a Personal Letter to a Leading Citizen of Saginaw, dated January 5, 1954," File 1953 Mar. 16, bx. 204, folder 1, Rollin M. Severance Collection, WHSM, Madison, Wisconsin, 2.

26. Examples of these arguments include E. H. Bronner and unknown, "Just One Turn on One Valve And!!/Spare the Pigs," ca. 1952, Wisc. Mss. 27 PB, folder "Anti-Fl. Material," Alex Wallace Collection, WHSM, Madison, Wisconsin; reprint of letter to the editor, *Catholic Mirror*, January 1952, by Bronner, and an anonymous letter to the editor, *Catholic Mirror*, March 1952; Western Minute Men USA, "Red Scheme for Mass Control: Some New Ideas on the Fluoridation Conspiracy," *American Mercury* 89 (1959): 135; "Current Information on the Chicago Situation . . . ," February 25, 1957, bx. 1, folder 11, Naturopathy Collec-tion (M0759), Series I, Stanford University, Stanford, California; "Can Flouridation [*sic*] of Your Water Supply Cause Cancer?" *Freemen Speak* 1, 1 (1955): 4.

27. Bureau of Public Information, "Comments"; Charles T. Betts, "This Poisoning of Our Drinking Water," ca. 1953, Wisc. Mss. 13 PB, folder 44, Mrs. Elmer P. Haubert Collection, WHSM, Madison, Wiscon-sin. This reprint notes that the article was originally published in *Herald of Health* in February but does not identify the year of publication.

28. Betts, "This Poisoning." Author's emphasis.

29. Bureau of Public Information, "Comments," 696–97; E. H. Bronner, "Stop Fluoridation before It Stops Us," March 1, 1953, Wisc. Mss. 13 PB, folder 47, James Mortier Collection, WHSM, Madison, Wisconsin.

30. Lee Foundation, "Price List."

31. Morris A. Bealle, "The Great Fluoride Hoax: Reprints from Issues of American Capsule News," n.d., bx. 1, folder 9, Naturopathy Collection (M0759), Series I, Stanford University, Stanford, California.

32. Frederick B. Exner, "Fluoride vs. Freedom," *National Health Federation Bulletin* 9 (1963): 31.

33. An example of this is Aileen S. Robinson, "PTA Leaders and Our 'Bill of Rights': Letter to the Edi-tor, *Tallahassee Democrat*," ca. 1953, unprocessed records #M71-022, Rollin M. Severance Collection, WHSM, Madison, Wisconsin.

34. Gladys Caldwell and Philip E. Zanfagna, *Fluoridation and Truth Decay* (Reseda, Calif.: Top-Ecol Press, 1974), 19.

35. James Rorty, "Introduction," in F. B. Exner and G. L. Waldbott, *The American Fluoridation Experi-ment*, ed. J. Rorty (New York: Devin-Adair Company, 1957), 8. Author's italics.

36. House Committee on Interstate and Foreign Commerce, *Hearings on H.R. 2341, a Bill to Protect the Public Health from the Dangers of Fluorination of Water*, 83rd Cong., 2d sess., 1954, 88; McNeil, *The Fight for Fluoridation*, 146.

37. McNeil, *The Fight for Fluoridation*, 145–50.

38. McClure, *Water Fluoridation*, 150; McNeil, *The Fight for Fluoridation*, 277–78.

39. It is not clear why Wier introduced the bill. Pro-fluoridationist historian Donald McNeil implied that he did it under pressure from vocal anti-fluoridationists from his district, and that he left all responsi-bilities for preparing for the hearings on bill in the hands of anti-fluoridationists. See McNeil, *The Fight for Fluoridation*, 187–88. Wier did not appear to have been active in the anti-fluoridationist movement be-yond introducing this bill, and in his testimony before the Wolverton committee Wier did not make any strong anti-fluoridation statements.

40. McClure, *Water Fluoridation*, 188–90; McNeil, *The Fight for Fluoridation*, 278–79.

41. House Committee, *Hearings on H.R. 2341*, 16–17, 49, 52, 152–55, 161, 172, 178–79, 184.

42. McNeil, *The Fight for Fluoridation*, 190.

43. House Committee, *Hearings on H.R. 2341*, 6.

44. "Confidential—The success of this venture depends upon the element of surprise," 1956, bx. 8, file "Waldbott, Mrs. G. L.," Donald R. McNeil Collection (M63-231), WHSM, Madison, Wisconsin.

45. Myron Allukian, Josephine Steinhurst, and James M. Dunning, "Community Organization and a Regional Approach to Fluoridation of the Greater Boston Area," *Journal of the American Dental Association* 102 (1981): 492.

46. McNeil, *The Fight for Fluoridation*, 190–91.

47. R. C. Faine et al., "The 1980 Fluoridation Campaigns: A Discussion of Results," *Journal of Public Health Dentistry* 41, 3 (1981): 138.

48. Leonard F. Menczer, "Fluoridation: Analysis of a Successful Community Effort—Challenge to State and Local Dental Societies," *Journal of the American Dental Association* 65 (1962): 673–79, and Leonard F.

Menczer, "The Petitionee Who 'Opposes' Fluoridation," *Journal of the American Dental Association* 65 (1962), 711–16, describe just this difficulty.

49. Cora Sharon Leukhart, "An Update on Water Fluoridation: Triumphs and Challenges," *Pediatric Dentistry* 1 (1979): 33.

50. David Rosenstein et al., "Fighting the Latest Challenge to Fluoridation in Oregon," *Public Health Reports* 93 (1978): 69; Leukhart, "An Update," *Pediatric Dentistry* 33; R. C. Faine, "An Agenda for the Eighties: Community and School Fluoridation," *Journal of Public Health Dentistry* 40 (1980): 259.

51. John M. Frankel and Myron Allukian, "Sixteen Referenda on Fluoridation in Massachusetts: An Analysis," *Journal of Public Health Dentistry* 33 (1973): 102.

52. An example of this is "For Fluoridation," n.d., 16G:114, ADA files, American Dental Association Archives, Chicago, Illinois.

53. Examples of this include Fanchon Battelle, "Fluoridation Unmasked," ca. 1952, Wisc. Mss. 13 PB, folder 43, Mrs. Merlin Meythaler Collection, WHSM, Madison, Wisconsin; Citizens Committee on Fluoridation, "Statement Opposing the Use of Public Funds for Adding Fluorine to the Public Water Supply of the District of Columbia," June 29, 1953, bx 2, folder "Miscellaneous Opposition Material," Donald R. McNeil Collection (M63-231), WHSM, Madison, Wisconsin.

54. Ethel H. Fabian, "Open Letter to President Nixon," *National Fluoridation News* 16, 1 (1970): 1.

55. "President Carter Sends Warm Greetings to Wrong Political Group," *National Fluoridation News* 23, 4 (1977): 2.

56. Ibid.

57. Cyril Echele, "How Presidential Candidates Stand," *National Fluoridation News* 22, 2 (1976): 1; House Committee, *Hearings on H.R. 2341*, 8–11.

58. Exner, "Why Not to Fluoridate," 2.

59. Examples of this include John E. Mueller, "The Politics of Fluoridation in Seven California Cities," *Western Political Quarterly* 19 (1966): 59; Easley, "The New Anti-fluoridationists"; Faine, "An Agenda."

60. Louis I. Dublin, "Water Fluoridation: Science Progresses against Unreason," *The Health Education Journal* 15 (1957): 250.

61. Paul Starr, *The Social Transformation of American Medicine* (New York: Basic Books, 1982), 284–85.

62. Monte M. Poen, *Harry S. Truman versus the Medical Lobby: The Genesis of Medicare* (Columbia: University of Missouri Press, 1979), 218–19.

63. W. D. Herrstrom, "*Americanism Bulletin* no. 18," October 1951, Wisc. Mss. 13 PB, folder 25, Edward A. Hansen Collection, WHSM, Madison, Wisconsin, 4.

64. Swendiman, "The Argument," 2.

65. W. D. Herrstrom, "*Americanism Bulletin* no. 22," February 1952, bx. 3, Donald R. McNeil Collection (M63–231), WHSM, Madison, Wisconsin, 3.

66. Beatrice J. Brown, letter to the editor, *National Fluoridation News* 12, 4 (1966): 3.

67. Phoebe Courtney, *How Dangerous Is Fluoridation?* (New Orleans: Free Men Speak, 1971), 112.

68. John R. Lilliendahl Jr., "Speaking Out," *National Fluoridation News* 9, 6 (1963–64): 4.

69. Daniel W. Schwartz, "The Right to Be Sick," *National Fluoridation News* 14, 5 (1968): 2.

70. Veronica Peterson, letter to the editor, *New York Times*, June 8, 1958 4.

71. Allen Walker Read, letter to the editor, *National Fluoridation News* 12, 3 (1966): 2.

72. Eva L. Collins, letter to the editor, *New York Times*, September 2, 1963, 14.

73. Robert N. Mayer, *The Consumer Movement: Guardians of the Marketplace* (Boston: Twayne Publishers, 1989), 17.

74. Royal Lee and John G. Frisch, "Letter to Dr. J. G. Frisch/Letter to Dr. Royal Lee," March 1951, Wisc. Mss. 13 PB, folder 25, from a scrapbook entitled "Reprints and Articles on Fluorine," Edward A. Hansen Collection, WHSM, Madison, Wisconsin.

75. Royal Lee and unknown, "Reprint of Royal Lee speech 'Fluorine and Dental Caries'/editorial entitled 'PTA Backs Fluorides,' " January 3, ca. 1952, Wisc. Mss. 13 PB, folder 25, Edward A. Hansen Collection, WHSM, Madison, Wisconsin, 4. Other examples include Royal Lee, "An Open Letter to All Public Officials Responsible for a Pure Water Supply," April 16, 1957, bx. 1, folder 6, Naturopathy Collection (M0759), Series I, Stanford University, Stanford, California, 2.

76. Caldwell and Zanfagna, *Fluoridation and Truth Decay*, 3.

77. "Pres. Carter and Sen. Kennedy Push for Fluoride," *National Fluoridation News* 25, 1 (1979): 1; Mayer, *The Consumer Movement*, 16, 18, 26.

78. Ferne Woodhull, "Letter to the Editor," *National Fluoridation News* 17, 5 (1971): 2.

79. The two parts of the *Consumer Reports* article were "Fluoridation: The Cancer Scare," *Consumer Reports* 43 (1978): 392–96, and "Six Ways," *Consumer Reports* 43 (1978): 480–82; Stephen Barrett, *The Health Robbers: How to Protect Your Money and Your Life* (Philadelphia: George F. Stickley Co., 1980), 209–19; Stephen Barrett and Sheldon Rovin, *The Tooth Robbers* (Philadelphia: George F. Stickley Co., 1980).

80. For articles on his comments against fluoridation, see "Nader Questions P.H.S. Policy," *National Fluoridation News* 16, 2 (1970): 1; "Fluoridation Lobby Unhappy with Nader," *National Fluoridation News* 16, 4 (1970): 1; Ralph Nader, "Nader Interview," *National Fluoridation News* 16, 5 (1970): 1; "Look Ma, Brown Stain," *National Fluoridation News* 17, 4 (1971): 1.

81. "Citizens Medical Reference Bureau Inc. Bulletin No. 477," 1954, Unprocessed Records, Donald R. McNeil Collection (M63-231), WHSM, Madison, Wisconsin, 1.

82. Caldwell and Zanfagna, *Fluoridation and Truth Decay*, 186.

83. House Committee, *Hearings on H.R. 2341*, 177.

84. Betty Gyneth T. Franklin, "Safe Water Department," *National Health Federation Bulletin* 13 (1967): 23–26.

85. Koziar, "Letter to the Editor."

86. Exner, "Government," 1.

87. James Rorty, "The Fluoridation-Resistance Movement," in F. B. Exner and G. L. Waldbott, *The American Fluoridation Experiment*, ed. J. Rorty (New York: Devin-Adair Company, 1957), 218; House Committee, *Hearings on H.R. 2341*, 155, 172.

88. Forrest J. Pinkerton, "Reprinted Letter to Mrs. G. J. Watumull," July 23, 1971, SC 923, Ethel B. Dinning Collection, WHSM, Madison, Wisconsin.

89. Eloise Dyer, "Letter to the Editor," *National Fluoridation News* 12, 5 (1966): 2.

90. Waldbott, *A Struggle with Titans*, 143–44.

91. Arnold Simmel and David B. Ast, "Some Correlates of Opinion on Fluoridation," *American Journal of Public Health* 52 (1962): 1269–73; William A. Gamson and Peter H. Irons, "Community Characteristics and Fluoridation Outcomes," *Journal of Public Health Dentistry* 17 (1961): 66–74; Chester W. Douglass and Dennis C. Stacey, "Demographic Characteristics and Social Factors Related to Public Opinion on Fluoridation," *Journal of Public Health Dentistry* 32 (1972): 128–34; C. J. Wallace, Ben J. Leggett, and Patricia A. Retz, "The Influence of Mass Media on the Public's Attitude Toward Fluoridation of Drinking Water in New Orleans," *Journal of Public Health Dentistry* 35 (1975): 40–46; John P. Kirscht, "Attitude Research on the Fluoridation Controversy," *Health Education Monographs* 10 (1961): 16–28; Jean P. Frazier, "Fluoridation: A Review of Social Research," *Journal of Public Health Dentistry* 40 (1980): 214–33; Donald B. Rosenthal and Robert L. Crain, "Executive Leadership and Community Innovation: The Fluoridation Experience," *Urban Affairs Quarterly* 1 (1966): 39.

92. John E. Mueller, "Fluoridation Attitude Change," *American Journal of Public Health* 56 (1968): 1876.

93. William A. Gamson, "The Fluoridation Dialogue: Is It an Ideological Conflict?" *Public Opinion Quarterly* 25 (1961): 536; William Kornhauser, "Power and Participation in the Local Community," in R. L. Warren, ed., *Perspectives on the American Community: A Book of Readings* (Chicago: Rand McNally, 1966), 491–93.

Engendering Alternatives

The author wishes to express her gratitude to Robert Johnston, Alan Marcus, Todd Savitt, Anne Kirschmann, and Taner Edis for their many helpful comments and suggestions. She also thanks Iowa State University for support in conducting this research.

1. Naomi Rogers, "Women and Sectarian Medicine," in Rima D. Apple, ed., *Women, Health, and Medicine in America* (New Brunswick, N.J.: Rutgers University Press, 1990), 273–302; Thomas Neville Bonner, *To the Ends of the Earth: Women's Search for Education in Medicine* (Cambridge: Harvard University Press, 1992). On the history of women's access to allopathic training, see Mary Roth Walsh, *Doctors Wanted, No Women Need Apply: Sexual Barriers to the Medical Profession, 1835–1975* (New Haven: Yale University Press, 1977), and Regina Morantz-Sanchez, *Sympathy and Science: Women Physicians in American Medicine* (New York: Oxford University Press, 1985).

2. James C. Whorton, *Nature Cures: The History of Alternative Medicine in America* (New York: Oxford University Press, 2002), 64; James C. Whorton, "The First Holistic Revolution: Alternative Medicine in the Nineteenth Century," in Douglas Stalker and Clark Glymour, eds., *Examining Holistic Medicine* (Buffalo, N.Y.: Prometheus Books, 1985), 37, 40. See also William G. Rothstein, *American Physicians in the Nineteenth Century: From Sects to Science* (Baltimore: Johns Hopkins University Press, 1972); Paul Starr, *The Social Transformation of American Medicine* (New York: Basic Books, 1982); and Norman Gevitz, ed., *Other Healers: Unorthodox Medicine in America* (Baltimore: Johns Hopkins University Press, 1988).

3. Whorton, *Nature Cures*, 40. For background, see John S. Haller Jr., *The People's Doctors: Samuel Thomson and the American Botanical Movement, 1790–1860* (Carbondale: Southern Illinois University Press, 2000), and Ronald L. Numbers, "Do-It-Yourself the Sectarian Way," in Guenter B. Risse, Ronald L. Numbers, and Judith Walzer Leavitt, eds., *Medicine without Doctors: Home Health Care in American History* (New York: Science History, 1977), 49–72.

4. Rogers, "Women," 300.

5. Edward Clarke, *Sex in Education: A Fair Chance for Girls* (Boston: Osgood, 1874); Londa Schiebinger, *Nature's Body: Gender in the Making of Modern Science* (Boston: Beacon Press, 1993); Ludmilla Jordanova, *Sexual Visions: Images of Gender in Science and Medicine between the Eighteenth and Nineteenth Centuries* (Madison: University of Wisconsin Press, 1989); Cynthia Eagle Russett, *Sexual Science: The Victorian Construction of Womanhood* (Cambridge, Mass.: Harvard University Press, 1989). See also Carroll Smith-Rosenberg and Charles E. Rosenberg, "The Female Animal: Medical and Biological Views of Woman and Her Role in Nineteenth-Century America," *Journal of American History* 60 (1973): 332–56.

6. Susan E. Cayleff, *Wash and Be Healed: The Water-Cure Movement and Women's Health* (Philadelphia: Temple University Press, 1987), 53, 66, 74; Whorton, *Nature Cures*. See also Jane B. Donegan, *"Hydropathic Highway to Health": Women and Water-Cure in Antebellum America* (Westport, Conn.: Greenwood Press, 1986).

7. Anne Taylor Kirschmann, "Adding Women to the Ranks, 1860–1890: A New View with a Homeopathic Lens," *Bulletin of the History of Medicine* 73, 3 (1999): 429–46; Anne Taylor Kirschmann, "A Vital Force: Women Physicians and Patients in American Homeopathy, 1850–1930," Ph.D. dissertation, University of Rochester, 1999.

8. Kristine Beyerman Alster, *The Holistic Health Movement* (Tuscaloosa: University of Alabama Press, 1989).

9. The Boston Women's Health Book Collective, *Our Bodies, Ourselves* (New York: Simon and Schuster, 1973), 2–3. See also Barbara Beckwith, "Boston Women's Health Book Collective: Women Empowering Women," *Women and Health* 10, 1 (1985): 1–7.

10. Boston Women's Health Book Collective, *Our Bodies, Ourselves* (1973), 236, 249–50. See also Barbara Ehrenreich, "Body Politics: The Growth of the Women's Health Movement," *Ms.*, May 1984.

11. Boston Women's Health Book Collective, *Our Bodies, Ourselves* (1973), 238–39.

12. The Boston Women's Health Book Collective, *Our Bodies, Ourselves*, 2nd ed. (New York: Simon and Schuster, 1975), 367–68.

13. Boston Women's Health Book Collective, *Our Bodies, Ourselves* (1975), 367–68; Boston Women's Health Book Collective, "When Yogurt Was Illegal," *Ms.*, July-August 1992.

14. As examples of this era's criticism of hospital childbirth and advocacy of alternatives, see Susanne Arms, *Immaculate Deception: A New Look at Women and Childbirth in America* (New York: Bantam Books, 1977); Sheila Kitzinger, *The Experience of Childbirth* (New York: Penguin Books, 1978); Raven Lang, *Birth Book* (Palo Alto, Calif.: Genesis Press, 1972); and Ann Oakley, *Women Confined: Towards a Sociology of Childbirth* (New York: Schocken Books, 1980).

15. For background, see Elizabeth Siegel Watkins, *On the Pill: A Social History of Oral Contraceptives, 1950–1970* (Baltimore: Johns Hopkins University Press, 1998), and Andrea Tone, *Devices and Desires: A History of Contraceptives in America* (New York: Hill and Wang, 2001).

16. Maryann Napoli, "Look Back in Anger: The DES and Dalkon Shield Scandals," *Ms.*, May-June 1996, 42; Morton Mintz, *At Any Cost* (New York: Pantheon, 1985).

17. Boston Women's Health Book Collective, *Our Bodies, Ourselves* (1975), 209.

18. Merilee Kernis, "Natural Birth Control: A Holistic Approach to Contraception," in Berkeley Holistic Health Center, *The Holistic Health Handbook: A Tool for Attaining Wholeness of Body, Mind, and Spirit* (Berkeley: And/Or Press, 1978), 307–15.

19. Ibid.

20. The Boston Women's Health Book Collective, *The New Our Bodies, Ourselves* (New York: Simon and Schuster, 1992), second edition 209.

21. Diana Dutton, *Worse than the Disease: Pitfalls of Medical Progress* (Cambridge: Cambridge University Press, 1988); Napioli, "Look Back in Anger."

22. Sue Rosser, *Women's Health—Missing from U.S. Medicine* (Bloomington: Indiana University Press, 1994); Eileen Nechas and Denise Foley, *Unequal Treatment: What You Don't Know about How Women Are Mistreated by the Medical Community* (New York: Simon and Schuster, 1994); Kathryn Graff Low et al., "Women Participants in Research: Assessing Progress," *Women and Health* 22, 1 (1994): 79–98; Joseph Palca, "Women Left out at NIH," *Science*, June 29, 1990, 1601; Carol Miller, "Women's Health: A Focus for the 1990s," *Bioscience* 40, 11 (1990): 817; "NIH Adjusts Attitudes toward Women," *Science*, September 21, 1990, 1374; "Is There Still Too Much Extrapolation from Data on Middle-Aged White Men?" *Journal of the American Medical Association* 263, 8 (1990): 1049–50. See also Michelle Oberman, "Real and Perceived Legal Barriers to the Inclusion of Women in Clinical Trials," in Alice Dan, ed., *Reframing Women's Health* (Thousand Oaks, Calif.: Sage 1994), 266–75; Paul Cotton, "Example Abound of Gaps in Medical Knowledge Because of Groups Excluded from Scientific Study," *Journal of the American Medical Association* 263, 8; (1990): 1051–2; and Marcia Angell, "Caring for Women's Health—What Is the Problem?" *New England Journal of Medicine* 329 4 (1993): 271–72. On gendered biology, see John Z. Ayanian and Arnold M. Epstein, "Differences in the Use of Procedures between Women and Men Hospitalized for Coronary Heart Disease," *New England Journal of Medicine* 325, 4 (1991): 221–25; Marsha Goldsmith, "Heart Research Efforts Aim at Fairness to Women in Terms of Causes, Care of Cardiac Disorders," *Journal of the American Medical Association* 264, 24 (1990): 3112–3; Jonathan Tobin et al., "Sex Bias in Considering Coronary Bypass Surgery," *Annals of Internal Medicine* 107 (1987): 19–25; and Richard M. Steingart et al., "Sex Differences in the Management of Coronary Artery Disease," *New England Journal of Medicine* 325, 4 (1994): 226–30.

23. Graff Low et al., "Women Participants in Research: Assessing Progress"; Paul Cotton, "Women's Health Initiative Leads Way as Research Begins to Fill Gender Gaps," *Journal of the American Medical Association* 267, 4 (1992): 469; "NIH Overwhelmed by Response to Women's Health Initiative," *Science*, May 10, 1991, 767; Ruth Kirschstein, "From the NIH: Largest US Clinical Trial Ever Gets under Way," *Journal of the American Medical Association* 270, 13 (1993): 1521; Joseph Palca, "NIH Unveils Plan for Women's Health Project," *Science*, November 8, 1991, 792; Committee to Review the NIH Women's Health Initiative, Institute of Medicine, *An Assessment of the NIH's Women's Health Initiative*, (Washington, D.C.: National Academy Press, 1993), 90; and Bernadine Healy, "A Medical Revolution," *Newsweek*, special issue on "Health for Life," spring-summer 1999: 64–65.

24. Cokie Roberts, "One Woman in Nine," *Washington Post*, February 23, 1992, A19; Susan M. Love with Karen Lindsey, *Dr. Susan Love's Breast Book* (Reading, Mass.: Addison-Wesley, 1995), 525; Christine Gorman, "Breast-Cancer Politics," *Time*, November 1, 1993, 74; Laura Bell, "Breast Cancer Research Boom," *Chicago Tribune*, August 27, 1995, 6, 8. For more on 1990s breast cancer activism, particularly in relationship to AIDS activism of the same era, see Amy Sue Bix, "Diseases Chasing Money and Power: Breast Cancer and AIDS Activism Challenging Authority," *Journal of Policy History* 9, 1 (1997): 5–32, and Barron H. Lerner, *The Breast Cancer Wars: Hope, Fear, and the Pursuit of a Cure in Twentieth-Century America* (Oxford: Oxford University Press, 2001). On the history of cancer research in general, see Richard A. Rettig, *Cancer Crusade: The Story of the National Cancer Act of 1971* (Princeton: Princeton University Press, 1977); James T. Patterson, *The Dread Disease: Cancer and Modern American Culture* (Cambridge, Mass.: Harvard University Press, 1987); and Robert Proctor, *Cancer Wars: How Politics Shapes What We Know and Don't Know about Cancer* (New York: Basic Books, 1995). For a broader look, see Stephen P. Strickland, *Politics, Science, and Dread Disease: A Short History of United States Medical Research Policy* (Cambridge, Mass.: Harvard University Press, 1972), and Victoria A. Harden, *Inventing the NIH: Federal Biomedical Policy, 1887–1937* (Baltimore: Johns Hopkins University Press, 1986).

25. Jane Brody, "What Women Can Do to Escape Heart Disease," *New York Times*, March 8, 1995, B6; Susan Ferraro, "The Anguished Politics of Breast Cancer," *The New York Times Magazine*, August 15, 1993, 24–27+; Gina Kolata, "Weighing Spending on Breast Cancer," *New York Times*, October 20, 1993, C14; ABC Nightly News, February 27, 1996; February 1996 fund-raising letter from the National Breast Cancer Coalition. See also James O. Mason, "A National Agenda for Women's Health," *Journal of the American Medical Association* 267, 4 (1992): 482, and Susan Jenks, "Cancer Experts Set Research Agenda for Women's Health in the 1990s," *Journal of the National Cancer Institute* 83, 20 (1991): 1443–4.

26. Susan Rennie, "Breast Cancer Prevention: Diet Vs. Drugs," *Ms.*, May-June 1993, 39–40, 42; Liane Clorfene-Casten, "The Environmental Link to Breast Cancer," *Ms.*, May-June 1993, 54; Liane Clorfene-Casten,

"Inside The Cancer Establishment," *Ms.*, May-June, 1993, 57; "Confronting Breast Cancer: An Interview with Susan Love," *Technology Review*, May-June 1993, 47–48; "Breast Cancer: Is It the Environment?" *Ms.*, April-May 2000; Sabrina McCormick, "Breast Cancer Activism," *Ms.*, summer 2002, 4–5; "Conflict Grows over Breast Cancer Strategy," *Nature*, March 3, 1994, 7.

27. David Plotkin, "Good News and Bad News about Breast Cancer," *Atlantic Monthly*, June 1996, 76; Julie Felner, "Dr. Susan Love Cuts through the Hype on Women's Health," *Ms.*, July-August 1997, 45; and Lindsy Van Gelder, "It's Not Nice to Mess with Mother Nature," *Ms.*, January-February 1989. See also Ellen Leopold, *A Darker Ribbon: A Twentieth-Century Story of Breast Cancer, Women, and Their Doctors* (Boston: Beacon Press, 1999).

28. The Boston Women's Health Book Collective, *Our Bodies, Ourselves for the New Century* (New York: Simon and Schuster, 1998), 622.

29. Katherine Eban Finkelstein, "Research for Your Life: Investigating Your Own Health Care," *On the Issues*, spring 1998, 38; "Newsmakers," *Newsweek*, April 2001, 43. For a historical examination of the popularity of alternative cancer cures, see Barbara Clow, *Negotiating Disease: Power and Cancer Care, 1900–1950* (Montreal: McGill-Queen's University Press, 2001).

30. David M. Eisenberg et al., "Unconventional Medicine in the United States: Prevalence, Costs, and Patterns of Use," *New England Journal of Medicine* 328 (1993): 246–52; David M. Eisenberg et al., "Trends in Alternative Medicine Use in the United States, 1990–1997," *Journal of the American Medical Association*, 280 (1998): 1569–75; and *Newsweek*, special issue on "Health for Life," spring-summer 1999, 13. On gender differences in attitudes toward health and health care, see Royda Crose, *Why Women Live Longer than Men . . . and What Men Can Learn from Them* (San Francisco: Jossey-Bass, 1997). See also Wayne B. Jonas, "Alternative Medicine—Learning from the Past, Examining the Present, Advancing to the Future," *Journal of the American Medical Association* 280 (1998): 1616–8; Roger Hand, "Alternative Therapies Used by Patients with AIDS," *New England Journal of Medicine* 320, 10 (1990); Robin Wilson, "Unconventional Cures," *The Chronicle of Higher Education*, January 12, 1996, A15–A16; "Weighing Alternatives," *Newsweek*, special issue on "Health for Life," spring-summer 1999, 92; Phil B. Fontanarosa, ed., *Alternative Medicine: An Objective Assessment* (New York: American Medical Association, 2000); Adrian Furnham, "Why Do People Choose and Use Complementary Therapies?" in Edzard Ernst, ed., *Complementary Medicine: An Objective Appraisal* (Oxford: Butterworth Heinemann, 1996); and Hans A. Baer, *Biomedicine and Alternative Healing Systems in America: Issues of Class, Race, Ethnicity, and Gender* (Madison: University of Wisconsin Press, 2001).

31. Dana Ullman, *The Consumer's Guide to Homeopathy: The Definitive Resource for Understanding Homeopathic Medicine and Making It Work for You* (New York: G. P. Putnam's Sons, 1995), 190.

32. Boston Women's Health Book Collective, *The New Our Bodies, Ourselves* (New York: Simon and Schuster, 1984): 54, 57; Boston Women's Health Book Collective, *Our Bodies, Ourselves for the New Century*, 101, 103–4, 106–7.

33. Boston Women's Health Book Collective, *The New Our Bodies, Ourselves*, 54, 57; Boston Women's Health Book Collective, *Our Bodies, Ourselves for the New Century*, 107, 108, 110, 115.

34. Dian Dincin Buchman, "A Natural Medicine Chest," *Ms.*, January-February 1994, 61; Adriane Fugh-Berman, "Having Our Soy," *Ms.*, January-February 1996, 30–31; Adriane Fugh-Berman, "Touch Me, Heal Me: What Can Body Work Do for You?" *Ms.*, September-October 1996, 38–39; "Profile; Janice Guthrie: Info-Power," *Ms.*, March-April 1997, 3.

35. Judith Orloff, *Dr. Judith Orloff's Guide to Intuitive Healing: Five Steps to Physical, Emotional, and Sexual Wellness* (New York: Times Books, 2000), 78; Kathleen F. Phalen, *Integrative Medicine: Achieving Wellness through the Best of Eastern and Western Medical Practices* (Boston: Journey Editions, 1998), 136.

36. Rosemary Gladstar, *Herbal Healing for Women* (New York: Simon and Schuster, 1993), 108; Jason Elias and Katherine Ketcham, *Feminine Healing: A Woman's Guide to a Healthy Body, Mind, and Spirit* (New York: Warner Books, 1997), xxii, 157, 179, 189–91. For background, see Jeffrey S. Levin and Jeannine Coreil, "'New Age' Healing in the U.S.;" *Social Science and Medicine* 23 (1986): 889–97.

37. Barbara Ehrenreich and Deirdre English, *For Her Own Good: 150 Years of the Experts' Advice to Women* (New York: Doubleday, 1978), 6; Margarete Sandelowski, *Women, Health, and Choice,* (Englewood Cliffs, N.J.: Prentice-Hall, 1981), 134.

38. Sandelowski, *Women, Health, and Choice*, 146, 149; Elias and Ketcham, *Feminine Healing*, xxii.

39. Sandra Harding, *The Science Question in Feminism* (Ithaca: Cornell University Press, 1986), 31, 125. As just a few examples from the literature on science and gender, see Londa Schiebinger, *Has Feminism*

Changed Science? (Cambridge, Mass.: Harvard University Press, 1999); Evelyn Fox Keller, *Reflections on Gender and Science* (New Haven: Yale University Press, 1985); Anne Fausto-Sterling, *Myths of Gender: Biological Theories about Women and Men* (New York: Basic Books, 1992); Carolyn Merchant, *The Death of Nature: Women, Ecology and the Scientific Revolution* (New York: Harper and Row, 1980); Donna Haraway, *Primate Visions: Gender, Race and Nature in the World of Modern Science* (New York: Routledge, 1989); Ruth Hubbard, *The Politics of Women's Biology* (New Brunswick: Rutgers University Press, 1990); Emily Martin, "The Egg and the Sperm: How Science Has Constructed a Romance Based on Stereotypical Male-Female Roles," *Signs* 16 (1991); and Sandra Harding, ed., *The "Racial" Economy of Science: Toward a Democratic Future* (Bloomington: Indiana University Press, 1993).

40. Gladstar, *Herbal Healing*, 24–25.

41. Karen Carlson, Stephanie Eisenstat, and Terra Ziporyn, *The Harvard Guide to Women's Health* (Cambridge, Mass.: Harvard University Press, 1996), 25; Elias and Ketcham, *Feminine Healing*, xix, 6.

42. Andrew Weil, *Eight Weeks to Optimum Health* (New York: Alfred A. Knopf, 1997), 210; Christiane Northrup, *The Wisdom of Menopause: Creating Physical and Emotional Health and Healing during the Change* (New York: Bantam Books, 2001), 84; Barbara Loecher, Sara Altschul O'Donnell, et al., *New Choices in Natural Healing for Women: Drug-Free Remedies from the World of Alternative Medicine* (Emmaus, Penn.: Rodale Press, 1997), 235.

43. Orloff, *Guide,* 34, 81–82, 100.

44. Ibid., xviii, 7, 8.

45. Ibid., 10–11, 32, 37–38, 98–99.

46. Loecher, O'Donnell, et al., 3, 214.

47. Orloff, *Guide*, 85–86; and Weil, *Eight Weeks*, 214.

48. Susan M. Williams, "Holistic Nursing," in Douglas Stalker and Clark Glymour, eds., *Examining Holistic Medicine* (Buffalo, N.Y.: Prometheus Books, 1985); Boston Women's Health Book Collective, *Our Bodies, Ourselves for the New Century*, 68. See also Philip E. Clark and Mary Jo Clark, "Therapeutic Touch: Is There a Scientific Basis for the Practice?" in Douglas Stalker and Clark Glymour, eds., *Examining Holistic Medicine* (Buffalo, N.Y.: Prometheus Books, 1985), 287–96, and Linda Rosa et al., "A Close Look at Therapeutic Touch," *Journal of the American Medical Association* 279 (1998): 1005–10.

49. Gladstar, *Herbal Healing*, 19. For background, see Lisa Corbin Winslow and David J. Kroll, "Herbs as Medicine," *Archives of Internal Medicine* 158 (1998): 2192–9, and Mary Ann O'Hara et al., "A Review of 12 Commonly Used Medicinal Herbs," *Archives of Family Medicine* 7 (1998): 523–36.

50. Anne McIntyre, *The Complete Woman's Herbal: A Manual of Healing Herbs and Nutrition for Personal Well-Being and Family Care* (New York: Henry Holt, 1994), 8–9.

51. Elias and Ketcham, *Feminine Healing*, 312.

52. Gladstar, *Herbal Healing*, 21, 23.

53. Kathi Keville with Peter Korn, *Herbs for Health and Healing: A Drug-Free Guide to Prevention and Cure* (Emmaus, Penn., Rodale Press, 1996), 152.

54. McIntyre, *Complete Woman's Herbal*, 9–10.

55. Gladstar, *Herbal Healing*, 55, 123, 218.

56. http://www.healinggarden.com.

57. Keville, *Herbs*, 284.

58. Loecher, O'Donnell, et al., *New Choices*, 51, 54.

59. Keville, *Herbs*; Emrika Padus, *The Woman's Encyclopedia of Health and Natural Healing* (Emmaus, Penn.: Rodale Press, 1981), 292. On the 1990s boom in herbal medicine marketing and consumerism, see John Greenwald, "Herbal Healing," *Time*, November 23, 1998, 58–67.

60. Katrina H. Berne, *Running on Empty: Chronic Fatigue Immune Dysfunction Syndrome (CFIDS)* (Alameda, Calif.: Hunter House, 1992), 30.

61. Susan Griffin, "The Internal Athlete," *Ms.*, May-June 1992, 37; Andrea Rudner, "Chronic Fatigue Syndrome: Searching for the Answers," *Ms.*, May-June 1992.

62. Berne, *Running on Empty*, 157, 163, 182, 197; Gary Null and Barbara Seaman, *For Women Only! Your Guide to Health Empowerment* (New York: Seven Stories Press, 1999), 168–69.

63. Null and Seaman, *For Women Only*, 169, 182.

64. Janice Strubbwe Wittenberg, *The Rebellious Body: Reclaim Your Life from Environmental Illness or Chronic Fatigue Syndrome* (New York: Plenum Press, 1996), 5, 236.

65. Ibid., 3, 5, 232, 236.

66. Robert A. Wilson, *Feminine Forever* (New York: M. Evans and Co., 1966). For background, see Amanda Spake, "The Menopausal Marketplace," *U.S. News and World Report*, November 18, 2002, 42–50; Elizabeth Siegel Watkins, " 'Doctor, Are You Trying to Kill Me?': Ambivalence about the Patient Package Insert for Estrogen," *Bulletin of the History of Medicine* 76 1 (2002): 84–104; Judith A. Houck, " 'What Do These Women Want?': Feminist Responses to *Feminine Forever*, 1963–1980," *Bulletin of the History of Medicine* 77, 1 (2003); and Patricia A. Kaufer and Sonja M. McKinley, "Estrogen Replacement Therapy: The Production of Medical Knowledge and the Emergence of Policy," in Ellen Lewin and Virginia Olesen, eds., *Women, Health, and Healing: Toward a New Perspective* (New York: Tavistock, 1985), 113–38.

67. Northrup, *Wisdom*, 3.

68. "A Beginner's Guide to Menopause," interview with Sandra Coney, *Ms.*, January-February 1995, 22. See also Carol Ann Rinzler, *Estrogen and Breast Cancer: A Warning to Women* (New York: Macmillan, 1993).

69. Northrup, *Wisdom*, 3.

70. Susan M. Love with Karen Lindsey, *Dr. Susan Love's Hormone Book: Making Informed Choices about Menopause* (New York: Random House, 1997), 35.

71. Ibid., 240, 277, 279.

72. Ibid., xvii.

73. Northrup, *Wisdom*, 190.

74. Timothy Gower, "New Answers to Menopause?" *Health*, January-February 2002, 76–82.

75. Elias and Ketcham, *Feminine Healing*, 253; and Nan Lu with Ellen Schaplowsky, *Traditional Chinese Medicine: A Woman's Guide to a Trouble-Free Menopause* (New York: Harper Collins, 2000), xii, xv, xx.

76. Northrup, *Wisdom*, 9, 20, 39, 97.

77. Paula Maas, Susan E. Brown, and Nancy Bruning, *The MEND Clinic Guide to Natural Medicine for Menopause and Beyond* (New York: Dell, 1997), 3–4.

78. Barbara Ehrenreich, "The Real Truth about the Female Body," *Time*, March 8, 1999, 69.

79. Northrup, *Wisdom*, 9, 38, 496–98.

80. Advertisement for "Menopause Relief Supplement," *U.S. News and World Report*, January 20, 2003, 21.

81. Amanda Spake, "Hormones on Trial," *U.S. News and World Report*, January 21, 2002, 54–56.

82. Jane E. Brody, "Sorting through the Confusion over Estrogen," *New York Times*, September 3, 2002; Denise Grady, "Risks of Hormone Therapy Exceed Benefits, Panel Says," *New York Times*, October 17, 2002. See also Gina Kolata, "Scientists Debating Future of Hormone Replacement," *New York Times*, October 23, 2002.

83. Denise Grady, "Weighing Risks and Benefits of Hormone Therapy," *New York Times*, April 30, 2002; Gina Kolata, "Cancer Risk of Hormones May Linger," *New York Times*, October 24, 2002. See also Isadore Rosenfeld, "My Advice on Estrogen," *Parade Magazine*, October 13, 2002, 6–8; Samantha Levine, "Tailor-made Treatments," *U.S. News and World Report*, November 18, 2002, 61–62; and Samantha Levine, "Hormones and . . . ," *U.S. News and World Report*, November 18, 2002, 63.

84. Gina Kolata, "Replacing Replacement Therapy," *New York Times*, October 27, 2002.

85. Gina Kolata, "Drug Agency Weighs Role of Hormone Replacements," *New York Times*, October 25, 2002; Kolata, "Cancer Risk"; Gina Kolata, "Menopause without Pills: Rethinking Hot Flashes," *New York Times*, November 10, 2002.

86. Claudia Kalb, "A Natural Way to Age," *Newsweek*, November 2, 2002, 64–65; Eric Nagourney, "Remedies: In Lieu of Hormones: Questions," *New York Times*, November 19, 2002, "A Natural Way through Menopause?" *U.S. News and World Report*, January 21, 2002, 56.

87. "The Estrogen Dilemma," *Newsweek*, special issue on "Health for Life," spring-summer 1999, 35–37.

88. "How Your Mind Can Heal Your Body," *Time*, January 20, 2003; "Health for Life: Inside the Science of Alternative Medicine," *Newsweek*, November 2, 2002, 45. See also Stephen Williams, "Another Road to Good Health," *Newsweek*, special issue on "Health for Life," spring-summer 1999, 90–91.

89. Tricia O'Brien, "The ABCs of Alternative Medicine: Curing What Ails You," *Family Circle*, September 18, 2001, 58–66.

90. Sarah Lyall, "Women Turn to Non-Traditional Methods to Find Refuge and Focus," *New York Times*, December 15, 2002.

91. Cathy Guisewite, *Cathy,* March 2, 2003.

92. Orloff, *Guide,* 61–62.

Inside-Out

The author thanks the staff of Health Records and Archives, Women's College Hospital.

1. "WCH Gets Its Day in Court," *Capsule Comments: Women's College Hospital* August 18, 1997, 1.

2. Hans Baer, *Biomedicine and Alternative Healing Systems in America: Issues of Class, Race, Ethnicity, and Gender* (Madison: University of Wisconsin Press, 2001); Robbie Davis Floyd and Gloria St. John, eds., *From Doctor to Healer: The Transformative Journey* (New Brunswick, N.J.: Rutgers University Press, 1998); Rosalind Coward, *The Whole Truth: The Myth of Alternative Healing* (London: Faber and Faber, 1989).

3. Diane Stein, *All Women are Healers* (Freedom, Calif.: Crossing Press, 1990).

4. Susan Reverby, "Thinking through the Body and the Body Politic: Gendering Health Policy, Historical Perspectives from the United States, 1940–1980," in G. Feldberg et al., eds., *Women, Health, and Nation: Canada and the United States Since 1945* (Montreal: McGill-Queen's University Press, 2003), 404–20.

5. Georgina Feldberg et al., "Why Borders Matter," in G. Feldberg et al., eds. *Women, Health, and Nation: Canada and the United States Since 1945* (Montreal: McGill-Queen's University Press, 2003), 15–42; Georgina Feldberg and Robert Vipond, "The Virus of Consumerism," in Daniel Drache and Terry Sullivan, eds., *Health Reform: Public Success, Private Failure* (London: Routledge, 1999), 48–64. For discussion of the ways in which social activism and the political trends of the 1960s shaped a revolution in American medicine, see also Davis Floyd and St.-John, *From Doctor to Healer,* esp. 85 and 111–12.

6. Chantalle Maillé, "The Women's Health Movement in Quebec Society: An Analysis for the Purpose of the Constitutional Debate," in David Schneiderman, ed., *Conversations among Friends: Proceedings of and Interdisciplinary Conference on Women and Constitutional Reform* (Edmonton, Alta.: University of Alberta Centre for Constitutional Studies, 1993), 43.

7. Feldberg et al., "Why Borders Matter"; Georgina Feldberg and Marianne Carlsson, "Organized for Health: Women's Activism in Canada and Sweden," in Linda Briskin and Mona Eliasson, eds., *Women's Organizing and Public Policy in Canada and Sweden* (Montreal: McGill-Queen's University Press, 2000), 347–74.

8. The early documents of the WHM lend themselves to criticism that can be found in more recent secondary works. For example, the original and even more recent editions of *Our Bodies, Ourselves* presumed that all women are fertile and concerned about conception. They overlooked the issues of minority women and disabled women who were sometimes sterilized against their will. They ignored issues of infertility. See also C. Lesley Biggs, "Rethinking Midwifery in Canada," in Ivy Bourgeault, Cecilia Benoit, and Robbie Davis-Floyd, eds., *Reconceiving Midwifery: The New Canadian Model of Care* (Montreal: McGill-Queen's University Press, in press).

9. Biggs, "Rethinking Midwifery in Canada."

10. Leslie J. Reagan, *When Abortion Was a Crime: Women, Medicine and the Law in the United States, 1867–1973* (Berkeley: University of California Press, 1997); Frances Jane Wasserlein, "An Arrow at the Heart: The Vancouver Women's Caucus and the Abortion Campaign, 1969–1971," M.A. thesis, Simon Fraser University, 1990; Shannon Stettner, "From Abortion Reform to Abortion Repeal: The Rise of Doris Anderson's *Chatelaine* in the Lives of Women Readers, 1959–1977," M.A. thesis, University of Waterloo, 2000; Janine Brodie, Shelley A. M. Gavigan, and Jane Jenson, *The Politics of Abortion* (Toronto: Oxford University Press, 1992).

11. Eileen Young, "The Montreal Health Press: Working to Empower Women," *Canadian Women's Studies/ Les Cahiers de la femme* 14, 3 (1994): 45–47.

12. Coward, *The Whole Truth,* 157.

13. See Biggs, "Rethinking Midwifery in Canada"; C. Lesley Biggs, "The Case of the Missing Midwives: A History of Midwifery in Ontario from 1795–1900," *Ontario History* 75 (1983): 21–35; Cecilia Benoit, *Midwives in Passage: The Modernization of Maternity Care* (St. John's, Newfoundland: Memorial University, 1991); Ivy Lynn Bourgeault, "Delivery Midwifery: An Examination of the Process and Outcome of the Incorporation of Midwifery in Ontario," Ph.D. thesis, University of Toronto, 1996; Robbie Davis-Floyd, *Birth as an American Rite of Passage* (Berkeley: University of California Press, 1992).

14. Barbara Ehrenreich and Deirdre English, *Witches, Midwives and Nurses: A History of Women Healers* (Old Westbury, N.Y.: Feminist Press, 1973), 3.

15. Later examples include Jeanne Achterberg, *Woman as Healer* (Boston: Shamhala Press, 1990), and Bobette Peronne, H. Henrietta Stockel, and Victoria Krueger, eds., *Medicine Women, Curanderas and Women Doctors* (Norman and London: University of Oklahoma Press, 1989). See also Judith Ochshorn, "Goddesses and the Lives of Women," in Karen L. King, ed., *Women and Goddess Traditions in Antiquity and Today* (Minneapolis: Fortress Press, 1997), 377–406, and Savina J. Teubal, "The Rise and Fall of Female Reproductive Control as Seen through Images of Women," in Karen L. King, ed., *Women and Goddess Traditions in Antiquity and Today* (Minneapolis: Fortress Press, 1997), 281–301.

16. See, for example, Gena Corea, *The Hidden Malpractice: How American Medicine Mistreats Women as Patients and Professionals* (New York: Morrow, 1977), and Barbara Katz Rothman, *In Labor: Women and Power in the Birthplace* (New York: Harper and Row, 1985).

17. Pamela E. Klassen, *Blessed Events: Religion and Home Birth in America* (Princeton, N.J.: Princeton University Press, 2001); see also Louise Erdrich, *The Blue Jay's Dance: A Birth Year* (New York: Harper-Collins, 1995).

18. For histories of Women Healthsharing, see Amy Gottlieb, "Saying Goodbye to Healthsharing," *Canadian Women's Studies/Les Cahiers de la Femme* 14, 3 (1994), and Enakshi Dua, ed., *On Women Healthsharing* (Toronto: Women's Press, 1994).

19. "Notes from the Collective," *Healthsharing* 1, 1 (1979): 3.

20. Rhonda Love, "The Power of Science and Medicine" *Healthsharing* 2, 2 (1981): 11.

21. Clara Valverde and Connie Clement, "Nurturing Politics and Health: Centre de Sante des Femmes du Quartier," *Healthsharing* 1, 1, (1979): 15–17.

22. Connie Clement, "Health Care Choices: Making Yours," *Healthsharing* 1, 2 (1980): 12.

23. Coward, *The Whole Truth*, 11.

24. Valverde and Clement, "Nurturing Politics," 15.

25. Evelyn Fox Keller, *A Feeling for the Organism: The Life and Work of Barbara McKlintock* (San Francisco: W. H. Freeman, 1983); Carol Gilligan, *In a Different Voice: Psychological Theory and Women's Development* (Cambridge, Mass.: Harvard University Press, 1982).

26. "Notes from the Collective," 3.

27. For a longer discussion of health activism and the consumer rights movement, see Feldberg and Vipond, "Virus of Consumerism."

28. "Notes from the Collective," 2.

29. Kathleen McDonnell, "The Women's Health Movement," in Kathleen McDonnell and Mariana Valverde, eds., *The Healthsharing Book* (Toronto: Women Healthsharing, 1985).

30. Ibid.

31. "Collective Notes," *Healthsharing* 2, 4 (1981): 4; Rhonda Love, "Women in Medicine: Will It Make a Difference?" *Healthsharing* 2, 4 (1981): 14–17.

32. See, for example, Martin Kendrick and Christa Slade, *The Spirit of Life: The Story of Women's College Hospital* (Toronto: Women's College Hospital, 1993); *Passing the Flame: The Legacy of Women's College Hospital* (Toronto: White Pine Films, 1998).

33. Jacalyn Duffin, "The Death of Sarah Lovell and the Constrained Feminism of Emily Stowe," *Canadian Medical Association Journal* 146, 6 (1992): 881–88; Constance Backhouse, *Peticoats and Prejudice: Women and Law in Nineteenth-Century Canada* (Toronto: Women's Press, 1991), 112–41.

34. Ontario Medical College for Women, *Annual Calendar*, 1903, 5, University of Toronto Archives P78–0122 (02).

35. See, for example, Toronto Women's Medical College, *Announcement of the 9th Session*, 1891–92, 5–6, Women's College Hospital Archives.

36. See, for example, Ontario Medical College for Women, *Announcement of the 10th Session*, 1892–93, 11. See also Ruth Compton Brouwer, *New Women for God: Canadian Presbyterian Women and the India Missions, 1876–1914* (Toronto: University of Toronto Press, 1990), and Margo Gewurtz, "Embodying Science: Images of Canadian Women Medical Missionaries and Their Chinese Assistants," in R. Shteir and B. Lightman, eds., *Visual Vocabularies of Gender and Science*, forthcoming.

37. Gewurtz, "Embodying Science."

38. Ontario Medical College for Women, *Annual Announcement*, 1898, 6; see also Kendrick and Slade, *Spirit of Life.*

39. Women's Medical College, *Annual Report* 1911, 3, Archives, Women's College Hospital.

40. Women's Medical College, *Annual Report* 1912, 6, Archives, Women's College Hospital.

41. Women's Medical College, *Annual Report*, 1911, 6, Archives, Women's College Hospital.

42. Women's College Hospital, *Annual Report*, 1915, 4, Archives, Women's College Hospital.

43. The quote is from "Remarks: Opening of Hospital at 125 Rusholme Rd, July 17, 1915," Archives, Women's College Hospital, 21-C18-10. See also Women's College Hospital, *Annual Report*, 1912 and 1914.

44. Women's College Hospital, "Women's Work for Women's Needs," *Annual Report of the Women's College Hospital and Dispensary*, 1914, 3.

45. WCH, *Annual Report*, 1914, 5.

46. Ibid.

47. "Remarks: Opening of Hospital at 125 Rusholme Rd, July 17, 1915," 2.

48. Kendrick and Slade, *Spirit of Life*, 118.

A Quiet Movement

I gratefully acknowledge, first, the priests who worked with me for many years; thank you. I also would be remiss if I didn't also thank Robert Johnston for patiently commenting on and editing this essay; this was a wonderful opportunity. I received generous funding for this research, and for the presentation of this research, from the Association for Feminist Anthropology, the University of Iowa student government, the Graduate Student Senate, the Central States Anthropological Society, and the Department of Anthropology and Graduate College of the University of Iowa. Lastly, I would like to thank my family, Dan and Dylan, who put up with their anthropologist wife and mother.

1. W. E. B. Dubois, *The Negro* (New York: Oxford University Press, 1970 [1915]), 113–14.

2. *Orisha*-based worship is known by many names throughout its many lands of practice. Although I refer to it, per my narrators, as Orisha, many others in the United States refer to it as Santería, "the religion," Lucumi, La Regla de Ocha (the Law of the Orisha), and Yoruba religion. In this paper, I differentiate between the religion (Orisha) and the deities (*orisha*). While I primarily work with African Americans, the larger community of belief and practice is both multiracial and multicultural. Further, it is important to remember that people of all races have entered the religion through different religious avenues (e.g., Orisha versus Santería) and that there are differences that exist between lines of initiation; not all people with whom I work subscribe to the political aspects of the religion.

3. Karen McCarthy Brown, "Afro-Caribbean Spirituality: A Haitian Case Study," in L. Sullivan, ed., *Healing and Restoring: Health and Medicine in the World's Religious Traditions* (New York: Macmillan, 1989), 257.

4. Olodumare is considered neither male nor female, although numerous authors use the masculine pronoun when discussing Olodumare's nature and existence. I attempt to get around this as much as I can by simply using the proper name. Olodumare is also referred to as Olorun (the owner of the sky/heavens).

5. Carl Hunt. *Oyotunji Village: The Yoruba Movement in America* (Washington, D.C.: University Press of America, 1979). Hunt's informant, quoted here, was Oba Oseijeman; see my discussion below of the political history of the religion in the United States. In all other instances, names are pseudonyms.

6. There are numerous other *orisha* that will be further introduced in their relation to healing later in the essay. The actual number of deities is unknown, with estimates ranging from two hundred to two thousand (see J. Omosade Awolalu, *Yoruba Beliefs and Sacrificial Rites* [London: Longman, 1979], 20). In my experience, although there are many *orisha* acknowledged as being involved in people's lives, I have encountered only about twenty or thirty of them in my fieldwork. This disparity may be in part due to the conglomerate of cultural and religious beliefs brought to this hemisphere during the slave trade. Also, some *orisha* are tied to specific places. Further, much was undoubtedly forgotten, amended, or otherwise altered in people's minds and practices while living in horrendously oppressive circumstances. See my discussion later in the essay of the roles that particular *orisha* play in healing.

7. George Brandon, *Santeria from Africa to the New World: The Dead Sell Memories* (Bloomington: Indiana University Press, 1993), 70ff.; Melville J. Herskovitz, *The Myth of the Negro Past* (Boston: Beacon Press, 1990 [1941]), 160ff.; Fernando Ortiz, "Los Cabildos Afro-Cubana," *Revista Bimestre Cubana* 16 (1921): 5–39.

8. See Brandon. *Santeria from Africa to the New World*, 82; Steven Gregory, *Santeria in New York City: A Study in Cultural Resistance* (New York: Garland Publishing, 1999), 26.

9. Marta Moreno Vega, *The Altar of My Soul: The Living Traditions of Santeria* (New York: One World Books, 2000), 130–31. For the legends regarding how Shango, a Yoruba king, became an *orisha*, see Awolalu, *Yoruba Beliefs and Sacrificial Rites*, 33–34; Judith Illsely Gleason, *Oya: In Praise of the Goddess* (Boston: Shambhala, 1987), 60.

10. See Robert A. Voeks, *Sacred Leaves of Candomble: African Magic, Medicine, and Religion in Brazil* (Austin: University of Texas Press, 1997), 52; Gayraud S. Wilmore, *Black Religion and Black Radicalism* (Maryknoll, N.Y.: Orbis Books, 1991), 21.

11. Barbara Bush, *Slave Women in Caribbean Society, 1650–1838* (Kingston: Heinemann Publishers, 1990), 160. Iyalosha Adegoke told me family stories that echo this amalgam of fear, respect, and oppression; see Velana Huntington, "Oya with a Sword at My Back: Women and Experience in an Orisha Community," M.A. thesis, University of Iowa, 1998. Also, although Bush is focusing on the role of women in slave societies, one must assume that enslaved men also were active participants in religious and cultural resistance.

12. Clarke aptly points out that many of the "traditions" that are followed in some sectors of Orisha worship are based on earlier anthropological and sociological accounts of the Yoruba peoples in Nigeria. She also reminds us that Yoruba "tradition" is a product not only of British colonialism but also of internal struggles of those indigenous to Nigeria over who will have the right to control and enforce the resources, norms, and meanings of "tradition." Maxine Kamari Clarke, *Genealogies of Reclaimed Nobility: The Geotemporality of Yoruba Belonging* (Ann Arbor: U.M.I. Dissertation Services, 1997), 117, 97–98.

13. Dunham, unpublished biography, quoted in Marta Moreno Vega, *Yoruba Philosophy: Multiple Levels of Transformation and Understanding* (Ann Arbor: U.M.I. Dissertation Services, 1995), 65.

14. Beatriz Morales, *Afro-Cuban Religious Transformation: A Comparative Study of Lucumi Religion and the Tradition of Spirit Belief* (Ann Arbor: U.M.I. Dissertation Services, 1990), 132.

15. A long and detailed history of Orisha worship in the United States is not possible in this essay; however, there are other scholars that trace Orisha's history throughout this century. See, for example, Hunt, *Oyotunji Village*.

16. See Hunt, *Oyotunji Village*; Marta Moreno Vega, *Yoruba Philosophy: Multiple Levels of Transformation and Understanding* (Ann Arbor: U.M.I. Dissertation Services, 1995).

17. Quoted in Hunt, *Oyotunji Village*, 28; see also Oseijeman O. Adefunmi, *Olorisha: A Guidebook into Yoruba Religion* (Oyotunji Village, Sheldon, S.C.: Great Benin Books, 1982), v.

18. Amiri Baraka, *The Leroi Jones/Amiri Baraka Reader* (New York: Thunder's Mouth Press, 1991), 167.

19. John Mason, *Four New World Yoruba Rituals* (Brooklyn: Yoruba Theological Archministry, 1985), 14.

20. This reclamation of Africa has been echoed throughout the Americas; see James T. Houk, *Spirits, Blood and Drums: The Orisha Religion in Trinidad* (Philadelphia: Temple University Press, 1995) for the revitalization of Orisha in Trinidad, and V. Prata, "Candomble Says No to Syncretism," *Jornal da Bahia*, July 29, 1983, for information on Brazilian Candomble.

21. Bob Blauner, *Black Lives, White Lives: Three Decades of Race Relations in America* (Berkeley: University of California Press, 1989), 234. Van Deburg contends that the Black Power movements were effectively squelched in the 1970s and 1980s due to a number of factors. The most important for Van Deburg was the systematic and violent use of White force, although changing gender relations within society and the movements, the age of the constituents (middle-aged), and dissenting voices within the movement also contributed to its demise. See W. Van Deburg, *New Day in Babylon: The Black Power Movement and American Culture, 1965–1975* (Chicago: University of Chicago Press, 1992).

22. Brown, "Afro-Caribbean Spirituality: A Haitian Case Study," 257.

23. Joseph M. Murphy, *Santeria: An African Religion in America* (Boston: Beacon Press, 1988), 62.

24. Zora Neale Hurston, *Mules and Men* (New York: Harper Perennial, 1990 [1935]), 183.

25. Houk, *Spirits, Blood and Drums*.

26. *Alaafia* is the Yoruba (originally Arabic) word meaning "peace, health, wealth, and prosperity [to you]." Its primary meaning has been kept intact, and it is further used as a greeting among the people with whom I work. Further, it is considered to be a state of being toward which one aspires.

27. These were two of the extreme cases in which the *orisha* were called upon to intercede on a person's (physical) behalf. Not all treatments and results are so dramatic, and I don't know the health status of these women today, but I heard that they were still healthy. A third case was Adegoke's own experience with her

daughter's birth wherein upon life-threatening complications rituals were done in Nigeria on her behalf. She and her daughter are fine.

28. See Olli Alho, *The Religion of the Slaves: A Study of the Religious Tradition and Behaviour of Plantation Slaves in the United States 1830–1865* (Helsinki: Academia Scientiarum Fennica, 1976); Karen McCarthy Brown, *Mama Lola: A Vodou Priestess in Brooklyn* (Berkeley: University of California Press, 1991); Velana Huntington, "The Good Life: Health and Healing in Orisa," paper presented at the annual meeting of the American Ethnological Society, March 25–28, 1999; Hurston, *Mules and Men.* One needs to keep in mind, however, that Oseijiman was attempting to remove all "slave" references and practices from Orisha practice, thus returning it to its "original" Yoruba form. I simply want to note that it shares commonalities with other African-based forms of worship throughout the Americas by virtue of the fact that they *are* African-based.

29. Herbal remedies and preparations constitute a large part of Orisha worship, from healing baths to mixtures used in initiations. Osanyin is the *orisha* that is associated with the collection and preparation of herbs and herbal mixtures and as such must duly be called upon when making these potions. Verger and Voeks have written extensively on the "sacred leaves" of Orisha worship and practice; see Pierre Verger, *Awon Ewe Osanyin* (Ife: Institute of African Studies, University of Ife, 1967); Robert A. Voeks, "Sacred Leaves of Brazilian Candomble," *Geographical Review* 80 (1990): 118–31; Voeks, *Sacred Leaves of Candomble.*

30. See Awolalu. *Yoruba Beliefs and Sacrificial Rites*, 20–45; Donna Daniels, *When the Living Is the Prayer: African-Based Religious Reverence in Everyday Life among Women of Color Devotees in the San Francisco Bay Area* (Ann Arbor: U.M.I. Dissertation Services, 1998), 96.

31. Alfred Metraux, *Voodoo in Haiti* (New York: Schocken Books, 1972 [1959]); Roger Bastide, *The African Religions of Brazil: Toward a Sociology of the Interpenetration of Civilizations,* translated by H. Sebba (Baltimore: Johns Hopkins University Press, 1978); Verena Martinez-Alier, *Marriage, Class and Color in Nineteenth Century Cuba: A Study of Racial Attitudes and Sexual Values in a Slave Society* (Ann Arbor: University of Michigan Press, 1989); Herskovitz, *The Myth of the Negro Past.*

The Politics and Poetics of "Magazine Medicine"

1. Robin Bunton, "Popular Health, Advanced Liberalism and *Good Housekeeping* magazine," In Alan Peterson and Robin Bunton, eds., *Foucault, Health and Medicine* (London: Routledge, 1997).

2. Peter Conrad. "Public Eyes and Private Genes: Historical Frames, News Constructions, and Social Problems," *Social Problems* 44, 2 (1997): 141–154.

3. Michel Foucault, *Technologies of the Self* (Amherst: University of Massachusetts Press, 1988).

4. Ayurveda refers to the complex of South Asian humoral therapeutics that were codified in classical texts as far back as 600 B.C.E. For a detailed description, see Dominik Wujastyk, *The Roots of Ayurveda: Selections from the Sanskrit Medical Writings* (New Delhi: Penguin, 1998). In its classical form, therapeutic treatment of illness in this system involved a systematic combination of dietetics (*kayachikitsa*), herbal medication (*dravyaguna*) and a set of radical manipulative therapies that included oil massages and elimination programs (*pancakarma*).

5. For a more extended discussion on New Age politics, see David Hess, *Science in the New Age: The Paranormal, Its Defenders and Debunkers, and American Culture* (Madison: Wisconsin University Press, 1993), appendix; and Mark Ivor Satin, *New Age Politics: Healing Self and Society: The Emerging New Alternative to Marxism and Liberalism* (New York: Delacorte Press, 1979), ch.1.

6. John B.Thompson, *Ideology and Modern Culture* (Stanford: Stanford University Press, 1991), 218.

7. See Conrad, "Public Eyes." For a public arenas model of news as a social problem, see Stephen Hilgartner and Charles L. Bosk, "The Rise and Fall of Social Problems: A Public Arenas Model," *American Journal of Sociology* 4 (1988), 53–78.

8. See, for instance, Niklas Rose, "Government, Authority and Medical Expertise in Advanced Liberalism," *Economy and Society* 22, 3 (1993): 238–98.

9. Anthony Giddens, *Modernity and Self-Identity: Self and Society in the Late Modern Age* (Cambridge: Polity Press, 1991); Rose, "Government, Authority and Medical Expertise,

10. Robert Crawford, "Healthism and the Medicalization of Everyday Life," *International Journal of Health Services* 10, 3 (1980): 365–88; Kenneth R. Dutton, *The Perfectible Body: The Western Ideal of Physical Development* (London: Cassell, 1995).

11. Wendy Farrant and Jill Russell, *The Politics of Health Information* (London: Institute of Education, 1986).

12. Margaret Beetham, *A Magazine of Her Own? Domesticity and Desire in the Women's Magazine, 1800–1914* (London: Routledge, 1996); Joke Hermes, *Reading Women's Magazines: An Analysis of Everyday Media Use* (Cambridge: Polity Press, 1995).

13. See Hermes, *Reading Women's Magazines*, 17–20.

14. J.B. Elliott, "A Content Analysis of the Health Information Provided in Women's Magazines," *Health Libraries Review*, 11 (1994): 96–103; Barry Glassner, *Bodies: Overcoming the Tyranny of Perfection* (Los Angeles: Lowell House, 1992); Deborah Lupton, *The Imperative of Health: Public Health and the Regulated Body* (London: Sage, 1995).

15. Robin Bunton, "More than a Woolly Jumper: Health Promotion as Social Regulation," *Critical Public Health* 3, 2 (1990): 4–11; Alan Peterson and Deborah Lupton, *The New Public Health: Health and Self in the Age of Risk* (London: Sage, 1996); Matthew Schneirov, *The Dream of a New Social Order: Popular Magazines in America 1893–1914* (New York: Columbia University Press, 1994).

16. Bryan S. Turner, "The Interdisciplinary Curriculum: From Social Medicine to Postmodernism." In *Regulating Bodies: Essays in Medical Sociology* (London: Routledge, 1992).

17. Ludwig Fleck, *Genesis and Development of a Scientific Fact* (Chicago: University of Chicago Press, 1979), 21.

18. See Hess, *Science in the New Age*; Paul Heelas, *The New Age Movement* (Oxford: Blackwell, 1996).

19. James Boon, *Other Tribes, Other Scribes* (Cambridge: Cambridge University Press, 1982)

20. Hess, *Science in the New Age*; Jean English-Lueck, *Health in the New Age: A Study of California Holistic Practice* (Albuquerque: University of New Mexico Press, 1990).

21. See Crawford, "Healthism and the Medicalization of Everyday Life," 366.

22. Hess, *Science in the New Age*, 7.

23. Robert Ellwood, *Alternative Altars* (Chicago: University of Chicago Press, 1979); *Eastern Spirituality in America: Selected Writings* (New York: Paulist Press, 1987).

24. Andrea Diem and James R. Lewis, "Imagining India: The influence of Hinduism on the New Age Movement," in J.R. Lewis and J.G. Gordon, *Perspectives on the New Age* (Albany: State University of New York, 1992).

25. Interestingly, Vivekananda never used the term "Ayurveda," referring only to the less specific "Indian medicine" as part of the larger categories of Indian philosophy and religion.

26. Diem and Lewis, *Imagining India*, 151.

27. See Vivekananda, *The Complete Works of Swami Vivekananda* (Calcutta: Advaita Ashram, 1972).

28. With the New Age as our guide, it becomes clear that the class dimension is not an entirely full or accurate description of Ayurvedic user demographics. Studies on the composition and size of the New Age movement are contradictory—whereas James Lewis claims its largest constituency comes from "single upwardly mobile urban adults," Meredith McGuire highlights their suburban roots, and Catherine Albanese emphasizes the strong component of working-class people with only average levels of education. See Lewis, "Approaches to the Study of the New Age Movement," in Lewis and Melton, *Perspectives on the New Age*; McGuire, *Ritual Healing in Suburban America* (New Brunswick: Rutgers University Press, 1988); Albanese, "The Magical Staff: Quantum Healing in the New Age," in Lewis and Melton, *Perspectives on the New Age*.

29. Hess, *Science in the New Age*, 180–81; James Levin and Jean Coreil, "New Age Healing in the U.S.," *Social Science and Medicine* 23, 9 (1986): 889–897.

30. "Return of the Rishi," book review, *East West*, March, 1989, 23–25.

31. "Traditional Herbs for Modern Times," *Vegetarian Times*, 4, 1995, 27.

32. "Ayurveda to Complement Biomedicine," *Natural Health*, September, 1998, 17–19.

33. Deepak Chopra, *Return of the Rishi: A Doctor's Story of Spiritual Transformation and Ayurvedic Healing* (Boston: Houghton Mifflin, 1988), viii

34. Deepak Chopra, *Quantum Healing: Discovering the Power to Fulfill your Dreams* (New York: Bantam, 1991).

35. Deepak Chopra, *Ageless Body, Timeless Mind: The Quantum Alternative to Growing Old* (New York: Harmony Books, 1993).

36. Diem and Lewis, *Imagining India*.

37. Lisa Lowe, *Critical Terrains: French and British Orientalism* (Ithaca: Cornell University Press, 1991).

38. Harvey Cox, *Turning East: The Promise and Peril of the New Orientalism* (New York: Simon and Schuster, 1977); David Kopf, *British Orientalism and the Bengal Renaissance* (Berkeley: University of California Press, 1984); Edward W. Said, *Orientalism* (New York: Vintage, 1979).

39. Sydney Ahlstrom, *A Religious History of the American People* (New Haven: Yale University Press, 1972).

40. Ellwood, *Eastern Spirituality*, 42.

41. See Catherine Albanese, *Nature Religion in America: From the Algonkian Indians to the New Age* (Chicago: University of Chicago Press, 1990); Albanese, "The Magical Staff."

42. David Kopf, *British Orientalism and the Bengal Renaissance*, 34

43. See Diem and Lewis, *Imagining India*.

44. Diem and Lewis, "Imagining India," 161.

45. Rick Fields, *How the Swans Came to the Lake* (Boston: Shambala Press, 1981).

46. Vivekananda, *Complete Works*, ch. 2.

47. On the New Age movement generally, see Heelas, *The New Age Movement*, introduction.

48. Gary Snyder, "Why Tribe," In *Earth House Hold* (New York: New Directions, 1969).

49. Hess, *Science in the New Age*; Lewis and Melton, *Perspectives on the New Age*, 14–25.

50. Ashis Nandy, *The Intimate Enemy: Loss and Recovery of Self Under Colonialism* (London: Oxford University Press, 1983).

51. See Lawrence Cohen's article on Ayurvedic *rasayana*, "The Epistemological Carnival: Meditations on Disciplinary Intentionality and Ayurveda," in Don Bates, ed., *Knowledge and the scholarly medical traditions* (Cambridge: Cambridge University Press, 1995).

52. "Wonder Cures from the Fringe," *East West*, November, 1991.

53. "Quantum Healing," *New Age*, March, 1990.

54. For interesting typologies of New Agers, see Andrew Ross, *Strange Weather: Culture, Science and Technology in the Age of Limits* (London: Verso, 1991) and Levin and Coreil, *Social Science and Medicine*, 23, 9 (1986): 889–897.

55. On the DHSEA, see Johnston, "Introduction: The Politics of Healing," in this volume.

56. See "Ayurvedic Herbs," *Utne Reader*, November, 1993; "Why Spa?" *Utne Reader*, March 1995; "The Whole Truth: Massages and Herbal Farms," *Utne Reader*, July, 1996.

57. "Healing Sanctuaries," *New Times*, Spring, 1991, 18.

58. Francis Zimmermann, "Gentle Purge: The Flower Power of Ayurveda," in Charles Leslie and Alan Young, eds., *Paths to Asian Medical Knowledge* (Berkeley: University of California Press, 1992).

59. See for instance "Ayurvedic Spas for Today's Girls," *Natural Health*, 1992, 5.

60. "Traditional Medicine and Cutting Edge Insights," *Vegetarian Times*, December, 1997.

61. "Guru on the Go," *Amhealth*, 1992, 5.

62. "Healthy Weight Loss," *Total Health*, March, 1995.

63. For an excellent overview of this topic, see Charles M. Leslie and Alan Young, ed. *Paths to Asian Medical Knowledge* (Berkeley: University of California Press, 1992).

64. "A New World Herbalism," *Natural Health*, March, 1992.

65. "Where East meets West," *Vegetarian Times*, August, 1994.

66. "The New Ayurveda," *Total Health*, April, 1993.

67. For more on this view, see Ross, *Strange Weather*, 16.

68. "Making Gold," *Whole Earth Review*, 1994.

69. "Natural Energy and Well-Being," *Shaman*, 1995, 6.

70. Anxiety over sexual vitality and performance is common among South Asian men and is a phenomenon that has been researched by psychiatrists such as Sudhir Kakar as well as by medical anthropologists like Lawrence Cohen. See Lawrence Cohen, *No Aging in India: Alzheimer's, the Bad Family and Other Modern Things* (Berkeley: University of California Press, 2000) and Sudhir Kakar, *Intimate Relations: Exploring Indian Sexuality* (Chicago: University of Chicago Press, 1990).

71. "Traditional Remedies for Sexual Satisfaction," *New Times*, March, 1992.

72. "Sexual Remedies for Loss," *Trikone*, 8, 1997.

73. See for instance Cohen, "Epistemological Carnival" for an anthropological perspective on this issue.

74. For a good history of New Thought, see Hess, *Science in the New Age*, ch. 1; and Beryl Satter, *Each Mind a Kingdom: American Women, Sexual Purity, and the New Thought Movement, 1875–1920* (Berkeley: University of California Press, 1999).

75. "Health and Wealth," *Better Nutrition*, December, 1997.

76. "Hot New Medicine from 1500 B.C.," *Businessweek*, March, 1997.

77. "How to create something out of nothing," *Money*, Summer, 1996; "Master your Economic Destiny," *Success*, 1994, 7.

78. For a general overview of Chopra's philosophy of material goals, see his *Creating Affluence: Wealth Consciousness in the Field of All Possibilities* (Navatos, CA: New World Library, 1993).

79. Glen Rupert, "Employing the New Age: Training Seminars," in Lewis and Melton, *Perspectives on the New Age*.

80. Michael S. Goldstein, *The Health Movement: Promoting Fitness in America* (New York: Twayne, 1992), 151.

81. J. Gordon Melton, "A History of the New Age Movement," in Robert Butler, ed. *Not Necessarily the New Age* (Buffalo: Prometheus Books, 1988), 35–53.

82. "Spiritual Guidance for Entrepreneurs?", *East West*, November, 1994.

83. "Living with Beauty," *Good Housekeeping*, December, 1994; "Beauty is Only Skin Deep," *Good Housekeeping*, August, 1995.

84. Pratima Raichur, "What's Your Dosha," *Amhealth*, July, 1995, 21; See also "Ayurvedic Skin Care," *East West*, September, 1991.

85. "Traditional Indian Beauty Care," *Glamour*, April, 1995.

86. "Natural Postpartum Practices," *Mothering*, 1993, 2, 58.

87. "Centered Cuisine," *Vegetarian Times*, July, 1997.

88. "Natural First Aid the Traditional Way," *Maitri*, Summer, 1993.

89. For the Indian case, see Partha Chatterjee "Colonialism, Nationalism and Colonized Women: The Contest in India," *American Ethnologist* 16 (1989): 622–33; for the Dutch case, see Ann L. Stoler, "Carnal Knowledge and Imperial Power: Gender, Race and Morality in Colonial Asia," in Micaela di Leonardo, ed., *Gender at the Crossroads of Knowledge: Feminist Anthropology in the Postmodern Era* (Berkeley: University of California, 1991).

90. Ashis Nandy, *The Intimate Enemy: Loss and Recovery of Self Under Colonialism* (London: Oxford University Press, 1983).

91. "Energy and Longevity," *East West*, November, 1997.

92. "Ayurveda for Aging Bodies," *Midlife, Summer*, 1997.

93. "Energetics of Western Herbs," book review, *Whole Earth Review*, August, 1994.

94. "Reversing Old Age," *Prevention*, 1996, 4.

95. "Natural Healing for the Elderly," *Natural Health*, March, 1997.

96. "Promoting Longevity," *Natural Health*, March, 1998.

97. "Restoring Memory Loss," *Prevention*, 1997, 6.

98. See "Natural Drugs," *Chem&Industry*, 1996, 5; "A Tonic a Day," *Chemdruggist*, August, 1997; "Why Ayurveda?" *Drug and Cosmetic Industry*, February, 1998.

99. "The Right Stuff," *Vitality*, March, 1997.

100. McGuire, *Ritual Healing in Suburban America*.

101. James Lewis, "Approaches to the Study."

CAM Cancer Therapies in Twentieth-Century North America

Prior research that provided the background for this essay was supported by a grant from the National Science Foundation, Societal Dimensions of Engineering, Science, and Technology, for research on the "Public Understanding of Science" (SBE9511543). Many people in the CAM cancer therapy movement generously granted time for interviews that are included in *Evaluating Alternative Cancer Therapies* (see note 5).

1. David Eisenberg et al., "Unconventional Medicine in the United States," *New England Journal of Medicine* 328 (1993): 246–52; David Eisenberg et al., "Trends in Alternative Medicine Use in the United States, 1990–1997," *Journal of the American Medical Association* 280, 18 (1998): 1569–75.

2. John Weeks, "Charting the Mainstream," *Townsend Letter for Doctors and Patients* 211/212 (2001): 20–21. The monthly column is one of the best and most concise sources of information on the topic; see also www.onemedicine.com and his newsletter *The Integrator for the Business of Alternative Medicine.*

3. Morris Beale, *Medical Mussolini* (Washington, D.C.: Columbia Publishing Co. , 1939).

4. Brian Berman and David Larson (co-chairs, editorial review board), *Alternative Medicine: Expanding Medical Horizons. A Report to the National Institutes of Health on Alternative Medical Systems and Practices in the United States* (Chantilly, Va.: Workshop on Alternative Medicine, U.S. Government Printing Office, 1992).

5. David Hess, *Evaluating Alternative Cancer Therapies* (New Brunswick, N.J.: Rutgers University Press, 1999).

6. John Beard, *The Enzyme Treatment of Cancer and Its Scientific Basis* (London: Chatto and Windus, 1911).

7. David Hess, *Can Bacteria Cause Cancer?* (New York: New York University Press, 1997), 10–16.

8. Herbert Oettgen and Lloyd Old, "The History of Cancer Immunotherapy," in V. DeVita Jr. et al., eds., *The Biologic Theory of Cancer* (New York: J. B. Lippincott, 1991), 97.

9. Lida Mattman, *Cell Wall Deficient Forms* (Boca Raton, Fla.: CRC Press, 1993).

10. Hess, *Can Bacteria Cause Cancer?* ch. 3.

11. Ibid., 17–24.

12. Brian Martin, ed., *Confronting the Experts* (Albany: State University of New York Press, 1996); Brian Martin, *Suppression Stories* (Wollongong, Australia: Fund for Intellectual Dissent, 1997), www.uow.edu.au/arts/sts/bmartin/dissent/documents/ss/.

13. David Hess, "Suppression, Bias, and Selection in Science: The Case of Cancer Research," *Accountability in Research* 6 (1999): 245–57.

14. Hess, *Can Bacteria Cause Cancer?* 10–24.

15. Barry Lynes, *The Cancer Cure That Worked* (Queensville, Ont.: Marcus Books, 1987).

16. Hess, *Can Bacteria Cause Cancer?* 24–29.

17. Ibid., 29–39.

18. Ibid., 42–47.

19. I am selecting here two of the most prominent of the midcentury period. Another therapy in this category that attracted widespread attention was an oxidation product known as gloxilide, developed by William Koch. After suppression in the 1950s he moved to Brazil, and in 1996 I interviewed his colleague, Dr. Jayme Treiger, while I was a visiting Fulbright scholar at the Universidade Federal Fluminense.

20. Patricia Ward, "Who Will Bell the Cat?" *Bulletin of the History of Medicine* 58 (1984): 28–52.

21. Ibid., 42.

22. Marcus Cohen, "Emanual Recivi, M.D.: Innovator in Nontoxic Cancer Chemotherapy, 1896–1997," *Journal of Alternative and Complementary Medicine* 4, 2 (1988): 140–45.

23. Emanuel Revici, *Research in Physiopathology as Basis for Guided Chemotherapy: With Special Application to Cancer* (Princeton, N.J.: D. Van Nostrand, 1961).

24. Michael Lerner, *Choices in Healing* (Cambridge, Mass.: MIT Press, 1994), 161; Lawrence LeShan, *Cancer as a Turning Point* (New York: Dutton, 1989).

25. Max Gerson, *A Cancer Therapy* (Bonita, Calif.: Gerson Institute, 1990; orig. New York: Whittier, 1958); Patricia Spain Ward, "History of the Gerson Therapy" (San Diego: Gerson Research Organization; orig. *Healing Journal* 8, 1–2 [1993]: 30–38).

26. William Kelley, *One Answer to Cancer* (n.p.: Kelley Research Foundation, 1969).

27. www.healthexcel.com.

28. www.dr.-gonzalez.com.

29. Kenny Ausubel, *When Healing Becomes a Crime* (Rochester, Vt.: Healing Arts Press, 2000), 12.

30. Ibid.

31. Ibid., 124–25.

32. Peter Chowka, "The Hoxsey Story," *Whole Life Times,* January–February 1984, and Peter Chowka, "Tijuana's Alt Med Clinics: Finally the End of an Era?" http://naturalhealthline.com, accessed August 15, 2001.

33. Richard Thomas, *The Essiac Report* (Los Angeles: Alternative Treatment Information Network, 1993), 23.

34. Ibid., 60.

35. David Hess, "From Suppression to Integration: Changing Patterns of the Politics of Complementary and Alternative Medicine for Cancer," invited presentation, International Conference on Spinal

Manipulation and Minnesota Chiropractic Association Annual Convention, Minneapolis, 2000, ms available from the author.

36. Michael Culbert, *Freedom from Cancer* (New York: Pocket Books, Simon and Schuster, 1974), 29ff.

37. Hess, *Evaluating Alternative Cancer Therapies*, 103.

38. Greg Field, "Flushing Poisons from the Body Politic: The Fluoride Controversy and American Political Culture, 1955–1965," in Juergen Heideking et al., ed., *The Sixties Revisited: Culture, Society, Politics* (Heidelberg: Universitätsverlag, 2001), 469–485.

39. Culbert, *Freedom from Cancer*, 30.

40. Ralph Moss, *The Cancer Industry* (Brooklyn, N.Y.: Equinox, 1996), 177.

41. Interview, in Hess, *Evaluating Alternative Cancer Therapies*, 103.

42. James Petersen and Gerald Markle, "The Laetrile Controversy," in D. Nelkin, ed., *Controversy: Politics of Technical Decisions*, (Beverly Hills, Calif.: Sage, 1979), 165.

43. Stephen Barrett, *The Unhealthy Alliance*, 1988, www.hcrc.org.

44. James Harvey Young, "Laetrile in Historical Perspective," in G. Markle and J. Petersen, eds., *Politics, Science, and Cancer: The Laetrile Phenonmenon* (Boulder, Colo.: Westview, 1980), 23.

45. Ibid.

46. Hess, *Evaluating Alternative Cancer Therapies*, 15–17.

47. Donald Markle and James Petersen, "Resolution of the Laetrile Controversy," in H. T. Engelhardt Jr. and A. Caplan, eds., *Scientific Controversies* (New York: Cambridge University Press, 1987), 325.

48. Hess, *Evaluating Alternative Cancer Therapies*, 17.

49. Young, "Laetrile in Historical Perspective," p. 24.

50. Herman Aihara, *Basic Macrobiotics* (New York: Japan Publications, 1985).

51. Lerner, *Choices in Healing*, 287.

52. Michio Kushi, *The Macrobiotic Approach to Cancer* (Wayne, N.J.: Avery, 1981); Anthony Sattilaro and Thomas Monte, *Recalled by Life* (Boston: Houghton Mifflin, 1982).

53. John Boik, *Cancer and Natural Medicine* (Princeton, Minn.: Oregon Medical Press, 1996).

54. Seminar, "Comprehensive Cancer Care 2001," Washington, D.C., October 2001.

55. Robert Houston, *Repression and Reform in the Evaluation of Alternative Cancer Therapies* (Washington, D.C.: Project Cure, 1987).

56. Arlin Brown, *What Is the Arlin J. Brown Information Center?* (Fort Belvoir, Va.: Arlin J. Brown Information Center, n.d.).

57. Moss, *The Cancer Industry*, 187.

58. Ewan Cameron and Linus Pauling, *Cancer and Vitamin C* (Philadelphia: Camino Books, 1993; orig. 1979).

59. O. Carl Simonton et al., *Getting Well Again* (New York: J. P. Tarcher/St. Martin's, 1978).

60. Judah Folkman, "Tumor Angiogenesis: Therapeutic Implications," *New England Journal of Medicine* 285, 21 (1971): 1182–6. John Prudden's work on bovine cartilage and cancer, which posits an immune system mechanism rather than an angiogenesis mechanism, has vied with Folkman's work for priority and recognition in the cartilage field. See the review by Vivekan Flint and Michael Lerner, *Does Cartilage Cure Cancer? The Shark and Bovine Controversy: An Independent Assessment* (Bolinas, Calif.: Commonweal 1996), www.commonweal.org.

61. Moss, *The Cancer Industry*, 296, 242.

62. Barrett, *The Unhealthy Alliance*. Senator Proxmire had also been a supporter of Krebiozen, as reported by Ward, "Who Will Bell the Cat?" 44.

63. Michael Cohen, *Complementary and Alternative Medicine: Legal Boundaries and Regulatory Perspectives* (Baltimore: Johns Hopkins University Press, 1998), 80.

64. Barrett, *The Unhealthy Alliance*.

65. Moss, *The Cancer Industry*, 242.

66. Edward T. Creagan et al., "Failure of High-Dose Vitamin C (Ascorbic Acid) Therapy to Benefit Patients with Advanced Cancer," *New England Journal of Medicine* 301, 13 (1979): 687–90; Evellen Richards, *Vitamin C and Cancer: Medicine or Politics?* (New York: St. Martin's, 1991).

67. Charles G. Moertel et al., "A Clinical Trial of Amygdalin (Laetrile) in the Treatment of Human Cancer," *New England Journal of Medicine* 306, 4 (1982): 201–6.

68. Moss, *The Cancer Industry*, ix.

69. Ibid., xvi.

70. Hess, *Evaluating Alternative Cancer Therapies*, 132.

71. Moss, *The Cancer Industry*, xxv.

72. Ibid., 3.

73. Ibid., 165.

74. David Hess, "Stronger versus Weaker Integration Policies," *American Journal of Public Health*, 2002 vol. 92, #10 12–14.

75. "Jury Indicts Texas Doctor on 75 Counts," *New York Times*, November 26, 1995, 29.

76. Peter Chowka, "Tijuana's Alt Med Clinics: Finally the End of an Era?" http://naturalhealthline. com, accessed August 15, 2001.

77. American Cancer Society operational statement on complementary and alternative methods of cancer management 1999; www.cancer.org.

78. www.cancercenter.com.

79. www.blockmd.com.

80. Hess, *Evaluating Alternative Cancer Therapies*, 67–78.

Beyond the Culture Wars

Jonathan David Geczik passed away September 24, 2001, from a sudden heart attack. His many friends will miss his wit, keen intelligence, and passion for life. Jon was an accomplished poet, wrote two screenplays, and had finished manuscripts on political theory as well as on the alternative health movement. I will miss our collaboration and our friendship, and I dedicate this contribution to him.
—Matthew Schneirov

1. The term "holistic health" is the preferred one for many members of this network who we interviewed. Also, this term is used by Fuller to refer to New Age healing practices and beliefs. See Robert Fuller, *Alternative Medicine and American Religious Life* (New York: Oxford University Press, 1989), 91–117.

2. The alternative food movement is discussed in Warren J. Belasco, *Appetite for Change: How the Counterculture Took on the Food Industry* (Ithaca: Cornell University Press, 1989). A valuable discussion of the roots of the "holistic health movement" in the sixties can be found in June S. Lowenberg, *Caring and Responsibility: The Crossroads between Holistic Practice and Traditional Medicine* (Philadelphia: University of Pennsylvania Press, 1989), 66–78.

3. David Eisenberg et al., "Unconventional Medicine in the United States," *New England Journal of Medicine* 328 (1993): 246–52, and "Trends in Alternative Medicine Use in the United States, 1990–1997: Results of a Follow-up National Survey," *Journal of the American Medical Association* 280 (1998): 1569–75.

4. A more detailed discussion of these two groups can be found in Matthew Schneirov and Jonathan David Geczik, "A Diagnosis for Our Times: Alternative Health's Submerged Networks and the Transformation of Identities," *The Sociological Quarterly* 37 (1996): 627–44 and Schneirov & Geczik, *A Diagnosis for Our Times: Alternative Health, From Lifeworld to Politics* (Albany: State University of New York Press, 2003).

5. Discussions of nineteenth-century challenges to orthodox medicine can be found in *Alternative Medicine*; James C. Whorton, *Crusaders for Fitness: The History of American Health Reformers* (Princeton, N.J.: Princeton University Press, 1982); and Paul Starr, *The Social Transformation of American Medicine* (New York: Basic Books, 1982), 30–78.

6. Fuller, *Alternative Medicine and American Religious Life*, 34–37.

7. Max Weber, *The Protestant Ethic and the Spirit of Capitalism* (New York: Scribner, 1958).

8. Overviews of new social movement theory and representative expressions of the theory can be found in Steven Buechler, "New Social Movement Theories," *The Sociological Quarterly* 36 (1995): 441–64; Jean L. Cohen, "Strategy or Identity: New Theoretical Paradigms and Contemporary Social Movements," *Social Research* 52 (1985): 663–716; Klaus Eder, "A New Social Movement?" *Telos* 52 (1982): 5–20; Enrique Larana, Hank Johnston, and Joseph Gusfield, eds., *New Social Movements: From Ideology to Identity* (Philadelphia: Temple University Press, 1994); Claus Offe, "'New Social Movements' Challenging the Boundaries of Institutional Politics," *Social Research* 52 (1985): 817–68; Alberto Melucci, "The New Social Movements: A Theoretical Approach," *Social Science Information* 19 (1980): 199–226; and Alberto Melucci, "The New Social Movement Revisited: Reflections on a Sociological Misunderstanding," in Lewis Maheu, ed., *Social Movements and Social Classes* (London: Sage, 1995).

9. Useful overviews of the literature on alternative health in medical sociology can be found in Michael S. Goldstein, *Alternative Health Care: Medicine, Miracle or Mirage?* (Philadelphia: Temple University Press, 1999).

10. Claus Offe, *Disorganized Capitalism: Contemporary Transformations of Work and Politics* (Cambridge, Mass.: MIT Press).

11. Herman E. Daly, *Beyond Growth: The Economics of Sustainable Development* (Boston: Beacon, 1996).

12. Christopher Lasch, *The True and Only Heaven: Progress and Its Critics* (New York: W. W. Norton, 1991).

13. Robert D. Putnam, *Bowling Alone: The Collapse and Revival of American Community* (New York: Simon and Schuster, 2000), 22–24.

14. A discussion of alternative health networks in the gay community can be found in Bonnie Blair O'Connor, *Healing Traditions: Alternative Medicine and the Health Professions* (Philadelphia: University of Pennsylvania Press, 1985), 109–60.

15. A more intensive discussion of alternative health regimes in light of Michel Foucault's notion of "care of the self" can be found in Matthew Schneirov and Jonathan David Geczik, "Technologies of the Self and the Aesthetic Project of Alternative Health," *The Sociological Quarterly* 39 (1998): 435–51.

16. Teresa Brennan, *Exhausting Modernity: Grounds for a New Economy* (London: Routledge, 2000), 75–118.

17. For a somewhat different view of the political implications of the "natural," see Andrew Ross, "New Age Technoculture," in Cary Nelson and Paula Treichler, eds., *Cultural Studies* (New York: Routledge, 1992). Ross, in contrast to our discussion, does not see any socially transformative potential in the New Age celebration of the natural and emphasizes its ideological potential.

18. On prefigurative politics, see Sara M. Evans and Harry C. Boyte, *Free Spaces: The Sources of Democratic Change in America* (New York: Harper and Row, 1986).

19. This quote is from Walter Benjamin, *Illuminations* (New York: Schocken, 1968), 257.

20. Daly, *Beyond Growth*.

21. A discussion of this intellectual sources of what Daly calls the "third paradigm" can be found in Daly, *Beyond Growth*, 1–24.

22. Elaine Scarry, *The Body in Pain: The Making and Unmaking of the World* (New York: Oxford University Press, 1985).

Contemporary Anti-Vaccination Movements in Historical Perspective

This essay has greatly benefited from comments based on versions given at the Medical Humanities and Social Sciences Program, University of Illinois College of Medicine; the Health, Culture, and Society seminar of the Department of Behavioral Sciences, Sackler Medical School, Tel Aviv University; the Health Law Society, Yale Medical School; and the National Vaccine Information Center's Second International Public Conference on Vaccination in Arlington, Virginia.

I am grateful to those who provided materials: above all, the staff of the National Vaccine Information Center, and also Paul Bass, Catherine Diodati, Greg Grandin, Lyssa Mudd, Michelle Nickerson, and Robert Wolfe. Edda West and Mary James introduced me to Annie Riley Hale, Lila Corwin and Dan Berman made sure I knew about the episode of *The Simpsons*, and Lis Pimentel connected me to *The X-Files*. Matt Guglielmi, Jay Nelson, and Amy Nickel provided excellent research assistance, and Bethany Moreton co-wrote the section on anti-anthrax vaccine advocates.

Various scholars, activists, and officials graciously agreed to talk with me about the vaccine safety movement. I wish especially to thank Barbara Loe Fisher of the NVIC, who invited me to speak at the 2000 NVIC conference, encouraged my work, and granted me a chance to talk with her about her life and work. Many others at the NVIC conference were equally eager to converse, and I thank in particular Dawn Richardson of Parents Requesting Open Vaccine Information (PROVE). I have also benefited from exchanges with Lynne Curry, Nadav Davidovitch, Greg Field, Leslie Reagan, Anne Johnston, Mark Liechty, Rahul Rajkumar, Paula Treichler, Linda Forst, Ed Marcuse, Ted Slutz, and many friends who have been willing to indulge my fascination with this subject. My former colleagues at the Yale Medical School, Sue

Lederer, Naomi Rogers, and John Warner, have always been particularly encouraging of my scholarship in a somewhat strange byway of the history of medicine.

1. "Mr. X," http://thesimpsons.com/mrx/flushots.htm.

2. "Herrenvolk," www.insidethex.co.uk/pdf/scrp401.pdf, 13–15.

3. This essay will focus on the United States; for related Canadian developments, see the website for the Vaccination Risk Awareness Network at www.vran.org.

4. Ceci Connolly, "Bush Smallpox Inoculation Plan Near Standstill," *Washington Post*, February 24, 2003, A6; Donald G. McNeil, Jr., "National Programs to Vaccinate for Smallpox Come to a Halt," *New York Times*, June 19, 2003; Connolly, "Focus on Smallpox Threat Revived: Experts Say Immunization Program Is Crucial to Homeland Security," *Washington Post*, July 17, 2003, A3; Joyce Howard Price, "Health Workers Resist Smallpox Vaccinations," *Washington Times*, December 20, 2002; Donald G. McNeil, Jr., "Health Care Leaders Voice Doubts on Smallpox Inoculations," *New York Times*, January 30, 2003.

5. Richard Moskowitz, "Vaccination: A Sacrament of Modern Medicine," *Homeopath* 12 (March 1992): 137–44.

6. Michael Bliss, *Plague: A Story of Smallpox in Montreal* (New York: HarperCollins, 1991) 207. Robert D. Johnston, *The Radical Middle Class: Populist Democracy and the Question of Capitalism in Progressive Era Portland, Oregon* (Princeton: Princeton University Press, 2003), 177–90, discusses the historical literature on anti-vaccination movements.

7. Johnston, *Radical Middle Class*, 181–84; Perry Miller, *The New England Mind: From Colony to Province* (Cambridge, Mass.: Harvard University Press, 1953), 361. The more primitive *inoculation* differed from *vaccination* in that the former involved the transmission of live smallpox virus into a patient, whereas the latter involves the much weaker cowpox virus.

8. Johnston, *Radical Middle Class*, 182–83, 207–10; Chapin quote in Donald R. Hopkins, *Princes and Peasants: Smallpox in History* (Chicago: University of Chicago Press, 1983), 292–93; Paul Adolphus Bator, "The Health Reformers versus the Common Canadian: The Controversy over Compulsory Vaccination against Smallpox in Toronto and Ontario, 1900–1920," *Ontario History* 75 (1983): 349–368. It is worth noting the even stiffer opposition in many Western countries, culminating in England's effective exemption of citizens from compulsion by 1907. See Johnston, *Radical Middle Class*, 184–85.

9. Paul Greenough, "Global Immunization and Culture: Compliance and Resistance in Large-Scale Public Health Campaigns," *Social Science and Medicine* 41 (1995): 606.

10. Johnston, *Radical Middle Class*, 202–03.

11. Johnston, *Radical Middle Class*, 185–90, 197–206. The bible of smallpox research, which contains considerable information about the risks of the vaccination, is Frank Fenner et al., *Smallpox and Its Eradication* (Geneva: World Health Organization, 1988).

12. Eric S. Juhnke, *Quacks and Crusaders: The Fabulous Careers of John Brinkley, Norman Baker, and Harry Hoxsey* (Lawrence: University Press of Kansas, 2002), 119, 52, 82, 139–40; Gretchen Ann Reilly, "'Not a So-Called Democracy,'" in this volume.

13. Annie Riley Hale, *The Medical Voodoo* (New York: Gotham House, 1935), 26, 320, 331, 325, 50, 252–58.

14. *The Guilty: Shall They Be Held Accountable?*, ca. 1953, flyer in author's possession; *At the Sign of the Unholy Three*, flyer reproduced in Judd Marmor, Viola W. Bernard, and Perry Ottenberg, "Psychodynamics of Group Opposition to Health Programs," *American Journal of Orthopsychiatry* 30, 331 (1960): 336; Jane S. Smith, *Patenting the Sun: Polio and the Salk Vaccine* (New York: William Morrow, 1990), 359–67; Naomi Rogers, *Dirt and Disease: Polio before FDR* (New Brunswick, N.J.: Rutgers University Press, 1992), 176–83. The one book from the 1950s that laid out the case against vaccination, Eleanor McBean's *The Poisoned Needle: Suppressed Facts about Vaccination* (Mokelumne Hill, CA: Health Research, 1957), was primarily apolitical, making a case against vaccination mostly on medical grounds, and then mainly by way of citing nineteenth- and early-twentieth-century anti-vaccination authorities.

15. Johnston, *Radical Middle Class*, 183; Wilson G. Smillie, *Public Health Administration in the United States*, 2nd ed. (New York: Macmillan, 1945), 118.

16. That said, there was clearly a skepticism in the air about vaccination among certain communities even before the 1982 formation of DPT. Probably the best index of this is a set of articles from the late 1970s and early 1980s in *Mothering* magazine, collected most conveniently in *Immunizations* (Santa Fe, N.M.: Mothering Magazine, 1987). *Mothering*'s roots were in the "back to the land" counterculture of the

late sixties and early seventies. For a reflection on *Mothering*'s history of covering the vaccination issue, as well as a plea to take both sides of the debate seriously, see the editor's introduction to a special issue devoted to "Vaccination: The Issue of Our Times": Peggy O'Mara, "Why a Vaccination Special?", *Mothering* no. 79 (Summer 1996): 8–9.

17. "TV Documentary Shocks America and Parents Organize," *Dissatisfied Parents Together News* (henceforth *DPT News*), 1 (Fall 1983): 1, 13. All DPT newsletters are in the possession of the author, who purchased them from the National Vaccine Information Center. They are available for purchase through the organization's website, www.909shot.com.

DPT received considerable favorable—as well as hostile—media attention from the time of its creation. In its first year, for example, DPT officials received respectful treatment on the *MacNeil-Lehrer Report*, the *Phil Donahue Show* and the *Charlie Rose Show*. "Television and Radio Coverage of DPT Story Grows," *DPT News* 1 (Fall 1984): 10–11.

18. "DPT Develops Grant Proposal," *DPT News* 1 (Fall 1983): 18; "A Grassroots Movement is Launched," ibid., 2; Jeff Schwartz, "Support for the Vaccine Damage Compensation Bill Grows," ibid., 10.

19. "Medical/Science News," ibid., 3; Barbara Loe Fisher, "Editorial," ibid., 17.

20. "Who's Who at DPT National Headquarters," ibid., 6; "DPT Holds State Leadership Conference; New DPT Board and Officers Elected," *DPT News* 3 (Summer/Fall 1987): 7; "Where Does Your Membership Money Go," *DPT News* 1 (Fall 1984): 14; Kathi Williams, "Spring Yard Sale is a Success," ibid., 16.

21. Jeff Schwartz, "Wyeth Drops Out of DPT Market Citing High Costs of Lawsuits," *DPT News* 1 (Fall 1984): 2, 15; Jeff Schwartz, "Legislative Stalemate Slows Vaccine Safety/Compensation Bill," *DPT News* 2 (Winter 1986): 5–6; "Ten Senators Attend July Hearings on Compensation Bill," ibid., 10.

22. "Ten Senators"; "President Reagan Signs Vaccine Injury Compensation Bill into Law," *DPT News* 3 (Spring 1987): 1.

23. Ibid., 1, 10–12.

24. *New York Times*, October 28, 1986, A1, A22; "President Reagan Signs," 1, 10–14. Reagan signed the bill "with mixed feelings," owing to his "serious reservations" over its vaccine provisions. The president was upset about the surcharge on vaccines that would fund the compensation system, which he considered a tax; he also objected to the "unprecedented arrangement" whereby the system would be administered by the judiciary, not by the executive branch. Reagan considered this unconstitutional. *New York Times*, November 15, 1986, A1.

Historian Jeffrey Baker notes that "extreme antivaccine groups" also opposed the legislation; see Aaron Levin, "Vaccines Today," *Annals of Internal Medicine*, 133 (October 17, 2000): 661. For some hint at the reasons why more radical anti-vaccination groups might have seen the bill as a dangerous compromise, see Harris L. Coulter and Barbara Loe Fisher, *DPT: A Shot in the Dark* (New York: Harcourt, Brace, Jovanovich, 1985), 384, 388–89.

25. Coulter and Fisher, *DPT*; "*DPT: A Shot in the Dark* Sparks Praise and Criticism," *DPT News* 1 (Summer 1985): 20–22. Harris Coulter later went on to publish a more extreme anti-vaccination book, *Vaccination, Social Violence, and Criminality: The Medical Assault on the American Brain* (Berkeley: North Atlantic Books, 1990). Even a physician who works closely with the NVIC gave the book an extremely negative review; Marcel Kinsbourne, review of Coulter, *Journal of Autism and Development Disorders* 22 (1992): 329–30.

26. Coulter and Fisher, *DPT*, 142.

27. Coulter and Fisher, *DPT*, 404–05; "Vaccine News Briefs," *NVIC News* 3 (October 1993): 12. Although *DPT: A Shot in the Dark* was, and is, considered outside the medical mainstream, it is not clear that this should be the case. For example, as early as 1967 one of the most influential of British vaccinologists, Sir Graham Wilson, commented: "The arguments for and against the use of this vaccine [smallpox] where the disease is no longer endemic but is continually subject to the risk of reimportation are very nicely balanced.... Much the same holds true of pertussis vaccine and, to a less extent, of BCG. Whooping-cough has now such a low mortality that the advisability of continuing vaccination against this disease must be seriously questioned, particularly when there is reason to believe that, as judged by the comparative mortality index before and after 1951, vaccination has played little part in bringing about its fall." Graham S. Wilson, *The Hazards of Immunization* (London: Athlone Press of the University of London, 1967), 281.

28. *People*, November 22, 1999; "Barbara Loe Fisher on the Costs of Vaccination," *New York Times Magazine*, May 6, 2001, 31.

29. Interview with Barbara Loe Fisher, Arlington, Virginia, September 10, 2000; "NVIC/DPT Elects New Board of Directors," *NVIC News* 3 (October 1993): 4; "New Vaccine Committee Meets in D.C. To Advise National Vaccine Program," *DPT News* 4 (Summer 1988): 6; "Hepatitis B Vaccine: The Untold Story," *The Vaccine Reaction* Special Report (September 1998): 16; "Polio Vaccine Policy May Change," *The Vaccine Reaction* 1 (May 1995): 3; "Flu Mist Comments," NVIC email, December 19, 2002, in author's possession.

30. Schwartz, "Support for Vaccine Damage Compensation," 10; "Parents Call for Congressional Investigation after Long-Hidden DPT Vaccine Revealed at Capitol Hill Press Conference," *DPT News* 1 (Summer 1985): 1, 4–5; "Press Coverage of Vaccine Dangers Increase," ibid., 14–16; "Press Coverage of Vaccine Damage Issue Varies in Quality," *DPT News* 2 (Winter 1986): 15–17; "Parents Demonstrate at CDC in Atlanta," *DPT News* 4 (Spring 1987): 5; "DPT Receives More than 4,000 Letters after DPT Show Airs on "Today Show,"" ibid., 7.

31. *The Vaccine Hotline* no vol. (January 2000): 1. Tapes of these shows, purchased from the NVIC, are in the author's possession. Specific dates are at times not available.

32. *20/20*, January 22, 1999; MSNBC *News with Brian Williams*, October 1999.

33. Patrick Tierney, *Darkness in El Dorado: How Scientists and Journalists Devastated the Amazon* (New York: Norton, 2000); Edward Hooper, *The River: A Journey to the Source of HIV and AIDS* (Boston: Little, Brown, 1999).

34. Tierney, *Darkness in El Dorado*, 55, 82, 59.

35. D. W. Miller, "Academic Scandal in the Internet Age," *Chronicle of Higher Education*, January 12, 2001; Judith Shulevitz, "Academic Warfare," *New York Times*, February 11, 2001. Most of the major contributions to the controversy can be accessed at www.tamu.edu/anthropology/Neel.html. The best treatment of the early debate is Miller, "Academic Scandal." The final report of the AAA is available at www.aaanet.org/edtf.

36. "Final Report of the AAA El Dorado Task Force," II, 53; I, 26–27, www.aaanet.org/edtf/; D.W. Miller, "Although Flawed, Book on Yanomami Research 'Served Anthropology Well,' Report Concludes," *Chronicle of Higher Education*, December 7, 2001.

37. www.wwnorton.com/trade/external/tierney; John Horgan, "Hearts of Darkness," *New York Times Book Review*, November 12, 2001. In turn, the review in *The Bulletin of the Atomic Scientists* by Geoffrey Sea declared that "the book is as insightful as it is important." *Bulletin of the Atomic Scientists* 57(January/February 2001). A generally sympathetic review that takes Tierney to task for his errors on the vaccination issue is Greg Grandin, "Coming of Age in Venezuela," *The Nation*, December 11, 2000.

38. The best source for the debate over *The River* is Australian sociologist Brian Martin's website on "suppression of dissent," at www.uow.edu.au/arts/sts/bmartin/dissent/documents/AIDS/River/index.html.

39. Hooper, *River*.

40. "AIDS and Polio Vaccine," and "AIDS: Another Vaccine Related Illness," *NVIC News* 2 (April 1992): 8; "NVIC/DPT Calls for Testing of Polio Vaccine for Link to Origin and Spread of AIDS," *NVIC News* 4 (August 1994): 2; "OPV Contamination with Monkey Retrovirus?", *The Vaccine Reaction* 1 (July 1995): 3; "Microbiologist Issues a Challenge to Science: Did the First Oral Polio Vaccine Lots Contaminated with Monkey Viruses Create a Monkey-Human Hybrid Called HIV-1?", *The Vaccine Reaction* 2(April 1996): 1–6; Robin A. Weiss, "Is AIDS Man-Made?," *Science*, 286 (November 12, 1999): 1305–1306; John P. Moore, "Up the River without a Paddle," *Nature* 401(September 23, 1999): 325–326; Charles Gilks, "Blame Me," *New Scientist*, November 13, 1999, 54–55. Crucial titles in the popular spread of these theories are Eva Lee Snead, *Some Call it Aids—I Call It Murder: The Connection Between Cancer, Aids, Immunizations, and Genocide* (Jamaica, N.Y.: Aum Publications, 1993) and Tom Curtis, "The Origin of AIDS," *Rolling Stone*, March 19, 1992, 54–59, 61, 106, 108.

Despite their compliments, it should be emphasized that almost all top level-scientific figures did continue to disagree with the most fundamental parts of Hooper's case. Even those most skeptical of Hooper's theory, however, showed great sympathy to a competing argument about the origins of AIDS that was less sensational in presentation but, if anything, even more damning of previous vaccination efforts. According to this rival hypothesis, formulated most systematically by Preston Marx and Ernest Drucker, HIV did indeed result from the evolution of SIV, but it was instead spread from body to body by unsterilized, reused syringes during the course of public health work in Africa during the 1950s. Many, if not most, of these needles would have been used during mass immunization campaigns, the primary purpose of which was to eradicate polio from the continent. William Carlsen, "Quest for the Origin of AIDS: Controversial Book Spurs Search for how the Worldwide Scourge of HIV Began," *San Francisco Chronicle*, January 14, 2001; Carlsen, "Did Modern Medicine Spread an Epidemic? After Decades, and Millions of Injections, Scientists are Asking the Chilling Question," *San Francisco Chronicle*, January 15, 2001. Hooper's latest ideas, including his response to the unsterilized needle hypothesis, appear in "Aids and the Polio Vaccine," *London Review of Books* 25(April 3, 2003).

The AIDS-vaccine connection seemed to receive some indirect support from the universal acknowledgment of the presence of Simian Virus 40 (SV40) in polio vaccine administered to nearly 100 million Americans between 1955 and 1963. A possible link between SV40 and cancer is suggestive but seemingly inconclusive. For an official perspective, see Institute of Medicine Report, *Immunization Safety Review, SV40 Contamination of Polio Vaccine and Cancer*, October 22, 2002, www4.nas.edu/news.nsf/isbn/0309086108?OpenDocument.

41. www.salon.com/health/books/1999/10/06/aids/; Lawrence K. Altman, "New Book Challenges Theories of AIDS Origins," *New York Times*, November 30, 1999, D1, D6; Helen Epstein, "Something Happened," *New York Review of Books*, December 2, 1999, 1; Roy Porter, "Tissue Wars," *London Review of Books* 22 (March 2, 2002).

42. Jane E. Brody, "For the Vaccine-Wary, a Lesson in History," *New York Times*, October 3, 2000, F8; Randy Cohen, "The Ethicist," *New York Times Magazine*, May 6, 2001, 42; Leon Jaroff, "This Will Only Hurt for a Minute," *Time*, October 2, 2000, 80.

43. Kathy Koch, "Vaccine Controversies," *CQ Researcher* 10 (August 25, 2000): 665. The best description of the historical changes in and the current workings of the compensation system is Arthur Allen, "Shots in the Dark," *Washington Post Magazine*, August 30, 1998. A top official in the program lays out his perspective in Geoffrey Evans "Vaccine Liability and Safety Revisited," *Archives of Pediatric and Adolescent Medicine* 152 (1998): 7–10. For the dissenters' viewpoint, see "Funding for Compensation Bill Stalled in Ways and Means," *DPT News* 3(Summer/Fall 1987): 4; "House Votes to Appropriate Funds to Compensate Children Injured by Vaccines before October 1988," *DPT News* 4 (Summer 1988): 1, 6; "New Vaccine Committee Meets in D.C. To Advise National Vaccine Program," *DPT News* 4 (Summer 1988): 6, 13; "Compensation System Begins to Pay Out Awards," *Vaccine News* 5 (Summer 1990): 2, 6; "Vaccine Victims Have Until January 31 to File for Compensation," *NVIC mini News* 1(November 1990): 1, 2; "NVIC Finds Doctors are Refusing to Report Vaccine Reactions," *NVIC mini News* 1(November 1990): 3; "HHS Failure to Publish Childhood Vaccine Information Brings on Lawsuit," *NVIC News* 1 (March 1991): 1; "Four Month Extension for Compensation Law Gives More Children a Chance for Support," *NVIC News* 1 (March 1991): 2; "NVIC/DPT Files Lawsuit; DHHS Secretary Petitioned," *NVIC News* 1 (October 1991): 3; "Advisory Commission Votes to Shut Down Compensation System; DHHS Assistant Secretary Pledges Support to Keep System Operating," *NVIC News* 1 (October 1991): 4; "How the Compensation System Works for Vaccine Injuries and Deaths after October 1988," *NVIC News* 1 (October 1991): 5; "$12 Million Left for Pre-1988 Federal Compensation Claims," *NVIC News* 2 (April 1992): 3; "PL 99–660 Required Brochure to Provide Vaccine Facts, Finally Realized," *NVIC News* 2 (April 1992): 5; James Mason, letter, *NVIC News* 2 (April 1992): 6; "Response to Dr. Mason's Letter to NVIC/DPT Families," *NVIC News* 2 (April 1992): 7; "Pre-1988 Federal Compensation Fund Broke," *NVIC News* 2 (August 1992): 1, 6; "CDC to Neutralize Vaccine Info," *NVIC News* 3 (October 1993): 10; "Shalala Takes Away Compensation for DPT Injured Children," *The Vaccine Reaction* 1 (March 1995): 1–2; "NVIC Takes Shalala to Court," *The Vaccine Reaction* 1 (May 1995): 1.

44. "The National Vaccine Information Center (NVIC), an Ally for Freedom of Choice," *The Chiropractic Choice*, June 2002, 6, 10, www.thechiropracticchoice.com/; "Chiropractic: A Natural Way to Restore and Maintain Health," *The Vaccine Reaction* 2 (Special Edition, 1997): 1.

45. Allen, "Shots in the Dark," explains well the issues relating to the different pertussis vaccines. See also "DPT Testifies at FDA Committee Meeting on Possible Licensure of Lederle Acellular Vaccine," *NVIC News* 1 (March 1991): 3; "IOM Finds Link Between Pertussis and Rubella Vaccines and Severe Reactions," *NVIC News* 1 (October 1991): 2; "Acellular Pertussis Vaccine Licensed for Older Children by FDA," *NVIC News* 1 (April 1992): 1; "Fallout from Washington: The IOM Report Continues to be Misinterpreted," *NVIC News* 2 (April 1992): 4; Kathi Williams, "Opinion: New DPT Vaccine Not a Cure for Past Problems," *NVIC News* 2 (April 1992): 9; "NVIC/DPT Investigation Shows that Doctors and Government Fail to Report and Monitor Vaccine Death and Injury Reports," *NVIC News* 4 (August 1994): 1, 4–5; Barbara Loe Fisher, "Editorial," *NVIC News* 4 (August 1994): 3; "Purified Pertussis Vaccine Finally Licensed for Babies," *The Vaccine Reaction* 2 (August 1996): 1–3.

46. Rob Eshman, "A Novel Approach to Medicine," www.jewishjournal.com/old/endpaper.1.7.0.htm, January 7, 2000; Allen, "Shots in the Dark"; John H. Menkes and Harvey B. Sarnat, *Child Neurology* 6ᵗʰ ed. (Philadelphia: Lippincott, Williams, and Wilkins, 2000); "Center Hosts International Scientific Workshop," *Vaccine News* 5 (Spring 1990): 1, 9; Jan Goodwin, "Was it Murder or a Bad Vaccine?", *Redbook*, September 2000, 161; Lisa Reagan, "Show Us the Science," *Mothering* no. 105 (March/April 2001): 52.

47. Walecia Konrad with Emily Harrison Ginsburg, "Who's Calling the Shots?", *Offspring: The Magazine of Smart Parenting*, June/July 2000, 100; "Science Update on Vaccines/Vaccine Policy," *NVIC News* 1 (October 1991): 10; "AAP Recommends All Newborn Infants be Vaccinated with Hepatitis B Vaccine," *NVIC News* 2 (April 1992): 12; "AAP and CDC Recommended Infant Hepatitis B Vaccine; Encounters Dissent from Pediatricians and Parents," *NVIC News* 2 (August 1992): 5; "IOM Study on Vaccine Reactions Acknowledges Vaccine Risks and Lack of Scientific Data," *NVIC News* 3 (October 1993): 1, 2; "Court Finds FDA Violated Safety Guidelines, Victims of Oral Polio Vaccine Awarded Damages," *NVIC News* 3 (October 1993): 14; "Statement to the National Vaccine Advisory Committee by Barbara Loe Fisher, Co-Founder and President, National Vaccine Information Center, September 26, 1994," *NVIC News* 4 (November 1994): 2–4; "Chicken Pox Vaccine Shipped Out," *The Vaccine Reaction* 1 (May 1995), 4; "Oral Polio Vaccine May be Phased Out," *The Vaccine Reaction* 1 (July 1995): 2–4; "Live Polio Vaccine Voted Out," *The Vaccine Reaction* 2 (August 1996): 3–4; "Hepatitis B Vaccine: The Untold Story," *The Vaccine Reaction* Special Report (September 1998): 1–15; Lisa Reagan, "What about Mercury? Getting Thimerosal out of Vaccines," *Mothering* #105 (March-April 2001): 54–55; Holcomb B. Noble, "3 Suits Say Lyme Vaccine Caused Severe Arthritis," *New York Times*, June 13, 2000; "Rotavirus Vaccine Taken off the Market," *The Vaccine Hotline* no vol. (January 2000): 6. One of the best sources for a dissenting view on the epidemiology of vaccines generally, with analysis of specific vaccines as well, is Catherine J.M. Diodati, *Immunization: History, Ethics, Law and Health* (Windsor, Ontario : Integral Aspects, 1999); see also Randall Neustaedter, *The Vaccine Guide: Risks and Benefits for Children and Adults* (Berkeley: North Atlantic Books, 2002). For the official view on particular vaccinations, see the National Partnership for Immunizations website at www.partnersforimmunization.org/vaccine.html and the CDC's National Immunization Program's website at www.cdc.gov/nip/. See also for basic information Stanley A. Plotkin, Walter A. Orenstein, and Richard Zorab, *Vaccines*, 3rd edition (Philadelphia: W. B. Saunders, 1999). Also still valuable are H.J. Parish, *A History of Immunization* (Edinburgh: E and S Livingstone, 1965) and Allan Chase, *Magic Shots: A Human and Scientific Account of the Long and Continuing Struggle to Eradicate Infectious Diseases by Vaccination* (New York: William Morrow, 1982).

48. Sandra Blakeslee, "Prevalence of Autism Growing, Study Finds," *New York Times*, December 31, 2002; "Autism and Vaccines: A New Look at an Old Story," *The Vaccine Reaction*, Special Report (Spring/Summer 2000): 1–16; Reagan, "Show Us the Science," 41, 44–45, 47, 50–51. For a record of Burton's hearings on autism, as well as on other vaccinations (especially anthrax), see www.whale.to/v/burton1.html. See also two very different articles: Arthur Allen, "A Recipe for Disaster," www.salon.com, August 2, 2000; and Allen, "The Not-So-Crackpot Autism Theory," *New York Times Magazine*, November 10, 2002; as well as the special issue of *Time* devoted to autism, May 6, 2002. The official scientific review of the literature, which argues against a population-level vaccine-autism link, is Institute of Medicine, *Immunization Safety Review: Measles-Mumps-Rubella Vaccine and Autism* (Washington, D.C.: National Academies Press, 2000), available at http://books.nap.edu/books/0309074479/html/index.html

49. "IOM Study on Vaccine Reactions Acknowledges Vaccine Risks and Lack of Scientific Data," *NVIC News* 3 (October 1993): 1; "Massachusetts and New York Parents Oppose Chicken Pox Vaccine Mandates," *The Vaccine Hotline* no vol. (January 1999): 5; untitled, *The Vaccine Hotline* no vol. (June 1998): 3.

50. "DPT Holds State Leadership Conference," 7; "NVIC/DPT Elects New Board of Directors," *NVIC News* 3 (October 1993): 5.

51. "DPT Holds State Leadership Conference," 3, 7; "NVIC/DPT Elects New Board," 4.

52. "Texas Moms Take on the State Health Department and Win Informed Consent Rights," *The Vaccine Hotline* no vol. (January 1999): 1–4. Richardson's website is www.vaccineinfo.net.

53. Unless otherwise noted, the information about Dawn Richardson comes from an interview with the author, conducted by phone on November 4, 2000.

54. "Texas Got Conscientious Exemption and Prohibition of Punitive Action for not Immunizing," PROVE email, June 2, 2003, in author's possession.

55. See, for example, the foreword by Republican Connecticut congressman Christopher Shays to Thomas S. Heemstra, *Anthrax: A Deadly Shot in the Dark: Unmasking the Truth Behind a Hazardous Vaccine* (Lexington, KY: Crystal Communications, 2002).

56. "Measles Vaccine Experiments on Minority Children Turn Deadly," *The Vaccine Reaction* 2 (June 1996): 1–3; "Houston Activists Protest Vaccine Mandate at Town Hall Meeting," *The Vaccine Reaction* 2 (December 1996): 4; "Black Children in Memphis Forced to Get Hepatitis A Vaccine—Parents Protest," *The Vaccine Reaction* 2 (June 1996): 4–6; "Purified Pertussis Vaccine"; "Dissenters Act Up at AIDS Conference," *The Vaccine Reaction* 2 (August 1996): 4–5.

57. On the blurred boundaries of left and right, see Johnston, "Introduction: The Politics of Healing," in this volume; David A. Horowitz, *Beyond Left and Right: Insurgency and the Establishment* (Urbana: University of Illinois Press, 1997); and Christopher Lasch, *The True and Only Heaven: Progress and its Critics* (New York: W.W. Norton, 1991).

58. Richard Leviton, *Phy.si.cian: Medicine and the Unsuspected Battle for Human Freedom* (Charlottesville, VA: Hampton Roads, 2000), 510–511. For just one example among many of an influential antivaccination website, see www.nccn.net/~wwithin/vaccine.htm. The NVIC's website, www.909shot.com, also provides a portal for a wide variety of vaccine websites, both pro and con. Articles that use the term "antivaccination" without much reflection are P. Davies, S. Chapman, and J. Leask, "Antivaccination Activists on the World Wide Web," *Archives of Disease in Childhood* 22 (2002): 22–25 (which contains a lengthy list of sites) and Robert M. Wolfe, Lisa K. Sharp, and Martin S. Lipsky, "Content and Design Attributes of Antivaccination Websites," *JAMA* 287 (July 26, 2002): 3245–3248. In a letter three months later, however, Wolfe, Sharpe, and Pinsky agreed that it would be "healthier" to use the label "vaccine safety activists" rather than "antivaccinationists." *JAMA* 287 (October 9, 2002); http://jama.ama-assn.org/issues/current/ffull/jlt1009–2.html, and Wolfe has adopted this term in "Vaccine Safety Activists on the Internet," *Expert Review of Vaccines* 1 (2002): 249–252.

59. "To Parents Concerned about DPT Shots," 1 (Summer 1985): 17; Ann Millan, "Opinion: Vaccination Campaign," *NVIC News* 2 (April 1992): 10; untitled, *The Vaccine Hotline* no vol. (June 1998): 2. My argument is opposed to Robert M. Wolfe and Lisa K. Sharp in their "Anti-Vaccination Activists, Past and Present," *British Medical Journal* 325 (August 24, 2002): 430–32. Wolfe and Sharp contend that the antivaccination movement has "changed little" since the nineteenth century. (430)

60. Richardson interview.

61. Ann Millan, "Opinion: Know the Risks," *NVIC News* 2(April 1992): 11; Coulter and Fisher, *DPT*, 315; "First International Public Conference on Vaccination Puts Vaccine Risks on the Record," *The Vaccine Reaction* 3 (November 1997): 2; "Conflict of Interest Charges Leveled Against Federal Vaccine Advisors," *NVIC News* 1 (October 1991): 1.

62. Information on the anthrax program in this and the following paragraphs comes from Arthur Allen, "A Cure Worse than the Disease?," www.salon.com, October 27, 2000; Pauline Jelinek, "Anthrax Vaccination Policy Reviewed," Associated Press, May 17, 2002; Barbara Loe Fisher, "Special NVIC Report: Biological Warfare and Anthrax Vaccine," December, 2001, www.909shot.com/Newsletters/spanthrax.htm. For more on the varieties, and effects, of the disease, see Jeanne Guillemin, *Anthrax: The Investigation of a Deadly Outbreak* (Berkeley: University of California Press, 1999), especially 1–7.

63. Mark Arax, "No Vaccine, No Glory, Navy Says," *Los Angeles Times*, June 21, 2003.

64. Seymour M. Hersh, *Against All Enemies: Gulf War Syndrome: The War Between America's Ailing Veterans and Their Government* (New York: Ballantine, 1998). The first mention (among many) by NVIC of Gulf War Syndrome is "Vaccine News Briefs," *NVIC News* 4 (August 1994): 7.

65. Information on subscribing to Anthrax-no is available at http://groups.yahoo.com/group/Anthrax-no/.

66. These observations come from an analysis of Anthrax-no from 1999 to 2003.

67. uucarolyn@nextdim.com, message 8, Anthrax-no Digest Number 383, October 5, 1999.

68. rdharrison@compuage.com, message 11, Anthrax-no Digest Number 363, September 19, 1999; rdharrison@compuage.com, message 3, Anthrax-no Digest Number 335, August 29, 1999.

69. loup@swva.net, message 12, Anthrax-no Digest Number 418, October 31, 1999.

70. Meryl Nass's website is one of the most important in the world of anti-vaccination as a whole; see www.anthraxvaccine.org.

71. Barbara Loe Fisher, "Editorial," *NVIC News* 3 (October 1993): 3; "Funding for National Health Identifier Number Stopped by Texas Congressman," *The Vaccine Hotline* no vol. (January 1999): 3–4.

72. The case for a bioterrorist smallpox threat is laid out most compellingly in Jonathan B. Tucker, *Scourge: The Once and Future Threat of Smallpox* (New York: Atlantic Monthly Press, 2001); see also Richard Preston, *The Demon in the Freezer: A True Story* (New York: Random House, 2002).

73. Ceci Connolly, "Homeland Bill Covers Smallpox Shot Liability," *Washington Post*, November 16, 2002; Barbara Loe Fisher, "Smallpox and Forced Vaccination: What Every American Needs to Know," *The Vaccine Reaction* Special Report (Winter 2002): 12.

74. Information in these paragraphs comes from Helen Dewar, "Homeland Security Bill Faces Senate Test," *Washington Post*, November 19, 2002; David Firestone and Richard A. Oppel, Jr., "The Fine Print: Special Concerns; Critics Say Security Bill Favors Special Interests," *New York Times*, November 19, 2002; Firestone, "Senate Votes, 90–9, to Set Up a Homeland Security Dept. Geared to Fight Terrorism," *New York Times*, November 20, 2002; Bob Herbert, "Whose Hands are Dirty?", *New York Times*, November 25, 2002; Jonathan Weisman, "A Homeland Security Whodunit," *Washington Post*, November 28, 2002; Sheryl Gay Stolberg, "A Capitol Hill Mystery: Who Aided Drugmaker?", *New York Times*, November 29, 2002 (quote); Jonathan Weisman, "In the Homeland Security Bill, A Quiet Bonus," *Washington Post*, November 29, 2002; "The Man Behind the Vaccine Mystery," CBS News, December 12, 2002, www.cbsnews.com/stories/2002/12/12/eveningnews/printable532886.shtml; Robert Pear, "Legal Risks: For Victims of Vaccine, Winning Case will be Hard," *New York Times*, December 14, 2002; Helen Dewar, "Senate to Repeal Law Shielding Drug Giants," *Washington Post*, January 11, 2003.

75. The quote comes from Firestone, "Senate Votes."

76. Barbara Loe Fisher, "Power Grab by Federal Government Sets Stage for Forced Vaccination in America," NVIC email, January 6, 2003, in author's possession; "Briefing Paper—Homeland Security and Vaccine Compensation," www.909shot.com/Issues/briefing_paper.htm.

77. "Homeland Security Bill Update," PROVE email, November 19, 2002, in author's possession.

78. Emily Martin, *Flexible Bodies: The Role of Immunity in American Culture from the Days of Polio to the Age of AIDS* (Boston: Beacon, 1994), 203.

79. Information about Wingspread comes from the chief summary document from the group's second full meeting, Roger H. Bernier, "Proposal for a Demonstration Project—The Vaccine Policy Analysis Collaborative (VPAC)," presented to the NVAC [National Vaccine Advisory Committee], June, 2003, available at www.cdc.gov/od/nvpo/meetings/june2003/bernier.ppt.

80. The philosophical foundations for Wingspread are well-articulated in a compelling article by Chris Feudtner and Edgar K. Marcuse of the University of Washington, "Ethics and Immunization Policy: Promoting Dialogue to Sustain Consensus," *Pediatrics* 107 (May 2001): 1158–1164. Feudtner and Marcuse argue that, given the recent breakdown in the consensus supporting immunization, the government must implement a more democratic public policy process that moves beyond a strictly medical/epidemiological cost-benefit analysis to include ethical considerations as well. In contrast to vaccine officials who fear that any criticism of vaccines will undercut immunization efforts, these two public health officials embrace public debate and honor the widely different perspectives that citizens have on this issue, arguing that the very process of debate provides legitimacy and furthers the possibility of consensus. Feudtner and Marcuse also admit what seems heresy in establishment vaccine circles, namely that personal freedom and family autonomy are in fact values worth upholding. Citizens and government officials might, in the end, determine that other values, especially collective epidemiological protection, might outweigh concerns about liberty and therefore warrant coercion, but such decisions must be reached only after open and honest debate. We would also do well, they contend, to move away from at least parts of the current one-size-fits-all policy, since "for each vaccine . . . considerations would differ, suggesting that a spectrum of policy enforcement strength is warranted, titrating the degree of coerciveness to the particular disease and vaccine-specific tradeoffs." (1163) Finally, the authors offer an opportunity to move away from polarized philosophical positions and toward more concrete ethical decision-making. Instead of arguing simply about whether it is right or just to compel vaccinations—or to evade them—an ethical discussion might instead fruitfully ask: if vaccines were only recommended, instead of mandated, *how many* parents would not have their children vaccinated, with what quantitative effects on public health? Right now, we simply do not have this crucial information. In the end, the authors effectively make the case that the only just, as well as the only truly effective, immunization policy must involve "as much political dialogue as epidemiology." (1163)

From Cultism to CAM

This chapter is an adaptation of material published in James C. Whorton, *Nature Cures: The History of Alternative Medicine in America* (New York: Oxford University Press, 2002).

1. *The New Yorker*, September 26, 1994, 85.

2. David Eisenberg et al., "Unconventional Medicine in the United States," *New England Journal of Medicine* 328 (1993): 251; David Eisenberg et al., "Trends in Alternative Medicine Use in the United States, 1990–1997," *Journal of the American Medical Association* 280 (1998): 1575.

3. Spalding Gray, *Gray's Anatomy* (New York: Vintage, 1994), 39.

4. *Journal of the American Medical Association* 280 (1998).

5. Matthew Ramsey, "Alternative Medicine in Modern France," *Medical History* 43 (1999): 289. The argument that the effort to suppress medical cults is a political act aimed at increasing majority practitioners' professional unity, social status, and cultural authority is made most fully by Susan Smith-Cunnien, *A Profession of One's Own: Organized Medicine's Opposition to Chiropractic* (Lanham, Md.: University Press of America, 1998).

6. For a survey of the evolution of unconventional medicine in America, see James Whorton," The History of Complementary and Alternative Medicine," in Wayne Jonas and Jeffrey Levin, eds., *Essentials of Complementary and Alternative Medicine* (Philadelphia: Lippincott Williams and Wilkins, 1999), 16–30. On the expression of Hippocratic tradition within alternative medicine, see René Dubos, "Hippocrates in Modern Dress," *Proceedings of the Institute of Medicine of Chicago* 25 (1965): 242–51.

7. Louis Reed, *The Healing Cults* (Chicago: University of Chicago Press, 1932), 2–3.

8. D. D. Palmer, *The Chiropractor's Adjuster: Text-book of the Science, Art and Philosophy of Chiropractic for Students and Practitioners* (Portland, Ore.: Portland Printing House, 1910), 101; Benedict Lust," The Principles and Program of the Nature Cure System," in B. Lust, ed., *Universal Naturopathic Encyclopedia Directory and Buyers' Guide Year Book of Drugless Therapy for 1918–19* (Butler, N.J.: Lust, 1918), 25; Arthur Forster, *The White Mark: An Editorial History of Chiropractic* (Chicago: National Publishing Association, 1921), 254–55, 301–2; R. L. Alsaker, "Do Germs Cause Disease?" *Physical Culture* 43, 2 (1920): 87.

9. Abraham Flexner, *Medical Education in the United States and Canada* (New York: Carnegie Foundation for the Advancement of Teaching, 1910), 156, 158, 160, 164, 233, 319.

10. George Dock, "A Visit to a Chiropractic School, *Journal of the American Medical Association* 78 (1922): 61; Thomas Duhigg, "Where Chiropractors Are Made," *Journal of the American Medical Association* 65 (1915): 2228–9; Arthur Seyse, "Chiropractic from the Inside," *New York State Journal of Medicine* 24 (1924): 550; "The Menace of Chiropractic," *Journal of the American Medical Association* 80 (1923): 715–16; Frank Jett and A. W. Cavins,"The Chiropractic Situation," *Journal of the Indiana State Medical Association* 26 (1933): 172, 230.

11. Reed, *The Healing Cults,* 66–69; Morris Fishbein, *The Medical Follies.* (New York: Boni and Liveright, 1925), 135; *Health Messenger*, February 1926, 21.

12. Benedict Lust, "Editorial Drift," *The Naturopath and Herald of Health* 3 (1902): 168–71; Lust cited by Paul Wendel, *Standardized Naturopathy* (Brooklyn, N.Y.: Wendel, 1951), 41; Herbert Shelton, "The Procrustean Bedstead," *Nature's Path* 32 (1927): 477; Edward Purinton, "Efficiency in Drugless Healing," in Benedict Lust, ed., *Universal Naturopathic Encyclopedia Directory and Buyers' Guide Year Book of Drugless Therapy for 1918–19* (Butler, N.J.: Lust, 1918), 102; Edward Purinton, "Where to Find Health," *The Naturopath and Herald of Health* 14 (1914): 284.

13. C. B. Atzen, "Creed vs. Science," *Journal of the American Osteopathic Association* 15 (1915–16): 151–52; Carl McConnell, "Osteopathic Diagnosis," *Journal of the American Osteopathic Association*" 8 (1908–9): 113; R. P. Beideman, "Seeking the Rational Alternative: The National College of Chiropractic from 1906 to 1982," *Chiropractic History* 3 (1983): 18.

14. Regular Allopathic Drug Doctors," *Herald of Health and Naturopath* 26 (1921): 138.

15. James Burrow, *Organized Medicine in the Progressive Era: The Move Toward Monopoly* (Baltimore: Johns Hopkins University Press, 1977), 52 (the campaign for a national health department is discussed on pages 100–2); Richard Bergen, "Cultist Therapy as Criminal Negligence," *Journal of the American Medical Association*, 196 (1966): 250; A. A. Erz, "Medical Laws vs. Human Rights and Constitution," *The Naturopath and Herald of Health* 18 (1913): 459.

16. J. T. Robinson, "The National Bureau of Health," *The Naturopath and Herald of Health* 15 (1910): 555–56; J. T. Robinson, "The Origin and Workings of the Medical Trust," *The Naturopath and Herald of Health* 17 (1912): 528–30; Robert Baker, "Fighting the Doctor-Drug Trust," *The Naturopath and Herald of Health* 17 (1912): 513–15.

17. A. A. Erz, "What Medicine Knows and Does Not Know about Rheumatism," *The Naturopath and Herald of Health* 17 (1912): 600; Palmer, *The Chiropractor's Adjuster,* 887–88.

18. Richard Shryock, *Medical Licensing in America, 1650–1965* (Baltimore: Johns Hopkins University Press, 1967).

19. Samuel Baker, "Physician Licensure Laws in the United States, 1865–1915," *Journal of the History of Medicine and Allied Sciences* 39 (1984): 173–97.

20. Henry Wood, "Medical Slavery through Legislation," *The Arena* 8 (1893): 687–88.

21. Champe Andrews, "Medical Practice and the Law," *The Forum* 31 (1901): 542–51, 547; E. R. Booth. *History of Osteopathy and Twentieth-Century Medical Practice*, 2nd edition (Cincinnati: Jennings and Graham, 1905), 213–24; Alexander Wilder, *History of Medicine* (New Sharon, Me.: New England Eclectic Publishing, 1901), 315, 456.

22. Benedict Lust, "History of the Naturopathic Movement," *Herald of Health and Naturopath* 26 (1921): 479–80; *The Naturopath and Herald of Health* 17 (1912): 610; Friedhelm Kirchfeld and Wade Boyle, *Nature Doctors: Pioneers in Naturopathic Medicine* (Portland, Ore.: Medicina Biologica, 1994), 188; Benedict Lust, "Medical Liberty versus Unconstitutional Health Laws," *Naturopath and Herald of Health* 33 (1934): 296–98; Vern Gielow, *Old Dad Chiro: A Biography of D. D. Palmer* (Davenport, Iowa: Bawden, 1981), 99–114.

23. Arthur Geiger, "Chiropractic: Its Cause and Cure," *Medical Economics* 19 (1942): 42; W. H. Rafferty, *Health and Love à la Chiropractic* (n.p.: n.p., n.d.), Kremers Reference Files, American Institute of the History of Pharmacy, University of Wisconsin, 63 (A) II; J. Stuart Moore, *Chiropractic in America: The History of a Medical Alternative* (Baltimore: Johns Hopkins University Press, 1993), 74; Norman Gevitz, *The D.O.'s: Osteopathic Medicine in America* (Baltimore: Johns Hopkins University Press, 1982), 40.

24. Gevitz, *The D.O.'s*, 42, 137; Moore, *Chiropractice in America*, 89–92; Wendel, *Standardized Naturopathy*, 35.

25. "Public Health League." *Medical Sentinel* 29 (1921): 40.

26. Channing Frothingham, "Osteopathy, Chiropractic, and the Profession of Medicine," *Atlantic Monthly* 130 (1922): 81; Norman Gevitz, " 'A Coarse Sieve': Basic Science Boards and Medical Licensure in the United States," *Journal of the History of Medicine and Allied Sciences* 43 (1988): 36–63.

27. "Results of Basic Science Examinations," *Northwest Medicine* 27 (1928): 206; Gevitz, " 'A Coarse Sieve,' " 47–48.

28. Gevitz, " 'A Coarse Sieve,' " 61–63.

29. Gevitz, *The D.O.'s*, 75–87, 107–10.

30. Erwin Blackstone, "The A.M.A. and the Osteopaths: A Study of the Power of Organized Medicine," *The Antitrust Bulletin* 22 (1977): 408–9.

31. Russell Gibbons, "The Rise of the Chiropractic Educational Establishment 1897–1980," in F. Lints-Dzaman, ed., *Who's Who in Chiropractic International*, 2nd ed., (Littleton, Colo.: Who's Who in Chiropractic International, 1980), 348–49.

32. Wendel, *Standardized Naturopathy*, 30, 135–36; Kirchfeld and Boyle, Nature Doctors, 203, 207–8; *Bastyr University Catalog 2000/2001*.

33. Blackstone, "The A.M.A. and Osteopaths"; Gevitz, *The D.O.'s*, 124, 134–36.

34. Gevitz, *The D.O.'s*, 124; Benedict Lust, editorial, *Herald of Health and Naturopath* 23 (1918): 524; W. J. Cohen. *Independent Practitioners under Medicare* (Washington, D.C.: Department of Health, Education, and Welfare, 1969), 142, 197.

35. Cohen, *Independent Practitioners*, 142, 197; Norman Gevitz, "The Chiropractors and the AMA: Reflections on the History of the Consultation Clause," *Perspectives in Biology and Medicine* 32 (1989): 292–93; American Medical Association, *Digest of Official Actions, 1959–1968* (Chicago: American Medical Association, 1971), 335; "How the New Ethics Code Affects You," *Medical Economics* 27 (October 1949): 56.

36. "AMAgrams," *Journal of the American Medical Association*, 216 (1971): 586; "A Call to Arms," *Journal of the American Medical Association* 217 (1971): 959; Walter Wardwell, *Chiropractic: History and Evolution of a New Profession* (St. Louis: Mosby Year Book, 1992), 166; William Jarvis, "Chiropractic: A Challenge for Health Education," *Journal of School Health* 44 (1974): 213; Ray Casterline, "Unscientific Cultism: Dangerous to Your Health," *Journal of the American Medical Association* 220 (1972): 1009; Moore, *Chiropractic in America,* 130.

37. Susan Getzendanner, "Permanent Injunction Order Against AMA," *Journal of the American Medical Association* 259 (1988): 81–82; Wardwell, *Chiropractic,* 11, 168–78; Moore, *Chiropractic in America,* 131–37.

38. Gevitz, "The Chiropractors and the AMA," 294–96.

39. Norman Cousins, "The Holistic Health Explosion," *Saturday Review*, March 31, 1979, 17–20; Ivan Illich, *Medical Nemesis: The Expropriation of Health* (New York: Pantheon, 1976), 4, 35; Thomas McKeown, *The Role of Medicine: Dream, Mirage, or Nemesis?* (London: Nuffield Provincial Hospitals Trust, 1976); Rick Carlson, *The End of Medicine* (New York: Wiley, 1975); Marcia Millman, *The Unkindest Cut: Life in the Backrooms of Medicine* (New York: Morrow, 1977).

40. John Burnham, "American Medicine's Golden Age: What Happened to It?" *Science* 215 (1982): 1475; Robert Moser, *Diseases of Medical Progress* (Springfield, Ill.: Charles Thomas, 1959), 8; "In England Now," *Lancet*, 1956 (ii), 1155. For fuller discussion of overprescribing of wonder drugs, see James Whorton, " 'Antibiotic Abandon': The Resurgence of Therapeutic Rationalism," in John Parascandola, ed., *The History of Antibiotics: A Symposium* (Madison: American Institute of the History of Pharmacy, 1980), 125–36.

41. Illich, *Medical Nemesis*, 1, 4; Editors of Consumer Reports, *Chiropractors: Healers or Quacks? Delaware Medical Journal* 49 (1977): 294.

42. Harry Dowling, "A New Generation," *Antibiotic Medicine and Clinical Therapy* 3 (1956): 26.

43. Carlson, *The End of Medicine*, 34.

44. Buda Keller, "The Laity's Idea of the Physician," *Illinois Medical Journal* 44 (1923): 15; Charles Rosenberg, "Holism in Twentieth-Century Medicine," in Christopher Lawrence and George Weisz, eds., *Greater than the Parts: Holism in Biomedicine, 1920–1950* (New York: Oxford University Press, 1998), 335–55; Frederick Stenn, "Thoughts of a Dying Physician," *Forum on Medicine* 3 (1980): 718.

45. John Millis, *The Graduate Education of Physicians* (Chicago: American Medical Association, 1966), 34; Burnham, "American Medicine's Golden Age"; Carlson, *The End of Medicine*, 24, 29.

46. Kristine Alster, *The Holistic Health Movement* (Tuscaloosa: University of Alabama Press, 1989), 136–55; June Lowenberg, *Caring and Responsibility: The Crossroads between Holistic Practice and Traditional Medicine* (Philadelphia: University of Pennsylvania Press, 1989), 53–80.

47. James Gordon, "Holistic Medicine: Toward a New Medical Model," *Journal of Clinical Psychiatry* 42 (1981): 117 (Gordon's article is one of the best condensed presentations of holistic philosophy); Edward Bauman et al., *The Holistic Health Handbook* (Berkeley: And/Or Press, 1978); Norman Cousins, *Anatomy of an Illness as Perceived by the Patient* (New York: Norton, 1979), 48; Edward Purinton, *The Laugh Cure*, advertised in Benedict Lust, *Universal Naturopathic Encyclopedia Directory and Buyers' Guide Year Book of Drugless Therapy for 1918–19* (Butler, N.J.: Lust, 1918), 1233; Herbert Shelton, "Phobiotherapy," *Naturopath* 31 (1926): 184–87.

48. McKeown, *The Role of Medicine*, 9–10; Keller, "The Laity's Idea," 16; Cousins, *Anatomy of an Illness*, 48.

49. Quoted by Alster, *The Holistic Health Movement*, 1; George Engel, "The Need for a New Medical Model: A Challenge for Biomedicine," *Science* 196 (1977): 129–36.

50. *Journal of Holistic Medicine* 2 (spring/summer 1980): 2; *Journal of Holistic Medicine* 3 (1981), 2.

51. James Gordon, "Holistic Health Centers," *Journal of Holistic Medicine* 3 (1981): 72–85.

52. Empathology handbill placed under windshield wiper, 1997; Arnold Relman," Holistic Medicine," *New England Journal of Medicine* 300 (1979): 313.

53. Wayne Jonas and Jennifer Jacobs, *Healing with Homeopathy: The Complete Guide* (New York: Warner, 1996), 98; James Harvey Young," The Development of the Office of Alternative Medicine in the National Institutes of Health, 1991–1996," *Bulletin of the History of Medicine* 72 (1998): 279–82.

54. Young, "Development," 290, 293; Robert Park and Ursula Goodenough, "Buying Snake Oil with Tax Dollars," *New York Times*, January 3, 1996, A11; John Weeks, "Major Trends in the Integration of Complementary and Alternative Medicine," in Nancy Faass, ed., *Integrating Complementary Medicine into Health Systems* (Gaithersburg, Md.: Aspen, 2001), 5; Kathleen Finn, "Seattle First to Open Natural Medicine Public Health Clinic," *Delicious!*, November 1995, 12–13; Timothy Egan, "Seattle Officials Seeking to Establish a Subsidized Natural Medicine Clinic," *New York Times*, January 3, 1996, A6.

55. Finn, "Seattle," 12; Mike Maharry, "Insurance Companies Study Their Alternatives," *Tacoma News Tribune*, January 1, 1996, A1; Eileen Stretch with Nancy Faass, "The Evolution of Integrative Medicine in Washington State," in Nancy Faass, ed., *Integrating Complementary Medicine into Health Systems* (Gaithersburg, Md.: Aspen, 2001), 32–35; Weeks, "Major Trends," 6.

56. The University of Arizona Program in Integrative Medicine, 1996 announcement; Weeks, "Major Trends," 11.

57. Purinton, "Efficiency in Drugless Healing." 165. On the challenges to integrating conventional and alternative medicine, see Nancy Faass, ed., *Integrating Complementary Medicine into Health Systems* (Gaithersburg, Md.: Aspen, 2001).

INDEX